Concepts in Immunology and Immunotherapeutics

Third Edition

American Society of Health-System Pharmacists

Any correspondence regarding this publication should be sent to the publisher, American Society of Health-System Pharmacists, 7272 Wisconsin Avenue, Bethesda, MD 20814.

Produced by the American Society of Health-System Pharmacists' Product Development Office.
Cover and Page Design: Hector L. Coronado

ISBN: 1-879907-71-2

Contents

Preface iv

Reviewers v

Part I

Chapter 1—Overview of the Immune System 3
by Marc G. Sturgill

Chapter 2—Cellular and Tissue Components of the Immune System 15
by Steven P. Smith

Chapter 3—The Major Histocompatibility Complex 35
by Janelle B. Perkins

Chapter 4—Hypersensitivity Reactions 53
by Jeffrey C. Delafuente

Part II

Chapter 5—Autoimmune and Immunodeficiency Diseases 71
by Jeffrey C. Delafuente

Chapter 6—Immunization 85
by Sian E. Bigora and Karen I. Plaisance

Chapter 7—Immunology of HIV Infection and AIDS 115
by Bonnie D. Purdy and Karen I. Plaisance

Chapter 8—Solid Organ Transplantation 149
by Kathleen D. Lake, Stephen J. Rossi, and Lawrence Chodoff

Chapter 9—Bone Marrow Transplantation 213
by Timothy R. McGuire

Chapter 10—Immunotherapy of Cancer 229
by Jill K. Bruton

Chapter 11—Monoclonal Antibodies 269
by Val R. Adams and Janet L. Karlix

Answers to Self-Assessment Questions 300

Glossary 302

Index 310

Preface

Many pharmacy practitioners have never had a formal course in basic or applied immunology. However, in everyday practice they are finding it necessary to understand the functions of the immune system, its response to disease processes, and the mechanisms by which it may be modulated to treat disease. *Concepts in Immunology and Immunotherapeutics*, now in its third edition, is designed for practicing pharmacists and post-graduate trainees (e.g., residents and fellows) and for pharmacy students to use as a primer or supplement to other texts.

The text is divided into two major parts. Part I reviews the basic principles of immunology, including the cellular and tissue components of the immune system. Part II concentrates on the clinical application of these concepts for preventing and treating specific disease states. All chapters have undergone extensive editing, and material has been updated to reflect current information. Information on solid organ and bone marrow transplantation has been significantly expanded in this edition. Relevant terminology is defined in the glossary, and the index provides easy reference.

August 1997

Reviewers

ASHP gratefully acknowledges the following individuals, who donated their expertise in reviewing chapters for this publication:

Wayne S. Burkle, Pharm.D.
Daniel T. Casto, Pharm.D.
Robert E. Dupuis, Pharm.D., B.C.P.S.
Brian D. Fontaine
S. Diane Goodwin, Pharm.D.
John D. Grabenstein, Ed.M., M.S., F.A.S.H.P.
Karen Heim-Duthoy, Pharm.D.
Motria M. Krawczeniuk, Pharm.D.
William J. McIntyre, Pharm.D.
James R. Minor, Pharm.D., F.A.S.H.P.
William P. Petros, Pharm.D.
Meade Pimler, Ph.D.
Thomas W. Redford, Pharm.D.
William G. Reiss, Pharm.D., B.C.P.S.
Ralph E. Small, Pharm.D.
Kathleen M. Tornatore, Pharm.D.
Cindy J. Wordell, Pharm.D.
Gary Yee, Pharm.D., F.C.C.P.
William C. Zamboni, Pharm.D.

Part I

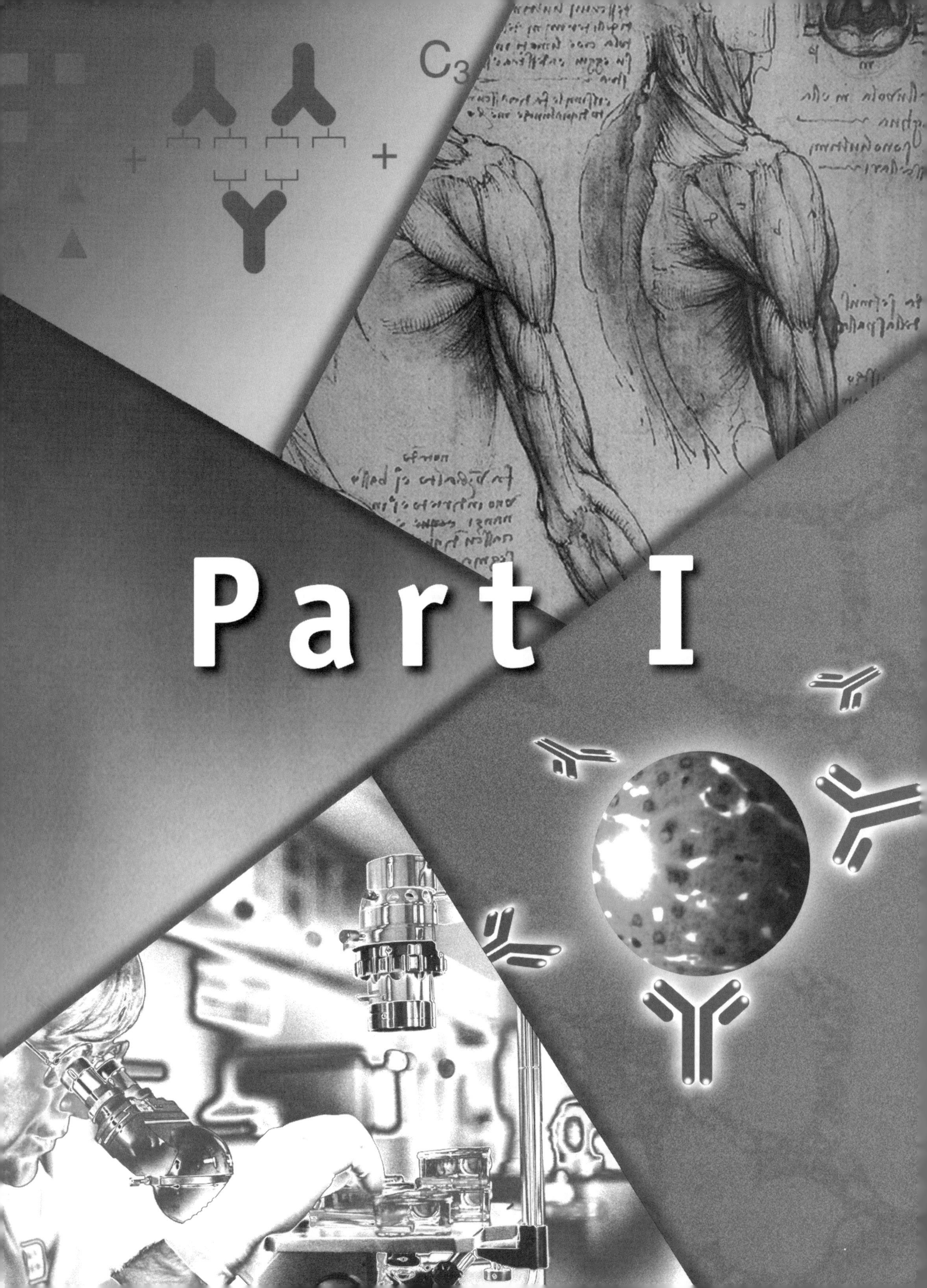

CHAPTER 1

Overview of the Immune System

Marc G. Sturgill, Pharm.D.
Assistant Professor
Department of Pharmacy Practice and Administration
College of Pharmacy
Rutgers, The State University of New Jersey
Piscataway, NJ

Organization of the Immune System 4
  Nonspecific (Innate) Immunity 4
    Physical and Chemical Barriers 4
    Phagocytosis 5
    Complement 5
  Antigen-Specific (Adaptive) Immunity 6
    Antigens and Antigen Presentation 6
    Antigen Recognition by B Lymphocytes 7
    Antigen Presentation to T Lymphocytes 7
  Humoral Immune Response 7
    Antigen Destruction by Antibodies 8
    Primary Versus Secondary Humoral Immune Response 8
  Cellular Immune Response 8
Inflammation and Hypersensitivity 8
The Immune System in Human Disease 10
  Autoimmunity 10
  Immunodeficiency 10
  Transplant Rejection 11
  Malignancy 11
Summary 11
References 11
Self-Assessment Questions 12

The human immune system is a sophisticated network of cells, tissues, and soluble factors capable of recognizing and responding to a vast array of potentially harmful agents. On initial exposure to an antigen (e.g., bacteria), the immune system mounts a two-pronged attack: a nonspecific inflammatory response that isolates the invader and, with the assistance of antigen-specific immune cells, ultimately destroys it. Components of the immune system specialized to "remember" the antigen then produce cells and circulating antibodies that will respond more rapidly and effectively on subsequent exposure to the same antigen.

Immune responses are not always beneficial to the host. Faulty regulation of the immune system can cause autoimmune disorders, such as rheumatoid arthritis, or hypersensitivity disorders, such as allergic rhinitis or allergic asthma. Transplant rejection is mediated by the same mechanisms that destroy a foreign antigen. Suppression of the normal immune response may also contribute to the appearance of certain types of cancer.

This chapter gives pharmacists a brief introduction to the components of the immune system, the properties that allow the immune system to recognize antigens, and the clinical consequences of immune dysfunction. After completing this introductory chapter, the reader should be able to:

1. Describe the general organization and function of the immune system.
2. Describe the innate immune response and the role this response plays in host defense.
3. Describe the components of the adaptive immune response and how this response leads to immunologic memory and immunity.
4. Describe the properties of antigens that label them as foreign, and how the various components of the immune system recognize these antigens.
5. Describe the four basic patterns of inflammatory response.
6. Describe briefly the consequences of immune dysfunction.

ORGANIZATION OF THE IMMUNE SYSTEM

The immune system can be broadly divided into three sets of organs: primary lymphoid organs, where young immune cells reproduce and mature; secondary lymphoid organs, where immune responses to antigens are generated; and tertiary lymphoid organs (any infected tissue in the body), where immune cells called effector cells complete the process of antigen destruction and removal.[1,2] A network of blood vessels and lymphatic channels connects these organs, and immunocompetent cells constantly circulate in this system, prepared to respond to the appropriate antigenic signal.

Immune responses can be antigen-nonspecific (innate) or antigen-specific (adaptive).[3] Innate immunity is the inherent ability of the host to resist infection and disease. This type of immunity is provided by physical and chemical barriers to infection, along with inflammatory cells and soluble mediators (circulating substances, such as complement proteins, that attract and stimulate inflammatory cells). In contrast to innate immunity, antigen-specific immunity, orchestrated primarily by T and B lymphocytes, adapts to the infectious agent, permitting subsequent infections to be more rapidly and effectively eliminated.[3,4]

Nonspecific (Innate) Immunity

Innate immunity is essential to host survival for two reasons.[3] First, on initial exposure to a particular antigen, nonspecific mechanisms provide the only line of defense until antigen-specific cells can be recruited and activated. Second, recruitment and activation of antigen-specific cells is mediated by soluble factors generated by antigen-nonspecific responses.[5]

Innate immunity also has two important disadvantages.[6] First, antigen destruction tends to occur only after tissue damage (inflammation) has already occurred, and because the cells that mediate inflammatory reactions are not capable of adaptation, this inflammatory response does not change with repeated exposure. Second, many microorganisms can mutate and eventually render such a rigid defense system ineffective.[5]

Physical and Chemical Barriers

Physical barriers, such as skin and mucous membranes, serve as the first line of defense against foreign invasion. Most microorganisms cannot penetrate intact skin because of the relative impermeability of the outer keratin-rich epidermal layer and the low pH of lactic acid and unsaturated fatty acids present in the underlying dermis.[3] Inner epithelial surfaces, such as the nasopharynx, lungs, and gut, are protected by a layer of adhesive mucus, which can effectively trap microorganisms until mechanisms such as ciliary movement, coughing, or peristalsis can remove them. These surfaces are also exposed to bactericidal chemicals, such as gastric acid in the stomach. Few microorganisms can survive both the acidic pH of the stomach and the alkaline pH of the small intestine.[3] The normal bacterial flora of the intestine also protect the host by competing with pathogenic microorganisms for essential nutrients and producing toxic metabolic by-products, such as lactic acid. Lysozyme, an enzyme present in saliva, tears, nasal mucus, and most other body secretions, kills bacteria by cleaving cell wall peptidoglycan.[3,5]

Phagocytosis

Once physical or chemical barriers are breached, white blood cells (WBCs) capable of phagocytosis (cellular ingestion and digestion of foreign particles) are rapidly attracted to the site of tissue invasion. These cells include granulocytes [polymorphonuclear leukocytes (PMNs), also called neutrophils, and eosinophils] and monocytes, which spend most of their lifespan as specialized cells called macrophages within tissue compartments.[7] Granulocytes, named for the granules of lytic enzymes in their cytoplasm, are more mobile than monocytes or macrophages, and large numbers are rapidly recruited once tissue injury has occurred. However, monocytes and macrophages are more efficient phagocytes, and they help initiate the antigen-specific immune response by acting as antigen-presenting cells (APCs). APCs trap and present antigenic particles to the T lymphocytes that orchestrate development of antigen-specific immunity and immunologic memory.[7] A detailed description of granulocytes and monocytes is provided in chapter 2.

Because phagocytes are antigen-nonspecific, their activity depends on chemotaxis and opsonization.[1] Chemotaxis is the migration of phagocytic cells toward chemical signals emitted at the site of tissue injury. Important chemotactic factors include bacterial metabolic by-products, collagen or fibrin fragments from damaged tissue, complement protein C5a, leukotriene B_4, prostaglandin D_2, and interleukin 8 (IL-8) released by activated macrophages.[7] Opsonization is the coating of the target cell by antibodies or complement proteins to facilitate attachment of phagocytic cells that express the appropriate receptors.

Phagocytosis begins when the phagocyte attaches to the antigen's cell membrane (Figure 1-1).[8] The phagocyte's membrane encloses the antigen as exposed portions of the opsonins are recognized and bound by receptors on the phagocyte's surface. The phagocyte eventually surrounds and internalizes the antigen, forming an intracellular vacuole called the phagosome. Lysosomes, cytoplasmic storage granules that contain potent hydrolytic enzymes, fuse with the phagosome to form a phagolysosome. The lysosome then degranulates, releasing the hydrolytic enzymes. Degraded antigenic particles may interact with class II major histocompatibility complex molecules (discussed below). This antigenic material–class II MHC molecule complex is then expressed on the cell surface to be presented to helper T cells (see chapter 2).

Phagocytic enzymes can also damage normal tissue, since degraded cellular debris and enzymes are normally released following phagocytosis. Extracellular degranulation occurs when the phagocyte is too small to engulf the entire antigenic particle, leading to secretion of degradative enzymes onto the surface of the antigen and into the surrounding environment.[3] Inflammation, characterized by warmth, swelling, redness, and pain, is the result of this tissue damage.[9] Many phagocytes die during the inflammatory response, especially if the reaction is prolonged or highly intense. Ensuing lysis of these cells exposes surrounding tissues to the effects of reactive enzymes. During infection with pyogenic bacteria, these processes form pus, which is composed of cellular debris generated by liquefaction of surrounding tissue.

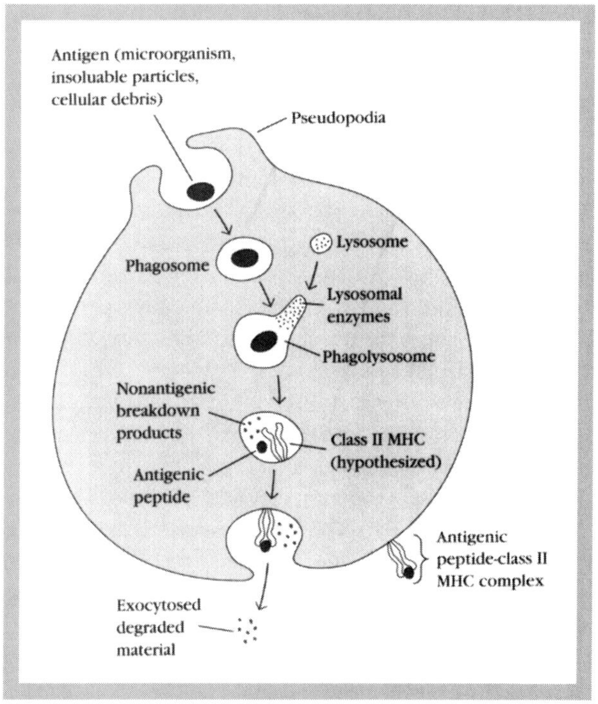

Figure 1-1. Phagocytosis and processing of exogenous antigen by macrophages. Following adherence of antigen to the macrophage membrane, long pseudopodia surround the attached material. Fusion of pseudopodia draws the material into the cell, forming a membrane-bound phagosome. Fusion of the phagosome with a lysosome produces a phagolysosome and results in release of the lysosomal contents. Most of the products from digestion of the ingested material are exocytosed. Some of the digested peptides are thought to interact with class II MHC molecules. The resulting antigenic peptide–class II MHC complexes then move to the cell surface, where they are presented to helper T lymphocytes.

SOURCE: *Reprinted with permission from Kuby J, editor.* Immunology. *2nd ed. New York: WH Freeman; 1994. p. 64.*

Complement

The complement cascade is a network of about 25 proteins that circulate unbound or are bound to cell surfaces. These proteins have three vital roles in maintaining host defense: opsonization of foreign material, direct cell lysis, and generation of inflammatory mediators.

The complement cascade can be activated by either the classical or the alternative pathway (Figure 1-2).[10,11] The classical complement cascade is initiated when an antigen-antibody complex (or "immune complex") comes into contact with the C1q domain of complement protein C1. Binding to a single immunoglobulin M (IgM) molecule or two immunoglobulin G (IgG) molecules activates C1, setting in motion a series of interactions with other complement proteins on the target cell surface.

In contrast, the alternative complement cascade is activated by the binding of C3b to activating surfaces (such as microbial cell walls) and so does not require the presence of preformed immune complexes (Figure 1-2). This pathway therefore has a vital role in defending against initial infection by a given bacteria: before the development of antigen-specific immunity and preformed immune complexes, it rapidly initiates chemotactic signals that attract antigen-nonspecific inflammatory cells.[10,11]

Once the complement cascade is set in motion, binding and cleavage of complement proteins generate various fragments that have biologic activity. For example, cleavage of C3 ultimately results in a complex that strongly opsonizes the target cell to monocytes and granulocytes that express C3b receptors.[12] In addition, cleavage of complement C5 releases C5a, an extremely potent chemotactic factor for monocytes and granulocytes.[10,12]

Many complement fragments with inflammatory activity are generated and released as the complement cascade proceeds. C4a, C3a, and C5a are called anaphylatoxins, because they stimulate smooth muscle contraction and increased vascular permeability.[10,13] Many clinical consequences of acute inflammation (pain, swelling, redness, and warmth) are initiated by complement activation.

Antigen-Specific (Adaptive) Immunity

Antigen-specific immunity is mediated by T and B lymphocytes.[4] Unlike granulocytes and monocytes, these cells have surface receptors that allow rapid recognition of antigens. In addition, these cells adapt to the antigen during initial exposure, permitting a more efficient response on subsequent exposures. Finally, B lymphocytes produce antigen-specific proteins called immunoglobulins that provide the host with immunologic memory. In some cases this memory persists for the life of the host.

Antigens and Antigen Presentation

Any substance capable of provoking an immune response is called an immunogen, whereas the target of the response is an antigen (i.e., it is "antibody-generating").[14] All immunogens are, by definition, antigenic, but an antigen may not be immunogenic. For example, haptens are small, antigenic chemical moieties that are not capable of eliciting an immune response unless coupled to a carrier mol-

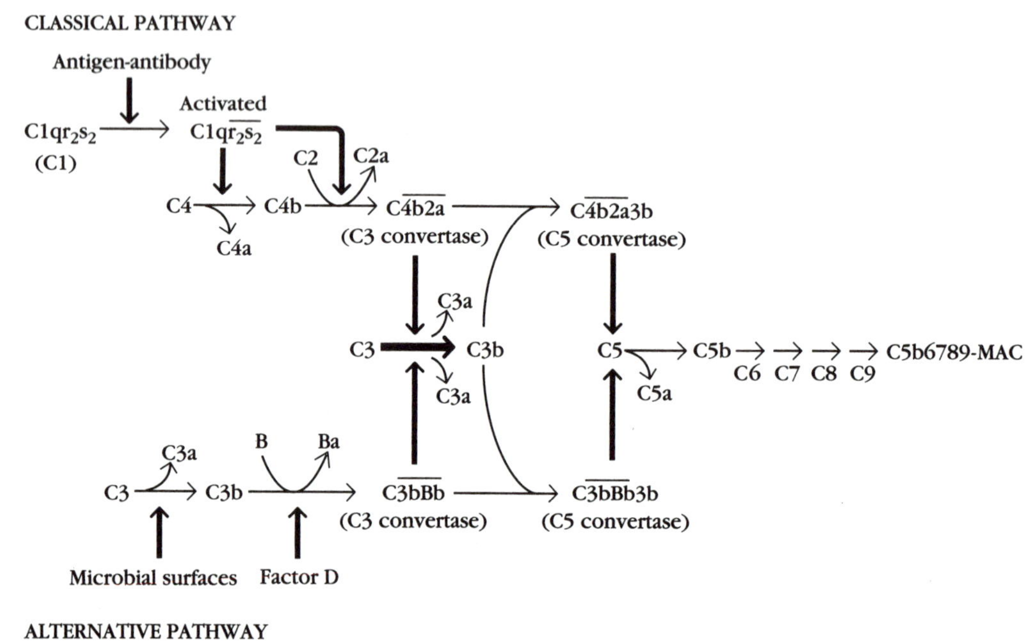

Figure 1-2. Classical and alternative complement pathways

SOURCE: *Reprinted with permission from Kuby J, editor.* Immunology. *2nd ed. New York: WH Freeman; 1994. p. 396.*

ecule.[14] The specific amino acid sequence of an antigen that is recognized and bound by antibody is called the antigenic determinant or epitope.[15] Most immunogens contain several distinct antigenic determinants, each capable of being recognized and bound by a different antibody.

Several physical, chemical, and topographical characteristics determine immunogenicity (Table 1-1). In general, proteins or polysaccharides of large molecular weight (molecular mass >10,000 daltons) are most likely to be immunogenic.[16] Structural complexity is important, probably because it determines the tertiary structure of the compound, so synthetic polymers of single amino acid or carbohydrate units are not immunogenic, regardless of molecular weight.[16] Other important factors include the ease with which the substance can be degraded and the dose and route of administration.[16] Large lipophilic molecules are more easily taken up and degraded by phagocytes than small lipophobic substances.[16] Finally, the genetic composition of the host ultimately determines whether an immune response is possible and how intense it will become.

Antigen Recognition by B Lymphocytes

Membrane-bound immunoglobulin (antibody) molecules on the surface of B lymphocytes recognize an antigen in its native three-dimensional conformation. Antibodies do not recognize the entire antigen but rather the six– to eight–amino acid or -oligosaccharide sequence of the epitope.[16] The tertiary or quaternary structure of an antigen is therefore important for several reasons. First, it determines the shape of the epitope, which in turn determines the shape required of the corresponding antibody paratope (the specific amino acid sequence that binds the epitope).[16] In addition, the epitope may not be a sequential amino acid sequence but may instead be composed of sequences from different parts of the antigen brought together by the folding of the protein.[15,17] Finally, the overall structure determines where the epitopes are located and whether they are accessible to antibodies. Peptide chains protruding from the globular surface of a protein are more likely to contain epitopes than regions buried within the globular structure.[16–18]

Because each individual immunoglobulin molecule recognizes only a single antigen, the immune system must be capable of constructing an extremely diverse set of antigen specificities to combat the array of antigens that confront the host. This variety is accomplished by the random manner in which immunoglobulin genes are assembled, transcribed, and translated.[19] A detailed description of immunoglobulins and B lymphocyte development is provided in chapter 2.

Antigen Presentation to T Lymphocytes

T lymphocytes contain membrane-bound T-cell receptors (TCRs), which, like immunoglobulins, are highly selective for a specific antigen. Random gene translocation during early T-lymphocyte development (analogous to that of immunoglobulin genes) permits production of a broad range of receptors.[20,21] TCRs only recognize small fragments of an antigen (perhaps no more than six to seven amino acids in length). This antigenic fragment must also be bound to a "self antigen"—a peptide or oligosaccharide on the host cell surface that identifies the cell as self. The genes that encode the production of these "self antigens" are referred to as the major histocompatibility complex (MHC);[16,22] these genes are called the human leukocyte antigen (HLA) complex in humans. Because the antigen must bind to both the T-cell and the HLA "antigen" (MHC restriction), it must have two binding regions. The epitope binds to the TCR, and a region called the agretope binds to the HLA "antigen."[16] See chapter 3 for a detailed description of the MHC.

Humoral Immune Response

Humoral immunity is conferred by soluble immunoglobulin molecules and can be transferred from one individual to another by serum transfusion, but its protection does not extend to the interior of cells. Because soluble immunoglobulin is central to humoral immunity, this type of immune response is specially designed to combat extracellular infections. Individuals with selective B-lymphocyte immune deficiencies are therefore prone to recurrent, severe bacterial infections. See chapter 2 for further discussion of B lymphocyte development.

Table 1-1. Properties of Immunogens[16]

	NONIMMUNOGENIC	IMMUNOGENIC
Molecular mass (Daltons)	<1000	>10,000
Chemical composition and structural complexity	Polymers of single amino acids or carbohydrates	Polypeptides or polysaccharides of sufficient molecular weight
Degradability	Polymers of D-amino acids (cannot be degraded within macrophages)	Lipophilic macromolecules of large molecular weight (more easily phagocytized)

Antigen Destruction by Antibodies

Immunoglobulin molecules are synthesized and displayed on the surface of B lymphocytes, but soluble immunoglobulins can only be produced and secreted by a specialized type of B lymphocyte called the plasma cell.[23] Once secreted by plasma cells, circulating antibodies seek out and bind to antigens and then orchestrate antigen destruction and removal. Antibody binding alone can inactivate some infectious processes, such as the release of bacterial toxins or the binding of certain viruses to host cells.[23] In most cases, however, antigen-antibody complexes stimulate destruction by antigen-nonspecific means.

As mentioned previously, the binding of either one IgM molecule or two IgG molecules to antigen can initiate the classical complement cascade.[10,11] Cellular lysis can then occur through formation of the membrane attack complex in the target cell membrane or by the release of chemotactic complement fragments that attract phagocytes. The binding of IgG to antigen also initiates two other types of destruction.[24] The IgG molecules act as opsonins, attracting phagocytes, such as neutrophils and macrophages, that express certain surface receptors. IgG can also initiate antibody-dependent cell-mediated cytotoxicity (ADCC). In this process, natural killer (NK) cells, large granular lymphocytes that also express those surface receptors, bind to IgG on the target cell membrane and release a series of enzymes that induce osmotic cell death (see chapter 2).[25]

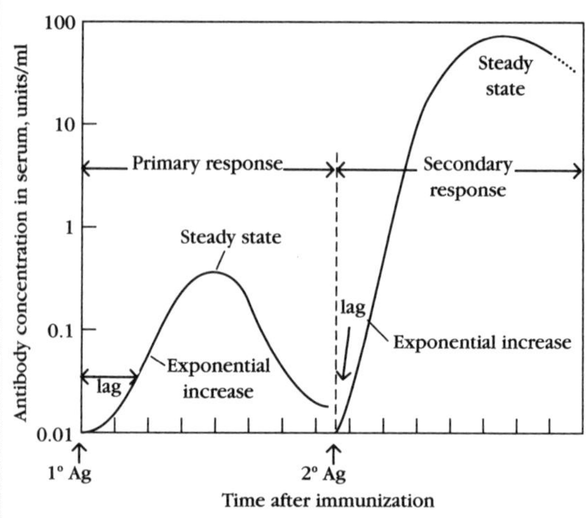

Figure 1-3. Primary and secondary humoral responses. Serum antibody concentrations following primary (1°) or secondary (2°) immunization with antigen. The antibody concentrations are plotted on a logarithmic scale. Time units are not specific because kinetics differ with the type of antigen, the route of administration, the presence or absence of adjuvants, and the species or strain of animal.

SOURCE: *Reprinted with permission from Kuby J, editor.* Immunology. *2nd ed. New York: WH Freeman; 1994. p. 325.*

Primary Versus Secondary Humoral Immune Response

Because of the many steps needed to produce plasma cells, a primary humoral immune response generally requires 5–10 days to fully develop (Figure 1-3).[23] In addition, this response is mediated initially by IgM antibodies of varying antigen affinities (the degree to which the antibody is attracted to its complimentary epitope). As the response continues, class switching leads to the generation of progressively more IgG antibody, and affinity maturation greatly enhances antigen affinity.[23,26] Because of the random nature of immunoglobulin gene rearrangement in developing B cells, some cells will produce lower-antigen-affinity antibodies. Through somatic hypermutation (an increased immunoglobulin gene mutation during the immune response), contact with antigen leads to selection of B cells expressing high-affinity antibody molecules. This process probably occurs as the concentration of available antigen begins to decrease; only those cells carrying high-affinity immunoglobulin will be able to obtain sufficient stimulus for activation.[26]

In contrast, subsequent exposure to the same antigen elicits a secondary humoral immune response, mediated primarily by antigen-specific memory B lymphocytes of high antigen affinity.[23,27] These cells can be activated by lower antigen concentrations, allowing a more rapid and intense humoral response. In addition, because of class switching and affinity maturation during the primary response, the immunoglobulin molecules in a secondary response are of high antigen affinity and are primarily from the IgG class.

Cellular Immune Response

In contrast to humoral immunity, which specializes in identifying and responding to extracellular pathogens, such as bacteria, the antigen-specific cellular immune response is designed to eliminate intracellular pathogens.[25] Cellular immunity is regulated by helper T lymphocytes, with effector functions provided by cytotoxic T lymphocytes and nonspecific cells, such as macrophages, NK cells, and granulocytes. Individuals with selective deficiencies of T lymphocyte–mediated immune responses are prone to severe infections with viruses, mycobacteria, or other intracellular organisms.[25] A detailed description of cellular immunity is provided in chapter 2.

INFLAMMATION AND HYPERSENSITIVITY

A successful immune response can be completely carried out by one component of the immune system (antigen-specific antibodies with complement-mediated lysis, for example). However, in most cases other components of the immune system are recruited into action (Figure 1-4).[9] Even when lymphocytes initiate the response, antigen destruction is usually done by nonspecific cells or soluble factors (e.g., interleukin 1 [IL-1], histamine, etc.). Antigen-nonspecific and antigen-specific components of the immune system must therefore act in a coordinated manner. In most cases the response is clinically undetectable. In certain cases, however, such as with chronic or repeated infection, the immune response is more intense and damage to surrounding tissues produces inflammation.[9,28]

Antigen-nonspecific granulocytes are the most rapidly mobilized cells, but they cannot respond until chemotactic factors are liberated at the site of tissue injury. Once an antigen has invaded blood or lymph, chemotaxis can be initiated by activation of the complement cascade, but when antigen is isolated in tissues, chemotaxis is generally stimulated by tissue mast cells, (granulocytic cells that produce potent inflammatory arachidonic acid metabolites).[9]

Mast cell degranulation also liberates histamine, which rapidly produces local vasodilation and increased vascular permeability.[29] Movement of intravascular fluid and protein (including fibrinogen) into the injured tissue results in swelling (edema), redness, and coagulation of interstitial fluid (induration). This response can cause clinical symptoms (including pain and fever), but it is vital to host defense because it helps limit the spread of bacteria, cellular debris, or toxic by-products of phagocytosis and mast cell degranulation. In genetically prone individuals, dysregulation of normal inflammatory mechanisms can lead to hypersensitivity (allergic) reactions or certain types of autoimmune disorders.[9,28]

The ultimate response to antigen follows one of four distinct patterns, depending on the cell type that mediates the response (Table 1-2).[9] In many cases, more than one type of inflammatory response can take place simultaneously, although one type tends to dominate the overall immune response. Hypersensitivity and autoimmunity (discussed in the next section) are natural extensions of these normal immune responses, representing situations in which control mechanisms that normally limit the immune response have failed.

Acute allergic inflammation, or immediate hypersensitivity, is mediated by degranulation of basophils and tissue mast cells, which liberates histamine.[30] These cells have receptors for immunoglobulin E (IgE), and on first exposure to the antigen the host produces antigen-specific IgE antibodies that coat these cells. On subsequent exposure to the antigen, degranulation rapidly occurs. Acute immunoglobulin-mediated inflammation is initiated when antigen binds to IgM or IgG antibodies,

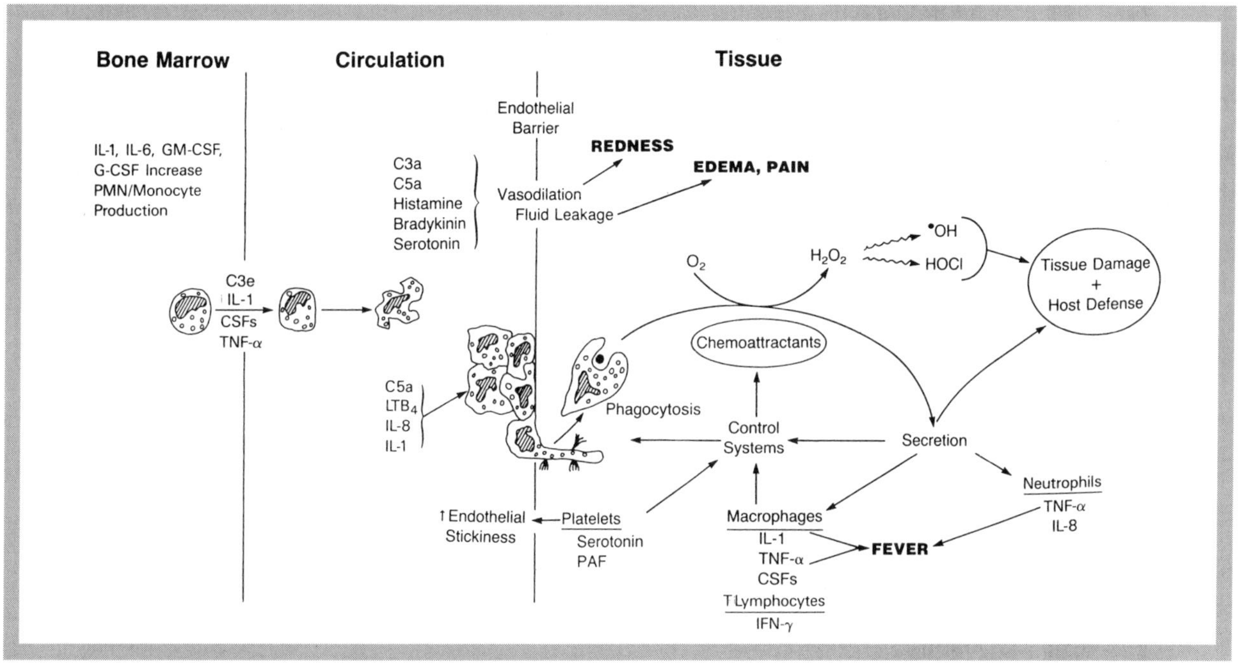

Figure 1-4. Coordinated inflammatory response. The four basic symptoms of inflammation are labeled in bold capital letters. G-CSF, granulocyte colony-stimulating factor; GM-CSF, granulocyte-macrophage colony-stimulating factor; IFN-γ, interferon gamma; IL-1, interleukin 1; LTB_4, leukotriene B_4; PAF, platelet-activating factor; TNF-α, tumor necrosis factor alpha.

SOURCE: *Reprinted with permission from Paul WE, editor.* Fundamental Immunology. *3rd ed. New York: Raven Press; 1993. p. 1016.*

Table 1-2. Categories of Inflammation

CATEGORY	IMMUNE RECOGNITION COMPONENT	SOLUBLE MEDIATORS	TIME COURSE	CELLULAR RESPONSE	CLINICAL EXAMPLE
Acute inflammation					
Allergic (reaginic)	IgE	Mast cell/basophil products (histamine, arachidonate products)	Seconds to minutes	Neutrophils, eosinophils; smooth muscle constriction	Atopy, urticaria anaphylaxis, asthma, seasonal rhinitis
Cytotoxic antibody	IgG, IgM	Complement	Hours to 1 day	Acute inflammation (neutrophils); lysis or phagocytosis of antigens	Autoimmune hemolytic anemia, thrombocytopenia associated with systemic lupus erythematosus
Immune complex	IgG, IgM	Complement	Hours to 1 day	Accumulation of neutrophils, eosinophils, and macrophages	Rheumatoid arthritis, systemic lupus erythematosus
Chronic inflammation					
Delayed hypersensitivity	T cells	Lymphokines, monokines	2–3 days	Lymphocytes, macrophages	Granulomatous diseases, tuberculosis, leprosy, sarcoidosis

SOURCE: *Reprinted with permission from Paul WE, editor.* Fundamental Immunology. *3rd ed. New York: Raven Press; 1993. p. 1017.*

forming immune complexes that then fix complement (activate the classical complement cascade).[31] Similarly, a third type of inflammation is caused by a failure to properly clear immune complexes from the body. These complexes can deposit in small blood vessels or well-perfused organs and fix complement, resulting in acute immune complex–mediated inflammation. A fourth type of inflammation, called chronic inflammation or delayed-type hypersensitivity, is mediated by T lymphocytes and macrophages.[30] A more detailed discussion of hypersensitivity is provided in chapter 4.

THE IMMUNE SYSTEM IN HUMAN DISEASE

The same processes that protect the host from infection can result in morbidity or mortality if normal regulatory mechanisms are lost, as illustrated by the development of hypersensitivity or autoimmune disorders. Similarly, lack of normal immune function predisposes the host to infection by pathogenic organisms. Proper function of the immune system therefore demands a delicate balance. The host must be able to rapidly and efficiently expand certain components of the immune system in response to foreign invasion while control mechanisms prevent the response from upsetting homeostasis.

Autoimmunity

The production of antibody paratopes and TCRs involves a random rearrangement of gene sequences and results in an almost infinite number of possible antigen specificities. All individuals are therefore thought to produce lymphocytes capable of interacting with "antigens" on normal host cells, yet the vast majority of these interactions fail to elicit an immune response.[32] Autoimmune disorders result from poorly understood disruptions in normal immune tolerance that lead to the production of antibodies reactive to normal host "antigens."[33] Autoimmune tissue damage occurs by one or more of the inflammatory mechanisms described previously. A detailed discussion of autoimmune disorders is provided in chapter 6.

Immunodeficiency

The coordinated efforts of complement, antigen-specific lymphocytes, and antigen-nonspecific phagocytes are crucial to an effective immune response. Failure of any component can predispose the host to infection by a variety of organisms. Immunodeficiency disorders can selectively involve one of these components or can affect multiple immune networks.[34] Moreover, they can be hereditary or acquired. Much of our knowledge of the roles of B and T lymphocytes and other components in host protection has been gained through the study of individuals with hereditary immunodeficiency disorders. See chapter 5 for a more detailed discussion of immunodeficiency disorders.

Transplant Rejection

The rejection of transplanted tissues or organs is a natural extension of the immune system response to invasion by antigens. Rejection is directed by recognition of antigens encoded by the HLA.[35] Donor and recipient matching at class I and class II HLA gene loci is vital in assuring graft success, but minor transplant antigens can also initiate rejection. Other important factors include the normal expression of class II HLA antigens on the grafted tissue, the degree to which the tissue is perfused by the blood supply (corneal transplants are protected from invasion by blood-borne T lymphocytes), and the competence of the recipient's immune response (illustrating the importance of post-transplant therapeutic immunosuppression).[35]

Acute rejection is a cellular immune response mediated by T lymphocytes, which are activated by APCs from the donor graft tissue.[36] In contrast, chronic rejection appears to be mediated primarily by deposition of immune complexes in graft blood vessels, with subsequent complement fixation.[37] A more detailed discussion of transplant rejection is provided in chapter 8.

Malignancy

For reasons that are poorly understood, certain types of cancer are more common in immunocompromised patients, whether the immune deficiency is congenital or acquired. Squamous cell carcinomas of the skin, cervical carcinoma, Kaposi's sarcoma, and non-Hodgkin's lymphomas are examples of cancers that occur much more commonly in patients with immune dysfunction.[38] One proposed explanation is that immunocompromise leads to failure of normal immune surveillance.

Malignant transformation induces expression of unique cell surface markers that allow the immune system to recognize these cells as foreign, thereby eliciting cell-mediated destruction.[39,40] Unfortunately, with the exception of tumors induced by viruses, antigens that are truly specific to tumor cells have been difficult to isolate.[39] Many tumor-associated antigens have been identified, including oncofetal antigens (carcinoembryonic antigen and alpha-fetoprotein) and differentiation antigens (T-lymphocyte markers such as CD5), but these markers can also appear on normal cells. Most spontaneous human tumor cells are very weak immunogens.[40] See chapter 10 for a more detailed discussion of tumor immunology.

SUMMARY

The human immune system provides the host with an efficient method of detecting and removing an enormous variety of potentially harmful environmental pathogens. Besides protecting the host on initial exposure, the immune system has components that learn from the experience and adapt themselves, becoming even more effective on subsequent exposure and conferring the host with immunologic memory.

Normal immune reactions can be detrimental to the host as well. Rejection of allografts is mediated by immune mechanisms identical to those operating in response to infection. Proper function of the immune system requires a delicate balance. Hypersensitivity reactions, autoimmune disorders, and immunodeficiency syndromes illustrate the morbidity that can result if immune system function becomes abnormally heightened or depressed. Immunodeficiency can also predispose the host to certain types of malignancy.

REFERENCES

1. Kuby J, editor. *Immunology*. 2nd ed. New York: WH Freeman; 1994. Cells and organs of the immune system; p. 47–84.
2. Picker LJ, Siegelman MH. Lymphoid tissues and organs. In: Paul WE, editor. *Fundamental Immunology*. 3rd ed. NewYork: Raven; 1993. p. 145–97.
3. Kuby J, editor. *Immunology*. 2nd ed. New York: WH Freeman; 1994. Overview of the immune system; p. 1–21.
4. Roitt I, editor. *Essential Immunology*. 8th ed. Cambridge, MA: Blackwell Scientific;1994. Specific acquired immunity; p. 22–39.
5. Janeway CA, Travers P, editors. *Immunobiology: The Immune System in Health and Disease*. New York: Garland; 1994. Basic concepts in immunology; p. 1.1–1.43.
6. Roitt I, Brostoff J, Male D, editors. *Immunology*. 2nd ed. New York: JB Lippincott; 1989. Adaptive and innate immunity; p. 1.1–1.10.
7. Parslow TG. The phagocytes: neutrophils and macrophages. In: Stites DP, Terr AI, Parslow TG, editors. *Basic and Clinical Immunology*. 8th ed. Norwalk, CT: Appleton & Lange; 1994. p. 9–21.
8. Greenberg S, Silverstein SC. Phagocytosis. In: Paul WE, editor. *Fundamental Immunology*. 3rd ed. New York: Raven; 1993. p. 941–64.
9. Gallin JI. Inflammation. In: Paul WE, editor. *Fundamental Immunology*. 3rd ed. New York: Raven; 1993. p. 1015–32.
10. Liszewski MK, Atkinson JP. The complement system. In: Paul WE, editor. *Fundamental Immunology*. 3rd ed. New York: Raven; 1993. p. 917–39.
11. Kuby J, editor. *Immunology*. 2nd ed. New York: WH Freeman; 1994. The complement system; p. 393–415.
12. Roitt I, editor. *Essential Immunology*. 8th ed. Cambridge, MA: Blackwell Scientific; 1994. Innate immunity; p. 3–21.

13. Hugli TE. Biochemistry and biology of anaphylotoxins. *Complement* 1986;3:11–127.
14. Roitt I, editor. *Essential Immunology*. 8th ed. Cambridge, MA: Blackwell Scientific; 1994. The primary interaction with antigen; p. 81–102.
15. Berzofsky JA, Berkower IJ. Immunogenicity and antigen structure. In: Paul WE, editor. *Fundamental Immunology*. 3rd ed. New York: Raven; 1993. p. 235–82.
16. Kuby J, editor. *Immunology*. 2nd ed. New York: WH Freeman; 1994. Antigens; p. 85–108.
17. Sela M. Antigenicity: some molecular aspects. *Science* 1969;166:1365–74.
18. Atassi MZ, Kazim AL. First consequences of the determination of the entire antigenic structure of sperm-whale myoglobin. *Adv Exp Med Biol*. 1978;98:19–40.
19. Parslow TG. Immunoglobulin genes, B cells, and the humoral immune response. In: Stites DP, Terr AI, Parslow TG, editors. *Basic and Clinical Immunology*. 8th ed. Norwalk, CT: Appleton & Lange; 1994. p. 80–93.
20. Imboden JB. T lymphocytes and natural killer cells. In: Stites DP, Terr AI, Parslow TG, editors. *Basic and Clinical Immunology*. 8th ed. Norwalk, CT: Appleton & Lange; 1994. p. 94–104.
21. Hedrick SM, Eidelman FJ. T lymphocyte antigen receptors. In: Paul WE, editor. *Fundamental Immunology*. 3rd ed. New York: Raven; 1993. p. 383–420.
22. Chen J, Alt FW. Gene rearrangement and B-cell development. *Curr Opinion Immunol*. 1993;5:194–200.
23. Kuby J, editor. *Immunology*. 2nd ed. New York: WH Freeman; 1994. Generation of the humoral immune response; p. 323–46.
24. Goodman JW. The immune response. In: Stites DP, Terr AI, Parslow TG, editors. *Basic and Clinical Immunology*. 8th ed. Norwalk, CT: Appleton & Lange; 1994. p. 40–9.
25. Kuby J, editor. *Immunology*. 2nd ed. New York: WH Freeman; 1994. Cell-mediated immunity; p. 347–68.
26. Gearhart PJ. Somatic mutation and affinity maturation. In: Paul WE, editor. *Fundamental Immunology*. 3rd ed. New York: Raven; 1993. p. 865–85.
27. DeFranco AL. B lymphocyte activation. In: Paul WE, editor. *Fundamental Immunology*. 3rd ed. New York: Raven; 1993. p. 505–29.
28. Kuby J, editor. *Immunology*. 2nd ed. New York: WH Freeman; 1994. Hypersensitivity reactions; p. 417–43.
29. Terr AI. Inflammation. In: Stites DP, Terr AI, Parslow TG, editors. *Basic and Clinical Immunology*. 8th ed. Norwalk, CT: Appleton & Lange; 1994. p. 137–50.
30. Kuby J, editor. *Immunology*. 2nd ed. New York: WH Freeman; 1994. Hypersensitivity reactions; p. 369–91.
31. Roitt I, editor. *Essential Immunology*. 8th ed. Cambridge, MA: Blackwell Scientific; 1994. Hypersensitivity; p. 312–36.
32. Kuby J, editor. *Immunology*. 2nd ed. New York: WH Freeman; 1994. Immune regulation and tolerance; p. 369–91.
33. Schwartz RS. Autoimmunity and autoimmune diseases. In: Paul WE, editor. *Fundamental Immunology*. 3rd ed. New York: Raven; 1993. p. 1033–97.
34. Roitt I, editor. *Essential Immunology*. 8th ed. Cambridge, MA: Blackwell Scientific; 1994. Immunodeficiency; p. 295–311.
35. Auchincloss H, Sachs DH. Transplantation and graft rejection. In: Paul WE, editor. *Fundamental Immunology*. 3rd ed. New York: Raven; 1993. p. 1099–1141.
36. Kuby J, editor. *Immunology*. 2nd ed. New York: WH Freeman; 1994. Transplant immunology; p. 559–78.
37. Roitt I, editor. *Essential Immunology*. 8th ed. Cambridge, MA: Blackwell Scientific; 1994. Transplantation; p. 337–62.
38. Ziegler JL. Cancer in the immunocompromised host. In: Stites DP, Terr AI, Parslow TG, editors. *Basic and Clinical Immunology*. 8th ed. Norwalk, CT: Appleton & Lange; 1994. p. 578–87.
39. Kuby J, editor. *Immunology*. 2nd ed. New York: WH Freeman; 1994. Cancer and the immune system; p. 579–604.
40. Schreiber H. Tumor immunology. In: Paul WE, editor. *Fundamental Immunology*. 3rd ed. New York: Raven; 1993. p. 1143–78.

SELF-ASSESSMENT QUESTIONS

Answers to these self-assessment questions can be found on page 300.

1. Immune system cells develop and mature in tissues referred to as:

   a. primary lymphoid organs.
   b. secondary lymphoid organs.
   c. tertiary lymphoid organs.
   d. bone marrow.

2. The inherent ability of the host to resist infection and disease is referred to as:

   a. inflammation.
   b. innate immunity.
   c. immunologic memory.
   d. humoral immunity.

3. Antigen-specific immune responses are mediated by:

   a. monocytes and macrophages.
   b. the classical complement pathway.
   c. polymorphonuclear leukocytes.
   d. T lymphocytes and B lymphocytes.

4. A bactericidal enzyme found in most body fluids, including saliva, tears, and nasal secretions, is called:

   a. peptidoglycan.
   b. lysosome.
   c. lactic acid.
   d. lysozyme.

5. Activation of the complement cascade prior to the development of an antigen-specific immune response occurs by the:

   a. alternative pathway.
   b. classical pathway.

c. binding of an immune complex to complement C1.
d. formation of the membrane attack complex.

6. Phagocytosis is a term that describes the engulfment and enzymatic destruction of pathogens by antigen-nonspecific effector cells. Antigen-nonspecific cells capable of phagocytosis include all of the following *except:*

a. neutrophils.
b. cytotoxic T lymphocytes.
c. eosinophils.
d. macrophages.

7. Phagocytosis of antigen by antigen-nonspecific cells often produces damage to surrounding normal tissue. This process, characterized by pain, swelling, redness, and tissue warmth, is called:

a. inflammation.
b. opsonization.
c. delayed-type hypersensitivity.
d. immune complex–mediated hypersensitivity.

8. The target of an immune response is referred to as a(n):

a. hapten.
b. immunogen.
c. paratope.
d. antigen.

9. B lymphocytes recognize antigen by means of membrane-bound immunoglobulin molecules. The specific amino acid sequence of the antigen that is recognized by the immunoglobulin is referred to as the:

a. paratope.
b. epitope.
c. mitogen.
d. hapten.

10. Small antigenic determinants that by themselves are unable to provoke an immune response are referred to as:

a. haptens.
b. carriers.
c. immunogens.
d. lysosomes.

11. Physical, chemical, and topographical characteristics that are important in determining immunogenicity include all of the following *except:*

a. molecular weight.
b. pKa.
c. tertiary structure.
d. ease with which the substance can be degraded.

CHAPTER 2

Cellular and Tissue Components of the Immune System

Steven P. Smith, Pharm.D., B.C.P.S.
Adult Oncology Clinical Specialist
Department of Pharmacy Services
Shands Hospital at the University of Florida
Gainesville, FL

Nonspecific Cellular Components 16
Myeloid and Lymphoid Cells 16
Mononuclear Cells 17
Polymorphonuclear Cells 19
Neutrophils 19
Eosinophils 19
Basophils 19
Mast Cells 20
Platelets 20
Specific Cellular Components 20
Lymphocytes 20
T Lymphocytes (Cell-Mediated Immunity) 20
Helper T Lymphocytes 20
Suppressor T Lymphocytes 20
Cytotoxic T Lymphocytes 21
Memory T Lymphocytes 21
T-Lymphocyte Subpopulation Markers 21
Monoclonal Antibodies 21
Sheep Erythrocyte Rosettes 22
B Lymphocytes (Humoral Immunity) 22
Antibody 23
Classification 23
Antigen-Antibody Interactions: Binding 24
Memory Cells 25
Non-B and Non-T Lymphocytes (Null Cells) 25
Communications: Soluble Mediators 25
Tissues of the Immune System 27
Bone Marrow 27
Thymus 27
Lymph Nodes 27
Spleen 28

*The contributions made by Tracey Waddelow, Michael Sneller, and Jim Koeller to this chapter are gratefully acknowledged.

Mucosal-Associated Lymphoid Tissue 28
High Endothelial Venule 29
Immune Regulation and Response 29
Memory 29
Immune Tolerance 30
Summary 30
References 31
Self-Assessment Questions 32

As discussed in chapter 1, the immune system is a complex network of cells, tissues, and soluble mediators that work together to elicit a variety of immune responses. Immunotherapeutics is the application of knowledge of the immune system's anatomy and physiology. Immunotherapy has practical application in immunization, allergy desensitization, and organ transplantation. Only by understanding the immune system's anatomy and physiology can one begin to shape the immunotherapy of a patient. This chapter describes the cellular and tissue components of the human immune system, a foundation for understanding how the immune system can be modulated. It first discusses myeloid and lymphoid cells and their roles in innate and adaptive immune responses. Cellular components involved in phagocytosis are discussed. An examination of T lymphocytes and their subpopulation markers follows. The characteristics and functions of B lymphocytes and antibodies are then discussed. The chapter concludes with a description of the tissues of the immune system. In addition to this chapter, the reader may find the following references helpful:

- Rich RR, Fleisher TA, Schwartz BD, Shearer WT, Strober W, editors. *Clinical Immunology: Principles and Practice*. St. Louis, MO: Mosby; 1996.
- Beutler E, Lichtman MA, Coller BS, Kipps TJ, editors. *Hematology*. 5th ed. New York: McGraw-Hill; 1995.
- Paul WE, editor. *Fundamental Immunology*. 3rd ed. New York: Raven; 1993.

After completing this chapter, the reader should be able to:

1. Describe the cells and tissues involved in immune response.
2. Describe the immunologic function of monocytes and macrophages.
3. Describe the immunologic function of polymorphonuclear granulocytes.
4. Describe the immunologic function of B and T lymphocytes.
5. Describe the structure and function of immunoglobulins.
6. Describe how the immune system is regulated.

NONSPECIFIC CELLULAR COMPONENTS

Myeloid and Lymphoid Cells

Most immune system cells are white blood cells (WBCs) that originate in the bone marrow. WBCs are broadly categorized as myeloid or lymphoid cells. Myeloid cells are the major components of the nonspecific (or innate) immune response, and lymphoid cells make up the specific (or adaptive) immune response. When a foreign substance (antigen) is first introduced into the body, the nonspecific immune response, including phagocytosis and inflammation, is initiated. Subsequent exposure to the same antigen triggers a specific immune response through B and T cells.

Myeloid cells grow to maturity in the bone marrow. Lymphoid cells differentiate and mature in lymphatic tissues, including bone marrow and the thymus, the primary lymphatic tissues. Some mature lymphoid cells circulate through secondary lymphatic tissues, such as the spleen and lymph nodes.

The maturation process of each of the different functional blood cells is depicted in Figure 2-1. All cells, myeloid or lymphoid, develop from a common pluripotent stem cell. The stem cell has the potential to become any mature cellular element in the blood. Unlike many cells that undergo simple mitosis, the stem cell must, by definition, undergo self-renewal and differentiation. Half the stem cells are eventually committed to differentiate into myeloid or lymphoid cells. The other half remain stem cells identical to their mother cells. In this way, the pool of stem cells is not depleted and a sufficient supply is shunted into the path of hematopoiesis, the generation or development of blood cells.[1]

In adults, hematopoiesis occurs predominantly in the bone marrow. The marrow contains a fertile microen-

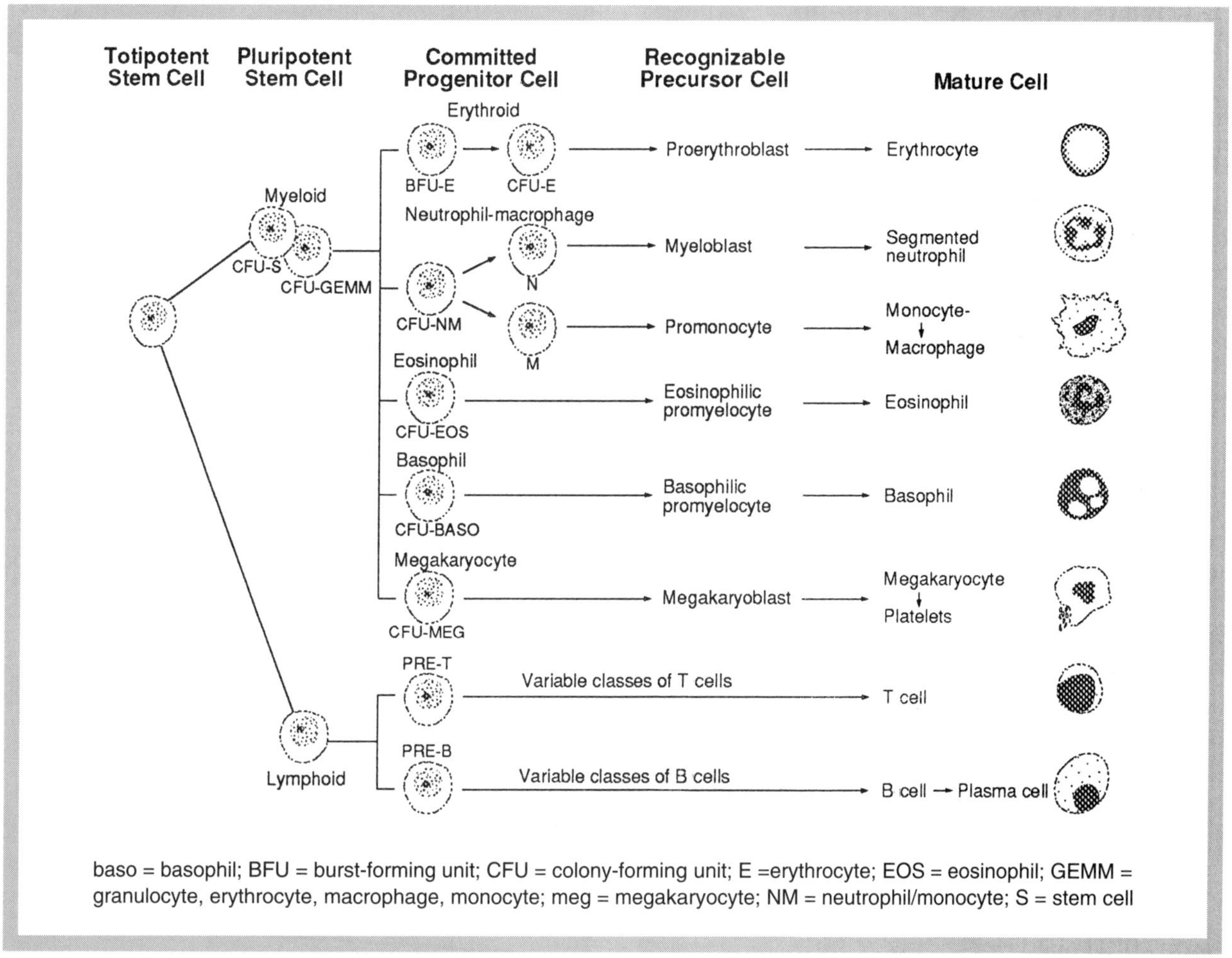

Figure 2-1. Hematopoiesis—the process of blood cell maturation from the stem cell to the active, functional blood cell

SOURCE: *Reprinted with permission from Chervenick PA. Hematopoiesis. In: Stein JH, editor.* Internal Medicine. *3rd ed. Boston, MA: Little, Brown; 1990. p. 946.*

vironment called the stroma. The stroma provides nutrients for growing cells and includes cells that produce colony-stimulating factors (CSFs). Each step in hematopoiesis is regulated by this array of CSFs.[2] Hematopoiesis produces six cell types in the myeloid family that are involved in the nonspecific immune response: mononuclear phagocytes, polymorphonuclear leukocytes (PMNs), eosinophils, basophils, mast cells, and platelets.[1]

In the nonspecific immune response, the most active cells are the phagocytes, which destroy antigens. The activity of these cells is unchanged by their interaction with the antigen (i.e., they are not antigen specific). Both mononuclear cells (macrophages) and polynuclear cells (neutrophils and eosinophils) are capable of phagocytosis.[3,4]

Mononuclear Cells

The function of monocytes and macrophages is based on the size, cellular morphology, and location of the cell. Monocytes develop from myeloid stem cells in the bone marrow and circulate through the bloodstream. Once the monocyte leaves the circulation and enters tissue, it becomes a macrophage, sometimes called a histiocyte. There are 3.5 times more macrophages in soft tissues than monocytes in the blood. The transformation in the soft tissues produces a cell 10 times the size of a monocyte. Because it has an increased supply of enzymes, lysosomes, and energy-producing mitochondria, the macrophage has increased phagocytic capacity. The collective pool of monocytes and macrophages found in the soft tissues, blood, and bone marrow has historically been referred to as the reticuloendothelial system.[5]

There are two types of macrophages, fixed and wandering. Fixed macrophages are described according to their location in tissue. For example, alveolar macrophages line the alveoli of the lung, reticular cells are in the spleen, microglial cells are in the brain, peritoneal macrophages patrol the abdominal cavity, mesangial cells inhabit the kidneys, Kupffer cells reside in the liver, osteoclasts are found in bone, and Langerhans cells exist in skin. Wan-

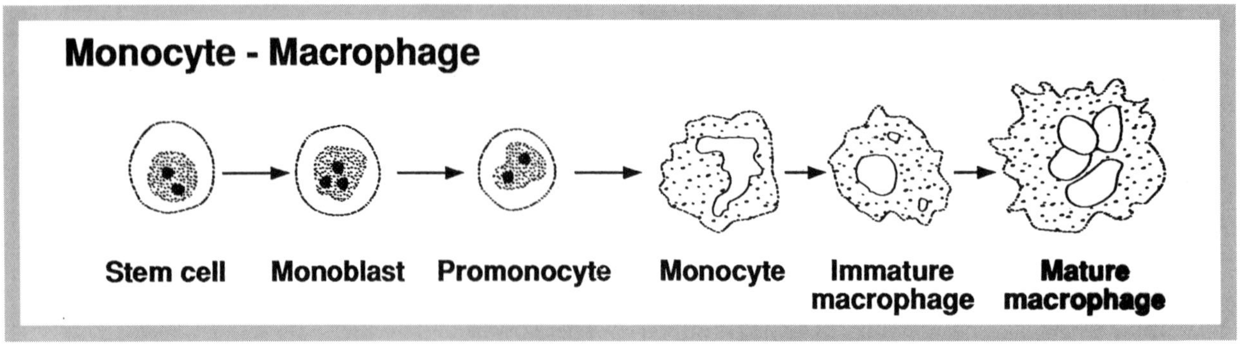

Figure 2-2. Mononuclear development

SOURCE: *Reprinted with permission from Hutton JJ, Cline MJ. Hematopoiesis and the red cell. In: Stein JH, editor.* Internal Medicine. *Boston, MA: Little, Brown; 1983. p. 1470.*

dering macrophages (monocytes) are found mostly in blood and only transiently in lymphoid tissue. Their function is to clear debris from tissue.[6,7]

The maturation process of the pluripotent stem cell to mature monocyte in the bone marrow takes seven days (Figure 2-2). Growth and development are controlled by interleukin 3 (IL-3), granulocyte-macrophage colony-stimulating factor (GM-CSF), and macrophage colony-stimulating factor (M-CSF). Monocytes live in the circulation for 8–72 hours before they leave the bloodstream and enter tissue to become macrophages. Monocytes adhere to the endothelial wall of the blood vessel by a process called margination. They then squeeze between the endothelial cells, into tissue, by a process known as diapedesis. Migration of the monocyte into tissues without the stimulation of inflammation is apparently a random event; inflammation increases capillary permeability, encouraging diapedesis. The average turnover rate for macrophages is seven million cells per hour per kilogram of body weight, and they are thought to live for months. Although macrophages are mature cells, they remain capable of cell division, a capacity neutrophils do not possess. Factors contributing to the death of these cells are not yet known. One hypothesis is that intense phagocytosis may lead to uncontrolled release of enzymes and other toxic chemicals into the cell's cytoplasm.[6,8]

Monocytes have two major functions, phagocytosis and antigen presentation. The outer membrane of a macrophage moves constantly. It is studded with microvilli, which help the macrophage attach to an antigen. The cell's interior has many small lysosomes containing digestive enzymes, such as acid hydrolases and peroxidase. When released into the phagocytic vesicle, these enzymes kill the invading organism. Two receptors on the cell's outer membrane promote binding of the macrophage to the invader: a receptor for the crystallizable fragment (Fc) portion of immunoglobulin, and a receptor for the C3b protein of complement. There are other receptors on the macrophage membrane that allow lymphokines to facilitate communication among cells.[6,8]

A normal resting macrophage is activated by lymphokines such as M-CSF, interferon gamma (IFN-γ), IL-3, and GM-CSF, which are all released from T lymphocytes. Once activated, macrophages release tumor necrosis factor (TNF) and interleukin 1 (IL-1), resulting in a more efficient killing cell. The activated macrophage increases in size, develops more pseudopods, and is better able to adhere to the antigen surface.[6,8] Other secretory products of macrophages are listed in Table 2-1.

Table 2-1. Macrophage Secretory Products

Enzymes
Elastase
Plasminogen activator
Collagenase
Lysozomal enzymes
Angiotensin-converting enzyme
Tissue procoagulant
Arginase
Cytokines and Growth Factors
G-CSF
GM-CSF
M-CSF
Tumor necrosis factor
Interleukins 1, 6, 8, 10, 12
Inflammatory Proteins
Complement C2, C3, C4, C5
Lysozyme
Interferon alpha
Interferon beta
Tissue Repair Factors
Platelet-derived growth factor
Fibroblast growth factor

SOURCE: *Adapted from Reference 8, Table 3, p. 116.*
G-CSF, granulocyte colony-stimulating factor; GM-CSF, granulocyte-macrophage colony-stimulating factor; M-CSF, macrophage colony-stimulating factor.

Macrophages also function as antigen-presenting cells (APCs). APCs process antigen biochemically to a more immunogenic form and then present it along with surface class II major histocompatibility complex (MHC) molecules on their cell surfaces to be recognized by specific, sensitized T lymphocytes. (A detailed discussion of the MHC is provided in chapter 3.) APCs initially activate helper T cells. The term APC is often used to designate a specific form of macrophage found in the skin or solid lymphoid organs.[4,8,9] Other cell types that function as APCs are dendritic cells, B lymphocytes, and microglial cells. APCs are primarily located in the skin (Langerhans cells), lymph nodes and spleen (follicular dendritic cells), central nervous system tissue (microglial cells), and thymus. Inside the lymph node, APCs are uniquely able to bind with more than one T cell, thereby presenting antigen to many cells at once.[8]

In addition to their roles as phagocytes and APCs, macrophages also serve in nerve regeneration and bone remodeling and aid in hematopoiesis.[6] Monocytes play an important part in tumor surveillance by seeking out tumor cell surface markers and then destroying the cell. Finally, monocytes and macrophages are reservoirs for pathogens such as the human immunodeficiency virus (HIV), mycobacteria, and some fungi.[10]

Polymorphonuclear Cells

Polymorphonuclear cells, or granulocytes, contain cytoplasmic granules that can be stained. The color, type, and number of the granules vary, depending on the stage of cell growth and development. Generally, the granules contain enzymes used in cellular functions such as respiration. The granulocyte family comprises neutrophils, eosinophils, basophils, and mast cells.

Neutrophils

The primary function of neutrophils is to phagocytize foreign particles. These specialized WBCs make up 60–70% of the total WBC count. Mature polymorphonuclear granulocytes are released into the bloodstream after a 14-day process of developing from pluripotent stem cells in bone marrow (Figure 2-3). Neutrophils reside in the bloodstream for approximately seven hours before they enter the tissues, where they survive for an additional 1–2 days. More than 100 billion neutrophils are produced each day.[11,12]

Neutrophils are an important part of the first-line defense against foreign substances. They phagocytize many different substances but are particularly important in defending against bacteria and certain fungal pathogens. Engulfed antigens are destroyed by digestive and hydrolytic enzymes released by neutrophils. Neutrophils are part of the general inflammatory response; neutrophilia (an increase in neutrophil count in the bloodstream) usually represents a normal response to bacteria or fungi. Corticosteroids cause demargination (movement of cells from the endothelial walls of blood vessels into circulation) of neutrophils and raise the counts in the blood. Neutropenia (decrease in neutrophil count) is a serious condition in which patients are susceptible to bacterial or fungal sepsis.[11,12]

Eosinophils

Eosinophils make up 1–3% of the total WBCs. Their granules are large and stain intensely red. They mature in the bone marrow for 3–6 days, then remain in the bloodstream for only minutes before entering the tissues for the remainder of their lives—approximately 12 days. Production of eosinophils is regulated by IL-1, IL-3, IL-5, GM-CSF, and granulocyte colony-stimulating factor (G-CSF).

Eosinophils have the capacity to phagocytize microorganisms, but not as efficiently as neutrophils and macrophages. Other immunologic roles include ingesting immune complexes and clearing parasitic organisms from the host. Eosinophils kill by attaching themselves to the foreign invader and releasing toxic granules. Eosinophils also temper hypersensitivity reactions by neutralizing histamine and stabilizing mast cell degranulation. (See chapter 4.) Eosinophilia (increased eosinophil count) has been associated with many disorders, including allergic reactions, asthma, parasitic infections, dermatitis, inflammatory gastrointestinal disorders, certain cancers, Addison's disease, and connective tissue disorders.[13]

Basophils

Basophils make up less than 1% of the total WBC count.

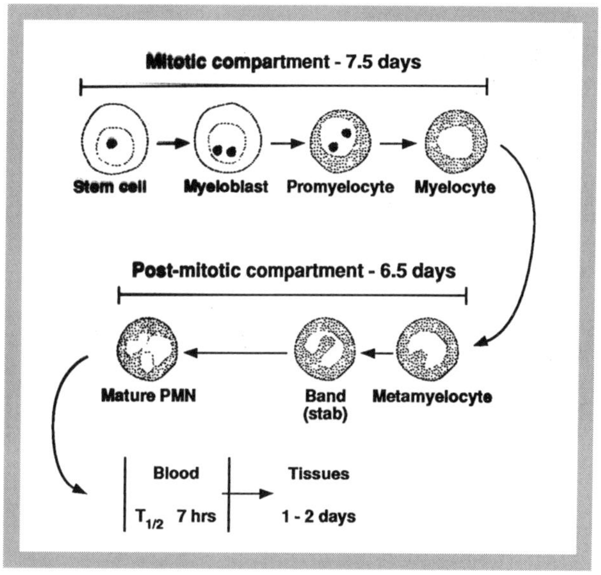

Figure 2-3. Neutrophil development. PMN, polymorphonuclear leukocyte (neutrophil); $T_{1/2}$, half-life.

SOURCE: *Reprinted with permission from Chervenick PA. Hematopoiesis. In: Stein JH, editor.* Internal Medicine. *2nd ed. Boston, MA: Little, Brown; 1987. p. 913.*

They are distinguished by their large, blue-staining, cytoplasmic granules, which contain histamine and other inflammatory mediators. Basophils have specific receptors on their surface that bind immunoglobulin E (IgE) antibody molecules secreted by B lymphocytes. When an antigen molecule interacts with these membrane-bound IgE antibodies, the basophil is triggered to release histamine and other inflammatory mediators. Histamine release increases vascular permeability, allowing deposition of antigen-antibody complexes. Basophilopenia (decrease in basophil count) has been associated with corticosteroid therapy, hypersensitivity reactions, and hyperthyroidism. Basophilia (increase in basophil count) has been seen in chronic myelogenous leukemia, inflammatory reactions, diabetes, hypothyroidism, viral infections, and iron deficiency.[14]

Mast Cells

Like basophils, mast cells stain blue, contain histamine and other inflammatory mediators in their granules, and are stimulated when IgE binds to their surface receptors. Mast cells leave the bone marrow more quickly than do basophils and then enter connective tissue, where they mature. The life span of most mast cells is 14–18 days. Mature mast cells still have the capacity to differentiate.

Two types of mast cells exist. Connective tissue–type mast cells are most commonly found around blood vessels, particularly in the skin, abdominal cavity, and lungs. They contain both heparin and histamine. Mucosal-type mast cells are plentiful in tissue exposed to the environment, such as the gastrointestinal tract and mucosal surfaces of the lungs. Mucosal-type mast cells contain histamine but lack heparin.[14,15]

Platelets

Much like basophils, platelets function as mediator cells, releasing chemicals that promote an immunologic or inflammatory response. They are cellular fragments from the large megakaryocytes in the bone marrow and have a life span of seven to nine days.[12] Platelets are involved primarily in blood clotting. They function immunologically during the inflammatory response by releasing factors that alter vascular permeability and activate complement components to draw other WBCs to the site (chemotaxis). The surface of platelets contains receptors for immunoglobulin G (IgG) and IgE as well as class I MHC products.[16]

SPECIFIC CELLULAR COMPONENTS

Lymphocytes

Lymphocytes make up 20% of circulating WBCs. The bone marrow and thymus produce one billion lymphocytes per day. The life span of a lymphocyte can be quite long, up to years for memory cells. Lymphoid cells are a heterogenous group that can be morphologically described as small lymphocytes or large granular lymphocytes. T lymphocytes, which mature in the thymus, are primarily responsible for cell-mediated immunity, B lymphocytes are responsible for what is historically known as humoral immunity (Figure 2-4), and null cells assist in antibody-dependent cell-mediated cytotoxicity (ADCC). Physically, these lymphocytes appear quite similar; T and B lymphocytes can be distinguished by cell surface markers.[4,9,17,18]

T Lymphocytes (Cell-Mediated Immunity)

T lymphocytes develop from stem cells in the bone marrow but differentiate in the thymus, where immature T cells are tested against thymus epithelial tissue to develop recognition of self from nonself. T cells that react to self are destroyed, and the rest develop into mature T cells.[12]

T cells spend their lives circulating between the bloodstream and the lymphatic system (lymph nodes and spleen). T-cell functions include regulating B cells, developing resistance to bacterial or viral invasion, and producing soluble cellular mediators, such as interleukins. T cells are the primary mediators of processes such as graft-versus-host disease, delayed hypersensitivity reactions, and solid organ or bone marrow graft rejection. These various aspects of T-cell function are collectively referred to as cell-mediated immunity.

The four classes of T cells are helper (inducer), suppressor, cytotoxic, and memory (delayed hypersensitivity).[9,19] Helper and suppressor T lymphocytes are also known as regulatory cells, cytotoxic T lymphocytes are called mediator cells, and memory T lymphocytes are referred to as effector cells.

Helper T Lymphocytes

The primary function of helper (inducer) lymphocytes is to orchestrate communication among the other cell types. This is why helper cells are generically referred to as regulatory cells. When an APC presents an antigen to a helper T cell, the T cell is stimulated to release IL-2, a lymphokine. IL-2 then stimulates other helper T cells as well as cytotoxic and memory T lymphocytes. A second lymphokine secreted by helper T cells, IFN-γ, stimulates natural killer cells and macrophages. In addition to establishing communication among T lymphocytes, helper T lymphocytes produce other lymphokines, such as IL-4, that stimulate the growth and differentiation of B cells.[20–22]

Suppressor T Lymphocytes

Controversy currently exists about whether suppressor cells or substances are responsible for the functions ascribed to them. In theory, suppressor T cells function as inhibitors rather than stimulators. Like helper T cells, suppressor T cells act on other T lymphocytes, inhibiting proliferation and stimulation of these cells.[23] The suppressor cell (or factor) also inhibits plasma cell functions and antibody production and participates in developing toler-

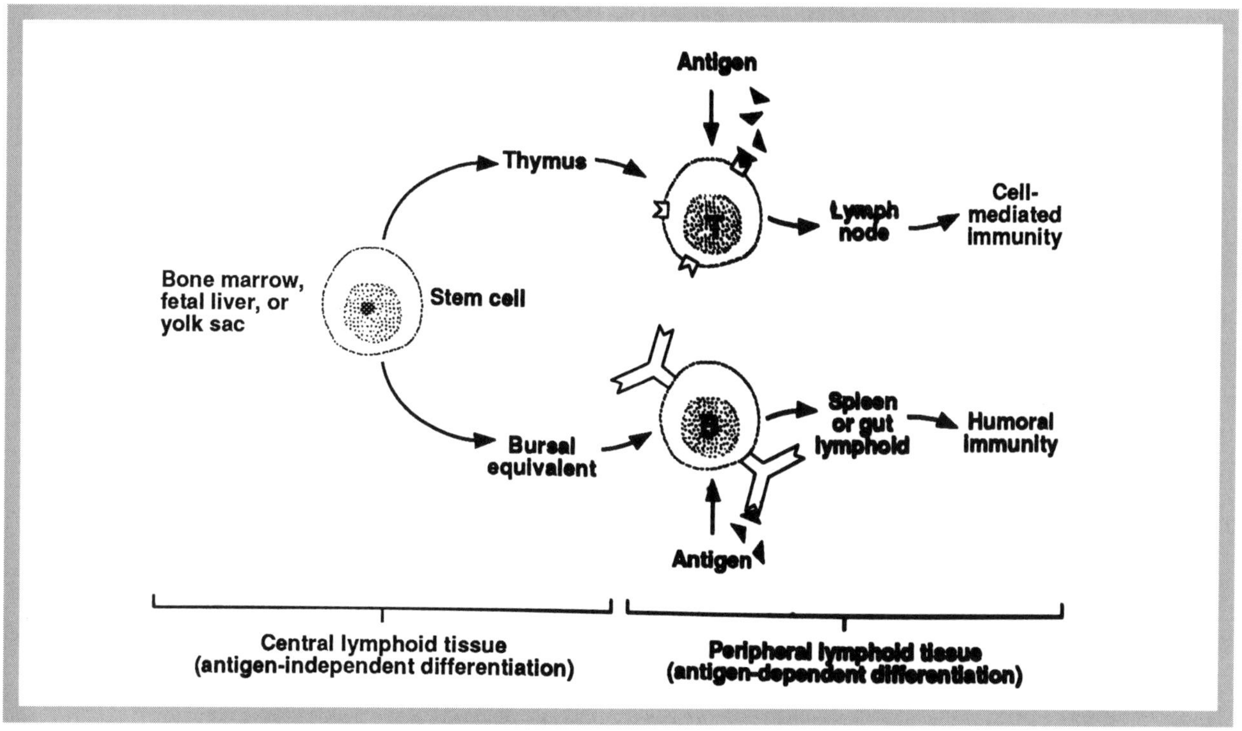

Figure 2-4. Lymphoid system

SOURCE: *Reprinted with permission from Bellanti JA, Kadiec JV. General immunobiology. In: Bellanti JA, editor.* Immunology III. *Philadelphia, PA: WB Saunders; 1985. p. 33.*

ance. Tolerance is the process by which the immune system learns what is foreign (i.e., self is distinguished from nonself). Tolerance prevents reactions to drugs and autoimmune diseases.

Cytotoxic T Lymphocytes

Cytotoxic T lymphocytes are the real warriors among the T lymphocytes. They attack cells bearing antigens on their membranes. Cytotoxic T lymphocytes bore holes through the invader's membrane, causing cell lysis and death. A single cytotoxic T cell can kill more than one target cell, which suggests that cytotoxic T cells are resistant to the lysing substances they contain.[24] Cytotoxic T lymphocytes are thought to be primarily responsible for graft rejection in transplants. (See chapters 8 and 9.) They also fight intracellular infections such as malaria and those caused by viruses, *Listeria monocytogenes*, and trypanosomes.[25] Cytotoxic T cells are also involved in autoimmune disorders, such as rheumatoid arthritis or multiple sclerosis.[25]

Because suppressor and cytotoxic T cells bear no surface markers that make it possible to distinguish between them, there has been speculation that they are the same cell type. They do have different functional activities, however, and are generally considered two different cell types.

Memory T Lymphocytes

These cells are more appropriately called delayed hypersensitivity cells because they play a pivotal role in inflammation associated with contact hypersensitivity. Memory T cells mediate delayed hypersensitivity reactions by releasing cytokines that activate macrophages and other phagocytic cells. IFN-γ, secreted by activated T cells, plays a central role in macrophage activation. IFN-γ enhances the ability of macrophages to migrate to sites of infection, phagocytize particles, and produce microbicidal oxygen metabolites. Other cytokines produced by T cells, such as IL-2 and GM-CSF, also function as macrophage activators. The delayed reaction occurs 24–48 hours after initial contact as cells accumulate, causing local tissue damage.[26,27]

T-Lymphocyte Subpopulation Markers

There are many T-cell surface markers, some more specific than others. The markers can be used to identify the developmental stage and functional capacity of the T cells. Surface markers also make it possible to isolate T cells or specific subtypes of T cells from other cells.[17,24] These markers may appear and disappear during T-cell development.

Monoclonal Antibodies

Monoclonal antibodies (MoAbs) are immunoglobulins produced by cloning a single cell, resulting in identical antibody molecules. MoAbs can be used as "lymphocyte

Table 2-2. Monoclonal Antibodies to Human T-Lymphocyte Surface Antigens

CLUSTER DESIGNATION[a]	COMMERCIAL MONOCLONAL ANTIBODIES	MOLECULAR WEIGHT OF MOLECULES	COMMENTS
Pan T cell			
CD2	Anti-T11, Leu-5, OKT11	50,000	Erythrocyte rosette-associated protein; adhesion molecule ligand for CD58.
CD3	Anti-T3 Leu-4 OKT3	20,000 22,000 28,000	Modulates antigen-specific T-cell responses; part of the T-cell receptor complex.
CD5	Anti-T1, Leu-1, OKT1	67,000	T- and B-cell marker; ligand for CD72.
T-cell subset			
CD4	Anti-T4, Leu-3a, Leu-3b, OKT4	60,000	$CD4^+$ T cells contain most inducer/helper functions; primarily class II MHC restricted; 50% to 65% of peripheral cells.
CD8	Anti-T8 Leu-2a, Leu-3b	30,000 32,000	$CD8^+$ peripheral T cells contain most suppresor/cytolytic functions; functions are class I MHC restricted; 25% to 35% of peripheral T cells.
CD25	Anti-tac	55,000	Recognizes low-affinity IL-2 receptor; blocks proliferation and IL-2 binding.

[a]MHC, major histocompatibility complex; IL-2, interleukin 2. Designations of clusters of differentiation (CDs) as assigned by the Fourth International Workshop and Conference on Human Lymphocyte Differentiation Antigens.

markers" to detect quantitative abnormalities of lymphocyte subsets in disease states. More sophisticated than separation of T versus non-T lymphocytes, MoAb technology can identify specific lymphocyte subtypes (Table 2-2) by specific cell surface markers called clusters of differentiation (CDs). Some CDs are found on many different cell types; others are specific to a certain cell type. MoAbs specific to each CD antigen exist, so the presence or absence of that antigen can be determined by the binding of the antibody.[4,17] (See chapter 11 for a detailed discussion of MoAbs.)

Sheep Erythrocyte Rosettes

One surface marker found on all T cells is a surface protein (CD2) that serves as an adhesion molecule, allowing T cells to bind to other cells. Sheep erythrocytes (SEs) express CD58, the ligand for CD2, and bind to the T cell at the CD2 surface marker. When combined, the T cells and the SEs form a visible rosette pattern. T cells can be detected by fluorescent stain of the nucleus, since mature SEs are not nucleated. This binding process can also be used to isolate T cells from non-T cells.[4,24]

B Lymphocytes (Humoral Immunity)

B lymphocytes are so named because they were first identified in the bursa of Fabricius, a specialized organ found in chickens. Stimulation of B lymphocytes results in immunoglobulin production. If serum containing certain antibodies is given to a host deficient in those antibodies, the host will be protected or become sensitized to the correlating antigens. Historically, serum was called humor; hence the term humoral immunity.[17]

B lymphocytes originate in the bone marrow from a common stem cell, as do the cells described earlier. B-cell maturation in the bone marrow occurs without antigen stimulation. Once cells have matured, they immediately leave the marrow to reside in peripheral tissues, where they are developed further by antigenic stimulation. After a mature B lymphocyte is stimulated by its complementary antigen, it may differentiate into the antibody-producing cell, the plasma cell (Figure 2-5). B cells that encounter their complementary antigen and are helped by a T lymphocyte may differentiate into memory (effector) cells with a much longer life span. (As stated earlier, effector cells can also be memory cells of T-cell origin.[17])

The membrane of the B cell bears a surface immunoglobulin that is specific for only one antigen. In addition, some B cells have membrane receptors for complement components (C3d and C3b), the Fc portion of immunoglobulin, interferons, and a B cell–stimulating factor called BSF-1 (recently renamed IL-4) that is produced

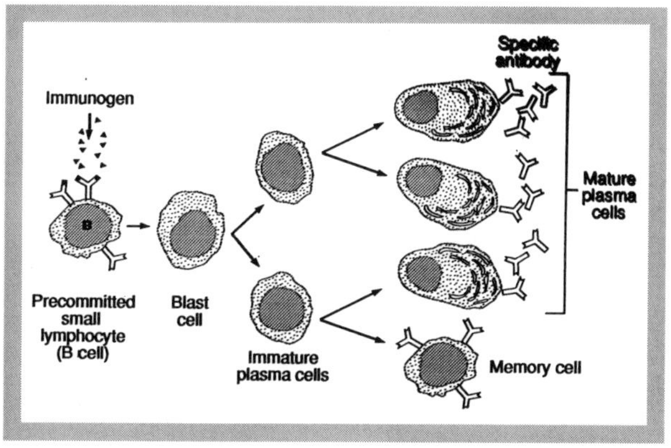

Figure 2-5. Humoral immune responses

SOURCE: *Reprinted with permission from Herscowitz HB. Immunophysiology: cell function and cellular interactions in antibody information. In: Bellanti JA, editor.* Immunology III. *Philadelphia, PA: WB Saunders; 1985. p. 125.*

by helper T cells and other cells. Activated B cells express other receptors used to modify growth and differentiation. Preliminary work on other B-cell markers has not produced more reliable or specific markers than surface immunoglobulin. Other cells, including T cells, carry Fc receptors, but not all B cells bear them.[17]

B-lymphocyte stimulation is a complex process that is only partially understood. One known mechanism is the specific antigenic activation of B lymphocytes with the help of T lymphocytes. Another mechanism uses T cells to produce nonspecific activation factors. Mitogens (substances such as lipopolysaccharide or bacterial endotoxin) induce T and B lymphocyte proliferation and may stimulate B cells nonspecifically. B cells may also be simply and directly stimulated by some large polymeric molecules (e.g., antigens such as dextran and polyvinylpyrolidone) without T-cell help. Once stimulated, B cells can differentiate into plasma cells, which produce the antibody.[28]

Antibody

The primary function of the plasma cell is to produce antibodies (immunoglobulins that interact with a specific antigen) against substances potentially harmful to the host. Figure 2-6 shows the basic structure of the IgG class of immunoglobulin.[29]

Four polypeptide chains make up the basic Y-shaped structure of immunoglobulin. The two smaller ones are identical light chains; the two larger ones are identical heavy chains. The heavy chains are roughly twice as long as the light chains, extending the full length of the Y-shaped molecule, whereas the light chains are found only along the two arms of the Y. The Fab (fragment of antigen binding) portion of the immunoglobulin contains variable regions of amino acids that allow the Fab molecule to recognize a specific antigen when it binds between the heavy and light chains of the Fab region. The Fc portion of the structure determines the effector function and class (IgG, IgM, IgA, IgD, or IgE) of the immunoglobulin.[29,30]

The immunoglobulin molecule can be divided into four regions. The hinge region is a flexible region at the base of the V that allows the two arms of the Y to move closer or further apart. Each arm of the Y is an independent antigen-binding site. The end portion of the V (amino terminal) is known to exhibit variation in amino acid sequence, hence the term variable region. Areas of greater variation within the variable region are referred to as hypervariable regions. The inner portion of the V (carboxy terminal) remains fairly consistent and is called the constant region.[29,30]

Classification

Antibodies are glycoproteins that can be classified into five distinct classes (IgG, IgA, IgD, IgE, or IgM) based on the type of heavy chain each contains. The distinguishing letters stand for gamma, alpha, delta, epsilon, and mu, respectively. IgA and IgG can be further subtyped as subclasses IgA1, IgA2, and IgG1 through IgG4. There are two types of light chains, kappa and lambda. Either may combine with one of the five different heavy chains, but both light chains are bound to each other by covalent and noncovalent bonds as well as disulfide linkages. IgG, IgD, and IgE all occur as single molecules. IgM occurs as a

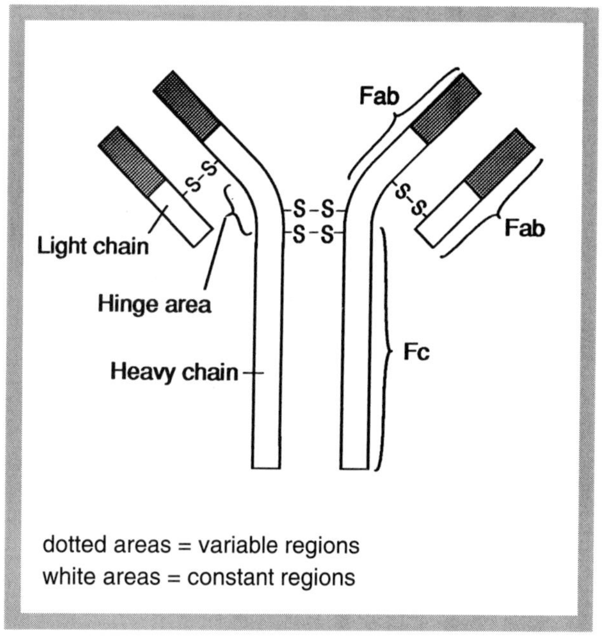

Figure 2-6. Basic immunoglobulin structure. Fab, fragment of antigen binding; Fc, crystallizable fragment

SOURCE: *Adapted with permission from Tami JA, Parr MC, Thompson JS. The immune system.* Am J Hosp Pharm. *1986;43:2485.*

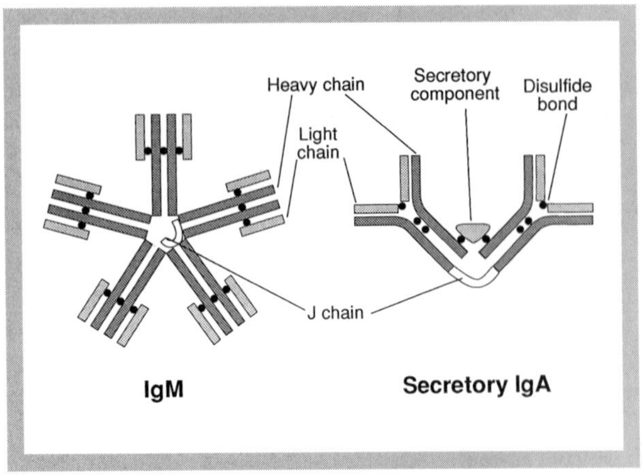

Figure 2-7. Immunoglobulin M (IgM) and immunoglobulin A (IgA) structure

SOURCE: *Reprinted with permission from Bernier GM. Antibody and immunoglobulins: structure and function. In: Bellanti JA, editor.* Immunology III. *Philadelphia, PA: WB Saunders; 1985. p. 93.*

pentamer in the circulation, but on the surface of a lymphocyte it occurs as a monomer. IgA occurs in monomeric and polymeric forms (Figure 2-7).[30,31]

The five immunoglobulin classes or isotypes differ in size, charge, amino acid sequence, and carbohydrate content (Table 2-3). Each class of immunoglobulin is heterogenous; this can be demonstrated electrophoretically.

Antigen-Antibody Interactions: Binding

Antigens are bound to antibodies by multiple noncovalent bonds at the antigen-binding site. These weak forces, such as hydrogen bonds and van der Waals forces, are so numerous that they contribute a great deal of binding energy. Close proximity between antigen and antibody is the primary force creating these noncovalent bonds. Structural characteristics lead to the proper fit between the antigen and antibody, maximizing bond formation and minimizing repulsive forces.[30]

The net result of attractive and repulsive forces between an antigenic determinant and one antibody binding site is termed affinity. In other words, affinity is an expression of the strength of one particular interaction

Table 2-3. Immunoglobulin Classification

	IMMUNOGLOBULIN CLASS				
VARIBLES	**IgG**	**IgM**	**IgA**	**IgE**	**IgD**
Heavy chain	Gamma	Mu	Alpha	Epsilon	Delta
Subclasses	Gamma 1, 2, 3, 4	Mu 1, 2	Alpha 1, 2	None	None
Extra chains	None	Joining	Joining and secretory	None	None
Serum concentration (approximate % of total Ig)	70	20	10	<1	<1
Plasma half-life (days)	IgG1 = 21 IgG2 = 20 IgG3 = 7 IgG4 = 21	5–10	6	2	3
Molecular weight	150,000 (polymer)	900,000 (polymer)	350,000	190,000	100,000
% carbohydrate	3	12	7	12	13
Placenta transfer	Yes	No	No	No	No
Major function	Primary or secondary response; fixes complement	Primary response; common antibody to blood group; fixes complement	Secretory response; bodily secretions, such as mucus lining the gastrointestinal tract	Allergic response	Membrane receptor

SOURCE: *Adapted with permission from Tami JA, Parr MC, Thompson JS. The immune system.* Am J Hosp Pharm. *1986;43:2485.*
Ig; immunoglobulin.

between antigen and antibody. The stronger the attractive forces, the higher the affinity and, probably, the better the "fit" between the antigen and antibody. Conversely, weaker attractive forces mean less affinity and imply a poorer fit.[32]

Avidity, on the other hand, describes the functional combined strength of all the interactions between an antibody and an antigen. One antigen often has many binding sites, which can boost the overall antigen-antibody interaction. Unlike affinity, which can be quantified, avidity is a more general term. Although avidity of the antibody for the antigen depends on the affinities at each binding site, avidity is not just the combined affinities of each binding site. Often, multiple bonds have a synergistic effect on binding, and the avidity exceeds the combined affinities.

Affinity and avidity are important in biologic reactions such as viral neutralization, enzyme inactivation, and complement fixation. High-affinity reactions are more desirable because high-affinity immune complexes are rapidly cleared from the circulation with little effect on renal function. Low-affinity complexes are cleared more slowly from the circulation and can be deposited on glomerular membranes, causing renal impairment.[32]

Specificity is the ability of the antibody to distinguish its target antigen from other antigens. The antibody's ability to interact with other related antigens is termed cross-reactivity.[32]

Memory Cells

Both T and B lymphocytes are capable of differentiating into memory (i.e., delayed-hypersensitivity and effector) cells. After initial contact between the T or B cells and the antigen, the lymphocytes are stimulated into proliferation and maturation. Some of the resulting progeny become the plasma cells that develop the antibodies used to fight the invader. Other lymphocytes are transformed into memory cells, which remain in circulation. On future stimulation by the specific antigen, these memory cells can more quickly mount a heightened immune response.[26,27]

Non-B and Non-T Lymphocytes (Null Cells)

Non-B and non-T lymphocytes—killer (K) and natural killer (NK) cells—cannot be identified by typical T- or B-cell surface markers and have been called third population cells or null cells.[33] K cells play a role in ADCC; they can recognize and kill only target cells that are coated with antibody.

NK cells are large granular lymphocytes that do not bear typical T- or B-cell surface markers. However, surface markers of NK cells have been described using MoAbs. The two most useful markers are CD56 and CD16, although not all CD56-positive or CD16-positive ($CD56^+$ or $CD16^+$) cells are NK cells. NK cells kill tumor and virally infected cells and help regulate hematopoiesis. They are found in the bone marrow, peripheral blood, spleen, liver, lung, and intestinal tract. In the liver, they are referred to as pit cells because they look like the pit of a fruit.[33]

Although it is accepted that NK cells originate from bone marrow precursors, their exact lineage is unclear. They may represent a third lineage similar to the T- and B-cell families. Little is known about the maturation process of NK cells. After escaping from the marrow cavity, NK cells are found primarily in the bloodstream or the spleen and have a life span of days to months. Mature NK cells still retain some capacity to proliferate.[33,34]

NK cells can kill tumor cells, virally infected cells, and bacterial pathogens through cell lysis without having first been sensitized to the target and without MHC recognition. In fact, increased MHC expression probably inhibits NK cell activity. NK cells are also capable of ADCC.[33]

NK cells destroy other cells by releasing perforins from cytoplasmic granules after contact with the target cell. Perforins—or, more descriptively, pore-forming proteins—are released as monomers but polymerize after inserting themselves into the target cell membrane, creating transmembrane holes that allow lysis by osmosis. NK cells also release TNF, which activates endonucleases and breaks DNA into smaller pieces. Through these lytic processes, NK cells play a role in removing malignant cells. Recently, NK cells have been described as mediators of the graft-versus-leukemia effect in bone marrow transplantation.[33]

NK cell regulation is mediated primarily by IL-2 but also by interferons. Interferons do not cause an increase in NK cell numbers, but all interferons enhance NK cell-induced lysis. The effect of IFN-α is greater than that of IFN-β, however.[33,34] The central cytokine mediator of NK cell activity is IL-2. Lymphocytes exposed to IL-2 in culture become lymphokine-activated killer cells capable of destroying tumor cells. The effect of IL-2 on NK cells has not been fully elucidated, but IL-2 does increase the quantity and size of lytic granules. NK cells produce IFN-γ, GM-CSF, and TNF-α.[33,34]

The role of NK cells in regulating hematopoiesis is still under investigation; depending on conditions, both hematopoietic stimulation and inhibition have occurred.[33] Cytokine release by NK cells tends to suppress granulocyte development and support erythroid and megakaryocytic generation.

Communications: Soluble Mediators

Many soluble substances are responsible for stimulating, suppressing, and orchestrating the activities of the immune system. The communications pathways among cells and tissues are the sites for the many commercially produced, natural, or recombinant immunologic agents, such

Table 2-4. Sources and Effects of Soluble Mediators[12,38–42]

SOLUBLE MEDIATORS	PRIMARY CELLULAR SOURCE	PRINCIPAL EFFECTS
Interleukins		
IL-1 (α, β)	Macrophages	Activates lymphocytes; increases WBC adhesion; induces pyrexia
IL-2	T cells	T-cell growth factor
IL-3	T cells	Multilineage CSF of stem cells
IL-4	T cells	B-cell growth factor
IL-5	T cells	B-cell growth and differentiation
IL-6	Leukocytes	B-cell growth and differentiation; acute phase response
IL-7	Bone marrow stromal cells	Early lymphocyte proliferation
IL-8	Endothelial cells, monocytes, T cells	Decreases adhesion of neutrophils to vascular endothelium; attenuates inflammatory events; chemotactic factor for neutrophils
IL-9	Activated T cells	Erythropoiesis
IL-10	Helper T cells	Regulates production of other cytokines
IL-11	Bone marrow stromal cells	Megakaryopoiesis; B-cell development
IL-12	B cells	Activates T lymphocytes and lymphokine-activated killer cells
IL-13	T cells	Stimulates immunoglobulin production and T-cell proliferation; inhibits monocyte inflammatory cytokine production
IL-14	T cells	Induces B-cell proliferation; inhibits immunoglobulin secretion
IL-15	Monocytes and macrophages	Stimulates T-cell proliferation; activates cytotoxic T cells, lymphokine-activated killer cells, and natural killer cells; induces activated B-cell proliferation; induces IgM, IgG1, and IgA secretion
Interferons		
IFN-α, -β	Leukocytes	MHC class I induction; antiviral IFN effects
IFN-γ	T cells	MHC class I and II induction; macrophage activation; increases lymphocyte adhesion
Colony-stimulating factors		
GM-CSF	Macrophages, T cells	Granulocyte and macrophage growth and differentiation
G-CSF	Macrophages	Granulocyte growth and differentiation
M-CSF	Monocytes	Monocyte and macrophage growth and differentiation
SCF (or MCGF)	Bone marrow stromal cells	Stimulates early hematopoietic progenitor cells
Tumor necrosis factors		
TNF-α	Monocytes and macrophages	Cachexia; increases activation of lymphocytes, granulocytes, and macrophages; increases cell adhesion
TNF-β (lymphotoxin)	T cells	Cytotoxicity (lymphotoxin)

MCGF, mast-cell growth factor; SCF, stem-cell factor; WBC, white blood cell.

as IFN-α. In general, these mediators are lymphokines, monokines, CSFs, B-cell growth factors, and other miscellaneous factors such as vasoactive substances and chemotactic factors (Table 2-4).[9,35–39]

Not all activities of these mediators have been definitely characterized, nor have all the interacting factors been identified. It should also be noted that the pathways may be affected by more than one mediator and may involve a complex response that subsequently influences other pathways. Chapter 10 gives further details about some of the more well-defined mediators of the immune system.

TISSUES OF THE IMMUNE SYSTEM

The structural cells of the lymphatic system are found in diffuse collections of tissues and as neatly packaged organs (Figure 2-8). There are two functional types of lymphatic tissue, primary and secondary. Primary lymphatic tissue (thymus and bone marrow) is centrally located within the body. This is the site of lymphocyte development, beginning with stem cells and resulting in mature, active lymphocytes. Secondary lymphatic tissue (lymph nodes and spleen) provides a site where lymphocytes, macrophages, and antigens interact.[12,40]

Bone Marrow

Throughout life, bone marrow is the source of stem cells of the immune system. The active portion of marrow in adults is found at the proximal ends of the long bones of the body and the sternum. Marrow consists mainly of stromal tissue and capillaries. Hematopoiesis occurs in the stroma, which is made up of endothelial cells, fibroblasts (collagen-producing cells), adipocytes (fat cells), and macrophages. Stromal cells produce collagen and adhesive proteins to locate maturing hematopoietic cells and anchor them in an environment rich with nutrients and CSFs. Once cells have matured, they squeeze across tiny pores into the circulation. After release from the bone marrow, each cell has its own life cycle in secondary lymphatic or other tissues.[40]

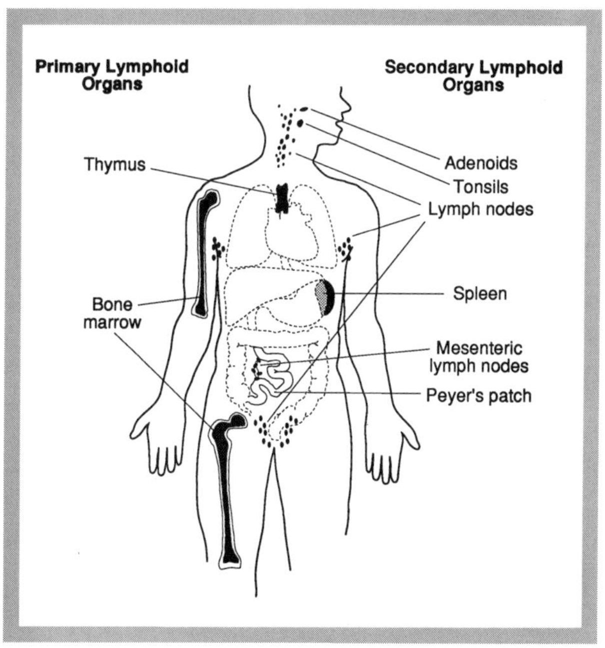

Figure 2-8. General overview of lymphatic tissue

Thymus

During the first three months of their gestation, immature T lymphocytes leave the bone marrow and travel through the bloodstream to the thymus. Located in the thorax, the thymus overlies the heart and great vessels (Figure 2-8). This organ is made up of small patches of tissue called lobules (Figure 2-9). The lobules have an outer layer of cells (the cortex), where immature T lymphocytes proliferate, and an inner layer of cells (the medulla), where more mature T cells are located. The thymus is made up of epithelial cells that probably support the lymphocytes through differentiation and help them develop the ability to recognize self. Theoretically, the thymus secretes hormones that support the development of T lymphocytes. The thymus also tests T cells against its own tissue, and cells that react against it (recognize self as nonself) are destroyed. Only 10% of the cells that enter the thymus survive.[12,40]

Lymph Nodes

Once the T cell matures, it emigrates out of the thymus to secondary lymphatic tissues. The major network of secondary lymphatic tissue consists of lymph nodes and lymphatic vessels (Figure 2-10). Lymph nodes are most prominent in the neck, axilla, abdomen (within the mesentery and along the spine), and groin (Figure 2-8). Lymph nodes filter tissue fluids (lymph), which are eventually returned to the thoracic duct and the bloodstream. Each lymph

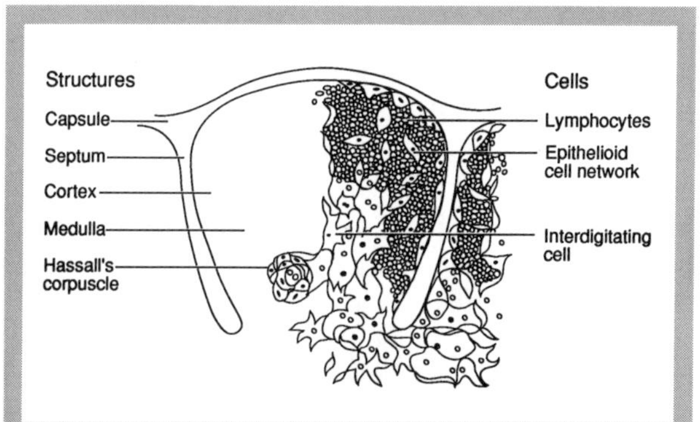

Figure 2-9. Structure of a thymus lobule

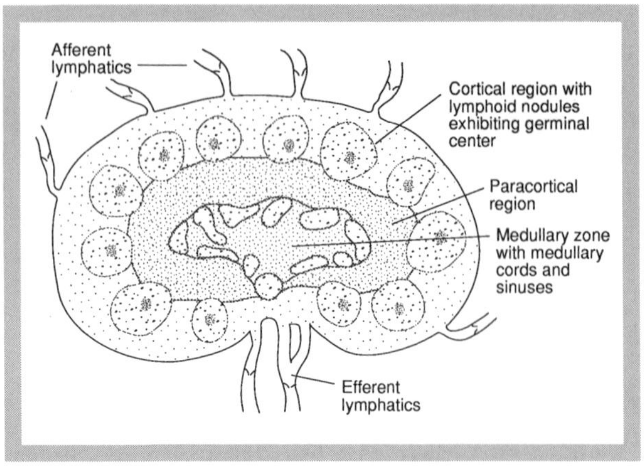

Figure 2-10. Lymph node

SOURCE: *Adapted with permission from Mota I. Tissues and cells of the immune system. In: Bier OG, da Silva W, Gotze D,* et al., *editors.* Fundamentals of Immunology. *Heidelburg, Germany: Springer-Verlag; 1986. p. 23.*

node is a complex, small (1–25 mm), ovoid organ. The outer cortex contains B lymphocytes, and the paracortex houses T lymphocytes and APCs. Some tissue from the outer two layers sends fibrous strands ("cords") through the inner tissue layer, the medulla, to form sinuses. The sinuses are lined with macrophages, which encounter antigens as the lymph flows through the node. Between these strands are B cells. When the node is antigenically stimulated, germinal centers are formed within a follicular structure. These are clusters of APCs, macrophages, T cells, and NK cells that play crucial roles in the development of the B cells, especially memory cells.[41]

Spleen

Located in the upper left abdomen behind the stomach, the spleen has two functions: filtering blood and trapping blood-borne antigens. The filtration process sorts cells, removes defective blood cells, and stores some cells. The spleen is also a place where lymphocytes, monocytes, and macrophages are exposed to immunogenic particles.

In addition, the spleen serves as another site of lymphocyte development. Red and white pulp are the two major tissue types of the spleen (Figure 2-11). White pulp makes up approximately 20% of the spleen, but this percentage varies with the immune status of the host. The lymphoid portion of the spleen is the white pulp, which is positioned around central arterioles. Both T and B cells are found within white pulp, with T cells clustered centrally around the arteriole and B cells slightly removed from the vessel. As in the lymph nodes, B cells may be present as unstimulated or stimulated cells in germinal centers, of which macrophages and APCs are also a part. Red pulp sinuses are lined with phagocytic cells and lymphocytes that have crossed over from the white pulp.[41,42]

Mucosal-Associated Lymphoid Tissue

Mucosal-associated lymphoid tissue (MALT) is a generic term for nonencapsulated lymphoid tissues. Mucosal linings of the body are constantly subjected to antigens, pathogens, and toxic substances and hence are the primary portals of entry for invaders. Areas where MALT can be found are the gastrointestinal, respiratory, and urogenital tracts. The nonencapsulated lymphoid tissues found within the gastrointestinal tract are often called gut-associated lymphoid tissue (GALT); a similar system in the lungs is called bronchial-associated lymphoid tissue (BALT). Because these areas are the primary sites of foreign invasion, they play a critical role in immunologic defense.

MALT, although existing as nonencapsulated cells, may be organized into discrete colonies, such as the tonsils, appendix, or Peyer's patches of the intestinal tract. Peyer's patches contain both mature B and T cells and are most numerous in the distal small intestine and the proximal large intestine. There are more than 200 Peyer's patches in the adult. The patch is much like the tissues already discussed, having lymphoid follicles and germinal centers. Hosts with minimal antigenic stimulation of the intestines have very small Peyer's patches. In addition to the microvilli of the intestinal lumen, the patch is covered by special epithelial cells that produce microfolds (hence the name M cell) over the surface of the patch.

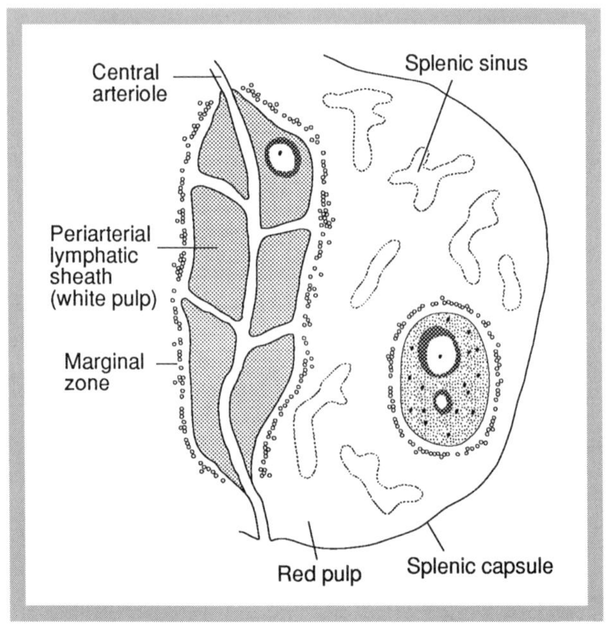

Figure 2-11. Spleen

The lymphocytes of the patch that are very close to the lumen have ready access to antigens. A large quantity of antigen is present in the intestine, and theoretically Peyer's patches are responsible for suppression of the immune response and development of tolerance; otherwise, the system would be overwhelmed. B cells in Peyer's patches are also responsible for secreting IgA into the bowel.[41]

High Endothelial Venule

Lymphocytes can enter the tissues of the lymphatic system through lymphatic vessels or the endothelial wall of a blood vessel. The particular region of blood vessels allowing this passage of lymphocytes, called the high endothelial venule (HEV), is made of columnar cells between which lymphocytes can pass. The HEV, a normal component of lymph nodes and Peyer's patches, can be stimulated by lymphokines (e.g., IFN-γ) and lymphocytes involved in an immune reaction in other tissues. Lymphocytes recognize the HEV with specific receptors. The migration process involves interactions of lymphocytes with various components of the extracellular matrix. Interaction results vary, but they include enhanced lymphocyte motility, increased lymphocyte adhesion, and T lymphocyte suppression.[43]

Lymphocyte traffic is the normal circulation of lymphocytes through the secondary lymphatic tissue and back into the bloodstream (Figure 2-12). Lymphocytes can cross blood vessel walls, moving into specific organs (MALT, spleen, bone marrow, lymph nodes, and thymus), where they may respond to antigenic stimuli. They then return to the general circulation, making their way through the major vessels of the lymphatic system to the thoracic duct, where they are emptied into the venous circulation.[43]

IMMUNE REGULATION AND RESPONSE

The host's first encounter with a specific antigen results in a primary response by the immune system (Figure 2-13). First, the new antigen must be processed and signals sent to the tissues and cells of the immune system to stimulate proliferation and maturation. The time between antigen introduction and host response varies, depending on the amount, route, solubility, and immunogenicity of the antigen and the physical status of the host. This interval is called the inductive or latent period (upper part of Figure 2-13). The isotype of antibody produced is IgM, followed by IgG. The rate and amount of antibody production depend on the number of cells that can be activated and on the metabolic rate, or half-life, of each antibody type.[40,44]

Memory

As shown in Figure 2-13, subsequent encounters between the host and the same antigen result in a more rapid and

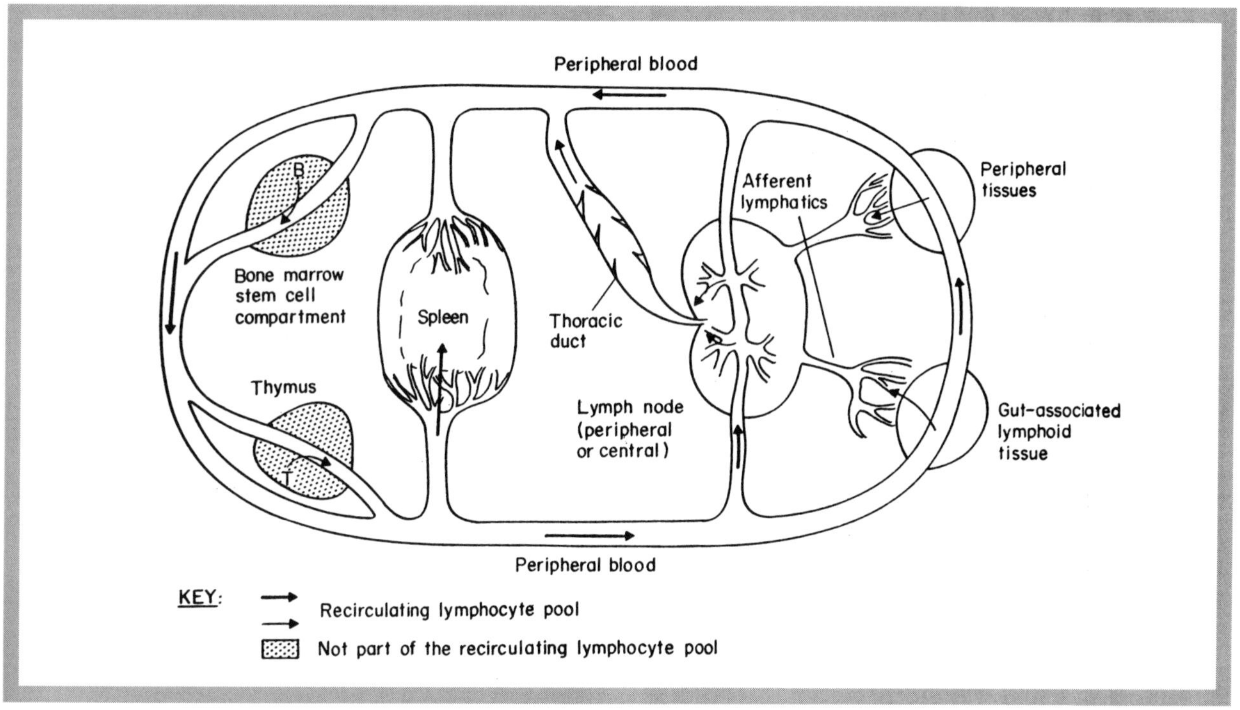

Figure 2-12. Lymphocyte traffic

SOURCE: *Reprinted with permission from McConnell I. Lymphocytes and the lymphoid system. In: Lachmann PJ, Peters DK, editors.* Clinical Aspects of Immunology. *Boston, MA: Blackwell Scientific; 1982. p. 90.*

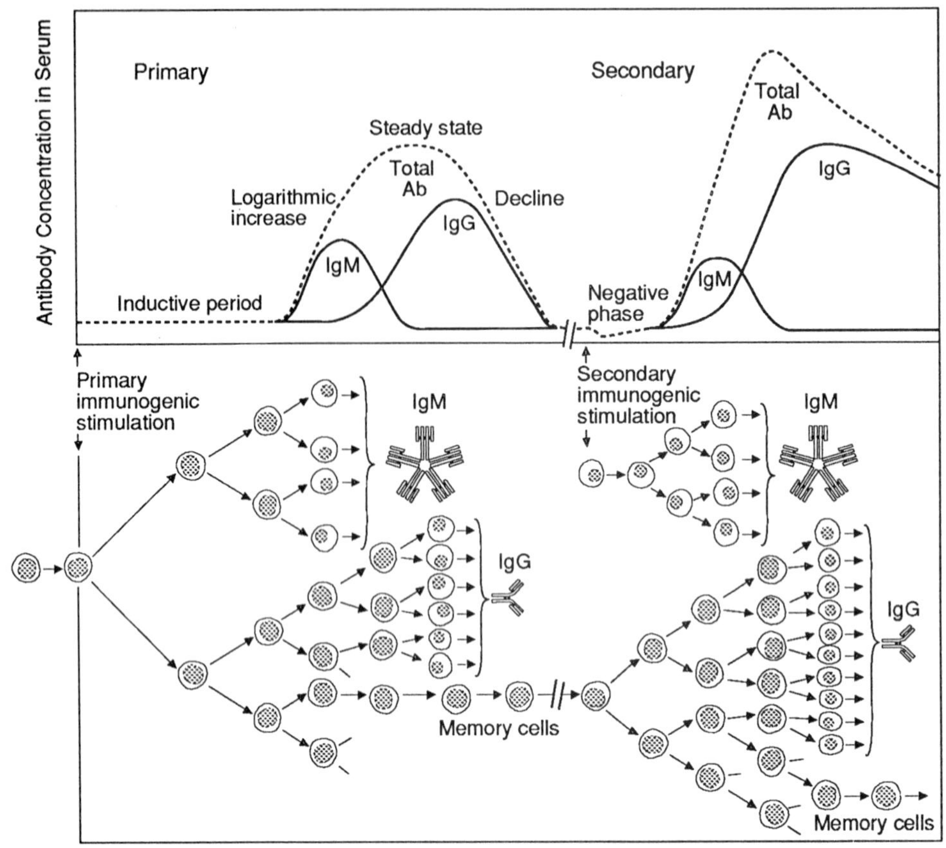

Figure 2-13. Primary and secondary responses of the immune system. Ab, antibody.

Reprinted with permission from Herscowitz HB. Immunophysiology: cell function and cellular interactions in antibody formation. In: Bellanti JA, editor. Immunology III. *Philadelphia, PA: WB Saunders; 1985. p. 120.*

enhanced response of the immune system. Memory cells produced by both T and B lymphocytes after the first antigenic exposure stimulate or generate more antibody-producing plasma cells. Antibodies already present react immediately when re-exposed to the antigen. A much smaller dose of antigen can evoke a secondary response; the amount of antigen required depends on the concentration of preformed antibody and on the length of time between the first and second exposures.[40,43]

Immune Tolerance

There are times when attenuation or elimination of the immune response benefits the host. Tolerance is the selective lack of response to an antigen that has previously been presented to the host. Generally, less mature cells are more likely to become tolerant. For example, a B lymphocyte becomes tolerant more readily than a mature plasma cell. If the host is repeatedly exposed to an antigen early in life, B-cell response may be lost. T lymphocytes may also become tolerant, but immature cells are no more susceptible than mature cells. Overall, T cells become tolerant at much lower doses of antigen than B cells do.[45]

Other factors in the development of tolerance are the antigen's dose, physical form (monomer versus polymer), and route of entry into the host. There are optimal doses of antigens for eliciting an immune response; exposure to doses at low or high extremes can result in tolerance. For example, intravenous doses of antigen can result in a more concentrated exposure to the antigen and therefore are more likely to induce tolerance than are doses introduced by other routes. In addition, monomeric forms of antigens are more likely to induce tolerance than are polymers.[45]

SUMMARY

The immune system is composed primarily of white blood cells that originate in the bone marrow and develop into myeloid or lymphoid cells. Myeloid cells include mononuclear phagocytes and granulocytes. Some granulocytes are phagocytic; others function as mediator cells. Phagocytosis is the process of attaching to and killing foreign particles or antigens.

Macrophages evolve from monocytes and are capable of cell division. Macrophages (as well as dendritic cells, B lymphocytes, and microglial cells) may also function as antigen-presenting cells. Granulocytes have granular nuclei and stain various colors; the granulocytes include neutrophils (which are polymorphonuclear), eosinophils, basophils, and mast cells. Platelets are myeloid cells that function as mediator cells and activate complement during the inflammatory process.

Lymphocytes include T, B, and null (killer and natural killer) cells. Subpopulations of T lymphocytes include helper T cells, suppressor T cells, cytotoxic T cells, and memory T cells. T cells are responsible for cell-mediated immunity, and B cells are responsible for humoral immunity. Null cells function in antibody-dependent cell-mediated cytotoxicity. Following activation, B cells may become plasma cells. Plasma cells produce antibodies (immunoglobulin), including IgG, IgA, IgD, IgE, and IgM. Both T and B lymphocytes can become memory cells.

The immune system comprises six tissues: bone marrow, thymus, lymph nodes, spleen, mucosal-associated lymphoid tissue, and high endothelial venule. Bone marrow is the source of immune cells. The thymus is the site where immature T lymphocytes develop. Lymphoid tissue filters foreign particles traveling through lymph; immune cells in the tissues are responsible for eliminating the foreign particles. The spleen filters blood for foreign particles and defective blood cells. Mucosal-associated lymphoid tissues are nonencapsulated tissues found in the gastrointestinal, respiratory, and urogenital tracts and are crucial to first-line immunologic defense. High endothelial venules are blood vessels that allow lymphocytes to pass through the immune tissues.

REFERENCES

1. Williams DA. Stem cell model of hematopoiesis. In: Hoffman R, Benz EJ, Shattil SJ, Furie B, Cohen HJ, Silberstein LE, editors. *Hematology: Basic Principles and Practice*. 2nd ed. New York: Churchill Livingstone; 1995. p. 180–92.
2. Abboud CN, Lichtman MA. Structure of the marrow. In: Beutler E, Lichtman MA, Coller BS, Kipps TJ, editors. *Hematology*. 5th ed. New York: McGraw-Hill; 1995. p. 25–37.
3. Newburger PE, Parmley RT. Neutrophil structure and function. In: Hoffman R, Benz EJ, Shattil SJ, Furie B, Cohen HJ, Silberstein LE, editors. *Hematology: Basic Principles and Practice*. 2nd ed. New York: Churchill Livingstone; 1995. p. 738–50.
4. Lewis DE, Harriman GR. Cells and tissues of the immune system. In: Rich RR, Fleisher TA, Schwartz BD, Shearer WT, Strober W, editors. *Clinical Immunology: Principles and Practice*. St. Louis, MO: Mosby; 1996. p. 15–38.
5. Lichtman MA. Classification and clinical manifestations of disorders of monocytes and macrophages. In: Beutler E, Lichtman MA, Coller BS, Kipps TJ, editors. *Hematology*. 5th ed. New York: McGraw-Hill; 1995. p. 878–80.
6. Faller DV, Mentzer SJ. Monocyte and macrophage development and function. In: Hoffman R, Benz EJ, Shattil SJ, Furie B, Cohen HJ, Silberstein LE, editors. *Hematology: Basic Principles and Practice*. 2nd ed. New York: Churchill Livingstone; 1995. p. 751–61.
7. Ganz T, Lehrer RI. Production, distribution, and fate of monocytes and macrophages. In: Beutler E, Lichtman MA, Coller BS, Kipps TJ, editors. *Hematology*. 5th ed. New York: McGraw-Hill; 1995. p. 875–7.
8. Unanue ER. Macrophages, antigen-presenting cells, and the phenomena of antigen handling and presentation. In: Paul WE, editor. *Fundamental Immunology*. 3rd ed. New York: Raven; 1993. p. 111–44.
9. Smith SP, Yee GC. Hematopoiesis. *Pharmacotherapy* 1992;12(2 Pt 2):11S–19S.
10. Lehrer RI, Ganz T. Biochemistry and function of monocytes and macrophages. In: Beutler E, Lichtman MA, Coller BS, Kipps TJ, editors. *Hematology*. 5th ed. New York: McGraw-Hill; 1995. p. 869–74.
11. Babior BM, Golde DW. Production, distribution, and fate of neutrophils. In: Beutler E, Lichtman MA, Coller BS, Kipps TJ, editors. *Hematology*. 5th ed. New York: McGraw-Hill; 1995. p. 773–8.
12. Newburger PE, Parmley RT. Neutrophil structure and function. In: Hoffman R, Benz EJ, Shattil SJ, Furie B, Cohen HJ, Silberstein LE, editors. *Hematology: Basic Principles and Practice*. 2nd ed. New York: Churchill Livingstone; 1995. p. 738–50.
13. Wardlaw AJ, Kay AB. Eosinophils: production, biochemistry, and function. In: Beutler E, Lichtman MA, Coller BS, Kipps TJ, editors. *Hematology*. 5th ed. New York: McGraw-Hill; 1995. p. 798–804.
14. Galli SJ, Dvorak AM. Production, biochemistry, and function of basophils and mast cells. In: Beutler E, Lichtman MA, Coller BS, Kipps TJ, editors. *Hematology*. 5th ed. New York: McGraw-Hill; 1995. p. 805–9.
15. Kline J. *Immunology*. Boston, MA: Blackwell Scientific; 1990. p. 26–7.
16. Plow EF, Ginsberg MH. Molecular basis of platelet function. In: Hoffman R, Benz EJ, Shattil SJ, Furie B, Cohen HJ, Silberstein LE, editors. *Hematology: Basic Principles and Practice*. 2nd ed. New York: Churchill Livingstone; 1995. p. 1524–35.
17. Kincade PW, Gimble JM. B lymphocytes. In: Paul WE, editor. *Fundamental Immunology*. 3rd ed. New York: Raven; 1993. p. 43–73.
18. Sprent J. T lymphocytes and the thymus. In: Paul WE, editor. *Fundamental Immunology*. 3rd ed. New York: Raven Press; 1993. p. 75–109.
19. Kipps TJ. Functions of T lymphocytes: T-cell receptors for antigen. In: Beutler E, Lichtman MA, Coller BS, Kipps TJ, editors. *Hematology*. 5th ed. New York: McGraw-Hill; 1995. p. 938–45.
20. Abbas AK, Singer GG. Regulatory and effector functions of $CD4^+$ T lymphocytes. In: Rich RR, Fleisher TA, Schwartz BD, Shearer WT, Strober W, editors. *Clinical Immunology: Principles and Practice*. St. Louis, MO: Mosby;

1996. p. 264–75.
21. Paul WE, Seder RA. Lymphocyte responses and cytokines. *Cell* 1994;76:241–51.
22. Swain SL, Weinberg AD, English M, *et al.* IL-4 directs the development of Th2-like helper effectors. *J Immunol.* 1990;145:3796–806.
23. Bloom BR, Salgame P, Diamond B. Revisiting and revising suppressor T cells. *Immunol Today* 1992;13:131–6.
24. Royer HD, Reinharz EL. T lymphocytes: ontogeny, function, and relevance to clinical disorders. *N Engl J Med.* 1987;317:1136–42.
25. Biddison WE. Cytotoxic T cell function. In: Rich RR, Fleisher TA, Schwartz BD, Shearer WT, Strober W, editors. *Clinical Immunology: Principles and Practice*. St. Louis, MO: Mosby; 1996. p. 276–80.
26. Berke G. The functions and mechanisms of action of cytolytic lymphocytes. In: Paul WE, editor. *Fundamental Immunology*. 3rd ed. New York: Raven; 1993. p. 965–1014.
27. Doherty PC. Immune responses to viruses. In: Rich RR, Fleisher TA, Schwartz BD, Shearer WT, Strober W, editors. *Clinical Immunology: Principles and Practice*. St. Louis, MO: Mosby; 1996. p. 535–49.
28. DeFranco AL. B lymphocyte activation. In: Paul WE, editor. *Fundamental Immunology*. 3rd ed. New York: Raven; 1993. p. 505–29.
29. Tami JA, Parr MC, Thompson JS. The immune system. *Am J Hosp Pharm*. 1986;43:2483–93.
30. Carayannopoulos L, Capra JD. Immunoglobulins: structure and function. In: Paul WE, editor. *Fundamental Immunology*. 3rd ed. New York: Raven; 1993. p. 283–314.
31. Potter KN, Capra JD. Immunoglobulin genes and proteins. In: Rich RR, Fleisher TA, Schwartz BD, Shearer WT, Strober W, editors. *Clinical Immunology: Principles and Practice*. St. Louis, MO: Mosby; 1996. p. 50–68.
32. Greenspan NS. Immunoglobulin function. In: Rich RR, Fleisher TA, Schwartz BD, Shearer WT, Strober W, editors. *Clinical Immunology: Principles and Practice*. St. Louis, MO: Mosby; 1996. p. 250–63.
33. Seaman WE. Natural killer cells. In: Rich RR, Fleisher TA, Schwartz BD, Shearer WT, Strober W, editors. *Clinical Immunology: Principles and Practice*. St. Louis, MO: Mosby; 1996. p. 282–9.
34. Spits H, Lanier LL, Phillips JH. Development of human T and natural killer cells. *Blood* 1995;85:2654–70.
35. Mulé JJ, Rosenberg SA. Catalogue of cytokines. *Biologic Therapy of Cancer Updates* 1992;2:1–11.
36. Mosmann T. Cytokines and immune regulation. In: Rich RR, Fleisher TA, Schwartz BD, Shearer WT, Strober W, editors. *Clinical Immunology: Principles and Practice*. St. Louis, MO: Mosby; 1996. p. 217–30.
37. Ambrus JL, Pippin J, Joseph A, *et al.* Identification of a cDNA for a human high-molecular-weight B-cell growth factor. *Proc Natl Acad Sci*. 1993;90:6330–4.
38. Carson WE, Giri JG, Lindemann MJ, *et al.* Interleukin (IL) 15 is a novel cytokine that activates human natural killer cells via components of the IL-2 receptor. *J Exp Med*. 1994;180:1395–1403.
39. Grabstein KH, Eisenman J, Shanebeck K, *et al.* Cloning of a T cell growth factor that interacts with the β chain of the interleukin-2 receptor. *Science* 1994;264:965–8.
40. Paul WE. The immune system: an introduction. In: Paul WE, editor. *Fundamental Immunology*. 3rd ed. New York: Raven; 1993. p. 1–20.
41. Weiss LP. Functional organization of hematopoietic tissues. In: Hoffman R, Benz EJ, Shattil SJ, Furie B, Cohen HJ, Silberstein LE, editors. *Hematology: Basic Principles and Practice*. 2nd ed. New York: Churchill Livingstone; 1995. p. 193–207.
42. Weiss L. Structure of the spleen. In: Beutler E, Lichtman MA, Coller BS, Kipps TJ, editors. *Hematology*. 5th ed. New York: McGraw-Hill; 1995. p. 38–42.
43. Anderson AO, Shaw S. Lymphocyte trafficking. In: Rich RR, Fleisher TA, Schwartz BD, Shearer WT, Strober W, editors. *Clinical Immunology: Principles and Practice*. St. Louis, MO: Mosby; 1996. p. 39–49.
44. Rich RR. The human immune response. In: Rich RR, Fleisher TA, Schwartz BD, Shearer WT, Strober W, editors. *Clinical Immunology: Principles and Practice*. St. Louis, MO. Mosby; 1996. p. 1–14.
45. Schwartz RH. Immunological tolerance. In: Paul WE, editor. *Fundamental Immunology*. 3rd ed. New York: Raven; 1993. p. 677–731.

SELF-ASSESSMENT QUESTIONS

1. The specific or acquired immune response to an antigen is the function of:

   a. stem cells.
   b. neutrophils.
   c. lymphocytes.
   d. eosinophils.

2. Which of the following cells are capable of phagocytosis and antigen presentation?

   a. monocytes/macrophages
   b. neutrophils
   c. B cells
   d. eosinophils

3. In the adult human, hematopoiesis occurs primarily in the:

   a. bone marrow.
   b. lymph nodes.
   c. thymus.
   d. spleen.

4. T lymphocytes mature in the:

   a. bone marrow.
   b. thymus.
   c. blood.
   d. spleen.

5. Neutrophils and monocytes/macrophages differ in that monocytes/macrophages:

a. present antigens to T cells.
b. are stimulated by GM-CSF.
c. are phagocytes.
d. develop in the spleen.

6. An antigen-presenting cell in the skin is called a(n):

a. osteoclast.
b. Langerhans cell.
c. melanocyte.
d. dendritic cell.

7. The function of neutrophils is:

a. to present antigen to T cells.
b. to phagocytose foreign particles.
c. to secrete G-CSF.
d. to regulate allergic reactions.

8. Common pathogens controlled by neutrophils include:

a. bacteria.
b. viruses.
c. protozoa.
d. mycobacteria.

9. Which group of drugs can artificially raise the neutrophil count by causing demargination?

a. diuretics
b. antipsychotics
c. corticosteroids
d. nonsteroidal anti-inflammatory analgesics

10. Neutropenia is serious because it leaves the patient susceptible to:

a. bacterial sepsis.
b. leukemia.
c. disseminated herpes simplex.
d. certain solid tumors.

11. Humoral immunity is orchestrated by:

a. B cells.
b. T cells.
c. neutrophils.
d. NK cells.

12. Solid organ graft rejection is believed to be due to:

a. B cells.
b. cytotoxic T cells.
c. memory cells.
d. NK cells.

13. The strength of attractive and repulsive forces between an antigen and antibody binding site is termed:

a. affinity.
b. specificity.
c. van der Waal forces.
d. steric hindrance.

14. Immunoglobulins are composed of:

a. long chain fatty acids.
b. carbohydrates.
c. lipoproteins.
d. glycoproteins.

15. IgE is important for its role in:

a. allergic reactions.
b. fungal infections.
c. bacterial infections.
d. graft-versus-host disease.

16. In general, the immune system is regulated by several:

a. soluble mediators.
b. pituitary hormones.
c. vitamins.
d. immunoglobulins.

17. Macrophage growth and development are influenced by:

a. IL-6.
b. G-CSF.
c. GM-CSF.
d. IL-11.

18. Fever can commonly be a biological effect of:

a. IL-1.
b. G-CSF.
c. IgG.
d. IgA.

19. B-cell growth and development is regulated by:

a. the thymus.
b. GM-CSF.
c. TNF-β.
d. several different interleukins.

CHAPTER 3

The Major Histocompatibility Complex

Janelle B. Perkins, Pharm.D., B.C.P.S.
Manager, Clinical Research Services, Bone Marrow Transplant Program
H. Lee Moffitt Cancer Center
Assistant Professor, Department of Internal Medicine
University of South Florida
Tampa, FL

Genetic Determination and Nomenclature of the MHC 36
Structure and Function of HLA Proteins 39
  Location and Structure 39
  Function 40
HLA and Disease 40
Histocompatibility Testing 42
  Serologic Assays 42
    Lymphocytotoxicity Assay 42
    Serologic Crossmatch 43
  Cellular Typing 43
  Molecular (DNA-Based) Methods 44
    Restriction Fragment Length Polymorphism 45
    Polymerase Chain Reaction 45
Blood Group Detection 45
  The ABO System 46
    Blood Typing 47
    Crossmatching 47
  The Rh System 47
    Methods of Rh Blood Group Detection 48
    Hemolytic Disease of the Newborn 48
Summary 48
References 49
Self-Assessment Questions 50

**The contributions made by Kelly A. Scott to this chapter are gratefully acknowledged.*

The major histocompatibility complex (MHC) is a cluster of genes found in all vertebrate species that encodes for cell-surface proteins. These proteins are responsible for the immune system's recognition of self and nonself. Recognition is an important function of the immune system because it protects the individual from diseases caused by microorganisms as well as damage from mutated or neoplastic cells. Without appropriate self-recognition mechanisms determined by MHC proteins, the immune system could no longer accurately determine self antigens, often resulting in autoimmune disease. Similarly, failure to recognize nonself antigens can lead to overwhelming infection or uncontrolled tumor growth. The MHC is also involved in induction of appropriate cellular and humoral immune response mechanisms and therefore plays a key role in the activation of cell-cell interactions involving macrophages, T cells, and B cells.[1,2]

Genetic determination, structure and immunologic function of the MHC products, and role of the MHC in autoimmune disease will be the primary subjects explored in this chapter. Methods of histocompatibility testing will also be discussed. The chapter concludes with an overview of blood group detection, including blood typing and Rh status determination.

After completing this chapter, the reader should be able to:

1. Describe the inheritance patterns and genetic components of the human MHC.
2. Describe the structures and functions of class I and class II human leukocyte antigen (HLA) molecules.
3. Explain the association between HLA type and selected autoimmune diseases.
4. Discuss the differences in HLA typing methods, including the rationale and limitations of the assays and interpretation of results.
5. Describe the immunologic determinants of the ABO and Rh blood systems.

GENETIC DETERMINATION AND NOMENCLATURE OF THE MHC

The existence of a human MHC was postulated in the 1950s and 1960s when antibodies that caused agglutination (clumping) of leukocytes were found in the sera of both transfused patients and multiparous women. The patterns of agglutination revealed the presence of definable antigenic proteins located on the surface of the leukocytes that became known as human leukocyte antigens (HLAs). International workshops met to categorize these serologic data and to standardize the definitions and nomenclature of HLAs. Shortly thereafter, HLAs were determined to be proteins encoded for by the MHC. With the application of molecular genetic techniques, scientists established the physical organization of the human MHC and identified individual genes responsible for specific HLA proteins. As shown in Figure 3-1, the human MHC consists of the class I genes (*HLA-A*, *-B*, and *-C*) and class II genes (*HLA-DR*, *-DQ*, and *-DP*).

The human genome consists of 23 pairs of chromosomes; within each pair, one chromosome is inherited from each parent. Each chromosome has a variety of loci where specific genes are found. An allele is one variation or alternate form of a given gene consisting of a different nucleotide sequence; alleles vary widely among individuals. The term haplotype describes the combination of alleles at each

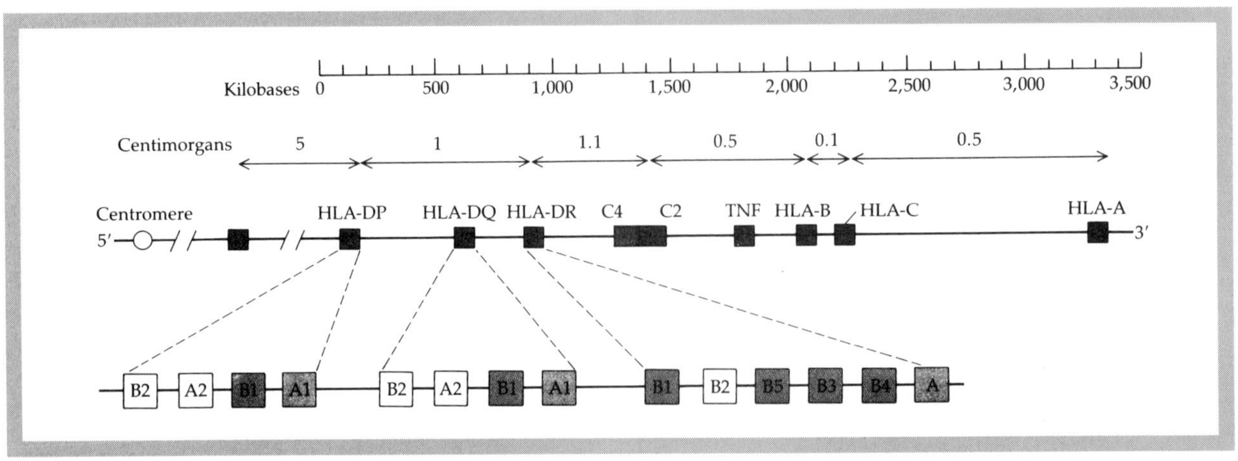

Figure 3-1. Genetic arrangement of the human major histocompatibility complex (MHC). An expansion of the class II region is shown in the lower portion of the figure. HLA, human leukocyte antigen; C2 and C4, complements 2 and 4; TNF, tumor necrosis factor.

SOURCE: *Reprinted with permission from Carpenter CB, David J. Histocompatibility antigens and immune response genes.* Sci Am Med. *1991;6(V):1.*

locus on a single chromosome; the haplotype is usually inherited as a unit. Each person has two haplotypes at each MHC locus, one inherited from each parent. Both haplotypes are expressed equally (codominance). Thus, the genetic composition (or genotype) of an individual is decided by the paternal haplotype and the maternal haplotype.

Based on Mendelian inheritance patterns, there is a 25% chance that two siblings will share both haplotypes (be HLA compatible), a 50% chance they will share only one haplotype, and a 25% chance they will share no haplotype (be completely HLA incompatible). HLA phenotype is a term used to indicate all the alleles detected in a given individual by serologic typing. HLA-matched siblings are said to be genotypically matched because they have inherited copies of the same maternal and paternal HLA alleles (i.e., the same genes and therefore the same HLA haplotype). In contrast, HLA-matched unrelated individuals carry HLA alleles that are phenotypically matched; they are not distinguishable by serologic typing methods but may have different HLA subtypes.[1,3]

Figure 3-2 shows an illustration of haplotype inheritance within the HLA complex. As mentioned previously, all of the alleles are codominant (both haplotypes are expressed to form an individual's genotype). For example, serological typing of offspring AC would reveal a phenotype of A1,2; B5,-; Cw1,-; Dw1,w2. The hyphen indicates that only one product of a particular locus can be typed because the individual either is homozygous (inherited the same allele from both parents) or possesses an antigen that cannot be typed because no appropriate reagents are available. Family studies distinguish between these two possibilities.[2]

The human MHC occupies a segment of approximately 3500 kilobases (thousand base pairs) on chromosome 6 and has been subdivided into classes of loci, each of which encodes for a group of structurally and functionally related proteins. The *HLA-A*, *-B*, and *-C* genetic loci encode for the class I proteins traditionally known as the classical major transplantation antigens. Further analysis of this region has revealed additional class I genes: *HLA-E*, *-F*, *-G*, *-H*, *-I*, and *-J*. Although these genes can po-

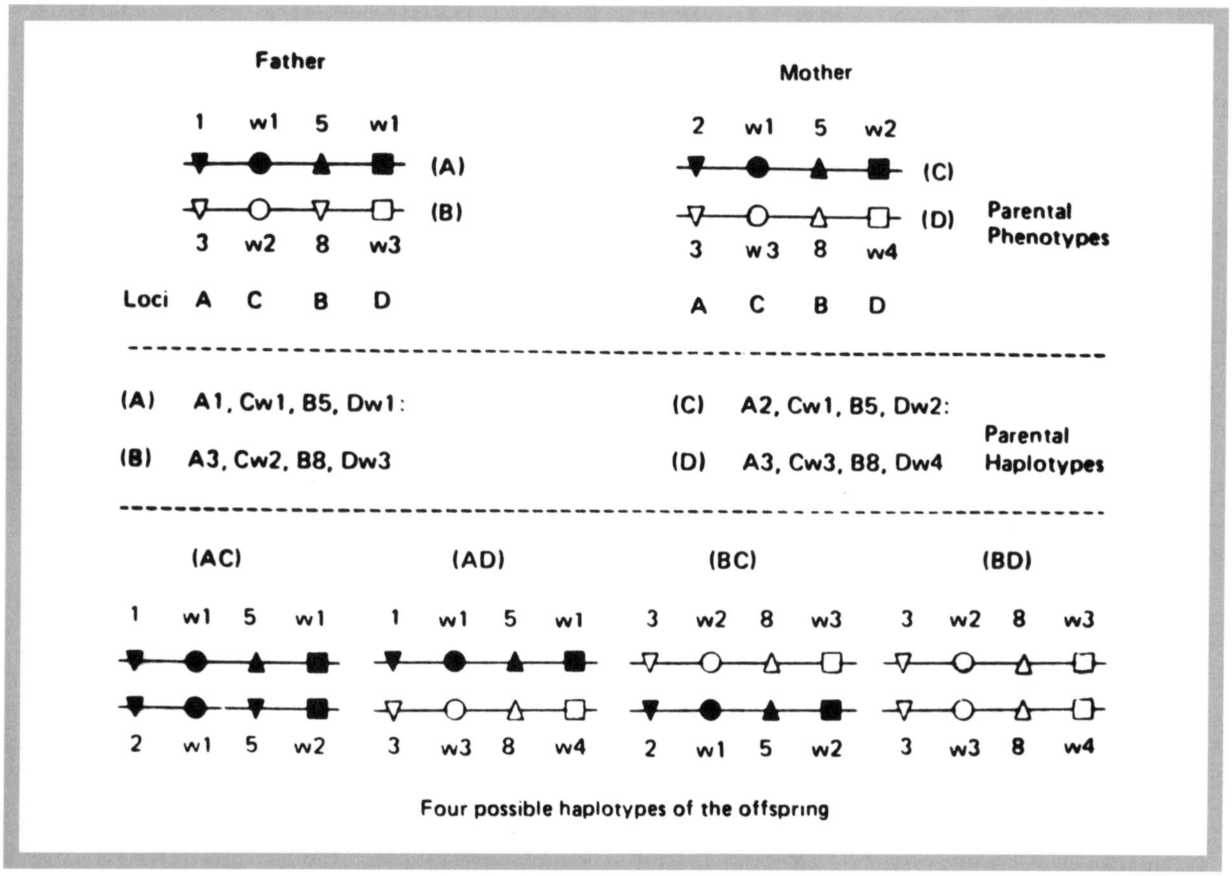

Figure 3-2. Diagrammatic representation of the genetic transmission of HLA haplotypes. Each parent has two haplotypes (one in each chromosome). Paternal haplotypes are designated A and B and maternal haplotypes, C and D. Each offspring receives one paternal haplotype and one maternal haplotype.

SOURCE: *Reprinted with permission from Goust JM. Major histocompatibility complex. In: Virella G, Goust JM, Fudenberg HH, editors.* Introduction to Medical Immunology. *2nd ed. New York: Marcel Dekker; 1990. p. 31–51.*

tentially direct the synthesis of class I proteins, the clinical significance of these proteins is unknown.[4] Class II genes are located in the *HLA-D* region; three loci—*DR*, *DQ*, and *DP*—encode the major products of the class II region. Other subregions identified in the *HLA-D* region include *DN* (formerly *DZ*), *DO*, *DMA*, and *DMB*. Neither the *HLA-DN* nor the *-DO* gene has been expressed in vivo, and the function of these genes is presently unknown. *HLA-DM* gene products are members of the immunoglobulin gene family and only distantly related to the class I and class II genes; further examination is required to learn their role as mediators of T-cell activation.[5]

Several other genetic regions are part of the human MHC. Genes coding for tumor necrosis factors alpha and beta are located between class I and class II genes.[2] The HLA class III region has been mapped between the *HLA-B* and *-DR* regions and contains genes for C2 and C4 of the classic complement pathway and properdin factors of the alternative pathway. Unlike class I and class II antigens, these proteins do not participate in any immunologic activity.[1] Recently, the *TAP* and *LMP* genes have been located within the class II region of the MHC. These genes encode transporter peptides responsible for carrying antigenic peptides to the HLA protein and proteases that generate short peptides from the antigens that bind to the HLA protein.[5]

Within each MHC locus, separate genes that correspond to the α and β peptide chains of the HLA protein have been identified. For class I proteins (HLA-A, -B, and -C), only the α chain is encoded by the genes in the MHC. For class II proteins (HLA-DR, -DQ, and -DP), both the α and β chains are encoded by the genes in the MHC. The *HLA-DR* family comprises a single gene (*DRA*) and up to four β genes (*DRB1*, *B3*, *B4*, and *B5*). All individuals express a *DRB1*-encoded peptide, which is found on the cell surface in association with the *DRA*-encoded peptide. The other functional class II *HLA-DRB* genes, *DRB3*, *DRB4*, and *DRB5*, encode peptides that are also found on the cell surface in association with a *DRA*-encoded peptide but at a lower level and only in certain class II haplotypes. *HLA-DQ* and *-DP* families each have one α and one β gene (*DPA*, *DPB*; *DQA*, *DQB*).[3,4]

The human MHC is extremely polymorphic, having multiple forms or alleles of the gene at each known locus. For example, there are at least 51 distinct alleles at the *HLA-A* locus, 102 at the *HLA-B* locus, and 35 at the *HLA-C* locus. Because of this extensive polymorphism, different individuals express different HLA proteins on their cell surfaces. This polymorphism leads to the antigenicity of different HLA proteins in different individuals, causing rapid graft rejection when tissue is transplanted between individuals who differ at their MHC loci (and therefore express different HLA proteins).[6]

Polymorphism is demonstrated in the naming system of the products of the class I and class II genes. The nomenclature of HLA proteins has been devised by the World Health Organization Nomenclature Committee for Factors of the HLA System. HLA types, determined using molecular methods of histocompatibility testing, are based on the locus encoding the protein, followed by an asterisk and a series of four numbers. The first two digits indicate the allele defined by serologic testing (serologic specificity), and the second two digits are assigned sequentially as the WHO recognizes each allele. For example, the allele *HLA-DRB1*0403* is from the *HLA-DRB1* locus, is associated with the HLA-DR4 serologic specificity, and was the third *HLA-DRB1*04* allele to receive official designation. With molecular-based typing methods reaching wider applicability, this nomenclature is currently used with a previously established system in which HLA proteins were named only according to serologic specificity.[7,8]

Because human matings are random, the frequency of finding a given allele at one HLA locus associated with a given allele at a second HLA locus should simply be the product of the frequencies of each individual allele in the population. However, because of a phenomenon known as linkage disequilibrium, certain combinations of HLA alleles (certain haplotypes) occur with a frequency much higher than expected. For example, the *HLA-B8* and *HLA-DR3* alleles are found in the North American white population with frequencies of 0.09 and 0.12, respectively. The expected frequency with which the *HLA-B8*, *DR3* haplotype should occur is 0.09 × 0.12, or 0.0108. However, this haplotype is found with a frequency of approximately 0.0740, almost seven times the expected frequency.[2] Linkage disequilibrium is expressed as the difference between the observed and the expected frequencies of the alleles. The alleles found in significant linkage disequilibrium vary within different racial groups, but in all racial groups examined, significant linkage disequilibrium has been observed.[2,8] Explanations for linkage disequilibrium include a selective advantage of a given haplotype, migration and admixture of populations, inbreeding, and random drift of the gene pool.[1]

Although the focus of this chapter is the MHC, minor histocompatibility genes are also present. Their protein products can be responsible for rejection phenomena in solid organ transplantation and graft-versus-host disease (GVHD) in bone marrow transplantation even when donor and recipient are matched at the MHC. Incompatibility of these minor histocompatibility proteins usually can be overcome by commonly used immunosuppressive agents.[8] In contrast, GVHD resulting from incompatibility of minor histocompatibility proteins can be more difficult to control because of related immune mechanisms. (See Chapter 8, "Solid Organ Transplantation," and Chapter 9, "Bone Marrow Transplantation.")

STRUCTURE AND FUNCTION OF HLA PROTEINS

Location and Structure

Class I proteins are located on all nucleated cells in the human body and were the first HLA proteins to be identified. They are particularly abundant on the surface of lymphocytes. HLA-A, -B, and -C proteins are two-chain, noncovalently linked structures consisting of a heavy α chain (MW 44,000) encoded for by the MHC and a β_2-microglobulin light chain (MW 11,500) not encoded by the MHC (Figure 3-3). The extracellular region of the class I protein is divided into α_1, α_2, and α_3 domains. Studies of the amino acid sequences of the α chain and of the nucleotide sequences of the class I MHC gene complex show that most of the differences between alleles occur in the α_1 and α_2 domains. Between the α_1 and α_2 domains is a groove or pocket that serves as the antigen-binding site (Figure 3-4). The antigen-binding site varies from one class I protein to another, and within given class I proteins it varies from allele to allele, binding only a limited number of antigenic peptides. The binding of the antigenic peptide to the α_1 and α_2 portions creates a ligand recognized by the T-cell receptor on CD8$^+$ (cytotoxic/suppressor) lymphocytes.[1] A critical step in T-cell activation results from the physical association between the CD8 antigen and the T-cell receptor; this association is facilitated by the T-cell receptor and CD8 antigen binding to the same class I molecule. When the T-cell receptor recognizes the α_1 and α_2 domains, the CD8 antigen interacts with the α_3 domain. Thus, all three domains of the class I molecule are important in binding to and activating CD8$^+$ T lymphocytes.[3] The α_3 domain shows much less genetic polymorphism and, with β_2-microglobulin, appears to support the more polymorphic α_1 and α_2 regions.[2]

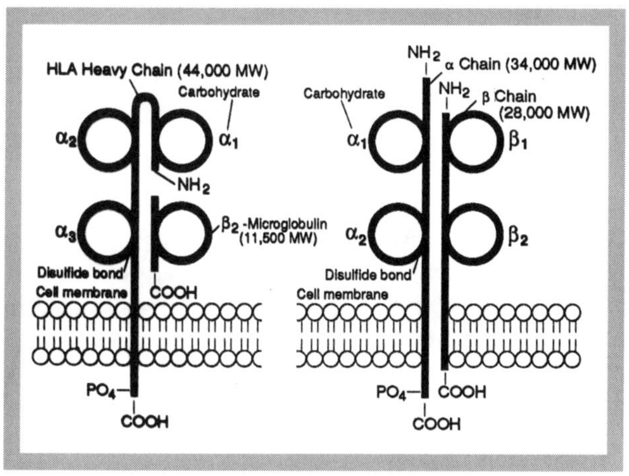

Figure 3-3. Structure of class I (left) and class II (right) histocompatibility antigens

SOURCE: *Reprinted with permission from Carpenter CB, David J. Histocompatibility antigens and immune response genes.* Sci Am Med. *1991;6(V):2.*

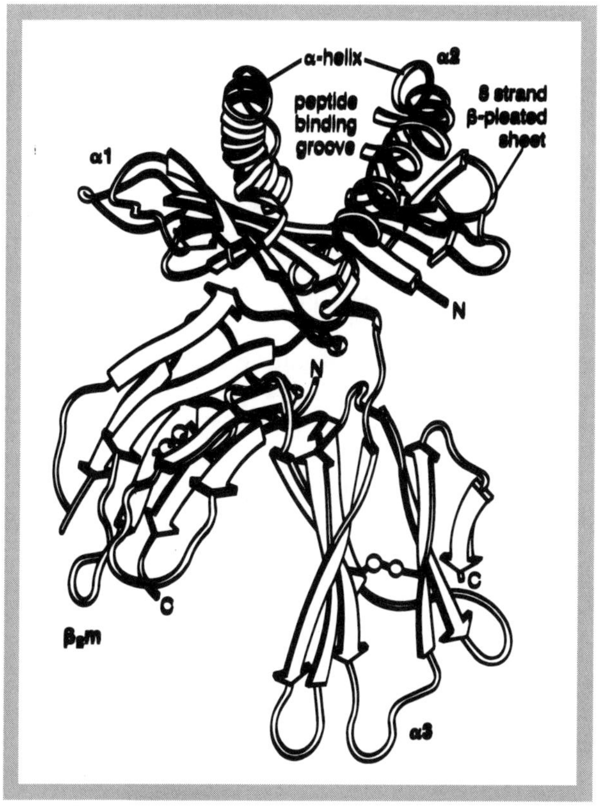

Figure 3-4. The diagrammatic crystalline structure of a class I MHC antigen (side view)

SOURCE: *Reprinted with permission from Stites DP, Terr AI.* Basic and Clinical Immunology. *7th ed. Norwalk, CT: Appleton & Lange; 1991. p. 47.*

Class II proteins are located on the surface of B cells, macrophages, Langerhans cells in the skin, Kupfer cells in the liver, microglial cells in the central nervous system, and interdigitating cells in the spleen. Other cells can be induced to express class II proteins. Except for activated suppressor T cells, T cells do not express class II proteins.[2] All cells expressing class II proteins simultaneously express class I proteins. Class II proteins consist of two peptide chains (α and β), both of which are encoded by genes within the HLA complex (Figure 3-3). The α chain (MW 34,000) and the β chain (MW 28,000) are bound noncovalently. The extracellular region contains two α domains (α_1 and α_2) and two β domains (β_1 and β_2) . The α_1 and β_1 domains form an interactive and hypervariable groove very similar to that created by the α_1 and α_2 domains of the class I protein. The polymorphism of the class II proteins is located in this groove, resulting in different antigen-binding sites for each class II protein. Thus, a given class II protein can bind only a limited number of antigenic peptides. The binding of a processed antigenic peptide to the groove creates a ligand recognized by the receptor on the CD4+ (inducer/helper) T cell.[2]

Function

The role of HLA proteins is to bind and present processed antigenic peptides to T cells that initiate both cellular and humoral immune responses. Class I proteins specifically bind peptides derived from endogenously synthesized proteins (e.g., viral and tumor peptides), present these antigenic peptides to CD8+ T cells, and restrict cell-mediated cytolysis to virus-infected cells. For an antigen to be recognized by a CD8+ T cell, the antigen must be recognized in combination with a class I protein. This phenomenon is termed HLA or MHC restriction. For example, viral proteins being synthesized in infected cells bind to HLA proteins inside the cell, and then the HLA protein–viral antigen complex is transported out of the cell, where it is recognized by CD8+ T cells as "self plus X." The antigen receptor of the CD8+ T cell recognizes a particular viral peptide only when the peptide is bound to a particular class I HLA protein. Once recognition occurs, the cytotoxic T cell kills the cell bearing the viral antigen.

Class II proteins also serve as receptors for processed peptides in a manner similar to that described for class I proteins; however, these peptides are derived predominantly from membrane and extracellular proteins (e.g., bacterial peptides) and are presented to CD4+ T cells (Figure 3-5).[4] Restrictions on the recognition of the class II antigenic peptide complex by CD4+ T cells are similar to those on the recognition of the class I antigenic peptide complexes by CD8+ T cells.[1]

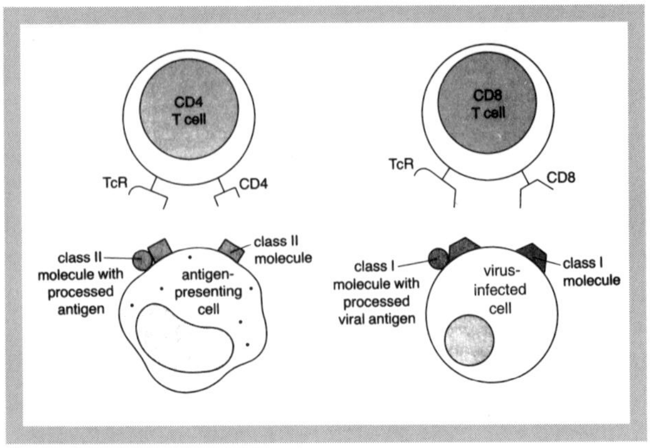

Figure 3-5. Antigen presentation. CD4+ T cells (left) recognize processed antigen in the context of class II molecules through the T-cell receptor (TCR) and recognize a portion of the nonpolymorphic region of the class II molecules through CD4. CD8+ cells (right) recognize processed antigen in the context of class I molecules through their TCR and a portion of the nonpolymorphic region of the class I molecules through CD8.

SOURCE: *Reprinted with permission from Schwartz BD. The human major histocompatibility human leukocyte antigen (HLA) complex. In: Stites DP, Terr AI, editors.* Basic and Clinical Immunology. *7th ed. Norwalk, CT: Appleton and Lange; 1991. p. 45–60.*

HLA AND DISEASE

A variety of diseases associated with specific HLA alleles have been described. Such associations are not absolute and imply only an increased risk (but not causality) of the disease when a certain allele is present. Most persons carrying one of these HLA alleles will not develop the associated disease, and the disease does occur in persons who lack the allele. Therefore, it seems that disease-associated HLA proteins play a permissive rather than a causative role in disease.[9] A list of diseases and their associated HLA alleles can be found in Table 3-1.

The degree of association of a particular disease with a particular HLA protein is quantitated by calculating the relative risk. Relative risk reflects the frequency of the disease in individuals with the disease-associated HLA protein compared with individuals who lack that protein. A relative risk greater than one suggests an association between the disease and the protein, and the higher the relative risk, the more frequent the association. The association of ankylosing spondylitis with HLA-B27 can be used to illustrate the meaning of relative risk. Ninety percent of Caucasian patients with ankylosing spondylitis in the United States possess HLA-B27, compared with approximately 9% of Caucasian controls (with HLA-B27, without ankylosing spondylitis). The relative risk of a Caucasian person with HLA-B27 developing ankylosing spondylitis is approximately 90 times that of a person without HLA-B27. Because of the strength of this association, HLA typing is now used in the differential diagnosis of this disease.[1,8]

Although ankylosing spondylitis is associated with a class I protein, most autoimmune diseases have been linked to class II proteins. An example of a class II protein–associated disease is rheumatoid arthritis (RA).[9,10] Approximately 80–90% of patients with seropositive RA carry either the HLA-DR1 or one of the three HLA-DR4 variant haplotypes. The strength of the association has varied considerably among studies, possibly due to the heterogeneity of the patients included. It has been suggested that the presence of the HLA-DR4 haplotype marks disease severity and susceptibility, with the frequency of DR4-subtype homozygosity increased in patients with more severe disease (i.e., a gene dose effect).[10]

Several hypotheses have been advanced to explain the mechanisms responsible for HLA-disease associations.[1,2,4,8–10] These include:

1. Particular HLA proteins act as receptors for etiologic agents, such as viruses, toxins, or other

Table 3-1. Diseases Showing Positive Human Leukocyte Antigen (HLA) Associations

DISEASE	HLA ANTIGEN	RELATIVE RISK[a]
Rheumatic		
Ankylosing spondylitis	B27	69.1
Reiter's syndrome	B27	37.0
Acute anterior uveitis	B27	8.2
Reactive arthritis (*Yersinia*, *Salmonella*, gonococcus)	B27	18.0
Psoriatic arthritis, central	B27	10.7
	B38	9.1
Psoriatic arthritis, peripheral	B27	2.0
	B38	6.5
Juvenile rheumatoid arthritis	B27	3.9
Juvenile rheumatoid arthritis (pauciarticular)	DR5	3.3
Rheumatoid arthritis	Dw4/DR4	3.8
Sjögren's syndrome	Dw3	5.7
Systemic lupus erythematosus	DR3	2.6
Gastrointestinal		
Gluten-sensitive enteropathy	DR3	11.6
Chronic active hepatitis	DR3	6.8
Ulcerative colitis	B5	3.8
Hematologic		
Idiopathic hemachromatosis	A3	6.7
	B14	26.7
	A13, B14	90.0
Pernicious anemia	DR5	5.4
Skin		
Dermatitis herpetiformis	DR3	17.3
Psoriasis vulgaris	Cw6	7.5
Psoriasis vulgaris (Japanese)	Cw6	8.5
Pemphigus vulgaris (Jews)	DR4	14.6
	A26	4.8
Behcet's anemia	B5	3.8
Endocrine		
Insulin-dependent diabetes mellitus (juvenile diabetes mellitus)	DR4	3.6
	DR3	4.8
	DR2	0.2
	BfF1[b]	15.0
Graves' disease	B8	2.5
	DR3	3.7
Graves' disease (Japanese)	B35	4.4
Addison's disease	Dw3	10.5
Subacute thyroiditis (de Quervain)	B35	13.7
Hashimoto's thyroiditis	DR5	3.2
Congenital adrenal hyperplasia	Bw47	15.4
Neurologic		
Myasthenia gravis (without thymoma)	B8	3.3
Multiple sclerosis	D/DR2	2.7
Manic-depressive disorder	B16	2.3
Narcolepsy	DR2	130.0
Schizophrenia	A28	2.3
Renal		
Idiopathic membranous glomerulonephritis	DR3	5.7
Goodpasture's syndrome (anti-GBM)	DR2	15.9
Minimal change disease (steroid responsive)	DR7	4.2
IgA nephropathy (French, Japanese)	DR4	3.1
Gold/penicillamine nephropathy	DR3	14.0
Polycystic kidney disease	B5	2.6
Infectious		
Tuberculoid leprosy (Asians)	B8	6.8
Paralytic polio	B16	4.3
Low vs. high response to vaccina virus	Cw3	12.7

SOURCE: *Reprinted with permission from Isselbacher KJ, Braunwald E, Wilson JD,* et al., *editors.* Harrison's Principles of Internal Medicine. *12th ed. New York: McGraw-Hill; 1991. GBM, glomerular basement membrane; IgA, immunoglobulin A.*

[a] *Relative risk* = $\dfrac{(\%\ \text{antigen-positive patients}) \times (\%\ \text{antigen-negative controls})}{(\%\ \text{antigen-negative patients}) \times (\%\ \text{antigen-positive controls})}$

[b] *BfF1 is an allele of the complement system that is HLA linked, but it is not antigen.*

foreign substances, allowing entry of the pathogen into the cell and rendering the individual more susceptible to infection;
2. The HLA protein in question has a stronger or weaker affinity for an antigen, resulting in an inappropriate immune response;
3. The T-cell antigen receptor is responsible for disease predisposition, but because T-cell recognition is restricted by an HLA protein, an apparent association is seen between the disease and HLA;
4. The disease-associated HLA protein is immunologically similar to the causative agent, leading either to an immune response directed not only against the agent but also against self (autoimmune disease) or the lack of an immune response because the pathogen is seen as self; and
5. Expression of the disease-associated HLA protein is linked to expression of the actual but unknown causative agent so that the two products are coexpressed.

Because HLA-associated diseases are a heterogeneous group, different mechanisms may be operating in different HLA-associated diseases, or perhaps more than one mechanism may be operating concurrently to produce a single disease.[1,2,5,8] Once mechanisms are more completely understood, specific approaches to prevention and treatment can be developed. For example, research suggests that specific peptides can be designed that, when bound to the disease-associated HLA protein, prevent T-cell activation. A peptide that binds to the associated HLA-DR protein and inhibits the activation of deleterious T-cell responses by the unknown triggering antigen could be used to treat RA. Another approach is the use of specific monoclonal antibodies (either anti-HLA or anti-T-cell receptor) that would prevent antigen presentation and T-cell activation.[10] The ideal intervention would be directed toward the specific autoantigen responsible for T-cell activation or the MHC-restricted activation of T cells. This intervention, in turn, must be protected from the immune response.[9] Further studies are necessary to clarify these issues.

HISTOCOMPATIBILITY TESTING

Transplantation of solid organs and bone marrow has become increasingly successful as the importance of histocompatibility and effective immunosuppression has been realized. Because successful transplantation (specifically, lack of rejection) can be predicted by the "likeness" of the donor and recipient with respect to HLA, methods for HLA typing and matching have developed rapidly over the past two decades. This discussion will focus on serologic, cellular, and molecular (DNA-based) methods of histocompatibility testing.

Serologic Assays

Serologic testing includes the lymphocytotoxicity assay and the serologic crossmatch. These assays are based on the fact that when lymphocytes are exposed to serum that contains antibodies to the HLA proteins expressed on the surface of the lymphocytes, complement is fixed and cells are lysed. If, on the other hand, the antibodies in the serum are not directed toward the HLA proteins found on the surface of those lymphocytes, no reaction occurs. Over the years, these assays have been refined so that they are reliable, reproducible, do not require sophisticated instrumentation, and provide results within a few hours. However, limitations do exist. These tests require live, healthy cells that express HLA proteins; these are rare in cancer patients undergoing chemotherapy or radiation therapy before a transplant. Because class II proteins are expressed only on B cells (found in limited number in the blood), typing of class II proteins is more laborious. Also, sera used for the lymphocytotoxicity assay are of a human source that may be limited in quantity and difficult to standardize. Finally, to be discussed at length later in this section, the lymphocytotoxicity assay cannot detect most of the HLA allelic variability.[3] Many attempts have been made to develop monoclonal antibodies with enough specificity for use as typing reagents. Although some monoclonal antibodies are currently available to type particular HLA proteins, the majority cannot fix complement, a vital component of most serologic assays.

Lymphocytotoxicity Assay

The sera used in the lymphocytotoxicity assay are of a human source and have high titers of antibodies directed at known HLA proteins (i.e., antisera). This assay is useful primarily to identify the presence of class I proteins, but it can also identify the presence of class II HLA-DR and -DQ proteins. The test is described in Figure 3-6. Lymphocytes from the donor are purified and added to antisera targeted against specific HLA proteins. Complement is added, and the lymphocyte-antisera mixture is incubated. If the HLA proteins on the lymphocyte surface match the HLA type of the antibodies, the lymphocytes are killed by the antibodies and complement. When a dye (such as eosin) is added, dead lymphocytes absorb the dye and appear red. Living lymphocytes do not absorb the dye. By examining the percentage of cells killed by each antiserum (patterns of reactivity), one can identify which antisera were specific for the donor lymphocytes and assign an HLA type. The procedure is then repeated with recipient lymphocytes. When this test is done with a battery of antisera, the HLA types of both donor and recipient can be established based on their reaction pat-

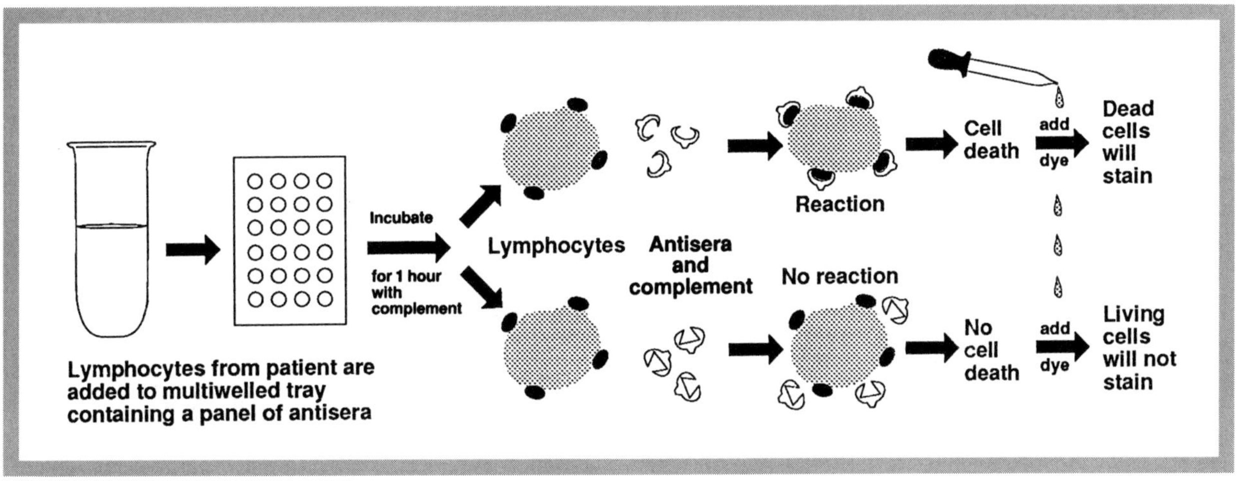

Figure 3-6. Complement-dependent lymphocytotoxicity assay for HLA molecules

terns. When the donor and recipient are siblings, a determination can be made about whether they have identical HLA haplotypes, semi-identical haplotypes, or nonidentical haplotypes. When the donor/recipient pair are unrelated, serologic testing can only determine whether they are phenotypically similar.

Serologic Crossmatch

Serologic crossmatch detects antibodies or other factors in the recipient's sera that would bind to donor HLA proteins and result in early graft loss. For renal transplantation, the crossmatch is a very important pretransplant procedure.[11] Several methods are used for crossmatching, including the complement-dependent cytotoxicity assay and the flow cytometry crossmatch. In the complement-dependent cytotoxicity assay, serum from the recipient is incubated with lymphocytes from the potential donor for 30 minutes, complement is added, the mixture is incubated, and dye is added. If the two individuals are HLA identical, no antibodies directed toward the donor's HLA proteins will be present in the recipient, and the crossmatch results would be negative. However, with HLA-nonidentical individuals, the recipient may have antibodies directed against the HLA proteins on the donor's lymphocytes, which would result in cell lysis and a positive crossmatch. The flow cytometry crossmatch is a more sensitive assay that does not rely on complement fixation but instead measures the binding of antibodies in the recipient sera to donor lymphocytes.[11]

In crossmatching patients' sera against donor cells, clinically irrelevant results can occur. One example is a positive reaction due to autolymphocytotoxic antibodies. These antibodies, mostly IgM, are cytotoxic to autologous lymphocytes in the presence of complement but are not damaging to renal allografts. However, not all IgM antibodies are autoantibodies, and these must be differentiated from IgM antibodies that are alloreactive. Autoantibodies can often be removed by a wash step, leaving behind alloantibodies.[11]

The clinical relevance of a positive crossmatch has changed with the recognition that antibody reactivity to T and/or B cells may result in different graft outcomes. Positive T-cell crossmatches are more clearly associated with graft failure than positive B-cell crossmatches are. The clinical relevance of positive crossmatches also has changed with improved immunosuppressive regimens (i.e., cyclosporine-containing regimens). More patients considered high risk by crossmatch results are now successfully receiving transplants with these more effective regimens.[11]

Cellular Typing

Cellular typing evaluates the interaction of donor and recipient lymphocytes. The premise of this kind of test is that lymphocytes that express different HLA proteins on their surface proliferate when mixed in vitro. This proliferation is known as the mixed lymphocyte reaction (MLR) and is measured by uptake of radioactive thymidine. If lymphocytes with identical HLA haplotypes are mixed, stimulation and proliferation do not occur and no MLR takes place. The mixed lymphocyte culture (MLC) technique uses the MLR to assess compatibility. The MLC technique measures the amount of proliferation and reflects the response of T cells to HLA proteins present on other lymphocytes. When HLA-A, -B, and -C are identical between the two sources of lymphocytes as assessed by serologic typing, then any proliferation that occurs is due to incompatibilities in the class II region. To identify which lymphocytes (donor or recipient) are proliferating, a test known as the one-way MLC is used. In this test, donor lymphocytes are exposed to either radiation or mitomycin-C before they are mixed with recipient lymphocytes. The donor lymphocytes cannot proliferate and act only as HLA protein bearers. Any proliferation (a positive

MLC) is the result of a response of the recipient's lymphocytes directed against the donor's HLA proteins, and the donor is considered incompatible.

The MLC test has four disadvantages. First, a prolonged time is necessary to obtain results; cultures take five to seven days. Second, the test requires sufficient numbers of live, healthy lymphocytes in the peripheral blood that express class II protein. Third, the test lacks specificity for *HLA-DR* allele subtypes. Finally, the assay is sensitive to environmental factors. Results can be difficult to interpret and are not consistently predictive of clinical outcomes, and standardization from lab to lab can be difficult.[3] In addition, this assay only decides MLR compatibility—that is, whether two cell types differ in HLA-D proteins; it does not give an actual HLA class II type. Many transplant centers no longer routinely perform MLCs because more specific DNA-based typing assays are available.

Molecular (DNA-Based) Methods

The isolation and characterization of the genes encoding for HLAs have allowed the development of tests that identify donor and recipient HLA genotypes by the DNA sequence of the alleles being expressed. This methodology was primarily developed for the class II genes because of the limitations of serologic and cellular typing methods. These limitations became apparent when the same HLA serologic type was assigned to HLA proteins that DNA sequencing showed were different. HLA proteins assigned the same serologic type (or specificity) often vary at positions that may influence peptide binding or T-cell recognition.[7] For example, the serologic specificity HLA-DR4 has been assigned to at least 15 HLA proteins with different antigen-binding sites. Figure 3-7 shows the serologic specificity associated with the WHO nomenclature assigned according to DNA-based methods and the actual amino acid sequence of the allelic product. All 15 allelic products type identically with serologic reagents, but T cells can distinguish many, if not all, of these 15 allelic products. This suggests that these allelic differences may be important in transplantation, especially when unrelated donors are considered.[3]

Comparisons of molecular and serologic HLA typing have usually concluded that serologic typing has a significant error rate. The major difference between serologic testing and most molecular typing is the quality of information, particularly the structural relationships of the

Serological Specificity	WHO Nomenclature	Amino acid sequence (1 10 20 30 40 50 60 70 80 90 100)
DR1	DRB1*0101	GDTRPRFLWQLKFECHFFNGTERVRLLERCIYNQEESVRFDSDVGEYRAVTELGRPDAEYWNSQKDLLEQRRAAVDTYCRHNYGVGESFTVQRRVEPKVTVY
DR15 (2)	DRB1*1501	----------P-R------------F-D-YF---------------F-------------------I---A--------------V---------Q------
DR16 (2)	DRB1*1601	----------P-R------------F-D-YF-----------------------------------F--D-------------------------Q------
DR17 (3)	DRB1*03011	--------EYSTS------------Y-D-YFH----N---------F-----------------------K-GR--N--------V---------H------
DR18 (3)	DRB1*0302	--------EYSTS------------F---YFH----N---------------------------------K-GR--N------------------H------
DR11 (5)	DRB1*11011	--------EYSTS------------F-D-YF-----Y---------F----------E--------F--D-------------------------H------
DR12 (5)	DRB1*1201	--------EYSTG--Y-------------HFH----LL--------F---------V--S------I--D--------------AV---------H------
DR13 (6)	DRB1*1301	--------EYSTS------------F-D-YFH----N---------F-------------------I--DE--------------V---------H------
DR14 (6)	DRB1*1401	--------EYSTS------------F-D-YFH----F-------------------A--H----------R---E-----------V--------********
DR7	DRB1*0701	---Q------G-YK----------QF---LF-----F-------------------V--S------I--D--GQ---V-----------------H-E----
DR8	DRB1*0801	--------EYSTG--Y---------F-D-YF-----Y-------------------S---------F--D---L------------****************
DR9	DRB1*09011	*****************--------Y-H-G------N-------------------V--S------F--R--E---V------------------H-E----
DR10	DRB1*1001	--------EEV------------------RVH----YA-Y-----------------------------R-------------------------Q------
DR4	DRB1*0401	--------E-V-H------------F-D-YF-H---Y---------------------------------K------------------------Y-E----
DR4	DRB1*0402	--------E-V-H------------F-D-YF-H---Y-----------------------------I--DE--------------V--------********
DR4	DRB1*0403	--------E-V-H------------F-D-YF-H---Y------------------------------------E-----------V---------Y-E----
DR4	DRB1*0404	--------E-V-H------------F-D-YF-H---Y--V---------Y-E----
DR4	DRB1*0405	--------E-V-H------------F-D-YF-H---Y-------------------S-------------------------------------********
DR4	DRB1*0406	--------E-V-H------------F-D-YF-H--E-----------V---------Y-E----
DR4	DRB1*0407	--------E-V-H------------F-D-YF-H---Y------------------------------------E--------------------********
DR4	DRB1*0408	*************------------F-D-YF-H---Y--***************
DR4	DRB1*0409	*************------------F-D-YF-H---Y-------------------S-------------K----------------***************
DR4	DRB1*0410	******--E-V-H------------F-D-YF-H---Y-------------------S----------------------------V---*************
DR4	DRB1*0411	******--E-V-H------------F-D-YF-H---Y-------------------S----------------E-----------V--------********
DR4	DRB1*0412	******--E-V-H------------F-D-YF-H---Y-------------------S---------I--D---L-----------V-------*********
DR4	DRB1*0413	****----E-V-H------------F-D-YF-H---Y---------------------------------K--------------V---*************
DR4	DRB1*0414	******--E-V-H------------F-D-YF-H---Y-----------------------------I--DE-----------------------********
DR4x11	DRB1*0415	****----E-V-H------------F-D-YF-H---Y--------------------E--------F--D---------***********************

Figure 3-7. Alignment of *HLA-DRB1* sequences. The *HLA-DRB1*0101* sequence is shown at the top using the single-letter amino acid code. The sequences of selected *HLA-DRB1* alleles (left) are listed below using a "-" for residues that are identical to *HLA-DRB1*0101* and the single-letter amino acid code for different residues. The top section contains sequences representative of each of the major serological specificities. The bottom section shows *HLA-DRB1*04* sequences that are recognized by the World Health Organization (WHO).

SOURCE: *Reprinted with permission from Baxter-Lowe LA. Molecular techniques for typing unrelated marrow donors.* Bone Marrow Transplant. *1994;14(Suppl 4):S42–S50.*

HLA proteins. In contrast to serologic specificities, most molecular methods provide specific information about the primary sequences of the HLA proteins, allowing comparison of donor and recipient at the level of the amino acid sequence.[7]

Restriction Fragment Length Polymorphism

The first DNA-based method developed was the restriction fragment length polymorphism (RFLP) assay. In this technique, genomic DNA is cut at specific nucleotide sequences by restriction enzymes (endonucleases), which bind to and cleave double-stranded DNA at sites within or next to a particular sequence known as the recognition sequence. The recognition sequences used for HLA typing are those known to contain variations that defined specific HLA alleles. Therefore, in RFLP typing the HLA locus is cleaved into DNA fragments of different lengths (restriction fragment lengths) containing individual alleles. These DNA fragments are then separated by size electrophoretically, transferred by Southern blotting onto a filter, fixed, and then hybridized to a DNA probe corresponding to the HLA allele of interest. Different alleles exhibit different binding (or hybridization) patterns, and thus a specific HLA type can be assigned. The principal advantages of this technique include easily readable and reproducible determination of class II alleles (often subdividing class II serotypes into subtypes) and no requirements for cell surface expression or cell viability (which are necessary for cellular methods). However, RFLP typing is cumbersome and time consuming and lacks sensitivity to differentiate all subtypes of the HLA-DR alleles.[3,11]

Polymerase Chain Reaction

The development of the polymerase chain reaction (PCR) in the 1980s marked the next major advancement of DNA-based HLA typing. During the PCR process, a segment of DNA containing the HLA allele from a particular locus is sequenced, and oligonucleotide primers (small segments of single-stranded DNA) are synthesized. These primers are complementary to each end of the HLA DNA segment. The HLA gene is then amplified through a series of reactions: denaturation of the HLA DNA segment into single strands, attachment of the oligonucleotide primers to each end of the HLA DNA segment, and extension of the primers by DNA polymerase to form new double-stranded DNA across the entire DNA segment. Over a few hours, this repetition of amplification generates millions of copies of the chosen DNA sequence. PCR thus enables very minute quantities of DNA to be amplified into quantities sufficient for HLA typing.[12]

The first PCR-based method for HLA typing, oligotyping, involves amplification of DNA from HLA alleles followed by hybridization with a panel of sequence-specific oligonucleotide (SSO) probes that can distinguish one allele or group of alleles from another. The initial step, low-resolution oligotyping, identifies groups of alleles that correspond to a serologically defined specificity. Low-resolution oligotypes can then be used to achieve amplification of individual alleles. Amplified DNA from a particular allele is subsequently hybridized with appropriate probes to distinguish each allele from all others. This second stage of oligotyping is called high-resolution oligotyping. Although the importance of HLA matching at the level of high-resolution oligotyping is not well established, it is likely that it may benefit at least some patients.[7]

Several PCR methodologies have evolved that are now being used for HLA class II (and, on a more limited basis, class I) typing. These methodologies differ in their post-PCR manipulations (probe-hybridization techniques, electrophoresis-based techniques, and conformational analysis). A list of these methods is found in Table 3-2 (see page 46). A discussion of each of these methods is beyond the scope of this text but can be found in reference 13. Many of these methods will probably remain reference or research tools because of the time involved or the type of equipment necessary; some, however, have been commercially developed into kits that are now being used regularly in clinical HLA-typing laboratories. Examples of those being used clinically include the PCR-SSO, reverse dot-blot PCR-SSO, PCR-oligonucleotide capture sandwich assay, and the PCR-SSP.[13]

BLOOD GROUP DETECTION

This section provides a brief history of the development of blood-grouping systems and discusses their application in clinical practice. There are many applications of immunohematology, not only in the medical field but also in law, genetics, and anthropology.

The history of blood transfusions dates back to the late 17th century. Initial attempts at blood transfusion for humans used sheep's blood, which led to many deaths and the subsequent outlawing of transfusion therapy in England. By the 1800s it was determined that blood could be transfused only between individuals of the same species.[14]

Blood transfusion can be thought of as a form of tissue transplantation. Not only is blood transfusion the safest form of allotransplantation, it is one of the most important lifesaving measures practiced in medicine. However, because severe hemolytic reactions can occur if incompatible blood is transfused, nomenclature and typing systems are essential.

Many systems are used to classify blood groups. Currently, there are at least 22 different blood-grouping systems that describe approximately 400 blood group antigens in humans. The two most widely used are the ABO system and the Rh system.

Table 3-2. PCR-Based HLA-Typing Methods

METHOD	MULTIPLE PCRs	MULTIPLE PROBES	POST-PCR MANIPULATION	APPLICATIONS DESCRIBED
Probe-hybridization techniques				
PCR-SSO dot blot	–	+	H,SW,AR/CD	HLA-A,B,DRB,DQA,DQB,DPB
PCR-SSO reverse dot blot	–	+	H,SW,CD	HLA-DRB,DQA,DQB,DPB
PCR-oligocapture sandwich assay	–	+	H,SW,CD	HLA-DRB
PCR-dual phase oligocapture	–	+	H,SW,CD	HLA-DRB
PCR-HPA	–	+	H,Hy,CD	HLA-DRB
Electrophoresis-based techniques				
PCR-RFLP	–	+	RE,AGE	HLA-DRB,DQA,DQB,DPA,DPB
PCR-SSP	+	–	AGE	HLA-A,C,DRB,DQA,DQB
PCR-nested SSP	+	–	AGE	HLA-DRB
PCR-SBT	–	–	DD,DP	HLA-A,B,C,DRB
Conformational analysis				
PCR-SSCP	–	–	NDP	HLA-DRB,DQB
PCR-heteroduplex analysis	–	–	NDP	HLA-DRB,DQA,DQB
PCR-UHG-heteroduplex analysis	–	–	CM,NDP	HLA-DPB

SOURCE: *Reprinted with permission from Bidwell J. Advances in DNA-based HLA typing methods.* Immunol Today *1994;15:303–7. PCR, polymerase chain reactions; SSO, sequence-specific oligonucleotide; HPA, hybridization protection assay; RFLP, restriction fragment length polymorphism; SSP, sequence-specific primers; SBT, sequence-based typing; SSCP, single-stranded conformational polymorphism; UHG, universal heteroduplex generator; H, hybridization; SW, stringent washing; AR autoradiography; CD, colorimetric or chemiluminescence detection; Hy, hydrolysis of ester; RE, restriction endonuclease digestion; AGE, agarose gel electrophoresis; DD, dideoxynucleotide (chain termination) sequencing; DP, denaturing polyacrylamide gel electrophoresis; NDP, nondenaturing polyacrylamide gel electrophoresis; CM, crossmatch of PCR products.*

The ABO System

At the turn of the 20th century, a relatively simple red blood cell (RBC) antigen-grouping system was designed. This system was based on the fact that there are two main immunogenic antigens associated with RBCs, A and B. A person may have one, both, or neither of these two antigens. A third RBC antigen was then described and was denoted as H. H is a precursor of both A and B antigens. People who have neither A nor B antigens have high titers of the H antigen.

The nomenclature of this ABO system is based on which antigen or antigens are present on an individual's RBCs. People with the A antigen are blood group A, those with B antigens are blood group B, those with both A and B are blood group AB, and those who have neither A nor B antigens but have high levels of H antigen are blood group O.[15] The ABO nomenclature system is summarized in Table 3-3.

It was also found that the serum of many people contains antibodies directed against whichever antigen or antigens are not expressed on their own RBCs. That is to say, A individuals have anti-B antibodies, B individuals have anti-A antibodies, AB individuals have no antibodies, and O individuals have both anti-A and anti-B antibodies. Table 3-3 summarizes the antibody distribution in the ABO blood-grouping system.

Blood grouping was first used as a prerequisite to blood transfusion in the early 1900s, and in 1949 the actual structures of the three ABO antigens were described. The presence of antigens on RBCs is genetically controlled; the inheritance of these ABO antigens follows simple Mendelian patterns. Each individual possesses two alleles at the *ABO* locus (located on chromosome 9 in humans), one derived from each parent. There are six possible *ABO* genotypes based on the three available antigens: *AA*, *AO*, *BB*, *BO*, *AB*, and *OO*. The genotypes determine people's blood types. For instance, people with genotype *AA* and *AO* have blood type A; those with *BB* or *BO* have blood type B; those with *AB* have blood type AB, and those with genotype *OO* have blood type O (Table 3-3).

The ABO antigens are present on virtually all cells and tissues of the body, with the exception of lymphocytes and cells of the spinal cord and brain. The matching of blood groups in medicine is useful primarily in transfusions, allografts, and diagnosing hemolytic disease of the newborn (HDN).

Before blood is transfused, compatibility between donor and recipient must be established by typing the blood of both individuals. In addition to determining blood type, tests must verify the absence of cytotoxic an-

Table 3-3. ABO Blood Group System

BLOOD GROUP PHENOTYPE	POSSIBLE GENOTYPES	ANTIGEN ON RED BLOOD CELLS[a]	ANTIBODY IN SERUM	INCIDENCE IN U.S. POPULATION (%)
A	AA, AO	A	Anti-B	42
B	BB, BO	B	Anti-A	10
O (H)	OO	Neither A nor B	Both anti-A and anti-B	45
AB	AB	Both A and B	Neither anti-A nor anti-B	3

SOURCE: *Reprinted with permission from Barrett J.* Textbook of Immunology. *5th ed. St. Louis, MO: CV Mosby; 1988. p. 233.*
[a]*Cells of all blood groups contain the H substance.*

tibodies in the recipient that may be targeted against the donor's RBCs. Most severe hemolytic reactions that occur after transfusion are due to ABO mismatches.

Blood Typing

In determining a patient's blood type, both the cells and the serum are tested. When the cells are typed, they are mixed with serum containing known antibodies, and agglutination reactions are assessed. This method of RBC antigen typing is referred to as forward grouping. In testing a patient's serum, the serum is mixed with RBCs containing known antigens, and agglutination reactions are assessed. This method is known as reverse grouping.[15] Because correct typing of ABO antigens is vital, both forward and reverse grouping are routinely done. Table 3-4 summarizes the agglutination reactions found in ABO blood typing.

Crossmatching

The crossmatch test is a very important pretransfusion test, second only to typing in importance. A physician ordering a *type and cross* would receive results of both of these testing methods. In crossmatching, the recipient's serum is incubated with the donor's RBCs to assess the presence of antibodies that could cause hemolysis. If the cells agglutinate after this procedure, antibodies are present and the donor and recipient are judged incompatible.

For situations in which the transfusion will probably not be needed within 48 hours, a *type and screen* may be performed. In this case, the patient's blood type is determined, and then the blood is screened for the presence of antibodies by being mixed with a variety of common RBC antigens. When the patient is actually ready to receive the transfusion, a crossmatch must be done between the recipient and the actual donor's blood.[16] The crossmatch must be performed within 24 hours of the proposed transfusion, because the antibody status of the recipient can change rapidly and unexpectedly.[14]

When available, only ABO- and Rh-matched blood should be transfused. It was previously believed that type O blood (containing "no" antigens) could safely be given to any patient, and type O patients were referred to as universal donors. Conversely, it was thought that AB patients (having "no" antibodies) could receive any blood and were referred to as universal recipients. This concept has now been abandoned, because patients who receive repeated transfusions can develop high titers of antibodies directed against antigens of various blood groups. Also, prior pregnancy or organ transplantation can prompt a patient to develop high titers. Thus, "universal" donor whole blood should be used only in emergency situations when typing and crossmatching are not possible. However, administering packed RBCs (from which the serum containing most of the antibodies is removed) is safer than administering whole blood in emergency situations.[17]

The Rh System

The Rh system is antigenically separate from the ABO system and is the most complex of all the RBC antigen systems. The nomenclature most widely used for the Rh

Table 3-4. Results of ABO Typing

BLOOD TYPE	RBCs PLUS ANTI-A SERUM	RBCs PLUS ANTI-B SERUM
A	+	0
B	0	+
AB	+	+
O	0	0

+, agglutination; 0, no agglutination.

system was developed by Fisher and Race. The Fisher-Race nomenclature system approved by the World Health Organization is the simplest and easiest to understand.

The Rh gene complex, located on chromosome 1 in humans, consists of three closely linked loci containing three pairs of allelic genes. The alleles are denoted as *C*, *c*, *D*, *d*, *E*, and *e*. (In reality, the "*d*" allele has never been isolated; and the notation "*d*" simply means that *D* is not present.) Because the gene loci of the Rh system are so closely linked, they are generally inherited as a gene complex. In contrast to the ABO system, no naturally occurring antibodies are directed against Rh antigens. The only way such antibodies can develop is from sensitization via blood transfusions, organ transplants, or pregnancy.[16]

Methods of Rh Blood Group Detection

The assignment of an Rh type is based on the use of antisera, which are obtained from sensitized humans. To determine an Rh type, the antisera are mixed with the patient's RBCs and agglutination is assessed. The presence or absence of the D antigen determines whether an individual is Rh positive (Rh^+) or Rh negative (Rh^-). In fact, the terms Rh^+ and D^+ are synonymous, as are the terms Rh^- and D^-.[14]

The D antigen is often called the Rh antigen, because it is the most clinically important and the most immunogenic of the Rh antigens. The D antigen often induces antibody production after blood transfusions, and it is also responsible for the maternal-fetal incompatibilities seen in HDN. The D antigen is the only Rh antigen that is crossmatched between donor and recipient, since the C, c, E, and e antigens are much less immunogenic.[17] Patients whose blood agglutinates with anti-D serum are termed Rh^+, and those exhibiting no agglutination are termed Rh^-.

In addition to the importance of Rh matching before blood transfusions, understanding the Rh system is critical in the management of HDN, also known as Rh disease. A brief review of the pathogenesis of this disease illustrates the importance of the Rh system.

Hemolytic Disease of the Newborn

HDN was first described in 1936, when it was found that mothers of some infants had antibodies in their serum directed against their newborns' RBCs. These destructive antibodies are primarily anti-D antibodies, which are responsible for 95% of cases of HDN. The development mechanism of the anti-D antibodies and HDN is as follows.

During normal pregnancy, fetal RBCs do not enter the maternal circulation. However, during the placental trauma that occurs at delivery or miscarriage, fetal RBCs may cross the placenta and enter the mother's bloodstream. If the mother is Rh^- and the infant is Rh^+, the fetal RBCs stimulate the mother to produce cytotoxic antibodies after birth or miscarriage. The firstborn child is spared any problems with HDN. However, during subsequent pregnancies, a strong secondary response occurs, and maternal antibodies could cross the placenta and destroy fetal Rh^+ RBCs.

The clinical features of HDN include anemia and jaundice developing within 24 hours of birth. High concentrations of bilirubin can cause permanent damage to the central nervous system. High circulating levels of erythroblasts (RBC precursors) are also seen, so this clinical syndrome is also known as erythroblastosis fetalis.

The best treatment for HDN is prevention. As a rule, all premenopausal women who are Rh^- should receive only Rh^- blood to avoid sensitization. If the father of the child is Rh^+, the likelihood of HDN increases. Therefore, all pregnant women should undergo prenatal screening for this disease with ABO and Rh blood grouping, testing of the mother's serum against paternal RBCs, and possible testing of the amniotic fluid.

In the first pregnancy, treatment is not necessary before delivery. The preferred treatment is administration of exogenous anti-D antibody (Rh immunoglobulin). Administered within 72 hours after the birth of the first child, it neutralizes the Rh^+ fetal RBCs, preventing the production of maternal anti-D antibodies and avoiding sensitization. If the mother has already been sensitized to Rh^+ RBCs through a previous pregnancy or an Rh^+ blood transfusion, the prenatal screening may show increased titers of anti-D antibodies, and treatment with Rh immunoglobulin would need to be started before the baby is delivered. Figure 3-8 illustrates the sequence of events in the development and prevention of HDN.

The pathogenesis of HDN graphically illustrates the importance of knowing a patient's Rh status. Fortunately, the use of Rh immunoglobulin has drastically reduced the incidence of HDN and has a success rate of approximately 99%.[15]

There are also nonmedical uses for the blood group systems. Use of ABO and Rh phenotypes can help solve crimes involving blood traces. Furthermore, the genetic determination of these phenotypes can solve cases of disputed parentage and baby mix-ups in nurseries.[17] The extensive polymorphism seen, especially in the Rh and HLA antigens, can also prove valuable to anthropologists studying relationships among human populations, including migration and breeding patterns.

SUMMARY

The discovery and elucidation of the human MHC has enhanced medical science in many ways. Details of the function of HLA in antigen recognition by T cells have allowed better understanding of the body's defense against infection and tumor. Immune response mechanisms and

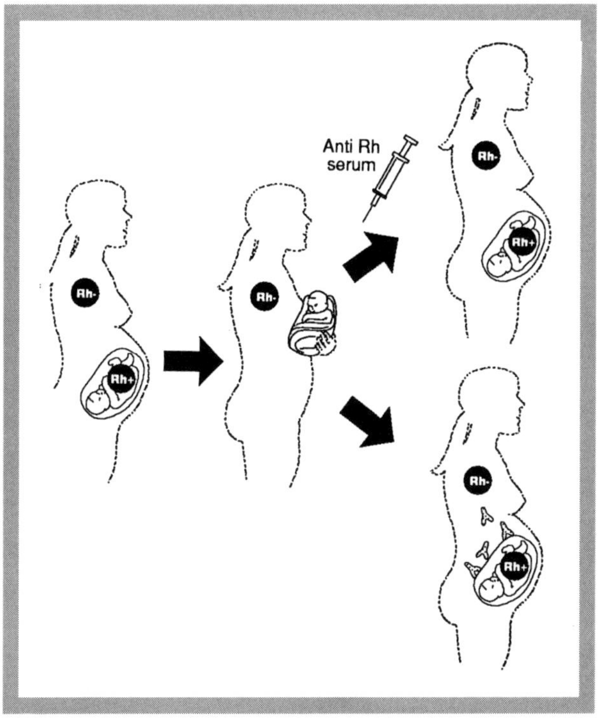

Figure 3-8. Development and prevention of hemolytic disease of the newborn (HDN). The Rh^- mother is exposed to Rh^+ antigens during the birth of her Rh^+ child. If passively immunized with anti-Rh sera immediately after delivery, the maternal anti-Rh immune response is suppressed. A subsequent Rh^+ fetus is uncomplicated by HDN (upper right). When passive immunization is not practiced, erythrocytes of an Rh^+ fetus are subject to destruction by maternal antibodies and complement (lower right).

SOURCE: *Reprinted with permission from Barrett J.* Textbook of Immunology. *5th ed. St. Louis, MO: CV Mosby; 1988. p. 339.*

their role in the pathogenesis of autoimmune disease are now better understood; this information is being used to develop specific therapies that may reduce the need for nonspecific immunosuppression. The setting in which knowledge of the MHC has had a major effect is transplantation. Mechanisms behind graft rejection and GVHD are now more fully described with respect to T-cell activation caused by HLA disparities. HLA-matching (along with more effective immunosuppression) has resulted in more successful outcomes that, in turn, have allowed more individuals the opportunity to receive this lifesaving form of therapy.

Important work continues to be done to determine the most clinically relevant means of typing. As PCR-based methods become more widely available and practical, the question of how critical matching on the genetic level is must be answered. In vitro and anecdotal clinical reports have suggested that HLA disparities resulting in differences in amino acid sequences within the antigen-binding groove may affect T-cell recognition and therefore clinical outcome. Further investigations are needed to decide which HLA genomic disparities are relevant when genotypically matched donors are not available. Once this is determined, the most cost-effective laboratory methods for HLA-typing can be defined.

The use of the ABO and Rh blood systems is very important in determining the antigenicity of blood products and the compatibility of donor and recipient before blood transfusion and organ transplantation and in maternal-fetal relationships. HDN demonstrates this importance and can be effectively treated with Rh immune globulin.

REFERENCES

1. Goodman JW. Antigen presentation and the major histocompatibility complex. In: Stites DP, Terr AI, Parslow TG, editors. *Basic and Clinical Immunology*. 8th ed. Norwalk, CT: Appelton & Lange; 1994. p. 58–65.
2. Goust JM. Major histocompatibility complex. In: Virella G, Goust JM, Fudenberg HH, editors. *Introduction to Medical Immunology*. 2nd ed. New York: Marcel Dekker; 1990. p. 31–51.
3. Begovich AB, Erlich HA. HLA typing for bone marrow transplantation. *JAMA* 1995;273:586–591.
4. Roitt IM, Brostoff J, Male D. *Immunology*. 4th ed. London: Mosby; 1996. p. 5.3–5.9.
5. Kelly A, Trowsdale J. Novel genes in the human major histocompatibility complex class II region. *Int Arch Allergy Appl Immunol*. 1994;103:11–15.
6. Benjamini E, Leskowitz S. *Immunology: A Short Course*. 2nd ed. New York: Wiley-Liss; 1991. p. 93–209.
7. Baxter-Lowe LA. Molecular techniques for typing unrelated marrow donors: potential impact of molecular typing disparity on donor selection. *Bone Marrow Transplant*. 1994;14(*Suppl* 4):S42–S50.
8. Hansen TH, Carreno BM, Sachs DH. The major histocompatibility complex. In: Paul WE, editor. *Fundamental Immunology*. 3rd ed. New York: Raven; 1993. p. 577–628.
9. Dalton TA, Bennett JC. Autoimmune disease and the major histocompatibility complex: therapeutic implications. *Am J Med*. 1992;92:183–188.
10. Nepom BS. The role of the major histocompatibility complex in autoimmunity. *Clin Immunol Immunopathol*. 1993;67:S50–S55.
11. Kerman RH. Relevance of histocompatibility testing in clinical transplantation. *Surg Clin North Am*. 1994;74:1015–1028.
12. Colombe BW. Histocompatibility testing. In: Stites DP, Terr AI, Parslow TG, editors. *Basic and Clinical Immunology*. 8th ed. Norwalk, CT: Appelton & Lange; 1994. p. 237–255.
13. Bidwell J. Advances in DNA-based HLA-typing methods. *Immunol Today* 1994;15:303–307.
14. Myrvik QN, Weiser RS. *Fundamentals of Immunology*. 2nd ed. Philadelphia, PA: Lea and Febiger; 1984.
15. Virella G, Goust JM, Fudenberg HH, editors. *Introduction to Medical Immunology*. New York: Marcel Dekker; 1986.

16. Davis M. Molecular genetics of T-cell antigen receptors. *Hosp Pract.* 1988;23(5):115–28.
17. Isselbacher KJ, Braunwald E, Wilson JD, *et al.*, editors. *Harrison's Principles of Internal Medicine.* 13th ed. New York: McGraw-Hill; 1994.

SELF-ASSESSMENT QUESTIONS

1. Which of the following terms accurately describes the expression of parental MHC haplotypes in offspring?

   a. autosomal dominant
   b. codominant
   c. autosomal recessive
   d. sex-linked

2. Based on Mendelian inheritance patterns, the chance that siblings will share both parental MHC haplotypes (i.e., be genotypically HLA identical) is:

   a. 25%.
   b. 50%.
   c. 75%.
   d. 100%.

3. Which of the following genetic loci *does not* belong to the class I family?

   a. *HLA-A*
   b. *HLA-B*
   c. *HLA-C*
   d. *HLA-D*

4. Which of the following class II gene loci located in the HLA-D region *does not* encode for a major expressed product?

   a. *HLA-DR*
   b. *HLA-DQ*
   c. *HLA-DP*
   d. *HLA-DO*

5. Class I antigens are found on:

   a. red blood cells.
   b. lymphocytes only.
   c. all nucleated cells.
   d. Kupfer cells in the liver.

6. Class I antigens bind endogenously synthesized antigenic fragments and present them to which lymphocyte subset for recognition?

   a. CD4
   b. CD8
   c. CD34
   d. CD56

7. Class II antigens are normally found on all of the following cells *except:*

   a. platelets.
   b. B lymphocytes.
   c. macrophages.
   d. Langerhans cells.

8. Class II antigens bind antigenic fragments derived predominantly from membrane and extracellular proteins and present them to which lymphocyte subset for recognition?

   a. CD4
   b. CD8
   c. CD34
   d. CD56

9. The phenomenon by which foreign antigens must be recognized by the appropriate T cell in the context of an HLA molecule is called:

   a. linkage disequilibrium.
   b. adaptive immune response.
   c. HLA (or MHC) restriction.
   d. immune tolerance.

10. Which of the following statements is true concerning HLA-associated diseases?

    a. HLA-B27 causes ankylosing spondylitis.
    b. A relative risk of less than one suggests an association between the disease and the HLA molecule in question.
    c. Most autoimmune diseases have been associated with class I antigens.
    d. One postulated mechanism responsible for HLA-disease associations is that the particular HLA molecule acts as a receptor for the actual etiologic agent.

11. Serologic assays for HLA typing include all of the following components *except:*

    a. radiolabeled thymidine.
    b. human sera containing anti-HLA antibodies.
    c. donor and recipient lymphocytes.
    d. complement.

12. Limitations to serologic typing include:

    a. the need for live, healthy macrophages that express class I HLA molecules.
    b. a more labor-intensive process for class II antigens.
    c. techniques that are unrefined.
    d. results that are difficult to reproduce.

13. Which of the following pretransplant procedures detects the presence of antibodies in the *recipient's sera* that, if the donor were HLA-incompatible, would cause cytolysis of *donor lymphocytes*?

    a. lymphocytotoxicity assay
    b. mixed lymphocyte reaction
    c. RFLP
    d. serologic crossmatch

14. The advantages of DNA-based typing over serologic typing include:

    a. less expensive equipment.
    b. shorter turnaround time for results.
    c. more specific information regarding HLA-DR subtypes.
    d. consistent results that are clinically relevant with respect to improved graft survival.

15. All of the following are DNA-based methods for HLA typing *except:*

    a. MLC.
    b. RFLP.
    c. PCR-SSO.
    d. PCR-SSP.

16. The ABO blood system's nomenclature is based on which of the following factors?

    a. A, B, and O antibodies are found on RBCs.
    b. A, B, and O antigens are found in the serum.
    c. A, B, and O antigens are found on RBCs.
    d. A, B, and O antisera are found on RBCs.

17. The RBCs of a patient with blood type A would agglutinate with which of the following antisera?

    a. Anti-A
    b. Anti-B
    c. Anti-O
    d. Both anti-A and anti-B

18. Which sequence of events best describes the development of hemolytic disease of the newborn?

    a. Maternal Rh^+ serum stimulates fetal antibody production.
    b. Maternal Rh^+ RBCs stimulate fetal antibody production.
    c. Fetal Rh^+ serum stimulates maternal antibody production.
    d. Fetal Rh^+ RBCs stimulate fetal antibody production.

CHAPTER 4

Hypersensitivity Reactions

Jeffrey C. Delafuente, M.S.
Professor and Associate Chairman
Department of Pharmacy Practice, College of Pharmacy
University of Florida
Gainesville, FL

Classification of Hypersensitivity Reactions 54
Anaphylactic Reactions 54
  Mechanism 55
    Allergens 55
    Role of IgE 55
    Mast Cell and Basophil Mediators 56
      Histamine 57
      Eosinophil Chemotactic Factor 57
      Neutrophil Chemotactic Factor 57
      Leukotrienes 57
      Prostaglandins 57
      Platelet-Activating Factor 57
  Prevalence and Incidence 58
  Diagnosis of Atopy 58
    Skin Testing 58
    In Vitro Testing 58
  Treatment 59
    Pharmacologic Therapies 59
      Antihistamines 59
      Sympathomimetic Agents 59
      Antiallergy Agents 59
      Corticosteroids 59
      Leukotriene Inhibitors and Antagonists 59
    Immunotherapy 60
Cytotoxic Reactions 60
  Mechanisms 60
  Drug-Induced Reactions 61
  Treatment 61
Immune Complex–Mediated Reactions 62
  Mechanisms 62
  Treatment 62

Cell-Mediated Reactions 63
Mechanisms 63
Treatment 64
Summary 65
References 65
Self-Assessment Questions 66

Hypersensitivity to drugs and other antigenic substances may result in reactions that require the use of pharmacologic agents to modulate inflammatory responses. The role of the pharmacist in preventing, identifying, and managing these problems requires an understanding of the pathogenesis of hypersensitivity reactions. Many acute and chronic pathologic states, including allergies, drug reactions, serum sickness, and organ transplant rejection, are caused by immunologically mediated hypersensitivity reactions.

This chapter discusses four types of hypersensitivity reactions—anaphylactic reactions, cytotoxic reactions, immune complex–mediated reactions, and cell-mediated reactions—and their mechanisms, diagnoses, and treatments. Each type of hypersensitivity is described in the context of its symptoms, causes, immune mechanism, prevalence and incidence, methods of diagnosis, and therapies. After completing this chapter, the reader should be able to:

1. Describe the mechanisms and treatments of the four types of hypersensitivity reactions.
2. Match examples of hypersensitivity reactions to one of the four types.
3. Describe the mediators of immediate hypersensitivity reactions.
4. Describe diagnostic techniques for immediate hypersensitivity reactions.

CLASSIFICATION OF HYPERSENSITIVITY REACTIONS

The immune system evolved as a mechanism for protecting the host against foreign substances. When normal immune mechanisms result in tissue damage to the host, the process is known as hypersensitivity. Many hypersensitivity reactions are heightened responses of normal immune functions, and they can often be described as inappropriate reactions.[1] The immunologic mechanisms involved in hypersensitivity reactions are often categorized in four types: type I, anaphylactic; type II, cytotoxic; type III, immune complex mediated; and type IV, cell mediated. This classification scheme was originally developed by Coombs and Gell[2] more than three decades ago.

The major immune constituents involved in hypersensitivity reactions are listed in Table 4-1. Type I reactions involve immunoglobulin E (IgE) and are responsible for many common allergic conditions (such as hay fever and hives) as well as life-threatening anaphylaxis from certain drugs or insect stings. Type II reactions, which often involve immunoglobulin G (IgG) or immunoglobulin M (IgM), cause many drug reactions involving destruction of blood cells. Examples of type II reactions involving drugs include penicillin-induced hemolytic anemia and chlorpromazine-induced agranulocytosis. Immune complexes are responsible for type III hypersensitivity reactions, which contribute to many rheumatic diseases, such as rheumatoid arthritis or systemic lupus erythematosus. Type IV reactions are primarily mediated by sensitized $CD4^+$ T lymphocytes, with participation by other cells, such as monocytes and macrophages. These reactions are responsible for delayed cutaneous hypersensitivity reactions, organ transplant rejection, and other immunologic phenomena.

Since the Coombs and Gell[2] system was developed, other immunologic mechanisms have been described that do not precisely follow this classification scheme, and the original classification has been modified to include newer findings.[3] For example, cells with Fc receptors can bind IgG-coated cells, leading to destruction of the antibody-coated cell. It has become evident that in many immunologically mediated diseases more than one type of hypersensitivity reaction is responsible for tissue damage. For example, mononuclear cell–derived factors and inflammatory cells (typical of type IV reactions) may have roles in some type I reactions, such as asthma or allergic rhinitis.[4,5] Also, type I mediators may have a role in diseases that are generally thought to be type III reactions.[6] Although supporting data is often lacking, many drug reactions probably have more than one type of hypersensitivity mechanism involved.

ANAPHYLACTIC REACTIONS

Type I (anaphylactic) reactions are immediate hypersensitivity reactions that are usually mediated by the inter-

Table 4-1. Immune Constituents of Hypersensitivity Reactions

HYPERSENSITIVITY REACTION	IG INVOLVED	COMPLEMENT INVOLVED	MAJOR IMMUNE CELLS INVOLVED	PRINCIPAL MEDIATORS
Type I				
Intermediate reactions				
Early-phase reactions	IgE	No	Mast cells	Histamine, leukotrienes
Late-phase reactions	None	No	Eosinophils, PMNs, lymphocytes	Multiple cytokines
Type II				
Cytotoxic reactions	IgG, IgM	Yes	None	None
	IgG	No	PMNs, NK cells, macrophages	
Type III				
Immune complex-mediated reactions	IgG, IgM	Yes	PMNs	Lysosomal enzymes
Type IV				
Cell-mediated reactions	None	No	T cells, macrophages	Multiple cytokines

Ig, immunoglobulin; PMNs, polymorphonuclear leukocytes; NK, natural killer.

action of mast cell–bound antigen-specific IgE and a specific antigen. These reactions develop within minutes of an IgE-antigen interaction. Clinical manifestations may be systemic, resulting in a shocklike state, or local, involving only one target site, such as the skin or nasal mucosa. Systemic reactions, known as anaphylaxis, can be life threatening. Within seconds to minutes after antigen exposure, the anaphylactic reaction begins. It can be manifested as respiratory distress, laryngeal edema, or vascular collapse. This state of shock is often fatal if not immediately treated. Other anaphylactic manifestations include pruritus, urticaria, and angioedema.

Mechanism

The type I hypersensitivity reaction is preceded by a precise sequence of events. Many factors play roles in this development.

Allergens

The term allergen usually refers to an antigen that elicits an allergic immune reaction. A few examples of allergens that cause type I hypersensitivity reactions are plant pollens, house dust mites, fungi spores, animal dander, foods, drugs, and insect venoms. The route of entry into the body can be inhalation (e.g., pollen, mold spores), ingestion (e.g., food, drugs), or injection (drugs, bee stings). Most allergens must have large molecular weights to bridge adjacent IgE molecules on mast cells. Substances of smaller molecular weight, such as drugs, become allergenic by covalently binding to protein molecules.[7] Small-molecular-weight substances that become immunogenic when conjugated to a carrier molecule are known as haptens.

Role of IgE

An individual must be sensitized for an immediate hypersensitivity reaction to occur. After the individual has been exposed to a particular antigen, antigen-specific IgE antibodies are produced. As with all immunoglobulin production, the antigen must be presented by an antigen-presenting cell, such as a macrophage, to a $CD4^+$ helper T cell. Through secretion of various cytokines, B lymphocytes then produce antigen-specific immunoglobulin. IgE is the isotype responsible for Type I reactions. An immediate reaction does not occur at this point. After antigen-specific IgE antibodies are produced, they attach to Fc receptors on mast cells and basophils. On subsequent exposure to the antigen, antigen-specific IgE on mast cells or basophils combines with the antigen to activate the cells, which then release inflammatory mediators. A clinical example of this phenomenon is a type I reaction to penicillin. Exposure to penicillin must have occurred at least once before to produce penicillin-specific IgE. The previous exposure allows mast cells to become sensitized, that is, coated with penicillin-specific IgE. On subsequent exposure to penicillin, the sensitized cells combine with penicillin to release mast cell mediators, such as histamine and leukotrienes, which are responsible for immediate reactions. The immediate hypersensitivity reaction is shown in Figure 4-1. Immediate reactions to penicillin range from local reactions, such as urticaria and pruritus, to fatal systemic anaphylaxis. The type of reaction de-

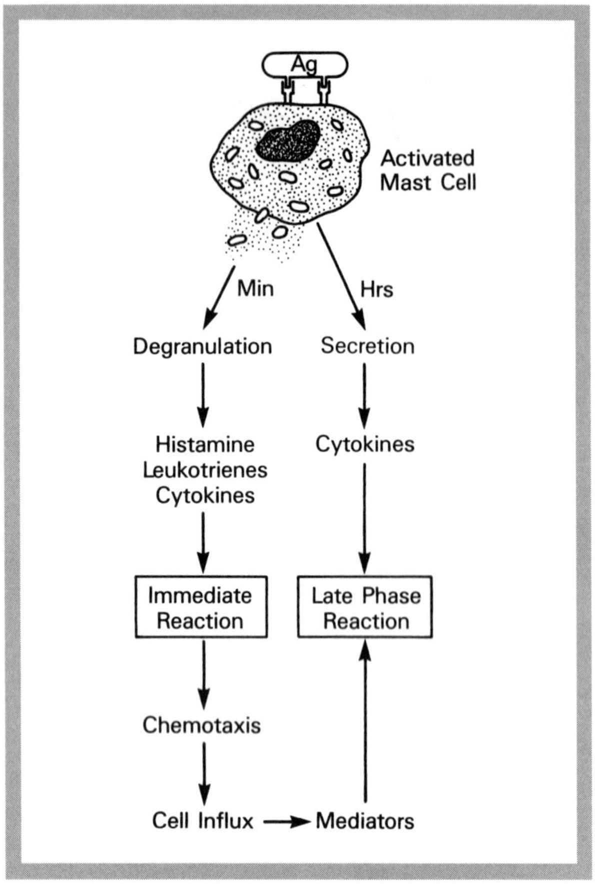

Figure 4-1. Mast cell–dependent immediate and late-phase reactions. Antigen (Ag) bridging two adjacent immunoglobulin E (IgE) molecules on a mast cell causes degranulation, as well as release and synthesis of mediators, resulting in an immediate reaction within minutes of antigen exposure. These mediators attract other inflammatory cells by releasing additional inflammatory cytokines, leading to a late-phase reaction hours after initial antigen exposure.

SOURCE: *Reprinted with permission from Goldstein RA, Paul WE, Metcalfe DD, Busse WW, Reece ER. Asthma.* Ann Intern Med. *1994;121:706.*

pends on the quantity and location of the sensitized mast cells interacting with the allergen.

Mast Cell and Basophil Mediators

Mediators derived from mast cells and basophils are responsible for type I reactions. Human mast cells are found in skin, synovium, and mesentery; around large and small blood vessels; in the mucosa of the respiratory tract; and in the subserosal and submucosal layers of the gastrointestinal tract.[8] Basophils make up 0.5–2% of circulating white blood cells. Both mast cells and basophils have surface receptors with a high affinity for the Fc portion of IgE. When an individual produces IgE, a large percentage of it is bound to the mast cell membrane. There are 100,000–500,000 IgE Fc receptors per mast cell, about 10% of which are occupied with IgE.[8] Basophils have approximately 40,000–100,000 IgE Fc receptors per cell.[9] Both mast cells and basophils contain mediators of inflammation. Antigen must bridge two adjacent antigen-specific IgE molecules for mediators to be released from these cells, as shown in Figure 4-1. After this step, cellular granules are secreted through the outer cell membrane. These granules contain preformed mediators as well as precursors for the generation of other mediators.[10,11] For example, arachidonic acid, which is liberated on activation of mast cells, is used to synthesize prostaglandins and leukotrienes. Table 4-2 lists mediators that are released or rapidly generated after mast cell activation.

Almost 20 years ago, researchers found that lymphocyte-derived cytokines are involved in cell-mediated reactions, but more recently it has been shown that human mast cells are also capable of producing some cytokines. These include interleukins (ILs) 4, 5, and 6, and tumor necrosis factor alpha (TNF-α).[12,13] These cytokines are most likely involved in perpetuating the allergic reaction. For example, IL-4 acts as a co-stimulatory growth factor for mast cells, inducing isotype switching of B cells into IgE-producing cells and promoting T-cell proliferation.[14,15] The production of more mast cells and more IgE-secreting B cells would provide more of the elements needed for type I reactions. IL-4–induced T-cell proliferation can then result in an additional source of inflammatory mediators, as described below in the section on cell-mediated immunity. IL-5 can enhance the allergic response because it is involved in B-cell differentiation and enhances growth and differentiation of eosinophils.

Table 4-2. Human Mast Cell Inflammatory Mediators

PREFORMED MEDIATORS
Histamine
Eosinophil chemotactic factor
Neutrophil chemotactic factor
Kininogenase
Arylsulfatase A
Exoglycosides
NEWLY GENERATED MEDIATORS
Leukotrienes
Prostaglandis
Thromboxanes
Platelet-activating factor
Monohydroxyeicosatetraenoic acids (HETE)
Hydroperoxyeicosatetraenoic acids (HPETE)

Eosinophils secrete numerous inflammatory mediators and are known to be involved in the pathogenesis of many allergic diseases, such as asthma. IL-6 is essential for antibody and IgE production. TNF-α may function as a costimulatory factor for activating T cells involved in the allergic reaction, producing inflammation. TNF-α is also a cofactor for stimulating B-cell antibody production. Together these cytokines perpetuate the allergic reaction by recruiting and activating inflammatory cells, leading to a late-phase reaction, as shown in Figure 4-1. If allergen exposure is continued, then chronic inflammation may occur.

Early events occurring after mast cell mediator release include increased vascular permeability, contraction of smooth muscle, and mucus secretion in the tissues in which mediator release occurred. Increased vascular permeability allows the leakage of intravascular fluid, causing edema, and serum proteins, such as antibodies and complement. Mast cell mediators also promote chemotaxis through the release of chemotactic mediators, which attract a variety of inflammatory cells. These cells may continue the inflammatory process hours after the initial release of mast cell constituents. Mast cell mediators involved in the pathogenesis of asthma have been well characterized.[17] Their roles in this disease are shown in Table 4-3. Some of the more important mediators of type I reactions are described in the following paragraphs.

Histamine

The best-known mast cell mediator is histamine. Histamine, stored in the granules of mast cells and basophils, is released by the granules after they have been released from the cells. Histamine is responsible for reactions such as smooth muscle contraction of bronchioles and small blood vessels, increased permeability of capillaries, and increased mucous secretion.

Table 4-3. Roles of Mast Cell Mediators in Asthma

PHYSIOLOGIC RESPONSE	MEDIATORS
Bronchospasm	Histamine Prostaglandins Leukotrienes Bradykinin Platelet-activating factor
Mucus secretion	Histamine Prostaglandins Leukotrienes Monohydroxyeicosatetraenoic acids (HETE)
Mucosal edema	Histamine Prostaglandins Leukotrienes Bradykinin
Airway inflammation	Neutrophil chemotactic factor Eosinophil chemotactic factor Platelet-activating factor Leukotrienes

Eosinophil Chemotactic Factor

Eosinophil chemotactic factor is another preformed mediator. After release from mast cells, this mediator attracts eosinophils to the area of allergic inflammation. Eosinophils are now thought to have a major role in the tissue damage seen in some allergic reactions.[18]

Neutrophil Chemotactic Factor

A high-molecular-weight neutrophil chemotactic factor (HMW-NCF) is released after mast cell activation.[19] This mediator has not been identified in human mast cell granules, and its site of synthesis is not certain. However, HMW-NCF is readily found in the serum of patients undergoing allergic reactions, and its presence in serum parallels that of histamine.[20] This mediator is a potent stimulus for attracting neutrophils (also called polymorphonuclear leukocytes, or PMNs). Although neutrophils contain numerous enzymes that can be destructive to normal host tissue, whether they participate in IgE-mediated allergic inflammation is still a matter of speculation. Neutrophils as well as other leukocytes produce factors capable of causing additional histamine release from the mast cells perpetuating the allergic response.[21]

Leukotrienes

Leukotrienes (LTs) are lipoxygenase metabolites of arachidonic acid that have potent bronchoconstricting and vasodilatory properties.[11,12] In allergic asthma, LTC_4, LTD_4, and LTE_4 have been identified as mediators of disease activity.[17] These mediators induce vasoconstriction, increase vasopermeability, enhance mucous secretion, and modulate the immune response. For example, LTD_4 enhances monocyte IL-1 production and can replace IL-2 as an inducer of interferon gamma (IFN-γ) by T cells.[22] Before leukotrienes were discovered, this mixture of leukotrienes identified in asthma was known as slow-reacting substance of anaphylaxis.

Prostaglandins

Prostaglandins (PGs) are cyclooxygenase metabolites of arachidonic acid generated after mast cell release. PGD_2 is formed from human lung mast cells and is a potent vasodilator.[13,23] The inflammatory cells attracted to the area of allergic inflammation, such as neutrophils and macrophages, produce additional bronchoconstricting and vasodilatory prostaglandins that further exacerbate the inflammatory reaction.

Platelet-Activating Factor

Platelet-activating factor (PAF) is a low-molecular-weight

substance released during certain type I reactions. It is the most potent bronchoconstrictor identified, and its effect on human airways is long-lived.[24] PAF stimulates the accumulation of eosinophils in the area of inflammation. Numerous inflammatory cells produce PAF, including platelets, macrophages, eosinophils, neutrophils, and perhaps mast cells.[10,23]

Prevalence and Incidence

Individuals with a predisposition for IgE-mediated allergic reactions are known as atopics. Approximately 20% of the population is atopic.[25] Some IgE-mediated allergic disorders include hay fever (allergic rhinitis), allergic asthma, urticaria, insect venom allergy, anaphylaxis, food and drug allergies, and atopic dermatitis (eczema). Of these, hay fever is the most common allergic disorder in the United States.

The onset of common allergies is usually in childhood, although an allergy can develop at any age. The prevalence of atopy increases with age during the first two decades of life and then gradually declines.[26] Symptoms depend on the target organ involved in the type I reaction. For example, rhinitis may be a symptom when only the upper respiratory tract is exposed to an allergen. If the allergen gets into the circulation, as with a bee sting, then anaphylaxis may occur. Symptoms may be seasonal (e.g., grass pollen allergy) or perennial (e.g., house dust mite hypersensitivity). Many patients with multiple allergies have perennial symptoms with exacerbations during pollen season. There is a genetic predisposition for developing allergies. If both parents are atopic there is a high probability of passing the trait on to their children.[23] The risk of atopy is much higher in children of atopic mothers than it is in children of atopic fathers.[27]

Diagnosis of Atopy

Allergies may be diagnosed in a variety of ways. None of the tests available supplant a good medical history and physical examination. The symptoms elicited during the medical history may be sufficient to diagnose an allergy. Variations in symptoms with the time of day, season, or environment give important information toward an accurate diagnosis. An occupational allergen may be suspected if an individual has symptoms only in the workplace; an allergy to cat dander may be suspected when symptoms consistently occur after exposure to cats. When a particular allergen cannot be identified by history or skin testing, in vitro testing may be carried out to aid in the diagnosis and treatment strategy.

Skin Testing

The mainstay for immediate hypersensitivity diagnosis is the skin test. Extracts of allergens are placed in the skin, and within minutes a reaction occurs. The reaction is caused by mast cell–bound allergen-specific IgE combining with the test allergen. Mast cells become activated and release histamine and other mediators. These mediators cause local vasodilation and increased capillary permeability, resulting in a wheal-and-flare reaction (hive-like reaction surrounded by redness), usually within 15 minutes. The preferred method of introducing the allergen into the skin is by prick testing.[28] In this procedure, a drop of the allergen extract is placed on the skin, and a needle is inserted through the solution, penetrating the external surface of the skin. Another method is intradermal allergen injection. Prick testing is associated with less discomfort, is less likely to cause systemic reactions, and correlates better with clinical sensitivity than does intradermal testing.[28] Antihistamine drugs decrease or block the development of the wheal-and-flare response; therefore, these drugs must be discontinued before skin testing.

Skin testing is the preferred procedure for most patients because there has been extensive experience with it, it is inexpensive and easy to administer, and the results are immediately available. However, skin testing is not without risk. Because the antigen is being injected, there is a possibility of a systemic anaphylactic reaction; resuscitation equipment and epinephrine should be readily available.

In Vitro Testing

Although in vitro tests for measuring total serum IgE and antigen-specific IgE are often useful in diagnosing allergy, their true place in allergy diagnosis is not well established.[29] For determining total IgE levels, a radioallergosorbent test (RAST) or paper radioimmunosorbent test is commonly used. These are radioimmunoassays that are highly specific and sensitive for detecting serum IgE. Enzyme-linked immunosorbent assay (ELISA) is now being used in some laboratories to measure IgE antibodies. Allergen-specific IgE can be semiquantitatively measured using RAST or ELISA, provided the antigen can be coupled to an insoluble matrix (e.g., plastic ELISA plate, filter paper, or dextran beads).

In vitro testing has some advantages over skin testing. There is no risk to the patient. Numerous in vitro allergen-specific assays can be done with a single venipuncture, whereas with skin testing multiple sites are needed. Antihistamine drugs do not interfere with in vitro tests and do not have to be discontinued before testing. In vitro tests are useful in infants and in patients with skin disorders such as eczema, in whom it may be difficult to find an unaffected area for skin testing.

There are also disadvantages to in vitro testing. The tests are considerably more expensive and less sensitive than skin testing, and they may produce false-negative results.[29] There is a lag in getting the results back from the laboratory. Because only a limited number of in vitro tests are available, commercial laboratories cannot test for all antigens that may be suspected of causing a patient's symptoms. The presence of antigen-specific IgE in serum does not give direct information about its pathogenic role.[29] Whereas a wheal-and-flare reaction from skin testing provides direct evidence of allergen hypersensitivity, a positive in vitro test detects only serum IgE, which may not be synonymous with hypersensitivity.

Treatment

Treatment of immediate hypersensitivity reactions depends on the clinical manifestations. The simplest treatment is avoiding the offending antigen. In the case of pollen allergy, total avoidance may be impractical; however, exposure to other allergens, such as animal danders, can be avoided. When eliminating the offending antigens is impossible, pharmacologic and immunologic therapies are alternatives.

Pharmacologic Therapies

Type I reactions can be blocked at various stages with antihistamines, sympathomimetic agents, and antiallergic agents.

Antihistamines

Antihistamine agents are helpful in treating symptoms of type I reactions. Unfortunately, because histamine is only one mediator involved in the pathogenesis of these reactions, blocking histamine receptors only partially alleviates symptoms. The H_1 histamine receptor is predominantly involved in allergic reactions, and H_1 antagonists are therefore used for these conditions. The second-generation H_1 antagonists, such as astemizole, loratadine, and fexofenadine, do not produce much sedation—a major advantage compared with many older antihistamines (e.g., diphenhydramine).[30] H_2-receptor antagonists, such as cimetidine, have no effect on type I reactions. However, for patients refractory to standard H_1-receptor antihistamines, the addition of an H_2-receptor antihistamine may be beneficial.[31] H_2 receptors are present in cutaneous vasculature, and the combination of H_1-receptor and H_2-receptor antihistamines has been most effective in certain urticarial syndromes.

Some H_1-receptor antagonists may also improve allergic symptoms via mechanisms unrelated to their histamine-blocking effects. The second-generation antihistamines azelastine and cetirizine inhibit the production of leukotrienes.[32] Terfenadine and loratadine can reduce the release of histamine and PGD_2.[30] More work is required to define the mechanisms of action of antihistamines; however, it is likely that many antihistamine drugs have multiple mechanisms of action beyond histamine antagonism.

Sympathomimetic Agents

Sympathetic nervous stimulation is useful to counteract some manifestations of mast cell degranulation. For example, stimulation of β_2-adrenergic receptors leads to bronchodilatation and may reverse some or all of the bronchoconstricting effects from allergen-induced asthma. α_1-Agonists, such as phenylpropanolamine and phenylephrine, constrict mucosal vasculature and are used predominantly as nasal decongestants. For systemic anaphylaxis, epinephrine is the preferred sympathomimetic agent because of its potent α- and β-adrenergic receptor–stimulating effects.

Antiallergy Agents

Antiallergy drugs are classified as noncorticosteroidal anti-inflammatory agents that can modify the acute and chronic tissue responses associated with type I reactions. Cromolyn sodium, the prototype drug in this class, can inhibit mast cell degranulation and prevent the clinical symptoms that follow antigen exposure. Cromolyn sodium also modulates the effector functions of neutrophils and eosinophils,[33] both of which may have active roles in many allergic reactions. Likewise, nedocromil sodium exhibits anti-inflammatory properties by modulating cellular components of inflammation, including eosinophils, neutrophils, macrophages, and mast cells.[34]

Corticosteroids

In many allergic conditions, such as asthma and allergic rhinitis, chronic inflammation is present. Corticosteroids do not relieve the acute allergic symptoms that follow allergen exposure, but they help suppress the inflammatory response seen in late-phase and chronic allergic reactions.

The mechanisms of action of corticosteroids are still unclear. Steroids do not prevent mediator release from mast cells. Among their many actions, they inhibit the actions of leukocytes, decrease edema by reducing vascular leakage, and prevent the influx of inflammatory cells into the area of mast cell degranulation. Corticosteroids can also increase the quantity of β-adrenergic receptors on tissues, enhancing the efficacy of β-agonists.

Corticosteroids can be given systemically or topically. Topical corticosteroids have proven to be effective for diseases such as asthma and hay fever. The use of inhaled and intranasal corticosteroids has circumvented many side effects of systemic administration.

Leukotriene Inhibitors and Antagonists

Because leukotrienes have a major role in type I hypersensitivity reactions, drugs that inhibit their synthesis or block their actions have been synthesized. Many drugs that inhibit the synthesis of leukotrienes by blocking the action of 5-lipoxygenase have been studied in allergic conditions. Clinical trials have shown that leukotriene receptor antagonists or synthesis inhibitors decrease bronchoconstriction in exercise-induced asthma and improve baseline pulmonary function, decrease symptoms, and decrease β-agonist use in moderate to severe asthmatics.[22] These agents have also been demonstrated to have clinical efficacy in allergic rhinitis. LTB_4 and LTD_4 antagonists have received the most study.

Two new agents that block the effects of leukotrienes are currently approved for clinical use. Zileuton, a 5-lipoxygenase inhibitor, is indicated for treatment of chronic asthma. Zafirlukast is a leukotriene receptor antagonist indicated for chronic asthma. Both of these agents have been shown to reduce the need for other medications to control the symptoms of asthma.[35] More data are needed to determine the therapeutic role of leukotriene antagonists and synthesis inhibitors in allergic inflammatory diseases.

Immunotherapy

Immunotherapy, also known as hyposensitization or desensitization, is an effective adjunct therapy for patients with seasonal allergic rhinitis, allergic asthma, or insect venom hypersensitivity.[35,36] Immunotherapy consists of injecting allergens subcutaneously in increasing doses over a prolonged period. Many controlled trials using immunotherapy have been carried out in patients with allergic rhinitis or asthma. Most studies demonstrate clinical improvement in 60–90% of patients.[36] Allergy immunotherapy results in reduction, not complete elimination, of symptoms. The selection of allergens for injection is based on positive skin test results, clinical history, and sometimes RAST when the other methods of diagnosis are inconclusive.

Immunotherapy is used mainly in patients whose symptoms are not adequately controlled by pharmacologic means and avoidance of the offending antigens. Immunotherapy usually begins with weekly injections of low concentrations of appropriate allergens. The dose of allergen administered is increased weekly until a maintenance dose is achieved. Under certain circumstances, rush immunotherapy has been used to achieve maintenance dose within a few days.[37] This form of therapy has been shown to result in a quicker IgG response.[38] Therapy then continues with monthly injections. Duration of treatment varies for each patient. Therapy should be discontinued if symptoms do not improve after two or three years of treatment.[36] The usual recommended length of treatment is three to five years, although some patients may require longer treatment periods.[36] There is always a risk of inducing an anaphylactic reaction with each injection. Because of this potentially severe risk, for a disease such as allergic rhinitis a combination of a second-generation antihistamine plus a topical corticosteroid may be the preferred therapy.[39] Immunotherapy should be used only after appropriate pharmacotherapy fails to improve symptoms satisfactorily.

The mechanisms by which hyposensitization reduces allergic symptoms are not clearly established. Skin test reactivity to the offending antigens decreases after a successful course of immunotherapy. Antigen-specific serum IgE levels diminish with a concomitant rise in antigen-specific serum IgG levels.[40] This IgG is thought to be a "blocking antibody" competing with mast cell–bound IgE for binding to the allergen. Immunotherapy has also been shown to induce suppressor T lymphocytes, which suppress the production of antigen-specific IgE.[41]

CYTOTOXIC REACTIONS

Type II hypersensitivity reactions are antibody-mediated cytotoxic reactions. Both IgG and IgM antibodies are involved in type II reactions. Cytotoxicity occurs when these antibodies are directed against intrinsic cell surface antigens or against antigens that have been absorbed on a cell surface. Some examples of clinically relevant type II reactions are hemolytic anemia from penicillin, thrombocytopenia from quinidine, erythroblastosis fetalis, Graves' disease, hemolytic anemia, idiopathic thrombocytopenia purpura (ITP), myasthenia gravis, and transfusion reactions.

Mechanisms

Several different mechanisms are involved in type II reactions. Antigen bound to IgG or IgM activates the complement cascade. Activation of complement at or near a cell membrane results in cell lysis and cell death (Figure 4-2).[3] Another mechanism of cytotoxicity involves

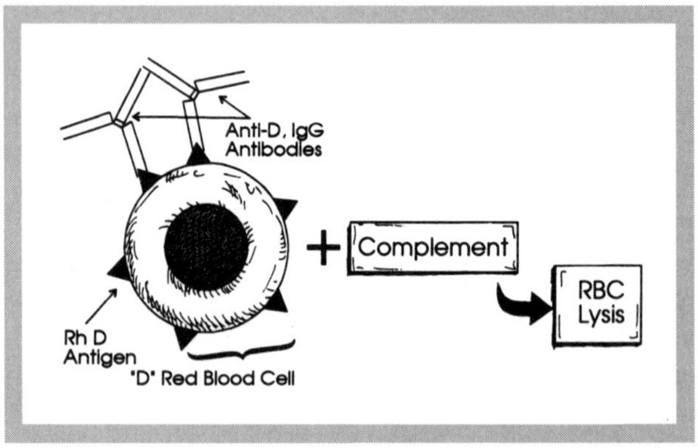

Figure 4-2. Type II hypersensitivity. Erythroblastosis fetalis is an example of a type II reaction in which the Rh antigen on the newborn's red blood cells are bound by maternal IgG antibodies against the Rh antigen. This cell-immune complex then activates the complement cascade, resulting in cell lysis.

SOURCE: *Reprinted with permission from Cruse JM, Lewis RE.* Illustrated Dictionary of Immunology. *Boca Raton, FL: CRC; 1995. p. 18.*

phagocytic cells, such as neutrophils, monocytes, and macrophages. These cells have Fc receptors for IgG. Once antigen-specific IgG has attached to cell surface antigens via its Fab region, the Fc region of IgG becomes available to bind phagocytic cell Fc receptors. The IgG-coated cell is then phagocytized and destroyed. Acute ITP is a good example of this type of mechanism. Approximately 90% of patients with this disorder have IgG anti-platelet antibodies. Phagocytic cells also have receptors for various components of activated complement proteins. After IgG or IgM attaches to cell surface antigens, complement is activated and deposited at the site of this antibody-antigen reaction (see chapter 1). Complement on a cell surface also leads to phagocytosis and destruction of the cell. The process of enhanced phagocytosis by IgG and complement is known as opsonization. IgG is also involved in cytotoxicity mediated by subpopulations of lymphocytes. Some T lymphocytes and natural killer cells have IgG Fc receptors.[3] IgG bound to cell surface antigens can also bind to these lymphoid cells, which lyse the IgG-bound cell. This process is called antibody-dependent cell-mediated cytotoxicity. Some tumor cells are destroyed by this mechanism.[42] (See chapter 9.)

Although type II reactions were originally described by Coombs and Gell as cytotoxic reactions, other noncytolytic antibody-mediated pathologic processes are now classified as type II reactions. For example, in some autoimmune diseases, antibodies directed against various receptors are produced.[43] These antibodies may stimulate a receptor to mimic a natural hormone, as in Graves' disease, or they may block receptor stimulation, as in myasthenia gravis, in which antibodies block acetylcholine from binding to its receptor. Noncytolytic antibodies may also protect a cell with foreign cell surface antigens from being destroyed by normal immunologic cytotoxic mechanisms. Antibodies can mask these foreign antigens, preventing them from being recognized by the immune system.

Drug-Induced Reactions

Many medications can cause type II reactions. The predominant feature is destruction of the formed elements of blood: red blood cells, white blood cells, and platelets. A few examples are listed in Table 4-4. The drug molecule or its metabolites may become antigenic by covalently binding to cell surface proteins, causing cell destruction by the mechanisms described above. The penicillins and cephalosporins are examples of drugs that cause this type of reaction. Other drugs cause type II reactions by forming antigen-antibody complexes in plasma. When these complexes become nonspecifically adsorbed to cell membranes, complement is activated, and cell lysis follows. This mechanism, called the innocent bystander reaction, is usually the reason some drugs cause hemolytic anemia.[44] Other drugs, such as methyldopa, induce autoantibodies against red blood cells. These autoantibodies destroy cells in the absence of the drug. Altered suppressor T-cell function caused by methyldopa has been implicated in the production of these autoantibodies.[45] Drug-induced type II reactions are usually reversible after the implicated drug is discontinued.

Treatment

The treatment for a type II immune reaction depends on the causes of the reaction and the clinical manifestations. If a medication is the cause, stopping the offending agent may be all that is necessary. For a disease such as chronic ITP, in which IgG antiplatelet antibodies lead to the destruction of platelets, treatment may involve corticosteroids or immunosuppressive drugs. These drugs most likely work by decreasing phagocytosis of antibody-coated platelets. Splenectomy is frequently performed, because the spleen is the primary location for platelet destruction by the reticuloendothelial system in this disease. High-dose intravenous immunoglobulin (1–2 g/kg) is also useful in therapy for chronic ITP and sometimes for acute ITP. It is thought that infused gamma globulin blocks the Fc receptors on macrophages, preventing phagocytosis of the IgG-coated platelets.[46] Immunosuppressive therapy is being tested for many autoimmune diseases characterized by type II mechanisms, such as diabetes mellitus.

Erythroblastosis fetalis (or hemolytic disease of the newborn, HDN) is a clinical example in which therapy is used to prevent type II reactions. During delivery of an Rh-positive (Rh^+) newborn to an Rh-negative (Rh^-)

Table 4-4. Examples of Drugs That Cause Cytotoxic Reactions

THROMBOCYTOPENIA[a]	HEMOLYTIC AMENIA[b]
Cephalothin	Cephalexin
Chloroquine	Chlorpropamide
Chlorpromazine	Ketoconazole
Codeine	Methyldopa
Isoniazid	Penicillin
Penicillin	Mitomycin
Propylthiouracil	Sulindac

Pathogenesis is only speculated for many of these drugs. Definitive data indicating a mechanism for an immunologically mediated drug reaction is often lacking.

[a]*Marcus AJ. Hemorrhagic disorders: abnormalities of platelet and vascular function. In: Wyngaarden JB, Smith LH Jr., editors.* Cecil Textbook of Medicine. *18th ed. Philadelphia, PA: WB Saunders; 1988. p. 1042–60.*

[b]*Spruill WJ, Wade WE. Anemias. In: DiPiro JT, Talbert RL, Hayes PE,* et al. Pharmacotherapy: A Pathophysiologic Approach. *3rd ed. Norwalk, CT: Appleton & Lange; 1997. p. 1857–75.*

mother, Rh^+ erythrocytes can enter the mother's circulation, sensitizing the mother to produce IgG anti-Rh antibodies. These anti-Rh antibodies can cause a hemolytic disease in subsequent Rh^+ newborns (see chapter 3). To prevent such reactions, Rh^- mothers of Rh^+ babies are given Rh_0(D) immune globulin within 72 hours of delivery. This treatment reduces the mother's risk of sensitization and the likelihood of developing IgG anti-Rh antibodies. The usual dose is 300 µg for full-term pregnancies and pregnancies terminated at 13 weeks of gestation or later. For pregnancies terminated before 13 weeks of gestation, a dose of 50 µg is given.

IMMUNE COMPLEX–MEDIATED REACTIONS

Mechanisms

Type III hypersensitivity reactions are immune complex (antigen-antibody complex) mediated. These reactions result when small circulating immune complexes (usually IgG or IgM) are deposited or lodge in the microvasculature or when the immunoglobulin is directed toward a tissue antigen. Immune complexes activate complement, which is chemotactic for neutrophils, as illustrated in Figure 4-3. As neutrophils phagocytize the immune complexes, they release lysosomal enzymes, which are destructive to normal host tissue and cause inflammation. Blood vessels and kidneys are frequent targets for immune complex deposition; the resultant clinical manifestation is vasculitis or glomerulonephritis, respectively. The antigens involved in the immune complexes may be bacterial, such as streptococci, resulting in post-streptococcal glomerulonephritis, or native DNA, as seen in systemic lupus erythematosus. Immune complexes have pathogenic roles in many disease states, such as rheumatoid arthritis, hypersensitivity pneumonitis, and the serum sickness prodrome of hepatitis B infection.[47] Many drug reactions have a type III pathogenesis.

Serum sickness reactions have been a useful model for increasing our understanding of type III hypersensitivity reactions. Before the advent of antibiotics, heterologous antiserum (usually from horses) was used to treat certain infectious diseases, and serum sickness reactions would ensue. Circulating immune complexes form and are deposited systemically in various tissue target sites, such as blood vessels, skin, and joints, causing inflammatory reactions. Signs and symptoms of serum sickness, which usually begin one to two weeks after exposure to the offending antigen, include fever, arthritis, arthralgias, rashes, vasculitis, lymphadenopathy, and splenomegaly. These symptoms are common to many multisystem, immune complex–mediated diseases.

Drugs, acting as haptens, can combine with drug-specific antibodies to form circulating immune complexes and cause serum sickness–like reactions. Penicillins, sulfonamides, cephalosporins, thiouracil, cholecystographic dyes, hydantoins, and streptomycin are common causes of these reactions.[45,48] Symptoms usually begin 7–10 days after therapy begins and may include serum sickness symptoms. Clinical manifestations may occur earlier if the patient has previously been exposed to the causative drug and should abate within a few days after discontinuing the drug.

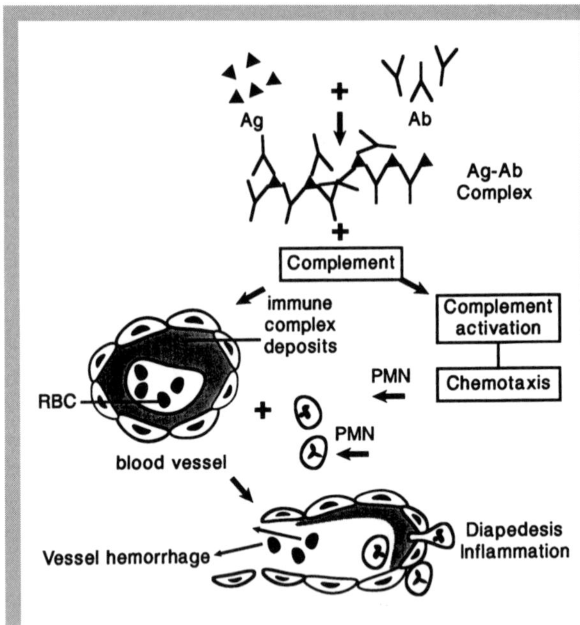

Figure 4-3. Immune complex–mediated reactions. Small antigen-antibody (Ag-Ab) immune complexes become deposited in blood vessels. Complement is activated, resulting in chemotaxis of neutrophils (polymorphonuclear leukocytes, or PMNs). As PMNs phagocytize the immune complexes, they release lysosomal enzymes, injuring the vessel wall, which manifests as vasculitis, hemorrhage, and local ischemia.

SOURCE: *Reprinted with permission from Cruse JM, Lewis RE.* Illustrated Dictionary of Immunology. *Boca Raton, FL: CRC; 1995. p. 27.*

Treatment

Clinical signs and symptoms determine the treatment for type III reactions. Therapy may range from a simple analgesic to treat pain associated with rheumatoid arthritis to potent immunosuppressive therapy for lupus nephritis. In general, drugs that suppress the inflammatory response caused by immune complex deposition are used. These drugs include corticosteroids, nonsteroidal anti-inflammatory agents, and immunosuppressive drugs, such as azathioprine, cyclophosphamide, cyclosporine, gold compounds, and methotrexate. Dosages and dosing schedules for these agents depend on the disease being treated and its severity. For patients with severe exacerbations or unrelenting disease, more than one agent might be used in an effort to decrease clinical manifestations. As symptoms improve, doses may be reduced and/or dosing intervals increased. Drug selection will depend on clinical symptoms and patient responses. Plasmapheresis is occasionally used to remove circulating immune complexes, although most studies have not shown this to be of lasting value.

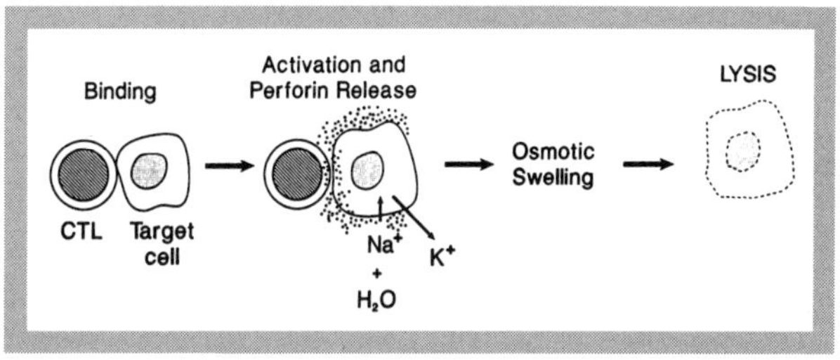

Figure 4-4. Cytotoxic T lymphocytes. Sensitized cytotoxic T lymphocytes (CTLs) recognize antigens on cells that have been infected with viruses or have become neoplastic. Following CTL recognition and binding of the target cell, CTLs generate cytokines, proteases, and perforins, which lead to target cell lysis.

SOURCE: *Reprinted with permission from Cruse JM, Lewis RE.* Illustrated Dictionary of Immunology. *Boca Raton, FL: CRC; 1995. p. 84.*

CELL-MEDIATED REACTIONS

CD4⁺ T lymphocytes are primarily responsible for cell-mediated (type IV) hypersensitivity reactions, also known as delayed hypersensitivity reactions. These reactions generally occur days after antigen exposure and are independent of antibodies and complement. The classic example of this type of reaction is the delayed cutaneous hypersensitivity (DCH) reaction used to identify individuals exposed to *Mycobacterium tuberculosis*. Purified protein derivative is injected intradermally, and a positive reaction (induration) slowly develops, reaching its maximum size 48–72 hours after the injection. In addition to delayed-type skin testing, other clinical examples of type IV reactions include contact dermatitis and organ transplant rejection (see chapter 8). Some antigen-sensitized CD8⁺ T lymphocytes are capable of cytolysis without involvement of immunoglobulin, as illustrated in Figure 4-4. This is another mechanism by which virus-infected and tumor cells can be destroyed.

Mechanisms

CD4⁺ T lymphocytes possess antigen-specific receptors and are activated when antigen is presented to them by macrophages along with appropriate cytokine signaling (see chapter 3). Within hours after appropriate antigen stimulation, T lymphocytes begin producing IL-2 and IL-2 receptors.[49] IL-2 can bind to the same cell that produced it in an autocrine fashion, as shown in Figure 4-5. DNA synthesis and cell mitosis occur once a sufficient number of IL-2 receptors have been bound with IL-2, causing clonal expansion of the activated cell. IL-2 secreted by antigen-activated T cells also activates non-antigen–specific T lymphocytes, which then participate in the type IV reaction. In addition to secreting IL-2, activated

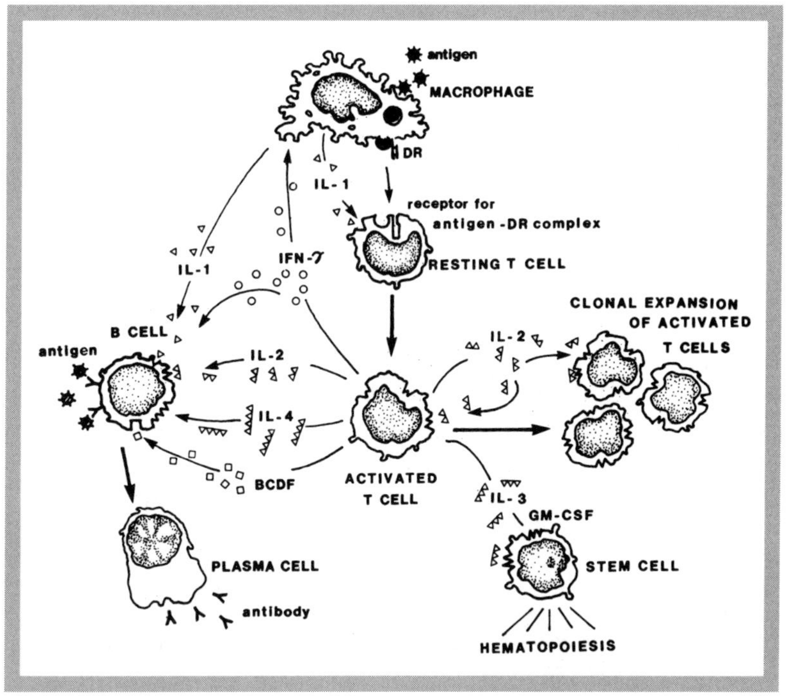

Figure 4-5. Roles of various lymphokines in hypersensitivity reactions. Beginning with the uptake of antigen by the macrophage, processed antigen is presented to the resting CD4⁺ T cell with the histocompatibility molecule (DR) and interleukin 1 (IL-1). The T cell becomes an activated T cell, producing interferon gamma (IFN-γ), IL-2, IL-3, IL-4, and B-cell differentiating factors (BCDF). The antigen also activates B cells through surface antibodies; under the influence of IFN-γ, IL-1, IL-2, IL-4, and BCDF, these cells become antibody-secreting plasma cells. Activated T cells also undergo clonal expansion under the influence of IL-2. IL-3 and granulocyte-macrophage colony-stimulating factor (GM-CSF), produced by activated T cells, induce hematopoiesis by stimulating the marrow stem cells.

SOURCE: *Reprinted with permission from Dinarello CA, Mier JW. Lymphokines.* N Engl J Med. *1987;317:942.*

Table 4-5. Selected Cytokines and Their Effects

CYTOKINE	EFFECTS
IL-1	Activates resting T and B cells; pyrogenic; induces IL-6 synthesis
IL-2	Growth factor for T and B cells; enhances NK cell function
IL-3	Mast cell growth factor; stimulates pluripotent stem cell proliferation
IL-4	Growth factor for activated B cells, resting T cells, and mast cells; induces isotype switching of B cells into IgE-producing cells
IL-5	Promotes B-cell differentiation; induces differentiation of eosinophils
IL-6	B-cell differentiation; essential for antibody production; induces acute phase reactant synthesis
IL-8	Involved in neutrophil chemotaxis
IL-9	T-cell growth factor
IL-10	Induces T-cell and mast cell growth; inhibits production of cytokines by Th1 cells
IL-12	Induces proliferation and cytokine production of B cells, NK cells, and monocytes
IL-13	Enhances IgE production
Colony-stimulating factors	Promotes neutrophil, eosinophil, and macrophage bone marrow colonies
IFN-γ	Antiviral activity; enhances cellular cytotoxicity; activates macrophage; augments IL-1 and TNF-α production
TNF-α	Cytotoxic for some tumor cells; pyrogenic

IL, interleukin; NK, natural killer; Ig, immunoglobulin; Th1, type 1 helper T cell; IFN-γ, interferon gamma; TNF-α, tumor necrosis factor alpha.

T lymphocytes also produce many other lymphokines. Activated T cells also produce IFN-γ, which also regulates cell-mediated cytotoxicity and activates macrophages.[50] Table 4-5 lists some cytokines that are responsible for the cellular infiltration and effector functions seen in type IV reactions as well as many antibody-mediated reactions. (See chapter 2 for additional information.)

In addition to the tuberculin skin test, DCH testing can be used to obtain information about a patient's prior exposure to other infectious agents, such as trichophyton, paramyxovirus (mumps), or coccidiodin. Induration (swelling), not erythema (redness), should be measured. Induration of 5–10 mm in diameter is usually considered a positive reaction. The individual antigens used, along with the concentration, determine the size of the induration considered positive. Multiple ubiquitous antigens are commonly used to evaluate a patient's cellular immunity, especially when an immunodeficiency syndrome is suspected.[51] Although DCH testing is a simple and useful procedure, there are problems associated with it. For example, a negative purified protein derivative test in a patient who might have impaired immunity cannot be properly interpreted without a positive control to indicate the presence of an intact immune system. Control antigens commonly used include *Candida albicans* (500 PNU/ml), tetanus toxoid (10 Lf/ml), and paramyxovirus (mumps) (40 CFU/ml).[52] A dose of 0.1 ml of each antigen is injected intradermally, and induration is measured at 48 hours. Some patients will have a maximum response between 48 and 72 hours after injection. About 95% of healthy adults respond to at least one antigen when using a panel consisting of purified protein derivative of tuberculin (PPD), *C. albicans*, paramyxovirus (mumps), and tetanus toxoid.[52]

The lack of DCH response, known as anergy, indicates a defective cellular immune response. However, anergy can often be misdiagnosed because skin tests are interpreted improperly. False-negative results can occur if too few antigens are used. To avoid this problem, four to six antigens should be used,[15,53] particularly in elderly patients.[54] If only one or two antigens are used, there is a possibility that the negative test results from lack of recent antigen exposure rather than from anergy.[51] Several investigators have shown that almost half of all negative DCH reactions to a variety of antigens convert to positive on repeat testing.[55,56] It is believed that the first test injection serves as a booster that enhances the sensitivity that had waned below the level of detection.[51] Therefore, serial testing may be useful to prevent a false diagnosis of anergy.

Treatment

As with the other types of hypersensitivity reactions, treatment of type IV reactions is dictated by the clinical situation. The goal of therapy is to suppress the activities of inflammatory cells at the pathologic site. Treatment may range from prednisone for contact dermatitis to combination potent immunosuppressive drugs to prevent organ transplant rejection. New therapeutic approaches are being tried as more knowledge is gained about the mechanisms of type IV reactions. Cytokine antagonists and monoclonal antibodies directed against selected cytokines and inflammatory cells are being investigated. (See chapters 5 and 8 for more thorough discussions of immunosuppressive drug therapy.)

SUMMARY

Hypersensitivity reactions can be categorized as type I (anaphylactic), type II (cytotoxic), type III (immune complex–mediated), and type IV (cell-mediated) reactions. The mechanism of type I reactions is an interaction among allergens, IgE, and mast cell and basophil mediators, such as histamine, eosinophil chemotactic factor, neutrophil chemotactic factor, leukotrienes, prostaglandins, and platelet-activating factor. Type I hypersensitivity can be detected with skin or in vitro testing and may be treated with antihistamines, sympathomimetic agents, antiallergy agents, corticosteroids, or immunotherapy. Type II reactions involve IgG and IgM antibodies and may be treated by administering corticosteroids or immunosuppressive drugs and sometimes by a splenectomy. Medications may cause type II reactions. Type III reactions involve circulating immune complexes. Their therapies depend on the clinical situation but generally utilize anti-inflammatory agents. Type IV hypersensitivity is a delayed reaction involving T lymphocytes and may range from contact dermatitis to organ transplant rejection. Causes and therapies vary, as with type III reactions, but continue to stress inflammation suppression.

REFERENCES

1. Roitt IM. *Essential Immunology*. Oxford, UK: Blackwell Scientific; 1994. p. 312–36.
2. Coombs RRA, Gell PGH. The classification of allergic reactions underlying disease. In: Gell PGH, Coombs RRA, editors. *Clinical Aspects of Immunology*. Philadelphia, PA: FA Davis; 1963. p. 317–37.
3. Rodnan GP, Schumacher R, editors. *Primer on the Rheumatic Diseases*. 8th ed. Atlanta, GA: Arthritis Foundation; 1983. p. 25–8.
4. Younger RE, Henry HG, Lieberman PL, *et al*. Characterization of mononuclear cell-derived histamine release enhancing factor. *J Allergy Clin Immunol*. 1987;80:547–57.
5. Frew AJ, Kay AB. Eosinophils and T-lymphocytes in late-phase reactions. *J Allergy Clin Immunol*. 1990;85:533–9.
6. Godfrey HP, Ilardi C, Engber W, *et al*. Quantitation of human synovial mast cells in rheumatoid arthritis and other rheumatic diseases. *Arthritis Rheum*. 1984;27:852–6.
7. DeSwarte RD. Drug allergy—problems and strategies. *J Allergy Clin Immunol*. 1984;74:209–21.
8. Marom Z, Casale TB. Mast cells and their mediators. *Ann Allergy* 1983;50:367–70.
9. Kulczycki A. Role of immunoglobulin E and immunoglobulin receptors in bronchial asthma. *J Allergy Clin Immunol*. 1981;68:5–14.
10. Peters SP, Schleimer RP, Naclerio RM, *et al*. The pathophysiology of human mast cells: in vitro and in vivo function. *Respir Dis*. 1987;135:1196–200.
11. Schleimer RP, MacGlashan DW, Peters SP, *et al*. Inflammatory mediators and mechanisms of release from purified human basophils and mast cells. *J Allergy Clin Immunol*. 1984;74:473–80.
12. Metcalfe DD. Mediators relevant in asthma and allergic diseases. In: Goldstein RA, moderator, Asthma. *Ann Intern Med*. 1994;121:698–708.
13. Abbas AK, Lichtman AH, Pober JS. *Cellular and Molecular Immunology*. Philadelphia, PA: WB Saunders; 1991. p. 283–97.
14. Lipsky PE. The control of antibody production by immunomodulatory molecules. *Arthritis Rheum*. 1989;32: 1345–55.
15. World Health Organization [WHO]. Primary immunodeficiency diseases [report of a WHO scientific group]. *Clin Exp Immunol*. 1995;99(*Suppl* 1):2–24.
16. Gosset P, Malaquin F, Delneste Y, *et al*. Interleukin-6 and interleukin-1α is associated with antigen-induced late nasal response. *J Allergy Clin Immunol*. 1993;92:878–90.
17. Friedman MM, Kaliner MA. Human mast cells and asthma. *Respir Dis*. 1987;135:1157–64.
18. Frigas E, Gliech GJ. The eosinophil and the pathophysiology of asthma. *J Allergy Clin Immunol*. 1986;77:527–37.
19. Lee TH, Nagy L, Nagakura T, *et al*. Identification and partial characterization of an exercise-induced neutrophil chemotactic factor in bronchial asthma. *J Clin Invest*. 1982; 69:889–99.
20. Belcher NG, Murdoch R, Dalton N, *et al*. Circulating concentrations of histamine, neutrophil chemotactic activity, and catecholamines during the refractory period in exercise-induced asthma. *J Allergy Clin Immunol*. 1988;81: 100–10.
21. White MV, Phillips RL, Kaliner MA. Neutrophils and mast cells: nedocromil sodium inhibits the generation of neutrophil-derived histamine-releasing activity (HRA-N). *J Allergy Clin Immunol*. 1991;87:812–20.
22. Henderson WR. The role of leukotrienes in inflammation. *Ann Intern Med*. 1994;121:684–97.
23. Frick OL. Immediate hypersensitivity. In: Stites DP, Stobo JD, Wells JV, editors. *Basic and Clinical Immunology*. 6th ed. Norwalk, CT: Appleton & Lange; 1987. p. 197–227.
24. Barnes PJ, Chung KF, Page CP. Platelet-activating factor as a mediator of allergic disease. *J Allergy Clin Immunol*. 1988;81:919–34.
25. Huang SH, Marsh DG. Immunogenetics of allergic disease. In: Middleton E Jr., Reed CE, Ellis EF, *et al*., editors. *Allergy: Principles and Practice*. St. Louis, MO: Mosby; 1993:60–72.
26. Marsh DG, Meyers DA, Bias WB. The epidemiology and genetics of atopic allergy. *N Engl J Med*. 1981;305: 1551–8.
27. Cookson W. The genetics of atopy. *J Allergy Clin Immunol*. 1994;94:643–4.

28. [Anonymous]. Allergen skin testing [position statement]. *J Allergy Clin Immunol*. 1993;92:636–7.
29. Terr AI. In vitro tests for immediate hypersensitivity. *Annu Rev Med*. 1988;39:135–45.
30. Simons FER, Simons KJ. The pharmacology and use of H_1-receptor-antagonist drugs. *N Engl J Med*. 1994;330: 1663–70.
31. Delafuente JC. Use of H_2 histamine antagonists in allergic disorders. *Clin Pharm*. 1988;7:422.
32. Naclerio RM. The effect of antihistamines on the immediate allergic response: a comparative review. *Otolaryngol Head Neck Surg*. 1993;108:723–30.
33. Kay AB, Walsh GM, Mogbel R, *et al*. Disodium cromoglycate inhibits activation of human inflammatory cells in vitro. *J Allergy Clin Immunol*. 1987;80:1–8.
34. Fink JN, Forman S, Silvers WS, *et al*. A double-blind study of the efficacy of nedocromil sodium in the management of asthma in patients using high doses of bronchodilators. *J Allergy Clin Immunol*. 1994;94:473–81.
35. Patterson R. Clinical efficacy of allergen immunotherapy. *J Allergy Clin Immunol*. 1979;64:155–8.
36. Rocklin RE. Clinical and immunologic aspects of allergen-specific immunotherapy in patients with seasonal allergic rhinitis and/or asthma. *J Allergy Clin Immunol*. 1983;72:323–34.
37. Horst M, Hejjaoui A, Horst V, *et al*. Double-blind, placebo-controlled rush immunotherapy with a standardized Alternaria extract. *J Allergy Clin Immunol*. 1990;85:460–72.
38. Weber RW. Allergen immunotherapy and standardization and stability of allergen extracts. *J Allergy Clin Immunol*. 1989;84:1093–6.
39. Bousquet J, Hejjaoui A, Michel FB. Specific immunotherapy in asthma. *J Allergy Clin Immunol*. 1990;86:292–305.
40. Patterson R. Allergen immunotherapy with modified allergens. *J Allergy Clin Immunol*. 1981;68:85–90.
41. Tamir R, Castracane JM, Rocklin RE. Generation of suppressor cells in atopic patients during immunotherapy that modulate IgE synthesis. *J Allergy Clin Immunol*. 1987;79: 591–8.
42. Greenberg PD. Mechanisms of tumor immunology. In: Stites DP, Terr AI, Parslow TG, editors. *Basic and Clinical Immunology*. 8th ed. Norwalk, CT: Appleton & Lange; 1994. p. 569–77.
43. Wilkin TJ. Receptor autoimmunity in endocrine disorders. *N Engl J Med*. 1990;323:1318–24.
44. Witte KW, West DP. Immunology of adverse drug reactions. *Pharmacotherapy* 1982;2:54–65.
45. Kirtland HH, Mohler DN, Horwitz DA. Methyldopa inhibition of suppressor-lymphocyte function. *N Engl J Med*. 1980;302:825–32.
46. Berkman SA, Lee ML, Gate RP. Clinical uses of intravenous immunoglobulin. *Ann Intern Med*. 1990;112:278–92.
47. Panush RS, Brestel EP, Delafuente JC, *et al*. Diagnostic studies for the rheumatic diseases. In: Panush RS, editor. *Principles of Rheumatic Diseases*. New York: J Wiley; 1981. p. 47.
48. Anderson JA. Allergic reactions to drugs and biological agents. *JAMA* 1992;268:2845–57.
49. Royer HD, Reinherz EL. T lymphocytes: ontogeny, function, and relevance to clinical disorders. *N Engl J Med*. 1987;317:1136–42.
50. Dinarello CA, Mier JW. Lymphokines. *N Engl J Med*. 1987;317:940–5.
51. Delafuente JC, Eisenberg JD, Hoelzer DR, *et al*. Tetanus toxoid as an antigen for delayed cutaneous hypersensitivity. *JAMA* 1983;249:3209–11.
52. Zweiman B, Levinson AI. Cell-mediated immunity in health and disease. In: Middleton E Jr., Reed CE, Ellis EF, *et al*., editors. *Allergy: Principles and Practice*. 4th ed. St. Louis, MO: Mosby; 1993. p. 963–89.
53. Decker EL. Skin testing for anergy: a review with proposed guidelines. *Hosp Formul*. 1980;15:369–74.
54. Delafuente JC, Meuleman JR, Nelson RC. Anergy testing in nursing home residents. *J Am Geriatr Soc*. 1988;36: 733–5.
55. Fereebee SH, Mount FW. Evidence of booster effect in serial tuberculin testing. *Am Rev Respir Dis*. 1963;88: 118–9.
56. Keystone EL, Demerieux P, Gladman D, *et al*. Enhanced delayed hypersensitivity skin test reactivity with serial testing in healthy volunteers. *Clin Exp Immunol*. 1980;40: 202–5.

SELF-ASSESSMENT QUESTIONS

1. Which is the most common atopic disease?
   a. urticaria
   b. eczema
   c. asthma
   d. hay fever

2. How quickly do type I hypersensitivity reactions develop?
   a. within minutes
   b. within hours
   c. within days
   d. within weeks

3. Which type of hypersensitivity reaction is independent of antibodies and complement?
   a. type I
   b. type II
   c. type III
   d. type IV

4. Which of the following is an example of a type IV hypersensitivity reaction?
   a. erythroblastosis fetalis
   b. eczema
   c. contact dermatitis
   d. systemic lupus erythematosus

5. Which of the following is an example of a type I hypersensitivity reaction?

   a. post-streptococcal glomerulonephritis
   b. insect venom allergy
   c. Graves' disease
   d. transfusion reactions

6. Which of the following mediators is responsible for increased permeability of capillaries during an immediate hypersensitivity reaction?

   a. eosinophil chemotactic factor
   b. leukotrienes
   c. histamine
   d. neutrophil chemotactic factor

7. Which of the following is the most potent bronchoconstrictor?

   a. platelet-activating factor
   b. histamine
   c. neutrophils
   d. prostaglandins

8. Which of the following is an advantage of in vitro testing over skin testing? It:

   a. is quicker.
   b. is safer.
   c. is more accurate.
   d. provides direct evidence of allergen hypersensitivity.

9. A radioallergosorbent test is used to detect what type of hypersensitivity?

   a. type I
   b. type II
   c. type III
   d. type IV

10. Which of the following can cause a fatal immunologic reaction within minutes of exposure in a predisposed person?

    a. contact dermatitis
    b. wasp sting
    c. serum sickness
    d. PPD skin test

11. Which of the following immunoglobulin isotypes is responsible for allergic reactions?

    a. IgA
    b. IgM
    c. IgE
    d. IgG

12. Interleukins are involved either directly or indirectly in which of the following hypersensitivity reactions?

    a. type I
    b. type III
    c. type IV
    d. all the above

13. All of the following mediators are involved in the pathogenesis allergic reactions *except:*

    a. histamine.
    b. leukotrienes.
    c. prostaglandins.
    d. epinephrine.

14. The preferred method of skin testing for type I hypersensitivity is which of the following?

    a. pricking the skin
    b. intradermal injection
    c. subcutaneous injection
    d. topical application

15. Which of the following have been identified as possible mechanisms of action for second-generation antihistamine medications?

    a. reducing the release of histamine
    b. reducing the release of prostaglandin D_2
    c. inhibiting leukotriene production
    d. all of the above

16. Cytotoxic reactions, such as hemolytic anemia, are caused by which type of hypersensitivity?

    a. IgE-mediated hypersensitivity
    b. antibody-mediated hypersensitivity
    c. immune complex–mediated hypersensitivity
    d. delayed hypersensitivity

17. For a drug-induced type II hypersensitivity reaction, the best treatment would be which of the following?

    a. Decrease the dose of the offending drug.
    b. Discontinue the offending drug.
    c. Do nothing; it will spontaneously resolve.
    d. Begin high-dose immunosuppressive therapy.

18. Which of the following drugs are often used to treat diseases with a type III hypersensitivity pathogenesis?

    a. nonsteroidal anti-inflammatory drugs
    b. immunosuppressive drugs
    c. steroidal anti-inflammatory drugs
    d. all of the above

19. A new approach to treating type IV hypersensitivity reactions resulting in disease is which of the following?

    a. histamine synthesis inhibitors
    b. low dose immunosuppressive agents
    c. cytokine antagonists
    d. second-generation antihistamines

20. How many skin tests should be used to avoid false-negative results in delayed cutaneous skin testing?

    a. one
    b. two
    c. two to three
    d. four to six

Part II

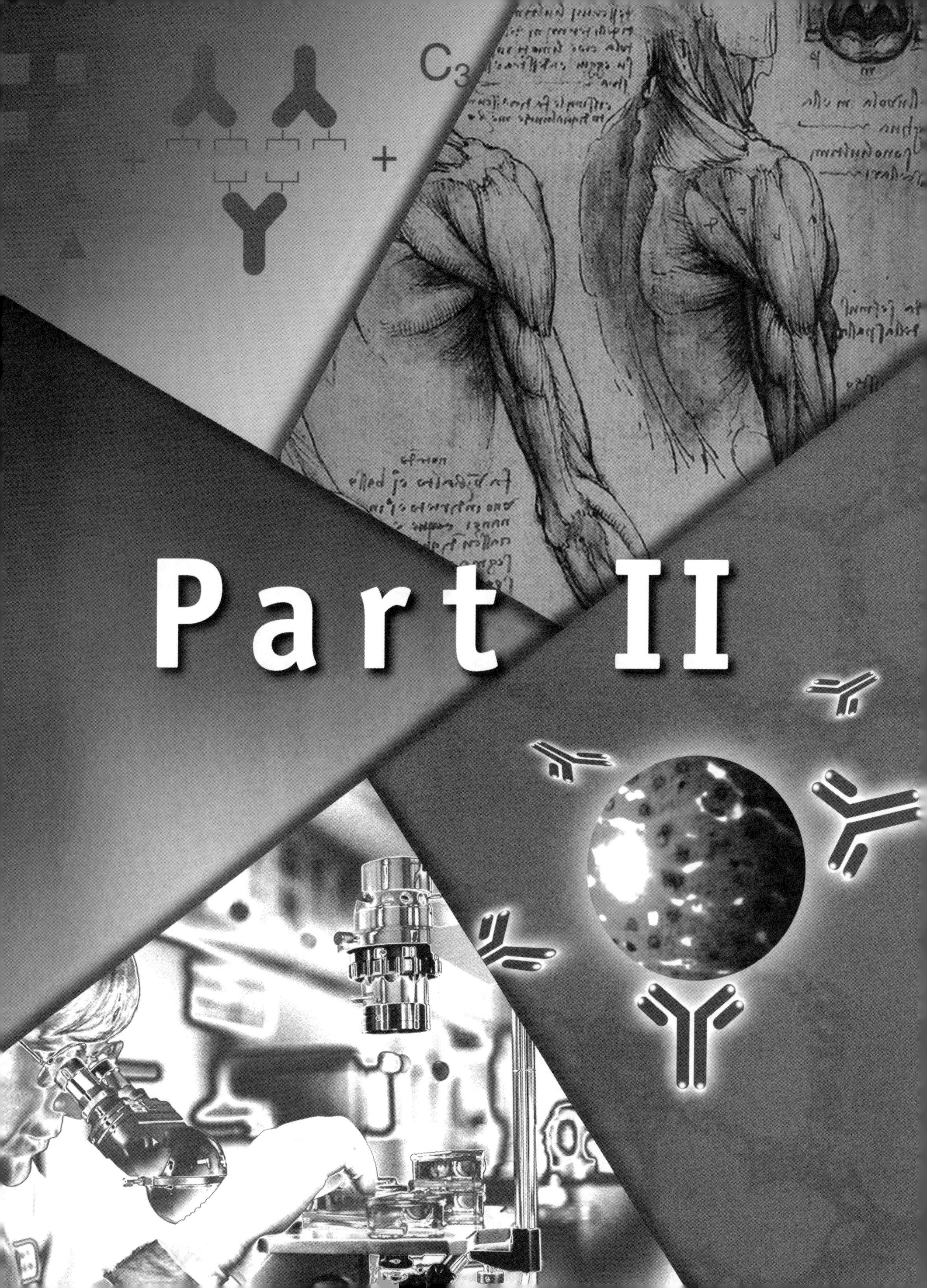

CHAPTER 5

Autoimmune and Immunodeficiency Diseases

Jeffrey C. Delafuente, M.S.
Professor and Associate Chairman
Department of Pharmacy Practice, College of Pharmacy
University of Florida
Gainesville, FL

Autoimmunity 72
Causes 72
Genetic Factors 73
Hormonal Factors 73
Infectious Factors 74
Immune Factors 74
Sequestered Antigens 74
Immunoregulatory T Cells 74
Cross-Reacting Antigens 75
Immunopathologic Mechanisms 75
Treatment of Autoimmune Diseases 75
Primary Immunodeficiency Diseases 76
Antibody Deficiency Diseases 76
X-linked Agammaglobulinemia 76
Common Variable Immunodeficiency 77
Selective IgA Deficiency 77
Therapy for Antibody Deficiencies 78
Combined Immunodeficiency Diseases 78
Cellular Immunodeficiency with Immunoglobulins 78
Severe Combined Immunodeficiency Disease 78
Therapy for Cellular Deficiencies 79
Complement Deficiencies 79
Secondary Immunodeficiency Diseases 79
Infectious Agents 79
Malignancy 79
Malnutrition 79
Aging 80
Drugs 80
Summary 81
References 81
Self-Assessment Questions 83

The immune system is designed to provide a complex response to an antigenic challenge. When it functions as it should, the immune system prevents and fights disease. However, sometimes the immune response does not function properly and mistakes self for nonself tissue. Autoimmune diseases are disorders caused by an immune response directed at self antigens in which the immune system attacks the patient's tissues. Autoimmune diseases are common, and pharmacists need to understand the pathophysiology of these diseases to select appropriate drug therapies. There are many new immunotherapies on the horizon that will make therapeutic interventions more complex.

Immunodeficiency diseases are characterized by abnormally weak immune responses and result in chronic opportunistic infections. Primary immunodeficiencies occur rarely, whereas secondary immunodeficiencies are much more prevalent. Primary immunodeficiencies are due to defects in the development or maturation of one or more of the components of the immune system. Treatment options are often limited. Secondary immunodeficiencies can be caused by medications or diseases that suppress the immune response. Removal of the offending medication or treatment of the underlying medical problem may correct the secondary immunodeficiency.

This chapter presents an introductory description of autoimmunity and its possible causes. A discussion of the immunopathologic mechanisms and treatment of autoimmune diseases follows. Primary immunodeficiency diseases are introduced next, with a discussion of antibody and cellular deficiency diseases and their therapies. The chapter also provides information about risk factors associated with secondary immunodeficiency diseases. After completing this chapter, the reader should be able to:

1. Describe pathogenic mechanisms involved in autoimmunity.
2. Describe principles of pharmacotherapy for autoimmune diseases.
3. Describe treatment modalities for antibody and cellular deficiencies.
4. List physical conditions that can impair the immune function.

AUTOIMMUNITY

Autoimmune diseases are caused by immunopathologic mechanisms that are destructive to host tissue. There are many autoimmune diseases. Some affect a single organ or tissue site, such as multiple sclerosis (MS), which affects the central nervous system. Others have multisystem effects, such as rheumatoid arthritis (RA), which can have extra-articular manifestations involving the heart, lungs, skin, and other sites. Treatment for these diseases depends on clinical manifestations and may range from simple nonsteroidal anti-inflammatory agents to potent immunosuppressive drugs.

Autoimmunity is the process of developing an immune response to self antigens (autoantigens). In the past two decades many investigators have repeatedly shown that the generation of sensitized T lymphocytes and immunoglobulins (antibodies) reactive to autoantigens is a normal process. This type of autoreactivity is necessary for T-lymphocyte receptors to recognize host major histocompatibility complex (MHC) antigens on macrophages and initiate both humoral and cellular immune responses to foreign antigens (see chapter 3). Other cell-cell interactions, such as those between B and T cells, also require recognition of self antigens to produce a proper immune response. Idiotypes are unique antigenic determinants in the variable region of antibodies responsible for antigen binding. Idiotypic and anti-idiotypic antibodies are required for immunoregulation and maintenance of homeostasis. Anti-idiotypes are antibodies reactive to the antigen-binding Fab portion of an immunoglobulin (i.e., antibodies against antibodies). The idiotypic and anti-idiotypic antibody interactions can serve as a negative feedback mechanism to suppress or turn off an immune response; this antibody interaction has also been shown to enhance immune responses. The idiotype–anti-idiotype network is a normal immunoregulatory mechanism. Autoreactive cells sensitized to host MHC antigens (e.g., T cell–macrophage interaction) and anti-idiotypic antibodies are beneficial forms of autoimmunity. Autoimmune diseases occur when there is uncontrolled production of autoantibodies or development of excessive autoreactive T lymphocytes resulting in tissue injury.

There are many autoimmune diseases and a wide spectrum of clinical manifestations. An autoimmune disease may be organ specific, affecting only one tissue or organ site (as in myasthenia gravis) or non–organ specific, causing systemic manifestations (as in systemic lupus erythematosus [SLE]). The autoantigens and pathogenetics involved in these diseases may vary among different disease processes. Table 5-1 lists some autoimmune diseases and associated autoantigens. No attempt is made in this chapter to describe each of these diseases in detail; however, a brief overview of many of these diseases can be found elsewhere.[1] Where applicable, selected diseases are used as examples to discuss research findings.

Causes

The etiology of autoimmune diseases is poorly understood, and no single concept can explain their causes and pathogeneses. Researchers have not yet identified the origin of an autoantibody or autoreactive T cell in an autoimmune disease.[2] Numerous theories have been generated and tested for many decades, and clearly the development of autoimmune diseases involves genetic, hormonal, infec-

Table 5-1. Autoantigens Associated with Diseases[3]

AUTOANTIGEN	AUTOIMMUNE DISEASES
Intracellular	
DNA	SLE, chronic active hepatitis, Sjögren's syndrome
RNA	SLE, Sjögren's syndrome
Nucleolus	SLE, PSS, polymyositis
Membrane receptors	
Thyrotropin	Graves' disease (stimulates), autoimmune thyroiditis (blocks)
Acetylcholine receptor	Myasthenia gravis (blocks)
Insulin receptor	IDDM (blocks)
Cell membranes	
Red blood cells	Autoimmune hemolytic anemia, SLE
Lymphocytes	SLE
Neutrophils	Autoimmune neutropenia, SLE
Platelets	ITP, SLE
Muscle	Polymyositis, RA, SLE
Islet Cells	IDDM
Plasma proteins	
Immunoglobulins	RA, SLE, Sjögren's syndrome
Complement	SLE, RA
Clotting factors	SLE
Hormones	
Insulin	IDDM
Thyroid hormones	Autoimmune thyroiditis
Glucagon	IDDM
Intrinsic factor	Pernicious anemia

SOURCE: *Adapted from Smith HR, Steinberg AD. Autoimmunity—a perspective.* Ann Rev Immunol. *1983;1:175–210.*
SLE, systemic lupus erythematosus; PSS, progressive systemic sclerosis; IDDM, insulin-dependent diabetes mellitus; ITP, idiopathic thrombocytopenia purpura; RA, rheumatoid arthritis.

tious, immunologic, environmental, and other factors acting singly or in combination.[3] Some of the more substantiated theories are discussed in this chapter.

Genetic Factors

Data from inbred strains of animals unequivocally show a genetic predisposition to the development of certain autoimmune diseases. In humans the data are not as convincing. Some families have a greater incidence of autoimmune disease than others, suggesting a genetic component to disease development.[4] In humans, there are correlations between certain autoimmune diseases and specific human leukocyte antigens (HLAs), particularly the *D* gene locus, which is closely linked to immune response genes (see chapter 3). Because genetic background determines how an individual reacts to a foreign antigen, it is possible that genes also determine how an individual reacts to autoantigens and, hence, disease susceptibility.[5] Table 5-2 lists HLAs associated with selected autoimmune diseases. The association of a particular HLA gene and an autoimmune disease does not necessarily mean that the gene is responsible for the disease. Many people have an associated HLA and never develop the disease, and some people with a particular disease may not have the associated HLA. However, possessing an associated HLA gene may predispose an individual to a disease, although perhaps only in combination with other etiologic factors. For example, in insulin-dependent diabetes mellitus (IDDM), with which certain HLAs are associated, there is an approximately 50% discordance rate in identical twins (i.e., one twin has IDDM and the other does not in 50% of twins in which one has IDDM).[6] These data strongly suggest that environmental factors may also have a role in disease susceptibility.[6,7]

Hormonal Factors

Sex hormones may play a role in the development of some autoimmune diseases. Many autoimmune diseases, such as RA, Graves' disease, and SLE, are much more prevalent in females. In animal models of SLE, estrogens have been shown to enhance disease development, whereas androgens inhibit the expression of autoimmunity.[8] Ab-

Table 5-2. Selected Autoimmune Diseases and Associated HLAs

DISEASE	ASSOCIATED HLA
Rheumatoid arthritis	Dw4, DR4
Systemic lupus erythematosus	DR2, DR3
Polymositis	DR3, DRw6
Sjögren's syndrome	DR2, DR3
Insulin-dependent diabetes mellitus	DR3, DR4
Hashimoto's thyroiditis	DR3, DR5
Graves' disease	DR3
Multiple sclerosis	DR2
Ankylosing spondylitis	B27

normal androgen metabolism has also been suggested as a contributing factor in SLE.[9] The exact role of sex hormones in human autoimmune diseases still needs to be determined, as current data are inconclusive.

Infectious Factors

Viral infections have been implicated in certain autoimmune diseases. Viruses may alter normal cell surface antigens, making them immunogenic. MHC antigens are likely targets in virus-infected cells, forming viral complexes that may serve as autoantigens.[4] Viruses may also induce expression of antigens normally repressed in host cells.[4] Infectious causes have been suggested in IDDM, MS, RA, SLE, and other autoimmune diseases.[7,10–12] Viruses implicated as causative agents in human autoimmunity include Epstein-Barr virus (EBV), myxoviruses, hepatitis viruses, cytomegaloviruses, Coxsackie viruses, retroviruses, and others.[12]

EBV has been associated with diseases such as RA. This virus may be important in autoimmunity because it is ubiquitous and persistent and can modulate the immune system.[12] EBV is a polyclonal activator of B lymphocytes, capable of inducing DNA and antibody synthesis, mitosis, and immunoglobulin secretion in B cells.[11] Although evidence suggests that EBV may be involved in the pathogenesis of autoimmune diseases, no direct connection has been proved. People may have EBV infections, such as mononucleosis, and never develop RA or other autoimmune diseases. This suggests that the virus is not the only factor in development of autoimmune disease.

Bacteria may also have a role in autoimmunity. It has been suggested that bacterial infections may activate clones of autoreactive T cells that cross-react with microbial heat shock proteins.[13] Heat shock proteins have been conserved throughout evolution in many prokaryotes and eukaryotes and can activate a subset of T cells. Microbial superantigens, toxins produced by numerous microbial pathogens, have been postulated to induce autoimmunity. They cause an abnormal helper T cell–B cell interaction that directly activates autoantigen-reactive T cells that otherwise would be inactive, which in turn activates B cells and induces monocyte cytokine production.[13,14]

Immune Factors

Host immunologic factors have a major role in autoimmune diseases. Many theories have been proposed to explain the role of the immune system in autoimmunity pathogenesis. A few of the more feasible theories are discussed here.

Sequestered Antigens

An immune response to most autoantigens does not occur under normal conditions because of tolerance to those antigens. Tolerance to autoantigens is acquired during embryonic development of the immune system, when autoantigens are in contact with developing immunoregulating mechanisms. However, some autoantigens do not normally come in contact with the immune system; when they do, these sequestered antigens may be seen as foreign. Autoantibodies are found in instances of tissue injury in which sequestered antigens become exposed to circulating T and B lymphocytes. For example, antibodies to sperm are detected after vasectomy. Also, antibodies to proteins of the crystalline lens have been found after eye injury, antibodies to cutaneous tissue may appear after a burn, and antibodies to heart muscle antigens after a myocardial infarction.[2,12] In all of these examples, the antigens eliciting an antibody response do not normally come in contact with immunocompetent cells. The autoantibody response usually subsides after tissue repair, and no sustained autoimmune pathology occurs.

Immunoregulatory T Cells

Many investigations have been conducted into the role of defective suppressor or helper T cells. Although defects in immunoregulation have been demonstrated in human autoimmune diseases, their role in autoimmunity is controversial. It seems likely that uncontrolled helper T-cell activity could result in the excessive generation of autoantibodies. Some animal models have demonstrated that helper T cells are the primary mediators of autoimmunity.[15] Likewise, diminished suppressor T-cell function could also account for disease activity. There is a correlation between suppressor T-cell activity and disease exacerbation in MS, suggesting that immunoregulation contributes to the pathogenesis. During periods of disease activity there are decreases in the number of suppressor T cells and in suppressor function.[10,16] Similar correlations between suppressor T-cell function and active disease have also been identified in SLE and rheumatoid arthritis.[17,18] The loss of suppressor cell function in SLE may be due to an immunoglobulin G (IgG) antisuppressor T-cell antibody.[19]

Cross-Reacting Antigens

Another reason for autoimmunity may be cross-reactivity between exogenous and autologous antigens. Complex foreign antigens may share an epitope (antigenic determinant) with the host tissue, resulting in cross-reactivity. A clinical example is rheumatic fever, a disease occurring after group A streptococcal pharyngitis. Patients with acute rheumatic fever may develop serum antibodies against group A streptococcal antigens that cross-react with antigens on organs affected by rheumatic fever (e.g., myocardium, heart valves, or joint capsules).[20] Animal models have shown that T lymphocytes sensitized to streptococcal antigens are cytotoxic for cardiac cells, lending further evidence that cross-reacting antigens may cause autoimmune disease.[20] More than 90% of individuals with ankylosing spondylitis have the *HLA-B27* gene. In ankylosing spondylitis, homology between amino acid sequences on the HLA-B27 molecule and various bacterial proteins has been identified, suggesting a possible cross-reacting link in this disease process.[21] When a microorganism elicits an immune response that cross-reacts with host constituents, the process is known as molecular mimicry. Although molecular mimicry may have a role in some disease states, such as rheumatic fever, in many other autoimmune diseases the autoantibodies produced do not cross-react with the microorganism or microbial product (e.g., toxin or cell wall) eliciting the autoimmunity.[2]

Immunopathologic Mechanisms

The immunopathologic mechanisms of tissue injury in autoimmune disease are described by Coombs and Gell.[22] Most autoimmune diseases involve IgG or IgM autoantibodies and elicit either type II or type III hypersensitivity reactions (see chapter 4).

Type I hypersensitivity reactions probably do not have a significant role in autoimmunity. However, IgE and mast cells have been implicated in some autoimmune diseases. Mast cells are believed to be involved in the pathogenesis of progressive systemic sclerosis, an autoimmune disease characterized by serum antinuclear antibodies and often seen in association with other autoimmune diseases.[23] Mast cells may also have a role in joint inflammation of RA.[24] IgE rheumatoid factor (IgE anti-IgG) has been isolated from synovial fluid in patients with RA and can cause in vitro mast cell degranulation when binding to IgG.[25]

Cytotoxic autoantibodies mediating type II reactions are commonly found in autoimmune diseases. These reactions are responsible for autoimmune hemolytic anemia, thrombocytopenia, neutropenia, and destruction of other formed elements of the blood. The endocrine system is particularly susceptible to autoimmune phenomena.[26] Autoantibodies to pancreatic beta cells are believed to be responsible for beta cell destruction resulting in IDDM. Autoantibodies can also bind to cell receptors to cause other diseases. For example, Graves' disease is manifested by autoantibodies to thyroid-stimulating hormone (TSH) receptors. These antibodies mimic the actions of TSH, activating the receptors to produce symptoms of hyperthyroidism.[27] In myasthenia gravis, antibodies to nicotinic acetylcholine receptors are produced. Antibodies binding to these receptors block the actions of acetylcholine and result in muscle weakness.[27]

Immune complexes, which are responsible for type III hypersensitivity reactions, are common to many autoimmune diseases. For example, DNA–anti-DNA complexes are frequently found in sera of patients with SLE, and immune complexes containing anti-IgG antibodies are prevalent in RA sera.[28] The multisystem involvement of these diseases reflects deposition of circulating immune complexes into various tissues as well as local production of immune complexes at the site of tissue injury.[29]

Type IV hypersensitivity reactions may account for some pathology in autoimmunity. Animal models have shown that sensitizing T cells to autoantigens results in autoimmune diseases.[30] In Hashimoto's thyroiditis, intradermal injection of thyroglobulin causes a type IV reaction, suggesting a lymphocyte-mediated pathogenesis.[30] Circulating activated T lymphocytes are found in IDDM, Graves' disease, and MS.[31,32] Activated T cells are also present in the lesions of affected target areas, such as the synovium in RA and the pancreas in IDDM. Because autoantibodies are often found in conjunction with sensitized T cells, it is difficult to know which pathologic mechanism predominates in disease activity; however, both are probably important.

Treatment of Autoimmune Diseases

The treatment of autoimmune diseases depends on the disease and clinical manifestations. Therapy may range from simple analgesics in RA to high-dose corticosteroids or cytotoxic drugs for life-threatening manifestations of SLE. Drug therapy will change as the disease improves or deteriorates, or as dictated by adverse drug reactions. In general, anti-inflammatory and immunosuppressive drugs are the cornerstones to pharmacologic management of autoimmune diseases.

Commonly used agents include nonsteroidal anti-inflammatory drugs, corticosteroids, immunosuppressive agents (such as gold compounds and hydroxychloroquine), and cytotoxic drugs (such as cyclophosphamide, azathioprine, chlorambucil, and methotrexate). Immunosuppressive agents such as cyclosporine look promising for many autoimmune diseases. All these drugs interfere with the inflammatory response, some affecting predominantly humoral immunity and some affecting cellular immunity. Immunosuppressive therapy has induced remission in IDDM, SLE, RA, MS, and other autoimmune diseases.[1,33–36] Many of these immunosuppressive and cytotoxic drugs are discussed in chapters 8 and 9.

New therapies that modulate the immune response are being investigated in many autoimmune diseases. Recent findings have implicated various cytokines in the pathogenesis of autoimmune diseases. For example, interleukin 1 (IL-1), interleukin 6 (IL-6), granulocyte-macrophage colony-stimulating factor, and tumor necrosis factor alpha (TNF-α) are present in high concentrations in inflamed joints.[37] It still remains uncertain if elevation in cytokine concentrations seen in selected autoimmune diseases are a cause of the disease or a result of the disease. However, experiments that examine the possible effectiveness of cytokine antagonists as therapeutic agents are ongoing. Natural antagonists of IL-1 and TNF-α have been identified and may have usefulness as therapeutic agents.[38] Some cytokines, such as transforming growth factor beta, suppress acute inflammation and may also some day prove therapeutically useful. Interferons beta-1A (INF-β1A) and beta-1B (INF-β1B) are now being used as a treatment of MS. Patients with MS have a deficiency in interferon production. The use of INF-β1B has made a marked difference in the therapy of this disease and has decreased the attack rate in patients.[39]

Another approach to immune modulation involves the use of monoclonal antibodies directed against cellular components of the immune system as well as inflammatory cytokines. For example, monoclonal antibodies targeted against cells containing CD4, CD7, CD25, CDw52, or CD54 cell surface antigens have been used in experimental settings to treat RA.[40] Also, monoclonal antibodies to IL-6 and TNF-α have been employed.[40] Although some of these investigations have not shown benefit, others have yielded encouraging results, with some patients showing clinical improvement after conventional therapies had failed to achieve therapeutic benefits. Lack of clinical improvement from some monoclonal antibody therapies may be related to a suboptimal dose or dosing interval, or, as in the case of CD4 monoclonal antibody used to treat RA, perhaps the antibody was directed against the wrong epitope on the CD4 molecule.[14,40]

PRIMARY IMMUNODEFICIENCY DISEASES

The causes of immunodeficiency diseases may be either primary (i.e., intrinsic) or secondary (i.e., resulting from an external source). Primary immunodeficiencies are rare and may involve humoral or cellular immunity, or both.

Immunodeficiencies are a diverse group of diseases with varying pathogeneses, causes, and clinical manifestations. More than 20 different forms of primary immunodeficiencies have been recognized since the first human immunodeficiency disease was described in 1952.[41] The World Health Organization has classified primary immunodeficiency diseases into three major categories: predominantly antibody deficiencies, combined immunodeficiency, and other well-defined immunodeficiency syndromes.[42] Table 5-3 describes some of these disorders. The pathogenesis of most of these diseases remains unknown, although the functional and cellular abnormalities of the various immunodeficiencies are well characterized. None of these diseases has been associated with an HLA, although many immunodeficiency diseases are associated with the X chromosome and therefore occur mostly in males.[43]

The exact incidence of the various immunodeficiency diseases is not known. Fortunately, these serious and often fatal diseases are rare. A few of the more common immunodeficiencies are discussed in this chapter, but even these diseases are quite rare.

Antibody Deficiency Diseases

Antibody deficiency diseases may be either congenital or acquired disorders, with deficiencies in all immunoglobulin classes or in just one class or subclass. The inability to form an antibody against a specific antigen or the absence of a subclass of immunoglobulin may be seen in patients with normal total serum immunoglobulin concentrations. Clinical attributes may range from asymptomatic, as in many patients with selective IgA deficiency, to severe recurrent pyogenic bacterial infections, as seen in X-linked agammaglobulinemia.[43]

Common clinical features of antibody deficiencies are recurrent pyogenic infections with encapsulated bacteria, chronic obstructive lung disease from recurrent infections, enteroviral infections, and low or absent antibodies in serum and secretions. B cells may be present in circulation.[43]

X-linked Agammaglobulinemia

This disease is also known as Bruton's disease and congenital, infantile, or sex-linked agammaglobulinemia. The term agammaglobulinemia is a misnomer, because small amounts of serum immunoglobulins are usually detectable. X-linked agammaglobulinemia occurs only in males. The diagnosis is suspected if serum IgA, IgG, and IgM are less than the 95% confidence limits for age- and race-matched controls.[43] A block in the maturation of pre–B cells to B cells appears to be the pathogenetic defect.[44] Normal numbers of pre–B cells are found in bone marrow, but there are few B cells in peripheral circulation.[43] Affected infants usually do well during the first six to nine months of life because maternal antibodies are still present. Recurrent pyogenic infections begin to appear during in-

Tables 5-3. Examples of Primary Immunodeficiencies[42,43]

DISORDER	FUNCTIONAL DEFICIENCIES	PRESUMED PATHOGENESIS	INHERITANCE
X-linked agammaglobulinemia	↓ all Ig isotypes	Defect in pre-B cell to B-cell differentiation	X-linked
IgA deficiency	↓ IgA	Failure of terminal differentiation	AR, unknown
Ig deficiency with ↑ IgM	↑ IgM, ↓ all other isotypes	Isotype switch defect	X-linked, AR, unknown
Transient hypogammaglobulinemia of infancy	↓ IgG, ↓ IgA	Differentiation defect: delayed maturation of helper function	Unknown
Common variable immunodeficiency	↓ various Ig isotypes, ↓ T cells	B cell defect, variable	AR, AD, unknown
Severe combined immudeficeincy	↓ Ig, ↓ B cells, ↓ T cells	Defective T- and B-cell maturation	AR, X-linked
Nezelof's syndrome	↓ T cells	Unknown, may involve thymus	AR, X-linked
Wiskott-Aldrich syndrome	↓ IgM, ↓ T cells	Cell membrane defect affecting stem cell derivatives	X-linked
Ataxia telangiectasia	↓ IgA, ↓ IgE, ↓ IgG, ↑ IgM	Disorder of cell cycle with chromosomal instability	AR
DiGeorge's syndrome	Normal or ↓ T cells, normal or ↓ Ig	Abnormal thymus development	Unknown

AD, autosomal dominant; AR, autosomal recessive; ↓, decreased; ↑, increased.

fancy and early childhood as maternal antibody levels decrease. Common infectious bacteria include *Streptococcus pneumoniae* and *Haemophilus influenzae*.[43,44] Sinusitis, pneumonia, otitis, meningitis, and septicemia are common infections. Chronic viral and fungal infections are not usually a problem, because cellular immunity remains functional.[43] These patients are at risk for developing vaccine-associated poliomyelitis and infections from certain enteric pathogens, such as echoviruses and *Giardia lamblia*.[44] Prognosis is good if immunoglobulin replacement therapy is initiated early.

Common Variable Immunodeficiency

This immunodeficiency can occur at any age in both males and females.[44] Its clinical presentation may be similar to that of X-linked agammaglobulinemia. In common variable immunodeficiency there is a high incidence of gastrointestinal abnormalities, often due to *Giardia lamblia* and gastrointestinal tumors. Recurrent bacterial infections of the sinuses and respiratory tract are common; frequently involved organisms include *H. influenzae*, *Pneumococcus pneumoniae*, *Streptococcus pyogenes*, and *Staphylococcus aureus*.[45] Pernicious anemia is a common feature, and bronchiectasis and lymphoreticular malignancies may also be concomitant diseases.

Normal numbers of circulating B lymphocytes are usually seen in common variable immunodeficiency, although some patients may have decreased B-cell numbers. As implied in the name of the disease, variable pathogenetic mechanisms are responsible for this immunodeficiency. The major defect is in the differentiation of mature B lymphocytes into antibody-secreting plasma cells.[43] Abnormal regulatory T-lymphocyte function may be a factor in some patients, with either an abnormality in helper T cells or overactive suppressor T cells.[44,46,47] Autoantibodies to lymphocytes may also be involved with this disease.[45]

Selective IgA Deficiency

The most common immunodeficiency in humans is selective IgA deficiency; the frequency is approximately 1 in 300 to 1 in 3040 people.[45] Many people are unaware that they have abnormally low serum IgA concentrations because they never develop any symptoms. Infections of the respiratory, gastrointestinal, and genitourinary tracts predominate in symptomatic patients. Encapsulated bacteria are usually responsible for recurrent infections; IgA is thought to prevent bacteria from attaching to mucosal surfaces. There is no evidence for increased susceptibility to viral infections. IgA deficiency may be associated with certain autoimmune diseases, such as RA, SLE, pernicious anemia, and thyroiditis.[48] It is not known why some individuals with this deficiency remain healthy while others become seriously ill.

There is no specific therapy for IgA deficiency other than appropriate treatment for concomitant infections. Replacing serum IgA is not useful, because it is not transported into secretions. Many of these patients have antibodies directed against IgA.[49] These patients should not receive any blood products containing IgA, because fatal anaphylactic reactions can occur. Extensively washing red blood cells to remove IgA prior to a blood transfusion or using plasma from an IgA-deficient donor will decrease the risk of an untoward reaction. Selective IgA deficiency may involve both IgA1 and IgA2. Abnormalities in both subclasses are sometimes accompanied by decreases in IgG2, IgG3, or IgG4. In addition, IgA deficiency may occur with only a single subclass of IgA being markedly decreased or absent.

Therapy for Antibody Deficiencies

The primary goal of therapy for immunoglobulin deficiencies is to control the frequency and severity of acute infections. Prophylactic long-term antibiotics may be needed for selected patients. The mainstay of treatment for most antibody deficiency diseases is replacement therapy with immunoglobulin administered either intramuscularly or intravenously. The intravenous route may be more effective at preventing infections[50] and also allows the large doses that are often needed in immunodeficiency diseases.

Problems associated with intramuscular therapy for primary antibody deficiencies include (1) acute pain at the injection site; (2) continued pain for several days because of prolonged distribution of the bolus from the injection site; (3) dose limitation due to small muscle mass (in infants and children); (4) immunoglobulin degradation by proteolytic enzymes at the injection site prior to absorption; (5) inadequate serum IgG concentrations; and (6) prolonged therapy required (one to two weeks) to reach peak serum concentrations.

Intravenous immunoglobulin (IVIG) has eliminated many of the problems associated with intramuscular administration and is now the preferred route for most patients. There is large interpatient variability in the pharmacokinetics of IVIG but little intrapatient variability. It is therefore necessary to establish a time-dose relationship for each patient. The goals of treatment are to maintain trough IgG concentrations above 500 mg/dl and prevent infections.[42,50] In most patients this can be achieved with doses of 200–400 mg/kg every three to four weeks.[50] Some patients will require as much as 600 mg/kg to maintain appropriate therapeutic immunoglobulin serum concentrations.[51] A description of IVIG products available for clinical use is provided in chapter 6.

Patients with selective IgA deficiency should cautiously receive any immunoglobulin preparation containing IgA because of the risk of a life-threatening allergic reaction. Many of these reactions are due to IgE anti-IgA antibodies. As stated above, some patients with selective IgA deficiency may also be deficient in IgG subclasses and need immunoglobulin replacement. The immunoglobulin preparation that contains the least amount of IgA should be selected for all patients with IgA deficiency. Also, patients with common variable immunodeficiency and undetectable IgA in their serum can develop IgE anti-IgA antibodies and experience an anaphylactic reaction.[52]

Combined Immunodeficiency Diseases

Combined immunodeficiency diseases have both a cellular and a humoral defect. The pathogenesis of combined immunodeficiencies is highly variable among affected individuals. Some patients may exhibit severe loss of both T- and B-cell function, whereas other patients may have only slightly impaired function of either cellular or humoral immunity.

The general clinical features of cellular immunodeficiency diseases are recurrent infections with opportunistic organisms, such as fungi, viruses, and *Pneumocystis carinii;* lack of delayed cutaneous hypersensitivity; high incidence of malignancy; and major developmental defects.

Cellular Immunodeficiency with Immunoglobulins

Cellular immunodeficiency with immunoglobulins, also known as Nezelof's syndrome, is characterized by lymphopenia. Patients have normal serum immunoglobulin concentrations, although they often fail to make a specific antibody in response to a foreign antigen. Patients with Nezelof's syndrome often present during infancy with recurrent or chronic infections of the lung, skin, genitourinary tract, and blood and failure to thrive.[43] Patients are anergic and their long-term prognosis is poor; most patients do not live into adulthood.

Severe Combined Immunodeficiency Disease

Severe combined immunodeficiency disease (SCID), which presents as a heterogeneous clinical entity, is the most severe form of immunodeficiency. The most common clinical symptoms are failure to thrive and severe illness in the first few months of life.[53] Persistent oral and perianal candidiasis, intractable diarrhea, and malabsorption are common.[53] Pneumonia from *P. carinii* is often seen.[44]

SCID is inherited as an autosomal recessive or X-linked recessive trait; about 75% of cases occur in males.[44,53] Both cellular and humoral immunity are affected. Patients are anergic and specific antibodies do not form in response to vaccinations.

The pathogenesis of this disease is very heterogeneous. In some patients there is a total absence of B lymphocytes, whereas others have markedly elevated numbers of circulating B cells.[54] Lymphocyte dysfunction is the result of defects in cellular differentiation.[55] In about 40% of SCID patients the immunologic defect is due to an absence of adenosine deaminase (ADA). Large amounts of deoxyadenosine, an ADA substrate, are found in these patients.[56] Deoxyadenosine is converted to a toxic compound in T cells, impairing their function. In addition, increased suppressor T-cell activity or decreased helper T-cell function may have a role in the pathogenesis of SCID.[54]

Therapy for Cellular Deficiencies

The most useful treatment for cellular deficiencies is immunologic reconstitution. Bone marrow transplantation can restore both cellular and humoral abnormalities in SCID.[57,58] If bone marrow transplantation is unsuccessful, death is almost certain in the first year of life. For patients with SCID due to ADA deficiency, an enzyme replacement product, polyethylene glycol-ADA (PEG-ADA), can be used. Most children receiving PEG-ADA have some clinical improvement, although some fail to respond.[59] The first gene transfer therapy tried in humans was done in a child with SCID. Gene transfer therapy using the ADA gene now has been performed experimentally in two SCID patients with ADA deficiency. Blood T-cell counts as well as many cellular and humoral immune responses normalized in these two patients. Blood ADA activity has lasted more than two years following the end of gene therapy, the patients' doses of PEG-ADA have been decreased by more than one-half since the gene transfer experiments began, and the patients have improved immune function.[56]

Complement Deficiencies

The complement system is important in the inflammatory response, in providing a mechanism of immunity to bacterial and viral infections, and in eliminating immune complexes. Deficiencies of most of the complement proteins have been described in humans. These deficiencies are mostly genetically transmitted and usually occur as individual complement component deficiencies. Because the complement system requires sequential activation, missing one component of the system can be very detrimental. Individuals with complement deficiencies are susceptible to infections and immune complex diseases. Unfortunately, there is no effective treatment for these disorders. The complement proteins are quickly catabolized, making replacement therapy impractical.

SECONDARY IMMUNODEFICIENCY DISEASES

The immunodeficiencies discussed previously are primary immunodeficiencies, all presumed to be due to intrinsic defects of the immune system.[42] Secondary immunodeficiencies can be caused by infectious agents, malignancies, malnutrition, aging, drugs, and a variety of disease processes. Both primary and secondary immunodeficiencies may present with similar clinical signs and symptoms. This section deals with some causes of secondary immune deficiencies.

Infectious Agents

An acute viral infection may cause a transient immunodeficiency, with lymphopenia, decreased cellular immunity, and a reversed ratio of helper T cells to suppressor T cells. In congenital rubella infection, cellular immunity may be depressed and hypogammaglobulinemia may be present. Measles infection causes a transient suppression of cellular immunity with normal humoral function.[60] These temporary conditions do not have any lasting detrimental effects. Persistent immunodeficiency can be caused by the human immunodeficiency virus (see chapter 7).

Malignancy

Many malignant neoplastic diseases are associated with secondary immunodeficiencies. In Hodgkin's disease, cellular immunity is suppressed and humoral immunity may also be impaired. Both acute and chronic leukemia may be associated with decreased cellular immunity, and variable immunoglobulin levels are seen in patients with these diseases. In myeloma there is an impairment in antibody responses. In addition to the effects of a malignancy on immune function, therapy for these diseases (such as chemotherapy and radiation therapy) can cause immune dysfunction by killing immunocompetent cells.

Malnutrition

Malnutrition can markedly impair immunologic function. Children with protein-calorie malnutrition show a high incidence of death from infections due to immunodeficiency states.[61] Common communicable diseases, such as mumps, can be fatal in these children. Replenishment with nutrients improves immunologic functions and decreases mortality. The effects of protein-calorie malnutrition on the immune system include thymic atrophy, decreased spleen weight, decreased circulating T cells, increased circulating non-T and non-B cells, impaired lymphokine production, anergy, decreased thymic hormone production, and impaired antibody formation.

Table 5-4. Effects of Single-Nutrient Deficiencies on Immue Function[62,63]

	PRIMARY IMMUNE SYSTEM COMPONENT AFFECTED			
NUTRIENT	T CELLS	B CELLS	MACROPHAGES	NEUTROPHILS
Vitamin A	+	+		
Thiamine		+		+
Vitamin B_6	+	+		
Vitamin B_{12}	+	+		
Riboflavin		+		
Biotin		+		
Pantothenic acid		+		
Folic acid	+	+		
Vitamin C	+		+	+
Vitamin D		+		
Vitamin E	+	+	+	
Niacin		+		
Iron	+	+	+	+
Magnesium		+		
Zinc	+		+	+
Selenium	+			

Single-nutrient deficiencies can also impair immune function.[62,63] This phenomenon has been studied mostly in animals because it is possible to deprive an animal of a single nutrient. Data from animal and human studies on nutrient deficiencies are summarized in Table 5-4.

Aging

Aging is associated with a decline in immune function. This decrease in immune function, referred to as immunosenescence, contributes to the high incidence of autoantibodies and neoplastic and infectious diseases seen in the elderly population.[64] Both cellular and humoral immunity may be affected. It is common to find decreased numbers of circulating T lymphocytes in elderly people. They often are anergic, and in vitro studies demonstrate depressed lymphocyte function. The ability to make specific antibody after an immunization may also be depressed, although enough antibody is usually made to offer some protection. Because immunosenescence abates immunologic responses, it is extremely important that elderly people receive proper immunizations to enhance their immunity to common infectious pathogens. Yearly influenza immunizations are recommended as well as pneumococcal immunization, which should be given only once.[65] Revaccination with pneumococcal vaccine six or more years after the initial vaccination should be considered in the elderly at high risk of pneumococcal disease due to chronic diseases or low antibody titers.[65]

Drugs

Many drugs used clinically can cause a secondary immunodeficiency. This may be a desired effect when a drug is used to suppress an autoimmune pathologic process or prevent organ transplant rejection. In other cases, such as cancer chemotherapy, it is an undesired effect. The effects of corticosteroids and immunosuppressive agents on the immune system can easily be explained on the basis of their pharmacology. Table 5-5 lists the effects of corticosteroids on various immune functions. Immunosuppressive drugs, such as gold compounds, azathioprine, cyclosporine, cyclophosphamide, and penicillamine, impair immune function by blocking the proliferation and activation of immunocompetent cells.[34] Drugs causing granulocytopenia or pancytopenia will also induce a sec-

Table 5-5. Immunologic Effects of Corticosteroids

Lymphocytes
↓ Cellular proliferation
↓ Lymphokine production and/or release
↓ Delayed cutaneous hypersensitivity reactions
Selective depletion from blood (T cells more than B cells)
Neutrophils
Blood neutrophilia
↓ Egress from circulation
↑ Release from bone marrow
↑ Circulating half-life
Blocked migration into inflammatory areas
Monocytes/Macrophages
Depletion from blood
Inhibition of mediator production and/or release
Blocked migration in response to cytokines
Eosinophils
Depletion from blood
Other effects
↓ Specific antibody formation
↓ Synthesis of prostaglandins

↓, decreased; ↑, increased.

ondary immunodeficiency. Phenytoin and penicillamine have been reported to decrease serum IgA concentration in some patients.[66,67] These patients may present with recurrent sinus and pulmonary infections. Apparently, phenytoin can induce suppressor cells, causing hypogammaglobulinemia.[66] This drug-induced effect resolves after the drugs are discontinued.

SUMMARY

Autoantibodies and lymphocytes sensitized to self antigens are necessary for maintaining normal homeostasis. Autoimmune diseases occur when this process becomes excessive and uncontrolled. There are numerous autoimmune diseases with a wide spectrum of clinical manifestations. The etiologies for these diseases remain unknown, but there are probably many factors involved, including genetic predisposition, environmental factors, and host immune responses. Tissue damage is mediated through sensitized cells or autoantibodies; both may play a role in some diseases. Generally, the treatment goal is to suppress the disease activity with anti-inflammatory and immunosuppressive drugs.

Clinical manifestations of the primary immunodeficiency diseases range from asymptomatic in some cases of IgA deficiency to chronic, severe infections. In many cases, the immunodeficiency is fatal. Fortunately, primary immunodeficiency diseases are rare. Treatment strategies usually focus on replacing the deficiency by administering immunoglobulin for antibody deficiency diseases or transplanting bone marrow for cellular deficiencies. Secondary immunodeficiencies may be iatrogenically caused by drugs or may result from a variety of disease states, including malignancies, malnutrition, viral infections, and some autoimmune diseases. Aging is also known to blunt the immune response.

REFERENCES

1. Condemi JJ. The autoimmune diseases. *JAMA* 1992;268:2882–92.
2. Atkinson JP. Some thoughts on autoimmunity. *Arthritis Rheum*. 1995;38:301–5.
3. Smith HR, Steinberg AD. Autoimmunity—a perspective. *Annu Rev Immunol*. 1983;1:175–210.
4. Cruse JM, Lewis RE. Contemporary concepts of autoimmunity. In: Cruse JM, Lewis RE, editors. *Autoimmunity: Basic Concepts; Systemic and Selected Organ-Specific Diseases*. Basel: Karger; 1985. p. 1–31.
5. Schattner A. Lymphokines in autoimmunity—a critical review. *Clin Immunol Immunopathol*. 1994;70:177–89.
6. Eisenbarth GS. Type I diabetes mellitus. A chronic autoimmune disease. *N Engl J Med*. 1986;314:1360–68.
7. Castaño L, Eisenbarth GS. Type-I diabetes: a chronic autoimmune disease of human, mouse, and rat. *Annu Rev Immunol*. 1990;8:647–79.
8. Steinberg AD, Raveche ES, Laskin CA, *et al*. Systemic lupus erythematosus: insights from animal models. *Ann Intern Med*. 1984;100:714–27.
9. Lahita RG, Bradlow HL, Ginzler E, *et al*. Low plasma androgens in women with systemic lupus erythematosus. *Arthritis Rheum*. 1987;30:241–48.
10. McFarlin DE, McFarland HF. Multiple sclerosis, parts 1 and 2. *N Engl J Med*. 1982;307:1183–8, 1246–51.
11. Tosato G, Steinberg AD, Blaese RM. Defective EBV-specific suppressor T-cell function in rheumatoid arthritis. *N Engl J Med*. 1981;305:1238–43.
12. Theofilopoulos AN. Autoimmunity. In: Stites DP, Stobo JD, Wells JV, editors. *Basic and Clinical Immunology*. 6th ed. Norwalk, CT: Appleton & Lange; 1987. p. 128–58.
13. Friedman SM, Posnett DN, Tumang JR, *et al*. A potential role for microbial superantigens in the pathogenesis of systemic autoimmune disease. *Arthritis Rheum*. 1991;34:468–80.
14. Schur PH. Arthritis and autoimmunity. The fifteenth Sigrid Juselius international symposium. *Arthritis Rheum*. 1994;37:1818–25.
15. Kumar V, Kono DH, Urban JL, *et al*. The T-cell receptor repertoire and autoimmune diseases. *Annu Rev Immunol*. 1989;7:657–82.
16. Reinherz EL, Weiner HL, Hauser SL, *et al*. Loss of suppressor T cells in active multiple sclerosis: analysis with monoclonal antibodies. *N Engl J Med*. 1980;303:125–9.
17. Sakane T, Steinberg AD, Green I. Studies of immune functions of patients with systemic lupus erythematosus. V. T cell suppressor function and autologous mixed lymphocyte reaction during active and inactive phase of disease. *Arthritis Rheum*. 1980;23:225–31.

18. Lau C, Budz-Tymkewycz S, Ramsden M, *et al.* Impaired release of a T-cell specific suppressor factor in rheumatoid arthritis. *Clin Exper Immunol.* 1985;61:489–95.
19. Sagawa A, Abdou NI. Suppressor-cell antibody in systemic lupus erythematosus: possible mechanism for suppressor-cell dysfunction. *J Clin Invest.* 1979;63:536–9.
20. Pope RM. Acute rheumatic fever and Jaccoud's arthropathy. In: Schumacher HR Jr., editor. *Primer on the Rheumatic Diseases.* 9th ed. Atlanta, GA: Arthritis Foundation; 1988. p. 156–60.
21. Tsuchiya N, Husby G, Williams RC, *et al.* Autoantibodies to the HLA-B27 sequence cross-react with the hypothetical peptide from the arthritis-associated Shigella plasmid. *J Clin Invest.* 1990;86:1193–203.
22. Coombs RRA, Gell PGH. The classification of allergic reactions underlying disease. In: Gell PGH, Coombs RRA, editors. *Clinical Aspects of Immunology.* Philadelphia, PA: FA Davis; 1963. p. 317–37.
23. Hawkins RA, Claman HN, Clark RAF, *et al.* Increased dermal mast cell populations in progressive systemic sclerosis: a link in chronic fibrosis. *Ann Inter Med.* 1985;102: 182–6.
24. Godfrey HP, Ilardi C, Engber W, *et al.* Quantitation of human synovial mast cells in rheumatoid arthritis and other rheumatic diseases. *Arthritis Rheum.* 1984;27:852–6.
25. Gruber B, Ballan D, Gorevic PD. IgE rheumatoid factors: quantification in synovial fluid and ability to induce synovial mast cell histamine release. *Clin Exper Immunol.* 1988;71:289–94.
26. Wilkin TJ. Receptor autoimmunity in endocrine disorders. *N Engl J Med.* 1990;323:1318–24.
27. Fraser CM, Venter JC. Anti-receptor antibodies in human diseases. *J Allergy Clin Immunol.* 1984;74:661–73.
28. Barnett EV, Knutson DW, Abrass CK, *et al.* Circulating immune complexes: their immunochemistry, detection, and importance. *Ann Intern Med.* 1979;91:430–40.
29. Halla JT, Schrohenloher RE, Volanakis JE. Immune complexes and other laboratory features of pleural effusions: a comparison of rheumatoid arthritis, systemic lupus erythematosus, and other diseases. *Ann Intern Med.* 1980;92:748–52.
30. Barrett JT, editor. *Textbook of Immunology: An Introduction to Immunochemistry and Immunobiology.* 4th ed. St. Louis, MO: CV Mosby; 1983. Autoimmunity. p. 402–31.
31. Jackson RA, Morris MA, Haynes BF, *et al.* Increased circulating Ia-antigen-bearing T cells in type I diabetes mellitus. *N Engl J Med.* 1982;306:785–8.
32. Hafler DA, Fox DA, Manning E, *et al.* In vivo activated T-lymphocytes in peripheral blood and cerebrospinal fluid of patients with multiple sclerosis. *N Engl J Med.* 1985;312:1405–11.
33. Bach JF. Insulin-dependent diabetes mellitus as an autoimmune disease. *Endocr Rev.* 1994;15:516–42.
34. Cash JM, Klippel JH. Second-line drug therapy for rheumatoid arthritis. *New Engl J Med.* 1994;330:1368–75.
35. Ebers GC. Treatment of multiple sclerosis. *Lancet* 1994;343:275–79.
36. Burlingame MB, Delafuente JC. Systemic lupus erythematosus and other collagen vascular diseases. In: DiPiro JT, Talbert RL, Yee GC, *et al.*, editors. *Pharmacotherapy: A Pathophysiologic Approach.* Stamford, CT: Appleton & Lange; 1997. p. 1661–74.
37. Rouveix B, Blin O. Pharmacological basis of immunotherapy in autoimmune diseases. *Clin Neuropharmacol.* 1993;16:104–12.
38. Arend WP, Dayer JM. Cytokines and cytokine inhibitors or antagonists in rheumatoid arthritis. *Arthritis Rheum.* 1990;33:305–15.
39. Goodkin DE. Role of steroids and immunosuppression and effects of interferon beta-1B in multiple sclerosis. *West J Med.* 1994;161:292–8.
40. Delafuente JC, Resman-Targoff BH. Monoclonal antibodies in the treatment of rheumatoid arthritis. *Ann Pharmacotherapy* 1994;28:650–4.
41. Bruton OC. Agammaglobulinemia. *Pediatrics* 1952;9: 722–7.
42. World Health Organization [WHO]. Primary immunodeficiency diseases [report of a WHO scientific group]. *Clin Exp Immunol.* 1995;99(*Suppl* 1):2–24.
43. Buckley RH. Immunodeficiency diseases. JAMA 1992;268:2797–806.
44. Rosen FS, Cooper MD, Wedgwood RJP. The primary immunodeficiencies, parts 1 and 2. *N Engl J Med.* 1984;311: 235–42, 300–10.
45. Huston DP, Kavanaugh AF, Rohane PW, *et al.* Immunoglobulin deficiency syndromes and therapy. *J Allergy Clin Immunol.* 1991;87:1–17.
46. Geha RS, Schneeberger E, Merler E, *et al.* Heterogeneity of "acquired" or common variable agammaglobulinemia. *N Engl J Med.* 1974;291:1–6.
47. Waldmann TA. Disorders of suppressor immunoregulatory cells in the pathogenesis of immunodeficiency and autoimmunity. *Ann Intern Med.* 1978;88:226–38.
48. Ammann AJ, Hong R. Selective IgA deficiency: presentation of 30 cases and a review of the literature. *Medicine* 1971;50:223–36.
49. Koistinen J, Heikkila M, Leikola J. Gammaglobulin treatment and anti-IgA antibodies in IgA-deficient patients. *Br Med J.* 1978;2:923–4.
50. Sneller MC, Strober W, Eisenstein E, *et al.* New insights into common variable immunodeficiency. *Ann Intern Med.* 1993;118:720–30.
51. Rosen FS, Cooper MD, Wedgwood RJP. The primary immunodeficiencies. *N Engl J Med.* 1995;333:431–40.
52. Burks AW, Sampson HA, Buckley RH. Anaphylactic reactions after gamma globulin administration in patients with hypogammaglobulinemia. Detection of IgE antibodies to IgA. *N Engl J Med.* 1986;314:560–4.
53. Gelfand EW, Dosch HM. Diagnosis and classification of severe combined immunodeficiency disease. *Birth Defects* 1983;19(3):65–72.
54. Pahwa SG, Pahwa RN, Good RA. Heterogeneity of B lymphocyte differentiation in severe combined immunodeficiency disease. *J Clin Invest.* 1980;66:543–50.
55. Pahwa RN, Pahwa SG, Good RA. T-lymphocyte differentiation in vitro in severe combined immunodeficiency. *J Clin Invest.* 1979;64:1632–41.
56. Blaese RM, Culver KW, Miller AD, *et al.* T lymphocyte-directed gene therapy for ADA$^-$ SCID: initial trial results after 4 years. *Science* 1995;270:475–80.
57. Reinherz EL, Geha R, Rappeport JM, *et al.* Reconstitution after transplantation with T-lymphocyte-depleted

HLA haplotype-mismatched bone marrow for severe combined immunodeficiency. *Proc Natl Acad Sci USA* 1982; 79:6047–51.

58. Reisner Y, Kapoor N, Kirkpatrick D, *et al.* Transplantation for severe combined immunodeficiency with HLA-A, B, C, D, DR incompatible parental marrow cells fractionated by soybean agglutinin and sheep red blood cells. *Blood* 1983;61:341–8.
59. Blaese RM. Development of gene therapy for immunodeficiency: adenosine deaminase deficiency. *Pediatr Res.* 1993;33(*Suppl*):S49–S53.
60. Ammann AJ. Immunodeficiency diseases. In: Stites DP, Stobo JD, Wells JV, editors. *Basic and Clinical Immunology*. Norwalk, CT: Appleton & Lange; 1987. p. 347–50.
61. Chandra RK. Nutritional regulation of immunity and infection: from epidemiology to phenomenology to clinical practice. *Pediatr Gastroenterol Nutr.* 1986;5:844–52.
62. Delafuente JC. Nutrients and immune responses. *Rheum Dis Clin N Am.* 1991;17:1–10.
63. Beisel WR, Edelman R, Nauss K, *et al.* Single-nutrient effects on immunologic functions. *JAMA* 1981;245:53–8.
64. Delafuente JC. Immunosenescence. In: Delafuente JC, Stewart RB, editors. *Therapeutics in the Elderly*. 2nd ed. Cinncinnati, OH: Harvey Whitney; 1995. p. 389–401.
65. Centers for Disease Control. Update on adult immunizations: recommendations of the immunization advisory committee. MMWR 1991;40(No. RR-12):1–94.
66. Cooper MD, Buckley RH. Developmental immunology and the immunodeficiency diseases. *JAMA* 1982;248: 2658–69.
67. Dosch HM, Jason J, Gelfand EW. Transient antibody deficiency and abnormal T suppressor cells induced by phenytoin. *N Engl J Med.* 1982;306:406–9.

SELF-ASSESSMENT QUESTIONS

1. The antigen to which autoantibodies are directed against in myasthenia gravis is:

   a. thyrotropin.
   b. acetylcholine receptor.
   c. intrinsic factor.
   d. DNA.
   e. RNA.

2. The antigen to which autoantibodies are directed against in pernicious anemia is:

   a. thyrotropin.
   b. acetylcholine receptor.
   c. intrinsic factor.
   d. DNA.
   e. RNA.

3. Which of the following cellular constituents can serve as autoantigens in systemic lupus erythematosus?

   a. neutrophils
   b. red blood cells
   c. lymphocytes
   d. platelets
   e. all of the above

4. The most common gene locus on the HLA gene associated with autoimmune diseases is which of the following?

   a. *HLA-A*
   b. *HLA-B*
   c. *HLA-C*
   d. *HLA-D*

5. Which of the following hormones is associated with enhancing some autoimmune diseases?

   a. progestins
   b. estrogens
   c. testosterone
   d. cortisol
   e. aldosterone

6. All of the following infectious agents have been implicated in autoimmune pathogenesis *except:*

   a. Epstein-Barr virus.
   b. hepatitis virus.
   c. group A streptococci.
   d. *Candida albicans.*
   e. cytomegalovirus.

7. When a microorganism elicits an immune response that cross-reacts with host constituents, the process is known as ______________.

8. Which of the following cytokines have been shown to suppress acute inflammation?

   a. transforming growth factor beta (TGF-β)
   b. interleukin 1 (IL-1)
   c. interleukin 2 (IL-2)
   d. granulocyte-macrophage colony-stimulating factor (GM-CSF)
   e. interleukin 4 (IL-4)

9. Which of the following cytokines is approved for therapy of multiple sclerosis?

   a. granulocyte-macrophage colony-stimulating factor (GM-CSF)
   b. interleukin 2 (IL-2)
   c. transforming growth factor beta (TGF-β)
   d. granulocyte colony-stimulating factor (G-CSF)
   e. interferon beta-1B (INF-β1B)

10. Drugs used to treat severe clinical manifestations of an autoimmune disease include all of the following *except:*

    a. azathioprine.
    b. prednisone.
    c. cisplatin.
    d. methotrexate.
    e. cyclosporine.

11. The most common type of immunodeficiency in humans is ______________.

12. The primary goal of therapy for immunoglobulin deficiencies is ______________.

13. The best route of administration of immunoglobulins for antibody deficiency diseases is ___________.

14. The goal for trough IgG serum concentrations in a patient receiving immunoglobulin replacement therapy in common variable immunodeficiency is ______________.

15. The average dose of immunoglobulin needed for immunoglobulin replacement therapy is ___________.

16. The first gene replacement therapy performed in humans was for which immunodeficiency disease?

17. List three causes of secondary immunodeficiency diseases.

18. Persons 65 years of age or older should receive which vaccine on a yearly basis?

19. Which of the following drugs have been reported to decrease serum IgA concentrations?

    a. penicillin
    b. valproic acid
    c. methotrexate
    d. phenytoin
    e. hydroxychloroquine

20. Corticosteroids act as immunosuppressive agents by which of the following mechanisms?

    a. decreasing lymphocyte proliferation
    b. decreasing neutrophil migration into inflammatory areas
    c. inhibiting inflammatory mediator release
    d. decreasing synthesis of prostaglandins
    e. all of the above

CHAPTER 6

Immunization

Sian E. Bigora, Pharm.D.
Senior Research Scientist
GloboMax LLC
Hanover, MD

Karen I. Plaisance, Pharm.D.
Associate Professor, Department of Pharmacy Practice and Science,
Pharmacokinetics-Biopharmaceutics Laboratory
University of Maryland School of Pharmacy
Baltimore, MD

Active Immunization (Vaccination) 86
Risks and Benefits of Vaccines 87
Allergenicity 87
Resurgence of Disease Without Vaccination: The Measles Vaccine 87
The Influence of Socioeconomic Benefits: The Varicella Vaccine 87
Legislation and Initiatives 89
Traditional Approaches to Vaccine Development 91
Attenuated Live Vaccines 91
Inactivated (Killed) Vaccines 94
HAV Vaccine 95
Conjugate Vaccines: *H. influenzae* 95
Biotechnological Approaches to Vaccine Development 96
Subunit Vaccines 96
Cloned Proteins 96
Synthetic Peptides 98
Attenuated Live Vaccines 99
Carrier Organisms: The Vaccinia Model 99
Approaches to Increasing Immunogenicity 100
Adjuvants 100
Anti-idiotypes 101
Passive Immunization 101
Intramuscular Immune Globulins 102
IMIGs in Toxin-Induced Diseases 102
IMIGs in Prophylaxis of Viral Infections 102
Hepatitis B Immune Globulin 103
Varicella-Zoster Immune Globulin 103
Intravenous Immune Globulins 103

**The contributions made by Kelly Scott to this chapter are gratefully acknowledged.*

IgG Subclasses 104
Subclass Deficiency 105
IgA Deficiency 105
Side Effects 105
Therapeutic Uses 106
Selection Variables 107
Summary 107
References 108
Self-Assessment Questions 111

Centuries ago, it was noted that people exposed to a particular pathogen never developed the disease a second time. This basic observation led scientists to investigate ways of artificially producing immunity against disease. Today, the widespread use of vaccines has led to the global eradication of smallpox, the elimination of polio from the United States, and dramatic reductions in the incidence of other infectious diseases.

Pharmacists can play a major role in the field of immunization. A knowledge of vaccine sources provides information necessary for product selection and storage. In addition, pharmacists can facilitate the selection of patients requiring either prophylaxis or treatment of disease with passive and/or active immunization techniques. Recent outbreaks of vaccine-preventable diseases were primarily the result of failure to vaccinate children at recommended ages. Pharmacists can take an active role in educating practitioners and the public about the need for accurate timing of vaccine administration. Because of the toxicity and potential long-term consequences of certain vaccines, pharmacists must also consider both clinical as well as legal risks and benefits of vaccine use and provide appropriate patient counseling while serving as patient advocates. Passive immunization and therapeutic intervention with intramuscular and intravenous immune globulins continue to be expanding fields in medicine.

This chapter is designed for pharmacists who want to gain a basic understanding of the immunization process. It highlights the results of early investigations into active immunization, followed by a discussion of both biotechnological and traditional approaches to modern vaccine development. Similarities and differences between active and passive immunization will be discussed. Finally, the principles of immunotherapy are presented, with a focus on the use of immune globulins for imparting passive immunity. For additional information, the following resources may be useful:

- Plotkin SA, Mortimer EA, Jr. *Vaccines*. 2nd ed. Philadelphia, PA: WB Saunders; 1994.
- Rabinovich NR, McInnes P, Klein DL, *et al.* Vaccine technologies: view to the future. *Science* 1994;265:1401–4.
- Ratko TA, Burnett DA, Foulke GE, *et al.* Consensus statement: recommendations for the off-label use of intravenously administered immunoglobulin preparations. *JAMA* 1995;273: 1865–70.

On completion of this chapter, the reader should be able to:

1. Describe risk factors associated with active immunization.
2. Discuss the risk-to-benefit relationship for active immunization with the newer vaccines.
3. Describe the development of traditional vaccines.
4. Discuss the biotechnological production methods of modern vaccines.
5. Describe the potential advantages and disadvantages of simultaneous administration of vaccines.
6. Discuss the therapeutic applications of intramuscular immune globulins.
7. Discuss considerations in the use of intravenous immune globulins.

ACTIVE IMMUNIZATION

Specific active immunity may be acquired naturally, through exposure to infectious agents, or it may be induced by means of immunization with inactivated (killed) or attenuated live organisms or toxoids. As described in chapters 1 and 2, the body's first contact with an organism (i.e., an antigen) stimulates immunologic memory so the body may effectively repel any later invasion by the same organism. This process explains why we rarely suffer twice from diseases such as mumps or measles, developing a complete and long-lasting immunity to those infections instead. Active immunization (vaccination) takes advantage of this basic process by exposing the body to a relatively harmless form of the antigen to imprint immunologic memory and stimulate the body's defenses against any subsequent exposure to the antigen.

Risks and Benefits of Vaccines

Although the purpose of vaccination is to establish adequate levels of memory cells and thus provide immunity upon renewed contact with the antigen, the first contact with the antigen during vaccination should not be harmful to the patient. The goal is to modify the pathogenic effect of the organism without losing the antigenicity.

The risk of complication from the vaccine must be balanced against the risk of contracting the disease. For diseases, such as smallpox, that have now been eradicated, the risk of untoward effects from vaccination outweighs the possible benefits. In contrast, the documented benefits of vaccines against other diseases, such as measles, far outweigh the small percentage of postvaccination complications. Factors to consider when assessing risks and benefits of vaccination include the risk of infection, the consequences of natural unmodified illness, the availability of a safe and effective vaccine, and the duration of vaccine effect.

The first written record of active immunization was variolation by a Chinese Buddhist nun around 1000 A.D. Her crude immunization attempts involved obtaining live smallpox organisms (variola) from the scabs of patients with the disease and introducing them into the nostrils of infants or children in an attempt to induce a mild form of the disease.[1] Unfortunately, this proved to be a relatively dangerous technique. However, even in today's era of technological advancement, certain vaccines still carry real, if rare, risks to the recipient. For example, vaccines for measles and rabies have been associated with postvaccination complications such as encephalitis, which has resulted in permanent brain damage.[2] The rate of postvaccination encephalitis with the measles vaccine is approximately one case per million vaccinations. This small incidence rate is approximately one-fifth to one-tenth the rate of encephalitis following natural measles. Since the introduction of the measles vaccine, the rate of postmeasles encephalitis has dropped 10-fold.[2,3] Therefore, the potential benefit from measles vaccination far outweighs the small risk of postvaccination encephalitis. The information documented in historical reports and postmarketing surveillance data provides the basis for making decisions concerning the risk-to-benefit relationship for currently used vaccines.

Allergenicity

Another risk is the potential for the vaccine to elicit an allergic response. This allergenicity usually results from the method of production, such as the use of chicken embryo culture media. When such methods are used in the production of a vaccine, complete purification may not be possible, and trace contaminants (such as egg protein) may persist in the final product. The use of human diploid cell lines as viral hosts, a method developed in the 1980s, has limited the risk of allergenicity.[4]

Resurgence of Disease Without Vaccination: The Measles Vaccine

It is clear that immunization is a vital component of pediatric and adult health care. Unfortunately, immunization is underutilized, even though it is one of the most cost-effective measures available for preserving and protecting health. The incidence rates of vaccine-preventable diseases in the United States has decreased dramatically since the mid-1950s, primarily because of the widespread public acceptance and availability of effective vaccines. However, the perception of a change in the risk-to-benefit relationship between disease and vaccine may lead to a resurgence of vaccine-preventable diseases.

Before the vaccine for measles became available in 1963, approximately 400,000 cases of measles were reported annually.[3] Figure 6-1 illustrates the rapid decline in measles cases following the introduction of the vaccine. Many cases prior to 1989 occurred in students in high schools and on college campuses, possibly reflecting the accumulation of measles-susceptible individuals resulting from either failure to immunize infants or from waning immunity.[5] Between 1989 and 1991, outbreaks occurred predominantly in preschoolers and infants (less than 15 months of age) in inner cities. Childhood measles vaccination of the mothers may have resulted in lower antibody levels than natural disease would have caused; these lower antibody levels may have led to lower maternal-fetal antibody transmission.[6] In areas where cases were occurring among infants, it was recommended that vaccination be given at 12 months of age. By 1993, a record low of 277 reported cases of measles was achieved in the United States.[7] Unfortunately, although the number of cases continues to be low, the disease still has not been eradicated. Three patterns have been observed with recent outbreaks: (1) a shift in age prevalence to the 5- to 19- year-old age group, (2) a rise in isolates that are genotypically similar to viruses from Europe and Japan, and (3) an increase in incidence in groups that do not accept vaccination because of religious or philosophical beliefs.

The Influence of Socioeconomic Benefits: The Varicella Vaccine

In early 1995, the Food and Drug Administration (FDA) approved the live attenuated varicella vaccine for use in individuals over the age of one year who have not had varicella.[8] Varicella-zoster virus (VZV) causes varicella (chickenpox), the primary infection, and zoster (shingles),

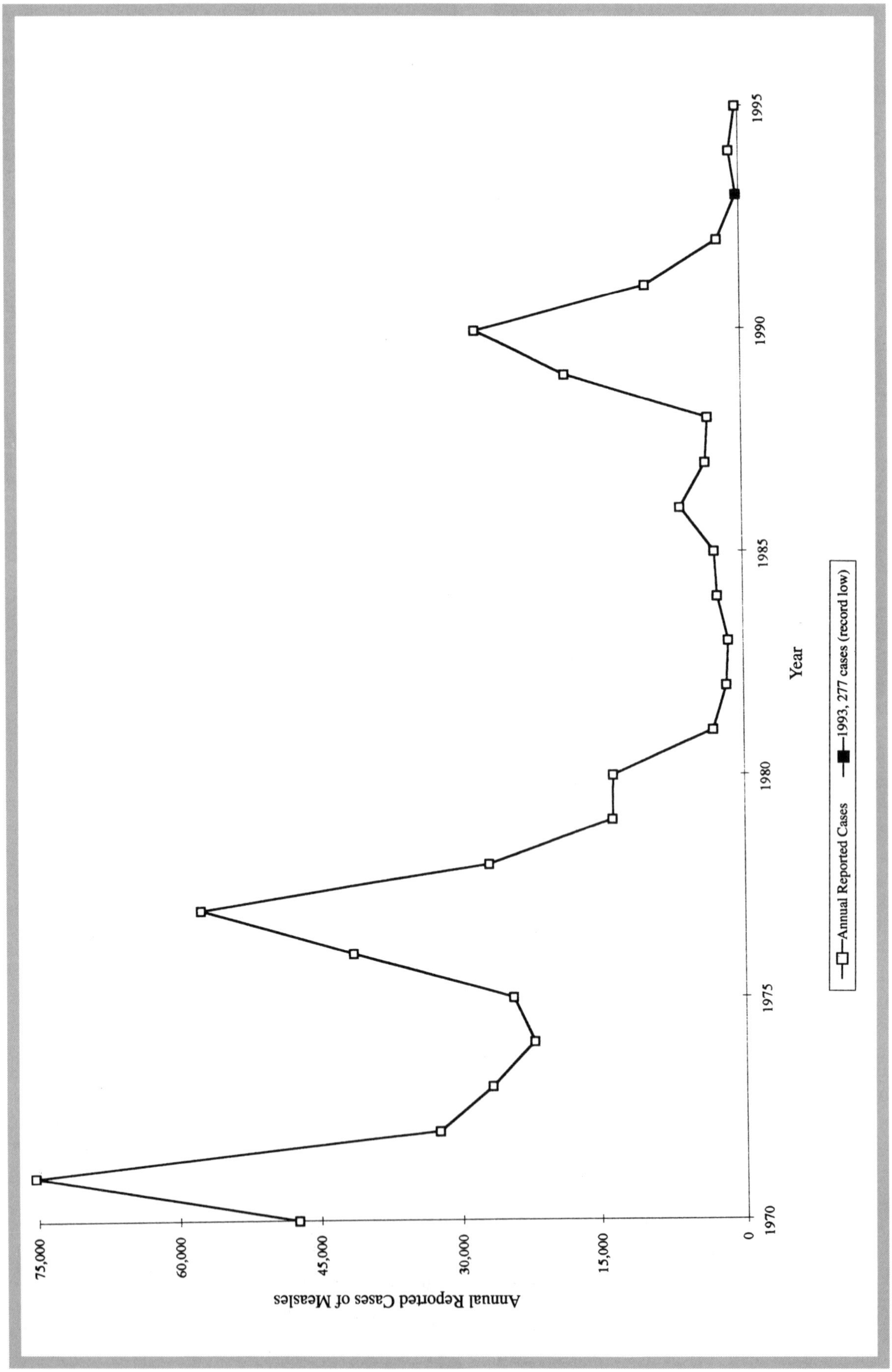

Figure 6-1. CDC-reported cases of measles (January 1970–October 1995)

a secondary infection caused by reactivation of the latent VZV. Varicella is generally a mild, self-limiting, but highly contagious childhood disease that, in most cases, provides lifelong immunity to varicella. During VZV infection, the VZV infects the sensory nerve ganglia. However, only 15% of patients will exhibit reactivation of VZV as zoster. Low VZV-specific cell-mediated immunity is associated with the development of zoster, especially in the elderly, immunocompromised, and infant populations.[8] Approximately 3.9 million cases of varicella occur in the United States each year. Usually these cases are uncomplicated, but infrequently they result in bacterial superinfection, Reye's syndrome, pneumonitis, encephalitis, glomerulonephritis, or arthritis. The mortality rate of varicella is estimated at 1.4 deaths per 100,000 cases in children but rises to 30.9 deaths per 100,000 cases in adults.[9]

Varicella also has a major socioeconomic impact. Because of the contagiousness of the disease, the child generally misses 7–10 days of school, and the parents generally lose several days of work. The estimated annual health care costs for varicella reach $399 million.[10] In 1994, a cost-benefit analysis related to the routine use of varicella vaccine estimated the vaccine would cost $384 million annually.[11] Based on these numbers, the net savings from routine vaccination would be $15 million. The major controversy surrounding the use of this vaccine is not related to its efficacy with regard to childhood varicella but to the issue of long-term protection against both varicella and zoster. It should be noted that the potential costs associated with lack of long-term protection were not included in the cost-savings for the vaccine.

In healthy children, 12 months to 12 years of age, a single dose results in a seroconversion rate of more than 95%.[12] In adults and adolescents, this rate was only 79–82% after one dose of vaccine but increased to 94% after the second dose. Because of the difference between the adult and child seroconversion rates, it is recommended that adults and children who are over 12 years of age receive two doses of the vaccine. Children 12 years of age or younger should receive only one dose.[8] In 95% of vaccine recipients, regardless of age, antibodies have been detected for as long as 10 years after immunization. The rate of chickenpox after vaccination is less than 5%, and vaccine recipients have a milder form of the disease, with fewer vesicles, lower fever, and more rapid recovery.[13,14] No severe or complicated cases of varicella have occurred in vaccine recipients, and their incidence of zoster is reduced.[15,16] In a subgroup analysis of 96 vaccinated children matched with 96 children who had natural varicella infections, there were 4 and 15 cases of zoster among the vaccinated and control groups, respectively.[17] After 13 years of follow-up in over 1500 vaccinated adults, no cases of vaccine-related zoster have been reported.[8]

Although these studies document the efficacy of the vaccine against varicella, it is unclear how this will affect the epidemiology of VZV infection. Will the incidence of zoster in middle age decrease because of a lower latency infection rate associated with the attenuated virus, or will waning immunity place older individuals at risk of VZV infection when the risks associated with varicella are higher?[17] Are the estimated cost-savings associated with routine pediatric vaccination still valid if the epidemiology of VZV infection changes? Are the risks associated with these unknowns worth the socioeconomic benefits? These questions will only be answered with continued surveillance of the varicella vaccine recipients. However, pharmacists should be aware of the benefits and risks associated with the vaccine to be able to advise patients, parents, and other health care providers.

Legislation and Initiatives

Companies that develop and produce vaccines carefully weigh all known risks associated with vaccination to minimize adverse effects on the patient. However, some adverse events occur in such a small percentage of patients that the incidence and severity of the effect may be unknown until mass production and vaccination are under way.

The 1976 nationwide "swine flu" immunization program provides a classic example of this problem.[2] A careful retrospective monitoring program revealed a fivefold increase in the development of Guillain-Barré syndrome after vaccination over its incidence in unvaccinated controls.[18] The rarity of this complication made it impossible to detect prior to widespread administration, illustrating the difficulty of predicting all risks of immunization. This experience also enforces the need for extensive postlicensure and postmarketing surveillance to identify and evaluate such adverse effects.

In an attempt to stabilize immunization programs following the swine flu epidemic and the increasing number of lawsuits being brought against vaccine developers during the early 1980s, the National Childhood Vaccine Injury Act (NCVIA) was enacted in 1986.[19] This act set guidelines to compensate people injured by certain vaccines. NCVIA mandated the reporting of adverse effects associated with vaccines. The Vaccine Adverse Event Reporting System (VAERS), an ongoing nationwide surveillance program, was instituted in accordance with NCVIA.[20] VAERS was established in late 1990 by the Department of Health and Human Services (DHHS) to centralize the collection and analysis of reports of adverse reactions to vaccines. DHHS has designated the Centers for Disease Control (CDC) and the FDA to implement VAERS.[19] Under this system, health care providers and vaccine manufacturers are required by law to report all suspected adverse events following vaccination with diphtheria, measles, mumps, pertussis, polio, rubella, or tetanus vaccines.[20] However, VAERS also includes reports of suspected adverse effects to any vaccine. Figure 6-2 shows a sample VAERS reporting form. Pharmacists should report adverse reactions to vaccines in accordance with their

VAERS

VACCINE ADVERSE EVENT REPORTING SYSTEM
24 Hour Toll Free Information 1-800-822-7967
P.O. Box 1100, Rockville, MD 20849-1100
PATIENT IDENTITY KEPT CONFIDENTIAL

For CDC/FDA Use Only
VAERS Number ______
Date Received ______

Patient Name: ______
Last First M.I.
Address ______
City State Zip
Telephone no. (___) ______

Vaccine administered by (Name): ______
Responsible Physician ______
Facility Name/Address ______
City State Zip
Telephone no. (___) ______

Form completed by (Name): ______
Relation to Patient ☐ Vaccine Provider ☐ Patient/Parent ☐ Manufacturer ☐ Other
Address (*if different from patient or provider*) ______
City State Zip
Telephone no. (___) ______

1. State
2. County where administered
3. Date of birth __/__/__ (mm dd yy)
4. Patient age
5. Sex ☐ M ☐ F
6. Date form completed __/__/__ (mm dd yy)

7. Describe adverse events(s) (symptoms, signs, time course) and treatment, if any

8. Check all appropriate:
☐ Patient died (date __/__/__ mm dd yy)
☐ Life threatening illness
☐ Required emergency room/doctor visit
☐ Required hospitalization (________days)
☐ Resulted in prolongation of hospitalization
☐ Resulted in permanent disability
☐ None of the above

9. Patient recovered ☐ YES ☐ NO ☐ UNKNOWN

10. Date of vaccination __/__/__ (mm dd yy) Time ______ AM PM

11. Adverse event onset __/__/__ (mm dd yy) Time ______ AM PM

12. Relevant diagnostic tests/laboratory data

13. Enter all vaccines given on date listed in no. 10

	Vaccine (type)	Manufacturer	Lot number	Route/Site	No. Previous Doses
a.					
b.					
c.					
d.					

14. Any other vaccinations within 4 weeks prior to the date listed in no. 10

	Vaccine (type)	Manufacturer	Lot number	Route/Site	No. Previous doses	Date given
a.						
b.						

15. Vaccinated at:
☐ Private doctor's office/hospital ☐ Military clinic/hospital
☐ Public health clinic/hospital ☐ Other/unknown

16. Vaccine purchased with:
☐ Private funds ☐ Military funds
☐ Public funds ☐ Other/unknown

17. Other medications

18. Illness at time of vaccination (specify)

19. Pre-existing physician-diagnosed allergies, birth defects, medial conditions(specify)

20. Have you reported this adverse event previously? ☐ No ☐ To health department ☐ To doctor ☐ To manufacturer

Only for children 5 and under
22. Birth weight ______ lb. ______ oz.
23. No. of brother and sisters

21. Adverse event following prior vaccination (check all applicable, specify)

	Adverse Event	Onset Age	Type Vaccine	Dose no. in series
☐ In patient				
☐ In brother or sister				

Only for reports submitted by manufacturer/Immunization project
24. Mfr./imm. proj. report no.
25. Date received by mfr./imm.proj.
26. 15 day report? ☐ Yes ☐ No
27. Report type ☐ Initial ☐ Follow-Up

Health care providers and manufacturers are required by law (42 USC 300aa-25) to report reactions to vaccines listed in the Table of Reportable Events Following Immunization Reports for reactions to other vaccines are voluntary except when required as a condition of immunization grant awards.

Form VAERS-1(FDA)

Figure 6-2. Vaccine Adverse Event Reporting System (VAERS) reporting form

institutional and departmental procedures and VAERS. The major limitation of VAERS is that the reports are essentially noncontrolled case reports, which makes a direct causal relationship difficult to determine. Controlled studies are necessary to evaluate any relationship raised by a VAERS report.

In general, manufacturers of vaccines are held legally and financially accountable for failure to comply with known safety standards in vaccine production methods. However, the threat of legal action based on unpredictable side effects could force private industry to either abandon research and development efforts or dramatically increase the price of vaccines to ensure financial survival.[21] To address this concern, Congress has passed laws to facilitate the settlement of lawsuits brought against vaccine manufacturers and to protect them from financial ruin. In this system, pharmaceutical companies put money into a central fund used to settle lawsuits against companies for adverse vaccine reactions that were not due to substandard manufacturing processes. In this way the incentive to pursue research and production efforts of these lifesaving therapeutic agents has been preserved.[2]

In response to the resurgence of measles cases, the Childhood Immunization Initiative (CII) was implemented in 1993. The goals CII intended to accomplish by 1996 were to: (1) eliminate indigenous cases of diphtheria, *Haemophilus influenzae* infection, measles, polio, rubella, and tetanus; (2) increase vaccination coverage of two-year-old children to 90% or greater; and (3) establish a system that maintains and further improves vaccination coverage levels.[22] This initiative also attempts to increase knowledge of vaccines and reduce vaccination costs to parents or guardians by the initiation of the "Vaccines for Children" program. This program, in effect from October 1994, provides free vaccinations to children who are not covered by health insurance. The most recent update from the national immunization survey addresses routinely recommended vaccination during 1995.[22a] This survey indicates that the 1995 CII interim coverage goals have been achieved or exceeded. During the last quarter of 1995, the 1996 interim national goals were also achieved. During this survey, vaccination levels were higher than ever recorded, and reported cases of diphtheria, tetanus, mumps, measles, rubella, poliomyelitis, and *H. influenzae* were at or near record low levels. Although national goals have been achieved for the individual vaccines, several states and urban areas did not achieve the 1995 interim goals. The completion of series of vaccinations still is more difficult to achieve than the goals for individual vaccines. Proven strategies for increasing vaccine coverage still need to be implemented in these areas.

Pharmacists can assist in meeting the goals of CII by encouraging parents to comply with vaccination recommendations from the CDC. They can also educate other health care workers about different vaccine products and administration schedules. Table 6-1 summarizes the current CDC-recommended immunization schedule for infants.[23] However, it is also the responsibility of pharmacists and physicians to advise the patient or patient's guardian about the risks of immunization, and it is the responsibility of all health care providers to use (i.e., store, dose, and administer) the vaccines in an appropriate manner. Pharmacists should ensure compliance with, and advocate, patient safety measures. In addition to compliance with infant immunization schedules, the pharmacist can act as an advocate for immunization in adults and special populations. The goals of CII that pertain to infants are attainable, but unless universal use of immunizations is implemented, the eradication of vaccine-preventable diseases will not be achievable.

Traditional Approaches to Vaccine Development

Active immunization traditionally uses either attenuated live microorganisms or inactived microbial products. For some diseases, such as poliomyelitis, both approaches have gained acceptance. Vaccines currently recommended for routine use in all age groups in the United States are summarized in Table 6-2.

Generally, live vaccines induce an immunologic response closely resembling natural infection. The organisms in attenuated live vaccines replicate logarithmically in the host until halted by the immunologic response to the vaccine. This multiplication of organisms produces a cumulatively greater antigenic load with live vaccines than with inactive vaccines, though the amount of antigen initially administered with inactived vaccines is generally greater. Vaccines containing attenuated live viruses (e.g., the oral polio vaccine) often generate long-lasting immunity with a single dose or a primary series of doses, and subsequent booster doses are often not required.[24–26]

An inactivated vaccine may contain killed whole organisms (e.g., pertussis), inactivated bacterial toxins (toxoids), or extracts of capsular material (e.g., *H. influenzae* type b) or other components (e.g., hepatitis B surface antigen). In contrast to attenuated live vaccines, inactivated vaccines usually do not provide permanent protection following a single dose; repeated vaccinations are generally necessary to maintain protective levels of antibody and to generate long-lasting immunity. Table 6-3 summarizes the characteristics of attenuated live and inactivated vaccines.[24–26]

The relative merits of inactivated vaccines have been debated. The controversy focuses on their relative immunogenicity, safety, ease of production, distribution, administration, stability, and cost.

Attenuated Live Vaccines

The pathogenicity of an organism must be reduced substantially to produce a safe vaccine, but for the vaccine to

Table 6-1. CDC Recommended Childhood Immunization Schedule[8,18]

<table>
<tr><th>Vaccine</th><th>Birth</th><th>2 months</th><th>4 months</th><th>6 months</th><th>12 months</th><th>15 months</th><th>18 months</th><th>4–6 years</th><th>11–12 years</th><th>14–16 years</th></tr>
<tr><td rowspan="2">Hepatitis B[a]</td><td colspan="2">HBV-1</td><td></td><td></td><td></td><td></td><td></td><td></td><td></td><td></td></tr>
<tr><td></td><td colspan="2">HBV-2</td><td colspan="4">HBV-3</td><td></td><td></td><td></td></tr>
<tr><td>Diphtheria, Tetanus, and Pertussis[b]</td><td></td><td>DTP</td><td>DTP</td><td>DTP</td><td colspan="3">DTP
or DTaP at >15 months</td><td>DTP
or DTaP</td><td colspan="2">Td</td></tr>
<tr><td>Haemophilus influenzae type b[c]</td><td></td><td>Hib</td><td>Hib</td><td>Hib</td><td colspan="2">Hib</td><td></td><td></td><td></td><td></td></tr>
<tr><td>Poliovirus[d]</td><td></td><td>OPV</td><td>OPV</td><td colspan="4">OPV</td><td>OPV</td><td></td><td></td></tr>
<tr><td>Measles, Mumps, and Rubella[e]</td><td></td><td></td><td></td><td></td><td colspan="2">MMR</td><td></td><td colspan="2">MMR</td><td></td></tr>
<tr><td>Varicella[f]</td><td colspan="9">Varivax</td><td>Varivax × 2</td></tr>
</table>

[a]*Infants born to hepatitis B surface antigen (HBsAg)–negative mothers should receive the second dose of hepatitis B virus (HBV) vaccine between 1 and 4 months, provided at least 1 month has elapsed from the first dose. The third dose can be given between 6 and 18 months. Infants born to HBsAg-positive mothers should receive hepatitis B immune globulin (HBIG) and HBV vaccine at different sites within 12 hours of birth. The second and third doses of HBV vaccine should be administered at 1 and 6 months of age, respectively.*

[b]*The fourth dose of diphtheria, tetanus, and pertussis (DTP) vaccine may be given at 12 months (or 6 months after the third dose). Combined DTP–*Haemophilus influenzae *type b (Hib) products can be administered at any of these times. Tetanus toxoid (Td) and diphtheria, tetanus, and acellular pertussis (DTaP) vaccines should only be used in children ≥15 months of age.*

[c]*OPV, oral poliovirus vaccine.*

[d]*Children who have received polyribosylribitol phosphate–meningiococcal protein conjugate (PRP-OMP) at 2 and 4 months of age do not require a dose at 6 months. Any of the licensed Hib products may be administered for the booster dose at 12–15 months of age.*

[e]*The second dose of measles, mumps, and rubella (MMR) vaccine should be administered at either 4–6 years or 11–12 years of age.*

[f]*Varicella vaccine (Varivax) should be given as one subcutaneous injection to children 12 years of age or younger. Adults and children 13 years of age or older should receive two doses 4–8 weeks apart. Dosing recommendation is from the American Academy of Pediatrics (AAP) and the Advisory Committee on Immunization Practice (ACIP) of the Centers for Disease Control (CDC).*

Table 6-2. Recommended Immunizations in the United States

PATIENTS	DTP	Td	MMR	OPV	Hib	Flu	HBV	PnV	OTHER
Infants	X		X	X	X		X		
Adolescents		X	a	b					
Healthy adults									
18–64 years old		X	a	b		c		c	
≥65 years old		X				X		X	
Pregnant women		X	d	b			e		
Health care workers		X	a			X	X		
Day care workers		X	X	X		X			
Veterinarians		X							rabies
Homosexual males		X					X		
Illicit drug users		X					X		
Prisoners		X					X		
HIV-infected patients		X	f			X	X	g	
Immunocompromised patients						g	h	g	
Splenectomized patients		X				X		X	

SOURCE: *Adapted from Guide for Adult Immunization, American College of Physicians, 1994. X signifies recommended immunization; Flu, influenza virus vaccine; PnV, pneumococcal vaccine; HIV, human immunodeficiency virus.*
[a]*All patients born after 1956 must have documentation of immunity to measles (vaccination or titers).*
[b]*Killed polio vaccine (IPV) may be given to nonimmune parents of children scheduled for OPV.*
[c]*Patients with chronic medical conditions as specified by ACIP.*
[d]*MMR is contraindicated in pregnancy.*
[e]*If mother is HBsAG-positive, the infant should receive HBIG and HBV vaccine.*
[f]*Patients <15 years old.*
[g]*Response is unpredictable.*
[h]*Chronic dialysis patients.*

Table 6-3. Characteristics of Vaccines

Characteristics of Vaccines
Attenuated live vaccines
Diminished pathogenicity
Both cell-mediated and humoral immunity
Longer lasting antibody protection
Ability to revert to pathogenic variant
Killed, inactivated vaccines
Nonreplicating and noninfectious
Need for multiple, booster administrations
Primarily humoral response

be effective, the organism must retain sufficient pathogenicity to infect the host. Various approaches to the attenuation of organisms are summarized in Table 6-4. These methods were developed, largely through trial and error, in the 1950s and 1960s with the goal of producing organisms that grow optimally under conditions different from those found in their natural host. Such organisms, though unable to reproduce in numbers adequate to result in disease, cause a subclinical infection sufficient to stimulate both cellular and humoral responses.[26] The general methods for attenuation that this section will focus on include adaptation to a foreign host (either species or tissue) and modification of optimal growth conditions.

The use of cowpox virus (vaccinia) to prevent smallpox (caused by the variola virus) is an example of a relatively nonpathogenic virus used to stimulate immunity to a closely related pathogen. More commonly, however, attenuated live vaccines have been produced by adaptation of virulent viruses to unnatural host cells. An example of this process is the attenuation of the Sabin poliovirus strain through growth in monkey kidney cells. Attenuated live measles, mumps, and rubella vaccines have been produced in a similar manner. The success of attenuation through adaptation depends on the characteristics of the organisms involved, the types of culture media and conditions, and the number of passages through laboratory culture. Although these procedures may be

Table 6-4. Traditional Approaches to the Development of Attenuated Vaccines

METHOD	EXAMPLE
Passage in cell culture (tissue adaptation)	MMR
Species adaptation	Smallpox
Temperature-selected mutants	Influenza

successfully applied to some viruses, problems may prevent application to even closely related viruses (e.g., poliovirus and foot-and-mouth disease virus). Mutations that occur during passage in culture are probably the cause of the problem, but the precise molecular effects of these mutations are not yet understood.[26]

Another classic approach to attenuation involves adaptation by growth at suboptimal temperatures. This approach can also be illustrated with poliovirus. When adapted to growth at 23°C in monkey kidney cell cultures, poliovirus had diminished neurovirulence and was unable to replicate at temperatures of 39–40°C. Procedures for attenuation by growth under suboptimal conditions vary dramatically, depending on the organisms involved.[26]

The infection caused by an ideally attenuated organism should provoke an immune response that mimics the response to the natural infection as closely as possible while producing little or no illness. The live virus should not be teratogenic, abortogenic, or oncogenic, and it should be unable to establish a latent infection. The organism's ability to disseminate throughout a population should be minimal. Finally, the attenuated organism must be genetically stable and incapable of reverting to a pathogenic form.[27]

The genetic stability of attenuated strains is an important concern. Even a minimal level of reversion, such as that producing one case of disease per 100,000 vaccinated subjects, is unacceptable if that case provides a focus of outbreak. The attenuated oral polio vaccine provides an example of genetic reversion.[26] The attenuated oral polio vaccine is usually preferred because of its ability to generate local immunity in the gastrointestinal tract. However, oral polio vaccine was associated with 76% of the 138 cases of paralytic poliomyelitis reported in the United States from 1973 through 1984 (although this incidence rate is decreasing).[27] In 1994, only one case of vaccine-associated poliomyelitis was reported in the United States.[28] The risk of disease associated with the vaccine appears to be much greater with the first dose of oral polio vaccine. In the United States, eradication of poliomyelitis is now approaching a reality, but that is not the case worldwide.[29] On September 29, 1994, the International Commission for the Certification of Poliomyelitis Eradication announced that wild poliovirus transmission has been interrupted in the Americas.[30] Although implementation of polio vaccination programs has dramatically decreased the worldwide incidence rate, polio immunization is still recommended in the United States because of the risk of imported disease.[27]

Inactivated (Killed) Vaccines

Inactivated, or killed, vaccines do not replicate and are generally less efficient in inducing an immune response than attenuated vaccines. Two or three doses of inactivated vaccine must usually be given to stimulate the primary and secondary responses necessary to produce long-lasting immunity. With attenuated live vaccine, the antigenic challenge increases over time. Therefore, a single dose of attenuated live vaccine is often sufficient.

The antigenic mass required for an inactivated vaccine to generate a protective immune response is often many times greater than the antigenic mass required for attenuated live vaccines. The differences in vaccine production procedures, cost, and administration created by this difference in dose size may be considerable. Furthermore, inactivated vaccines prepared from infected cell or tissue cultures may contain large amounts of extraneous material, increasing the possibility of adverse reactions.

Because inactivated vaccines do not replicate within the host, they cannot revert to a pathogenic variant and cause clinical disease. However, outbreaks of polio in 1955 have been attributed to incomplete inactivation of the virus in the vaccine product.[31] Several approaches have been used to produce inactive vaccines. These strategies and examples of vaccines produced through these methods are listed in Table 6-5. The classic approaches to producing inactivated vaccines employ techniques of biochemical purification and biophysical inactivation, such as physical inactivation of whole viruses or bacteria, use of inactivated toxoids produced by bacteria, purification of surface components of viruses or bacteria, and conjugation of purified surface components to other immunogens. Two recent additions to the vaccine armamentarium,

Table 6-5. Traditional Strategies for the Development of Inactivated Vaccines

METHOD	EXAMPLE
Inactivate whole pathogens	Pertussis
Inactivate toxins (toxoids)	Diphtheria, tetanus from pathogens
Purify surface components	Hepatitis B
Conjugate surface components	*Haemophilus influenzae* type b

hepatitis A virus (HAV) and *H. influenzae* type b (Hib) vaccines, illustrate the traditional and conjugate approaches to inactivated vaccine development.

HAV Vaccine

In early 1995, the FDA approved the licensure of a new inactivated HAV vaccine. This vaccine results in a more prolonged period of protection than the three to six months conferred by immune globulin.[32] This new vaccine is purified, inactivated with the use of formaldehyde, and then adsorbed onto aluminum hydroxide. Protective efficacy is estimated to be 94%.[32] The vaccine is currently recommended for individuals at high risk of developing HAV infection, such as travelers to endemic areas, American Indians, and Native Alaskans.

Vaccination of targeted groups may not be sufficient to eradicate this disease. More than 50% of patients with HAV infection will have no identifiable risk. Contact with these individuals may result in transmission of the disease. Universal immunization of infants should eliminate transmission to susceptible individuals.[33]

Conjugate Vaccines: *H. influenzae*

Before Hib vaccines were available, Hib was the leading cause of invasive pediatric bacterial diseases in the United States, accounting annually for an estimated 12,000 cases of meningitis and an additional 8000 cases of other invasive diseases, such as epiglottitis, cellulitis, and primary bacteremia.[34] The majority of Hib disease occurs in children younger than two years old.[34] Since the introduction of Hib conjugate vaccines in 1988, the incidence of invasive disease in infants and children has declined dramatically.[35] From 1987 to 1993, the incidence rate for Hib disease decreased by 95%, from 41 cases per 100,000 in children less than five years old to 2 cases per 100,000. The incidence rate among people more than five years old also declined from 1989 to 1993 by 89% (from 57 to 6 cases per 100,000).[36]

Type b capsular polysaccharide (polyribosylribitol phosphate, or PRP) vaccine, licensed in 1985, became the first vaccine available for the prevention of Hib disease. Because polysaccharide vaccines are generally T-cell independent, children less than 24 months old respond poorly, antibody levels wane rapidly, and repeated doses of PRP vaccine fail to induce booster responses.[37,38] The best responses were seen in children more than 24 months old and adults, but there was considerable variability in immunogenicity. Even in children more than 24 months old, the vaccine was not completely protective. The results of protective efficacy studies reflect the poor immunogenicity of the purified PRP. In case-controlled studies, the protective efficacy of this vaccine ranged from 45 to 88%.[39]

When the poorly immunogenic PRP is combined with a protein carrier, the immunologic response to PRP is enhanced. Conjugate vaccines employ a highly immunogenic protein carrier that is covalently linked to the PRP antigen. The antigenicity of the protein is incorporated in the immune response to the protein-PRP conjugate. PRP has been conjugated to a diphtheria toxoid (PRP-D), a nontoxic mutant diphtheria toxin (HbOC), tetanus toxoid (PRP-T), and the outer membrane protein of *Neisseria meningitidis* (PRP-OMP). These conjugate vaccines have three advantages. First, they produce a T cell–dependent immune response that is quantitatively enhanced, particularly in younger children. Second, repeat administrations of conjugate vaccines elicit booster responses. Third, a greater proportion of anti-PRP antibodies produced through vaccination are of the IgG class. The conjugate vaccines currently available in the United States are listed in Table 6-6. Although these vaccines have the same purpose, there are important differences in immunologic response among them. These differences are reflected by their respective immunization schedules.

Figure 6-3 shows the responses in children 15–24 months old immunized with PRP or PRP-D vaccine. Antibody responses to PRP-D are at least 10 times greater than those to PRP, and they are less dependent on age. Young infants will respond to PRP-D, although multiple doses are required. Furthermore, conjugate vaccines, such as PRP-D, induce booster responses.[40] An evaluation of the clinical efficacy of PRP-D was conducted in Finland. This open trial enrolled 60,000 newborns who were vaccinated at 3, 4, 6, and 14 months of age. After an average follow-up time of 9 months, there were 3 cases of invasive Hib infection among those who had received three doses of PRP-D and 20 cases among the controls, indicating 87% protective efficacy. Only minor adverse effects were reported.[41] However, limited efficacy (35%) with PRP-D

Table 6-6. *Haemophilus influenzae* Conjugate Vaccines Licensed in the United States

VACCINE	CARRIER	AGE ADMINISTERED (MONTHS)
HibTITER®	Mutant diphtheria toxin	2, 4, 6, and 12
ProHIBit®	Diphtheria toxoid	≥12
PedvaxHIB®	Outer membrane protein of *Neisseria meningitidis*	2, 4, and 12
ActHIB®, OmniHIB®	Tetanus toxoid	2, 4, 6, and 12

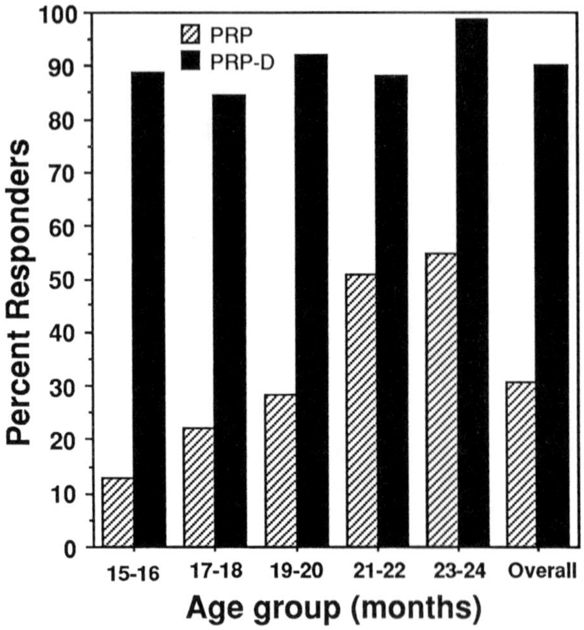

Figure 6-3. Immune responses to polyribosylribitol phosphate (PRP) and PRP-diphtheria toxoid (PRP-D)

SOURCE: *Reprinted with permission from Ward J. Newer Haemophilus influenzae type B vaccines and passive prophylaxis.* Pediatr Infect Dis J. *1987;6:799–803.*

in young infants of Native Alaskan heritage has been observed.[42] The difference in age distribution of Hib infection between the Finnish children and the Native Alaskan children may have contributed to this apparent difference in efficacy between the two populations. Although the majority of reported Hib disease in Native Alaskan children occurred before one year of age, this age group only accounted for 28% of the reported illness in Finland.[43] PRP-D is approved for use only in children more than one year old.

Both the HbOC and PRP-OMP conjugates, licensed for use in infants in 1990, were immunogenic in two-month-old infants.[44,45] It appears that PRP-OMP elicits a stronger antibody response than HbOC, but the antibody response to HbOC appears more prolonged than that to PRP-OMP.[43] In a large study conducted in the United States, the protective efficacy of three doses of HbOC was 100% (no cases in 20,800 children). There were 22 cases of Hib disease in 30,680 unvaccinated children and 3 cases in 4919 children who received only one dose of the vaccine.[44] Finally, a randomized trial that vaccinated Navajo infants with PRP-OMP at two and four months of age demonstrated an efficacy of 93%, with 1 case of invasive disease in the children completing the two-dose series and 14 cases in placebo recipients.[43] Further studies continue to document the efficacy of the three conjugate vaccines against Hib disease in infants.[34,46–48] Following the licensure of PRP-OMP, several lots used in the Navajo trial were found to be of relatively low immunogenicity.[34] A case-controlled efficacy trial in the Navajo children showed that the overall efficacy of Hib conjugate vaccines was 96–99%. The efficacy of PRP-OMP was 96% overall and 89% with the low-immunogenicity lots, suggesting that even the low-immunogenicity lots provided protection against Hib disease. The dramatic decrease in Hib disease is a result of the high efficacy of the vaccine and the reduced exposure of children to Hib as a result of the vaccine-related decrease in Hib nasopharyngeal colonization.[49]

In 1993, Tetramune®, a product that combines HbOC and DPT (diphtheria, pertussis, and tetanus toxins) in a premixed liquid formulation, was licensed. The safety profile of this product is similar to that of the individual products.[50] New products that combine the Hib vaccine with DPT and inactivated poliomyelitis vaccine are being investigated.[50–52] The ability to simultaneously administer these vaccines without affecting the immunogenicity of the individual vaccines should enhance compliance with vaccine administration schedules and help bring about the eradication of these vaccine-preventable diseases.

Biotechnological Approaches to Vaccine Development

Biotechnology provides safer, more efficient methods of vaccine production. An understanding of molecular genetics enables the development of attenuated vaccines with well-defined mutations rather than an accumulation of random mutations. In addition, recombinant DNA techniques allow the cloning and efficient expression of proteins for use in vaccines that contain a few precisely defined antigens. These strategies offer the promise of vaccines without the potential to revert to pathogenic variants as well as vaccines with fewer contaminants and, therefore, fewer side effects. These techniques also make possible the development of vaccines against organisms, such as *Treponema pallidum*, that are difficult to grow. Finally, biotechnological methods for creating cancer vaccines (see chapter 10) and vaccines against the human immunodeficiency virus (see chapter 7) are under evaluation.

This section addresses various biotechnological methods used in vaccine development, including subunit approaches (both cloned proteins and synthetic peptides), attenuation approaches, and approaches using carrier organisms. These methods are summarized in Table 6-7.

Subunit Vaccines

There are two types of subunit vaccines: those made with cloned proteins and those made with synthetic peptides.

Cloned Proteins

Genes that encode a specific antigen can be cloned and expressed in a variety of vectors. An example of an ap-

Table 6-7. Biotechnological Methods of Developing Vaccines

METHOD	VACCINE EXAMPLE
Subunit approaches	
Cloned proteins	Hepatitis B, malaria
Synthetic peptides	Hepatitis B, malaria
Attenuated organisms	
Eliminating virulence factor	Cholera
Delete metabolic factor	Typhoid
Vaccinia carriers	Herpes simplex, rabies
Anti-idiotypic vaccines	Hepatitis B, rabies

proach using cloned proteins is the genetically engineered vaccine for hepatitis B.

The incidence of reported hepatitis B virus (HBV) infection has increased steadily over the last decade, even after an effective plasma-derived vaccine became available. Globally, hepatitis B is associated with acute and chronic hepatitis and primary liver cancer. The incidence of acute HBV infection in the United States is now estimated at 200,000–300,000 cases per year, and more than 1 million people are chronically infected.[53]

The crucial immunogen in the HBV vaccine is the surface polypeptide antigen HBsAg. The gene encoding this peptide has been cloned and expressed in yeast, *Escherichia coli*, and mammalian cells. The first licensed recombinant vaccine for HBV was approved by the FDA in July 1986. Currently, there are two recombinant HBV vaccines licensed in the United States.

These vaccines are produced by inserting the gene containing the HBsAg subtype adw into a plasmid and inserting the plasmid into the yeast *Saccharomyces cerevisae*. The recombinant antigen forms spherical aggregate particles 17–25 nm in diameter, similar to the purified antigen from the plasma-derived HBV. Although as much as 25% of the plasma-derived antigen is glycosylated, the antigen expressed in yeast is not. The absence of glycosylation does not affect the ability to stimulate neutralizing antibodies. In addition, up to 5% of this final product may consist of yeast-derived proteins, though no yeast DNA is detectable.[54,55] No adverse consequences related to the development of antibody to these yeast proteins were observed during clinical trials.[54] Mammalian cells (Chinese Hamster ovary [CHO] cells) have also been used as vectors for production of recombinant HBV vaccine.[56] Both yeast and CHO-derived vaccines confer excellent antibody response in volunteers, with minimal adverse reactions.

The immunogenicity of the recombinant HBV vaccine is comparable to that of the plasma-derived product. More than 90% of healthy adults demonstrate protective antibodies to HBsAg (more than 10 IU/L) after a series of three 10-μg doses of the recombinant vaccine; equal rates of seroconversion have been demonstrated after three doses of either the plasma-derived vaccine (20 μg per dose) or recombinant vaccine (10 μg per dose).[57–59] Older adults demonstrate a lower antibody response than younger adults to either vaccine. In studies using three 5-μg doses of recombinant vaccine for children less than 12 years old, more than 99% of the recipients developed protective levels of antibodies.[54] Field trials conducted in the United States suggest that recombinant vaccines are 80–95% effective in preventing infection and clinical disease in susceptible individuals.[54,55] In studies of infants born to hepatitis B envelope antigen (HBeAg)- and HBsAg-positive mothers, the combination of hepatitis B immune globulin (HBIG) (0.5 ml at birth) and recombinant HBV vaccine (5 μg in each of three doses) was shown to protect 95% of these infants from developing the chronic carrier state; this efficacy equals that of HBIG plus plasma-derived vaccine.[60] However, hemodialysis patients develop a poorer response to the recombinant vaccine than do healthy adults, as shown by one study in which only 64% of hemodialysis patients developed protective levels of antibodies after receiving three 40-μg doses of recombinant HBV vaccine.[54]

Because the genes that encode for HBsAg are the only part of the HBV genome present in the yeast vector, no infectious HBV DNA can be produced. Adverse reactions to recombinant HBV vaccine during prelicensure trials were similar in extent and variety to those observed with the plasma-derived vaccine.[54]

Major risk factors for the transmission of HBV include multiple sexual partners and intravenous drug use. Universal immunization of adolescents would result in a reduction of HBV transmission and infection, because this is the age group currently most at risk for acquiring HBV infection.[53] However, lack of access to health care and generally poor compliance with vaccine schedules in these populations has limited use of the vaccine. Universal immunization of infants is part of an initiative for controlling HBV infection. The development of new vaccine products that will allow simultaneous vaccination for HBV, DPT, and/or Hib will help integrate HBV vaccine into the current immunization schedule. Although this should have a major impact in the future, immunization of older children and high-risk groups still needs to be implemented. The full duration of protection induced by the initial HBV vaccine series administered in infancy has not yet been determined. Studies in adults and infants have documented protection for periods up to 9 years.[53] The need for booster doses will be assessed as individuals are followed for 10 or more years after primary immunization.

The development of malaria vaccines is another example of a potentially useful application of the subunit approach. Malaria is a major public health problem, particularly in third world countries, afflicting 300 million people and causing 1–2 million deaths every year. Developing a vaccine against this disease is more difficult than developing an HBV vaccine because the causative agent, *Plasmodium falciparum*, expresses different antigens at different life cycle stages (Figure 6-4). Because of this difficulty, recombinant DNA methods are being used to develop an effective vaccine, which may serve as a prototype for vaccines against other diseases.

The life cycle of *P. falciparum* begins in the human host when the sporozoite form of the parasite is injected into the host's bloodstream by a mosquito bite. Within minutes, the sporozoites invade the hepatocytes, where they are protected from the body's defenses. Once inside the liver cells, the sporozoites reproduce until the hepatocytes burst, releasing thousands of merozoites. These merozoites invade red blood cells (RBCs), where they undergo repeated cycles of intracellular asexual multiplication, resulting in RBC lysis, release of more merozoites, and infection of other RBCs. A few merozoites differentiate into sexual forms called gametocytes, which are ingested by a mosquito feeding on the host's blood. The cycle begins again as the gametocytes are released from RBCs into the mosquito's stomach, eventually resulting in the production of thousands of sporozoites.

Developing a vaccine against malaria is complicated by the expression of different antigens at each stage in the *P. falciparum* life cycle. The first attempts at developing a vaccine were directed against the sporozoite stage; however, the time from sporozoite injection to invasion of the hepatocyte is very short. Clinical disease could result if even one sporozoite escapes the antibodies engendered by a vaccine. On the other hand, merozoite vaccines may ameliorate clinical illness but cannot prevent infection.

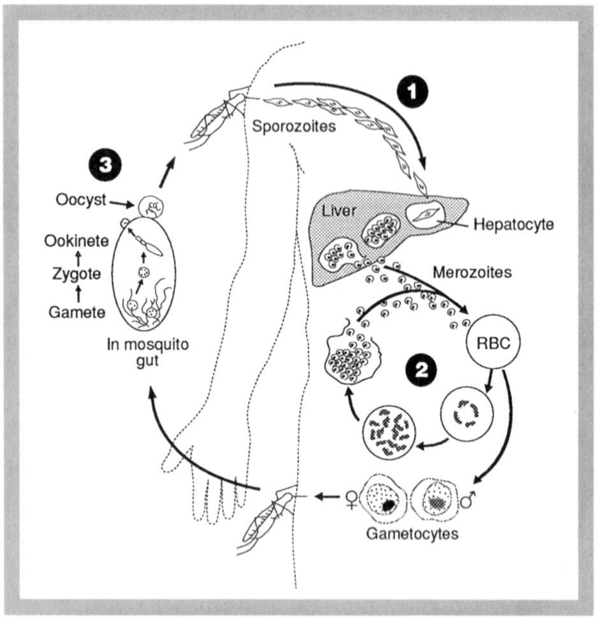

Figure 6-4. Life cyle of malaria. 1) Sporozoites; one sporozoite develops into 20,000 merozoites within a hepatic cell. 2) Merozoites rupture hepatic cells and invade red blood cells (RBCs). 3) Cycle in mosquito.

SOURCE: *Reprinted with permission from Miller LH, Howard RJ, Carter R, et al. Research toward malaria vaccines.* Science *1986;234:1349–56.*

A recombinant vaccine composed of the dominant epitope of the circumsporozoite (CS) protein, which coats the sporozoite, has been expressed in *E. coli*.[61] Volunteers immunized with this vaccine developed antibodies to *P. falciparum* sporozoite antigen. The efficacy of the vaccine was tested by exposing volunteers to mosquitoes infected with virulent *P. falciparum*. Only one subject was completely protected from parasitemia; two others were partially protected, and no protection was conferred to the remaining three subjects.[62] Such results are far from optimal, but they do suggest that higher doses of this sporozoite vaccine, perhaps in combination with merozoite antigens, may be a potentially useful strategy.

Synthetic Peptides

Synthesizing peptide antigens suitable for vaccination is an alternative to purifying antigens cloned in *E. coli*, yeast, or mammalian cells. The DNA sequence of the gene that encodes the critical immunogen forms the basis for the chemical synthesis of these peptides. An advantage of this approach is that multiple related peptides may be synthesized, incorporating variations found between strains. Peptide synthesis may also be directed at conserved, rather than variable, regions of the genome.

In one study, investigators working with epitopes of influenza virus synthesized 20 peptides corresponding to 75% of the influenza hemagglutinin. Antibodies directed at 85% of these peptides bound to influenza virus, suggesting that a peptide may stimulate an antibody response capable of binding the virus. In addition, a peptide synthesized from a region conserved in both influenza types A and B produced neutralizing antibodies for the different viral subtypes, indicating that synthetic peptide vaccines may provide protection for organisms with antigenic variability.[63]

As an alternative to the cloned protein approach, synthetic peptides have been used as antigens in a vaccine for the prevention of malaria. This sporozoite vaccine contains the major epitope of the CS protein, a sequence of four amino acids (asparagine-alanine-asparagine-proline) repeated in tandem 37 times. Nussenzweig and associates developed a synthetic vaccine consisting of three repeats of this sequence.[64] This peptide was conjugated to tetanus toxoid with aluminum hydroxide as an adjuvant and administered to volunteers. The vaccinated subjects were challenged by mosquitoes harboring virulent *P. falciparum*. The results were similar to those seen with the cloned CS vaccine: one volunteer was completely protected from parasitemia, and two others showed a significant delay in parasitemia.[65] This synthetic vaccine appears to be immunogenic, stimulating the production of biologically active antibody. Nevertheless, in the doses evaluated thus far, the vaccine did not protect against parasitemia. SPf66, a chimeric protein vaccine, contains 45 amino acids derived from the sporozoite epitope.[68] This new vaccine was evaluated in a randomized, placebo-controlled study of 586 children in Tanzania. No severe side effects were observed with the vaccine, which was highly immunogenic. The incidence of clinical malaria was decreased in the SPf66-receiving group, but the incidence of parasitemia was similar in both groups. The estimated efficacy of the vaccine was 31% (95% confidence interval, 0 to 52). Although for most infections an efficacy rate of 31% would be unacceptable, a reduction in morbidity of 31%, especially if mortality were also reduced, may be acceptable at this time with malaria.[67] The development of an effective vaccine against malaria appears to be in the near future. However, it may be necessary to combine peptides from both sporozoite and merozoite epitopes to increase the efficacy of the vaccine.[68]

These studies indicate that it is possible to elicit protective antibody responses in humans with subunit vaccines. These results with both cloned proteins and synthetic peptides are important not only for the development of malaria and HBV vaccines but also because they validate this approach to vaccine design.

Attenuated Live Vaccines

Recombinant DNA techniques allow a more defined approach to the rational design of attenuated organisms. DNA sequence analysis and viral genetics may be used to identify regions of the viral genome where alteration reduces the pathogenicity of the organism. In vitro site-directed mutagenesis allows point mutations into, or deletions from, any piece of cloned DNA in a selected, predefined position. The approach to genetically engineered attenuated live vaccines contrasts with the approach taken with subunit vaccines, in which recombinant technology is used to produce large amounts of a critical antigen isolated from the organism. Site-directed mutagenesis alters genes that encode a critical virulence or growth factor, retaining the organism as a vaccine.[26,69] Cholera and typhoid fever vaccines are examples of two different approaches to attenuated live vaccines. In the first approach, the gene that encodes for a critical virulence factor (e.g., cholera toxin) may be altered or deleted so that the organism survives and multiplies but does not produce disease.[70,71] In the second approach, a metabolic factor is modified so that the organism does not survive long enough to result in disease. This second approach has been used to develop a vaccine for *Salmonella typhimurium* in which the deletion of two genes has created additional growth requirements.[72] Because the vaccines are produced by eliminating a key region in the genome, the vaccine strains are incapable of reverting to pathogenic variants.

Carrier Organisms: The Vaccinia Model

In 1980, following global eradication of smallpox, the World Health Organization (WHO) suspended the use of the wild-type vaccinia virus vaccine. However, vaccines may be produced using vaccinia or other DNA viruses as carriers for one or more foreign antigens.[69] The vaccinia genome may be modified to incorporate foreign genetic material, producing a vaccine directed against a variety of dissimilar infectious agents. There are a number of examples in which foreign genes encoding pertinent antigens have been expressed by vaccinia virus. Animals inoculated with these recombinant viruses responded with serologic evidence of successful immunization, and in some cases, protection of these vaccinated animals against subsequent challenge with the infectious agent has been demonstrated.[73] Figure 6-5 outlines the basic strategy for creating recombinant vaccinia carriers through the introduction of foreign DNA sequences into infectious vaccinia virus.

Foreign genetic material is isolated and inserted into a cloned fragment of the vaccinia genome at a region that is not essential to vaccinia replication (e.g., thymidine kinase [TK] activity). It is crucial that the flow of genetic information essential for virus replication not be interrupted by insertion of this fragment. Next, this donor DNA is introduced into tissue culture that has been co-

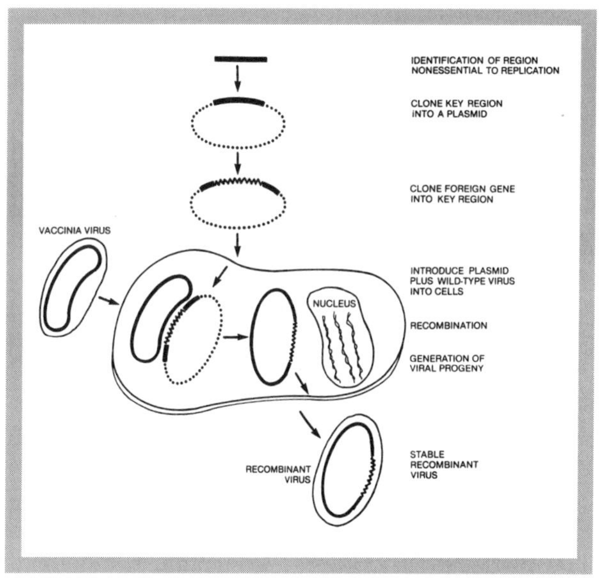

Figure 6-5. Strategy for creating recombinant vaccinia carriers

SOURCE: *Reprinted with permission from Ellis RW. New technologies for making vaccines. In: Plotkin SA, Mortimer EA Jr., editors.* Vaccines. *Philadelphia, PA: WB Saunders; 1988. p. 570.*

infected with vaccinia virus. In vivo recombination occurs between the vaccinia DNA sequences flanking the foreign DNA and the homologous DNA sequences on the wild-type replicating vaccinia, resulting in recombinant progeny virus.[73] Genes encoding for rabies glycoprotein, HBsAg, human immunodeficiency virus envelope glycoprotein, influenza hemagglutinin, herpes simplex glycoprotein D, and *P. falciparum* CS protein have all been cloned into the TK gene under transcriptional control of the vaccinia promoter.[69]

The vaccinia virus is attractive as a vector because, unlike the DNA from other animal viruses, the naked DNA of vaccinia is noninfectious and does not integrate into the host chromosome. In addition, a large amount of foreign DNA can be stably integrated into vaccinia. Thus, a number of foreign genes can be expressed in a single recombinant vaccinia virus, providing a live polyvalent vaccine that may be capable of eliciting immunity against a number of unrelated pathogens. The ability of the human immune system to respond adequately to such an antigenic intrusion, however, remains to be established, as does the relative immunogenicity of, and potential interferences among, the various antigens.[73]

Whether a recombinant vaccinia vaccine will be able to induce an immunologic response in an individual previously immunized against smallpox is a critical question. Vaccination usually involves administration of an antigen, the immune response being influenced by the vaccine components. With a vaccinia vector, however, the vaccine's immunogenicity may depend on the antibody status of the host to vaccinia as well as the response to the recombinant antigen. Since smallpox immunization was discontinued, the populations of vaccinia-naive children and adults with waning immunogenicity are increasing. Infants with variable transplacental antibodies to vaccinia may be candidates to receive polyvalent vaccinia recombinant vaccines. Given the complexity of this epidemiologic setting, assessing the efficacy of recombinant vaccinia vaccines may be difficult.[74] Nevertheless, encouraging results have been observed in studies of previously vaccinated animals. These animals, already vaccinated with recombinant vaccinia virus, were revaccinated with a second vaccinia recombinant expressing a new foreign antigen. The second vaccination resulted in antibodies to both the new antigen and vaccinia; however, no increase was observed in antibody response to the initial foreign antigen expressed by the first vaccinia recombinant.[73]

The manipulation of vaccinia virus illustrates the potential of carrier organisms to generate immunity against a broad spectrum of viral, parasitic, or bacterial pathogens. Multiple antigens may be cloned into vaccinia, as demonstrated by antibody response to three distinct antigens in animals vaccinated with a trivalent vaccinia recombinant.[75] Polyvalent vaccinia vaccines may reduce the number of immunizations required, perhaps allowing a combination of vaccines against the childhood diseases in a single vaccination.

Although the benefits of such vaccines appear to outweigh the risks, the safety of these vaccines must be addressed. Wild-type vaccinia has been associated with severe, although infrequent, reactions. Recombinant vaccinia vaccines must be evaluated for the propensity for such reactions from the vaccine. The pathogenesis of vaccinia encephalitis (caused by neurotropic vaccinia) is poorly understood. The impact, if any, that the introduction of foreign antigens may have on tissue tropism is of concern. Finally, the safety of these vaccines in immunosuppressed patients must be evaluated.[69]

Other carrier models are also under investigation. Avipoxviruses, a group of avian viruses related to vaccinia virus, hold some potential.[76] Because avipoxviruses are strongly host restricted to avian species, they cannot infect humans. A disadvantage with avipoxviruses is low immunogenicity, which would require repeated doses. Rabies and measles vaccines using this vector are being evaluated. Adenoviruses and polio viruses are also under investigation as vaccine vectors.

Approaches to Increasing Immunogenicity

Adjuvants

Adjuvants, such as aluminum salts, have been useful in enhancing the immune response to some vaccines or toxoids. Although the mechanism of potentiating antigenicity needs further clarification, it is known that a soluble antigen may become particulate when combined with an adjuvant. This property may be essential for synthetic vaccines, which tend to be water soluble and poorly immunogenic.[77] In addition, adjuvants prolong the release of antigen and mobilize phagocytes at the site of antigen deposition.[24] The only adjuvant approved for use in the United States is aluminum salt (hydroxide or phosphate), which is used in diphtheria, tetanus, HAV, and HBV vaccines.[76] Aluminum salts are not effective with all antigens, and they do not stimulate cell-mediated immunity.

Many of the structural components of microorganisms are themselves antigenic and may be suitable for use as adjuvants. For example, Freund's complete adjuvant (FCA) contains killed mycobacteria dispersed in a water-in-oil emulsion. Although this adjuvant usually stimulates high-level, prolonged immunity, local reactions preclude its use in humans. The minimal structure that can replace the adjuvant activity of mycobacteria in FCA is synthetic *N*-acetyl-muramyl-L-alanyl-D-isoglutamine, called muramyl dipeptide (MDP). Unlike other mycobacterial components, the adjuvant properties of MDP are present when administered either parenterally or orally in an aqueous medium. MDP exerts activity on several cell lines, including T cells, macrophages, and B cells. The essential mediators of this adjuvant effect appear to be T lymphocytes, as shown in transfer experiments and by stimulation of helper T-cell function in various carrier-hapten systems.[73] Depletion and even removal of macrophages do not reduce the adjuvant effect of MDP. B lymphocytes reconstituted with a monokine and interleukins can be stimulated by MDP, perhaps through enhanced differentiation of B cells into antibody-producing cells.[78]

Adjuvants may also be capable of suppressing the immune response. Immunosuppression has been described with Bacillus Calmette-Guérin (BCG) and lipopolysaccharide adjuvants and may occur with large doses of MDP. The antibody response to both particulate and soluble antigens is depressed in mice pretreated with high doses of MDP. T lymphocytes may mediate the suppressive effect of MDP. The capacity of MDP to inhibit the production of interleukin 2 and to increase the secretion of prostaglandins and oxygen metabolites may also play a role in its immunosuppressive effect. Because cell-mediated immunity is regulated by MDP, treatment of mice with a water-in-oil emulsion of MDP may induce nonspecific suppressor T cells.[78]

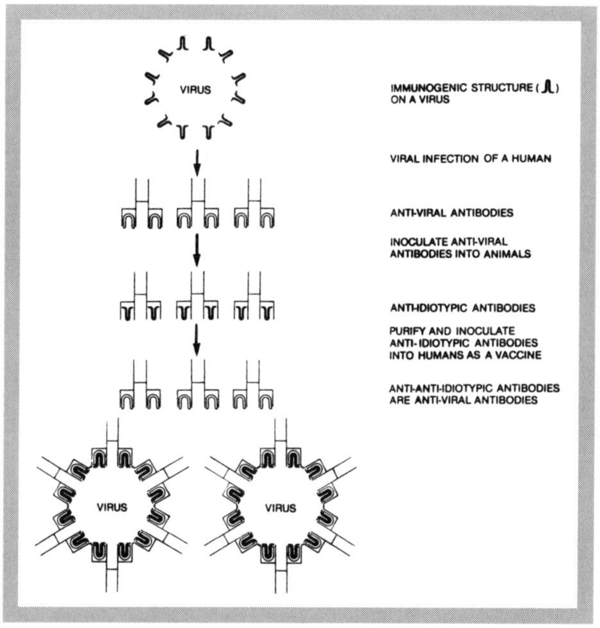

Figure 6-6. Development of anti-idiotypic antibodies as vaccines

SOURCE: *Reprinted with permission from Ellis RW. New technologies for making vaccines. In: Plotkin SA, Mortimer EA Jr., editors.* Vaccines. *Philadelphia, PA: WB Saunders; 1988. p. 574.*

Anti-idiotypes

Idiotypes are unique epitopes located either within the variable regions of immunoglobulin molecules produced by each individual B-cell clone or within T-cell receptors on each individual T-cell clone. Antibodies bear a structural image of their primary antigen at the antigen-binding site (the idiotype). Therefore, antibodies directed at these antibodies (anti-idiotypes) must have antigen-binding sites similar to the antigen. Administration of an anti-idiotypic antibody would stimulate an anti-anti-idiotypic antibody, which should be identical to the primary antibody (Figure 6-6). This strategy is analogous to making a negative from a photographic negative to produce a positive image.

In vaccination experiments, anti-idiotypic antibodies have been increasingly used, either alone or in combination with vaccinating antigens. In one study, pretreatment of mice with anti-idiotypic antibodies two weeks before vaccination enhanced the immune response to HBsAg. These anti-idiotypic antibodies were produced in rabbits that were administered monoclonal antibody to mouse HBsAg.[79] Thus, the anti-idiotypic antibodies represented an internal image of the HBsAg.

The protective effect of anti-idiotypes was first demonstrated by Sacks and associates, using a major surface glycoprotein (VAT 1.1) of a clone of *Trypanosoma rhodesiense* as the antigen.[80] Monoclonal antibodies against VAT 1.1 were used to prepare the anti-idiotypic antibodies. Pretreatment with anti-idiotypic antibodies four to five weeks before infection with the VAT 1.1 clone of trypanosomes prevented initial VAT 1.1 parasitemia.

Anti-idiotypes may also be useful in induction of an immune response when the corresponding antigens are not easily available. In addition, anti-idiotypes should enhance the induction of an immune response in young recipients of vaccines or when the antigens are poorly immunogenic. The use of anti-idiotypes may provide an opportunity to avoid the use of adjuvants; however, at present, most anti-idiotypes are produced in animals. Because animal-derived anti-idiotypes might result in extraneous antibody responses, human anti-idiotypes produced through monoclonal antibody technology may be needed. The potential risks of anti-idiotypes, such as immunosuppression and the generation of antireceptor autoantibodies or immune complexes, also need to be evaluated.

PASSIVE IMMUNIZATION

In active immunization, a patient receives a relatively harmless antigenic form of an organism to impart memory to the immune system, thereby stimulating production of endogenous antibodies (chapter 2 reviews the function of memory cells). In contrast, passive immunization protects a susceptible individual by directly administering exogenous replacement or supplemental immunoglobulins obtained from an immune donor. The means by which an individual acquires specific passive immunity may be either natural or induced. An example of natural passive immunity is that provided by the immunoglobulins newborns receive from their mothers in breast milk; an example of induced passive immunity is that imparted by the administration of exogenous animal or human immune globulins.

It was first recognized in the late 1800s that certain diseases (e.g., diphtheria and tetanus) are caused by specific toxins secreted by organisms. Soon after, researchers discovered that animals that survived exposure to these toxins had antibodies in their serum that were the source of this immunity, and the serum containing these antibodies came to be known as antitoxins.

Table 6-8. Currently Available Animal Antisera for Passive Immunization

DISEASE	PRODUCT	SOURCE
Black widow spider bite	Antivenin	Equine
Botulism	Botulism antitoxin	Equine
Diphtheria	Diphtheria antitoxin	Equine
Snakebite	Antivenin polyvalent; antivenin	Equine

Intramuscular Immune Globulins

Humoral immunity can be transferred from a sensitized person to a nonsensitized person through antibodies. Passive immunity is conferred on the fetus by placental transfer of maternal antibodies. The source of antibody for induced passive immunization may be immune globulin in serum from immunized animals (heterologous) or it may be antigen-specific or nonspecific pooled human immune globulin (homologous). Tables 6-8 and 6-9 list the animal antisera and human immune globulin products, respectively, currently available for passive immunization.

Passive immunization often involves injection of a specific immunoglobulin that targets a specific antigen. This process is referred to as seroprophylaxis or serotherapy. Serotherapy provides only temporary protection against an antigen because it does not promote the formation of protective antibodies by the recipient. Normal body catabolism and the rapid depletion of antibody as it combines with antigen contributes to the short duration of protection of exogenous immunoglobulin.[23,81]

Immunoglobulins for serotherapy are derived from either animal or human sources. Although antitoxins derived from active immunization of animals (i.e., horses and rabbits) will neutralize the same toxins in humans, they are less desirable than those from human sources. Animal sera frequently cause anaphylactic or serum sickness reactions because the human immune system recognizes the foreign proteins and forms IgE or IgG in response. Therefore, human immunoglobulin should be used whenever possible.

When human sources are not available, animal sera may be given in life-threatening situations. However, patients or their relatives must be carefully assessed by the pharmacist or other health care provider for pre-existing hypersensitivity to animal sera and possible type I hypersensitivity reactions (see chapter 4). A history of atopy or hypersensitivity greatly increases the likelihood of such a reaction. This history, along with concomitant skin testing, is critical to patient safety.

Serotherapy may provide immediate protection to a naive or specific antibody-free patient and has a variety of theoretical uses, but the number of current clinical uses is limited. Its primary use is as prophylaxis in patients exposed to diseases such as hepatitis and rabies.[81] Serotherapy is especially useful when the anticipated incubation period of the disease is shorter than the onset of protection with standard vaccination techniques (7–10 days).[2,82] The effectiveness of passive immunization depends on prompt administration of the antibodies, which must be given early in the incubation period to avoid the clinical illness. For instance, diphtheria antitoxin should be given within one hour of symptom onset to prevent any irreversible damage.[83] The effectiveness of the antitoxin rapidly decreases as the period between the onset of symptoms and administration increases.

The current uses of intramuscular immune globulins (IMIGs) outlined here include their use in treating established toxin-induced illnesses and in prophylaxis of viral infections.

IMIGs in Toxin-Induced Diseases

The role of IMIGs in treating toxin-induced diseases is primarily limited to antitoxins and antivenins used to prevent onset of disease in exposed patients. Toxin-induced diseases that can be treated with IMIGs include botulism, diphtheria, and black widow spider or snake bites. All IMIGs for this use are derived from horse sera (see Table 6-8).

IMIGs in Prophylaxis of Viral Infections

WHO currently recommends using IMIGs only for patients exposed to hepatitis A, hepatitis B, varicella-zoster, measles, rubella, or rabies. This use of IMIGs is much more common than use for toxin-induced diseases. IMIGs are useful for the prophylaxis of viral infections because they can decrease the severity or modify the effects of the diseases. As can be seen in Table 6-9, these immune globulins are antigen-specific: hepatitis B immune globulin

Table 6-9. Currently Available Immune Globulins for Passive Immunization

DISEASE	PRODUCT
Cytomegalovirus	Cytomegalovirus immune globulin IV (CMV-IVIG)
Hepatitis A	Immune globulin IM
Hepatitis B	Hepatitis B immune globulin (HBIG) IM
Hypogammaglobulinemia	Immune globulin IM, immune globulin IV
Measles	Immune globulin IM
Rabies	Rabies immune globulin IM
Rh isoimmunization	Rh_0(D) immune globulin IM
Rubella	Immune globulin IM
Tetanus	Tetanus immune globulin IM
Varicella	Varicella-zoster immune globulin (VZIG) IM
Vaccinia	Vaccinia immune globulin IM

IM, intramuscular; IV, intravenous.

(HBIG), rabies immune globulin, varicella-zoster immune globulin (VZIG). Antigen-specific immunoglobulins are derived from donors with very high circulating levels of a particular antibody. For example, VZIG is specific for varicella because it is derived from the serum of convalescent patients with zoster.[2] However, nonspecific human IMIG is used for other infections, such as hepatitis A, measles, and rubella. The two specific types of IMIGs that will be highlighted in this section are HBIG and VZIG.

Hepatitis B Immune Globulin

HBIG is the agent of choice in postexposure prophylaxis against hepatitis B. Active immunization with HBV vaccine is the most effective preventative tool for those at risk for HBV exposure, such as health care workers. However, if an unvaccinated person is accidentally exposed, vaccination alone is inadequate because of its delayed onset of protection.[84] HBIG provides high levels of anti-HBV antibody immediately. Because of its greater antigen specificity, it is more effective than and preferred over nonspecific human IMIG, which provides only minimal anti-HBV antibodies.[84] HBIG should be administered intramuscularly as soon as possible after exposure (preferably within 24 hours) to people exposed to materials contaminated with HBV virus, such as blood from a patient with hepatitis B.[54, 84–86] As was discussed earlier, prompt serotherapy will provide immediate protection until vaccination can impart active immunity to the exposed individual.

HBIG administered alone may not completely prevent the disease, but it does attenuate the clinical illness by lengthening the incubation period.[84] The Advisory Committee on Immunization Practice (ACIP) of the CDC therefore recommends coadministration of HBV vaccine and HBIG for postexposure prophylaxis in susceptible (unvaccinated) people who have perinatal or needle stick exposure to HBV-infected patients or their blood.[55] Infants born to HBsAg-positive mothers should receive HBV vaccine and 0.5 ml HBIG within 12 hours of birth and a second HBV vaccine at one month.[9] Thus a combination of active (HBV vaccine) and passive (HBIG) immunization is recommended for postexposure and prevention of HBV infection.

Varicella-Zoster Immune Globulin

VZIG is prepared from the plasma of adults who have high titers of anti-VZV antibodies. In contrast to HBIG, the use of VZIG is directed at immunocompromised patients with a significant exposure to VZV who are at high risk of developing complications. VZIG use is restricted because of cost considerations and limited supply. It is manufactured solely by Massachusetts Public Health Biologic Laboratory and distributed through the American Red Cross.[15] VZIG may be a lifesaving measure in certain high-risk patients who contract VZV, including neonates and those who are immunocompromised by disease, drugs, or radiation.[87] Table 6-10 lists the ACIP guidelines for patients who should receive VZIG. Despite VZIG administration, one-third to one-half of immunocompromised people exposed to VZV will develop clinical disease.[15] Passive immunization with VZIG will not necessarily prevent the onset of chickenpox, but it will act to modify the clinical course of the disease by decreasing its severity.[87,88] As with all serotherapy, VZIG must be administered promptly (within 96 hours) after exposure to VZV to be effective.[87,89,90] When used within this time frame in exposed immunodeficient children, VZIG significantly decreased the expected severity of chickenpox and significantly decreased mortality and the incidence of encephalitis and pneumonia to less than 25% of the expected rate without treatment.[91]

Intravenous Immune Globulins

An important development in passive immunization in the past decade is the introduction of immune globulin suitable for intravenous use. Before the mid-1970s, no immune globulin products could be given intravenously

Table 6-10. Guidelines of the Advisory Committee on Immunization Practices of the Centers for Disease Control for the Use of Varicella-Zoster Immune Globulin (VZIG)

Patients must meet all four of these criteria:

1. Persons susceptible to varicella-zoster.
2. Persons with significant exposure within 96 hours of VZIG administration.
3. Persons <15 years old (administration to immunocompromised adolescents and adults and to other older patients on an individualized basis).
4. Persons with one of the following underlying illnesses or conditions:
   a. Neoplastic disease (e.g., leukemia or lymphoma).
   b. Congenital or acquired immunodeficiency.
   c. Drug- or radiation-induced immunosuppression.
   d. Newborn of mother who has onset of chickenpox within five days before delivery or within 48 hours after delivery.
   e. Premature infant (gestation period >28 weeks) whose mother lacks a history of chickenpox.
   f. Premature infant (gestation period <28 weeks or birth weight ≤1000 g) regardless of maternal history.

because they caused IgG aggregate formation, anticomplement activity, and anaphylactic reactions. Aggregate formation was linked to the method of production. Reformulation has eliminated these problems, and now intravenous immune globulin (IVIG) products are available in the United States.[92]

IVIGs are derived from IgG isolated from pooled human serum. Although it contains primarily IgG, other antibody classes (IgE, IgM, and IgA) as well as other serum proteins may be present in trace amounts.[93] The larger the donor pool, the wider the spectrum of IgG antibodies contained in the serum. In fact, the WHO recommends that all IVIG products be derived from pools of at least 1000 donors.[93]

The intravenous route for administering immune globulins has many advantages over the intramuscular route. The greatest advantage is that IVIGs can be given in much larger doses than IMIGs. Other advantages include an immediate rise in blood levels, greater bioavailability, ease of and relatively painless administration, fewer severe adverse reactions, and a half-life more closely resembling that of endogenous IgG.[85,94]

All plasma donor units must be free of HIV, hepatitis C virus (HCV), and HBsAg. All IVIG products should contain not less than 90% of their immunoglobulin content as gamma globulin (as recommended by the WHO). Table 6-11 lists the currently licensed IVIG products available in the United States.

IgG Subclasses

There are four different subclasses of IgG present in IVIG products (IgG1, IgG2, IgG3, and IgG4) as well as in normal human serum. These subclasses differ both structurally and functionally, and their differences are important because they relate to disease etiology. Table 6-12 lists some of the presumed functions of each IgG subclass.

The clinical impact of an IgG subclass deficiency depends on the role of the subclass in the normal human immune system. Patients with an IgG subclass deficiency may be asymptomatic or prone to severe infections. The deficiency may be in a single subclass or in multiple subclasses. Most patients lack two subclasses; the predominant pattern is a lack of IgG1 and IgG3, followed in incidence by a deficiency of IgG2 and IgG4.[95] Among infection-prone adult patients with a single subclass deficiency, IgG3 accounts for the major deficiency; in children, IgG2 deficiency clearly dominates.[96,97]

Recent studies have shown that clinically relevant subclass deficiencies are under-recognized. Because total IgG consists of more than 70% IgG1, a subclass deficiency

Table 6-11. Intravenous Immune Globulin (IVIG) Products Licensed in the United States

PRODUCT	MANUFACTURER	FORMULATION
Gamimune® N	Bayer	Liquid in 10% maltose
Gammagard® S/D	Hyland	Lyophilized powder*
Gammar®-PIV	Centeon	Lyophilized powder
Iveegam®	Immuno-US	Lyophilized powder
Sandoglobulin®	Novartis	Lyophilized powder
Venoglobulin®-I	Alpha Therapeutic	Lyophilized powder
Venoglobulin®-S	Alpha Therapeutic	Solution*
Polygam® S/D	Hyland	Lyophilized powder*

**Solvent/detergent in manufacturing process.*

Table 6-12. Functions of Immunoglobulin G (IgG)

SUBCLASS	PRESUMED FUNCTIONS
IgG1	Tissue protection, complement fixation, response to antigen
IgG2	Response to bacterial polysaccharides
IgG3	Complement fixation, virus neutralization
IgG4	Protection of the respiratory tract by harnessing mast cells and basophils

of IgG2, IgG3, or IgG4 may not be identified if only total IgG is measured. In fact, a documented subclass deficiency, especially IgG2, occurred in 24% of patients who had abnormal susceptibility to infections, normal total IgG levels, and no clear pre-existing evidence of an immunodeficiency syndrome.[95] Therefore, measurement of each subclass in the workup of patients with frequent infections and a suspected immunodeficiency may be necessary to document an IgG subclass deficiency.

Subclass Deficiency

Commercially available IVIG products are useful in treating symptomatic patients with subclass deficiency. To more closely mimic normal serum, any IVIG product used should contain a proportion of each subclass similar to that found in normal serum. The WHO has recognized a "reference plasma" to act as a guideline for subclass distribution. The percentage of each subclass in currently available IVIG products, in comparison with the WHO reference, is presented in Table 6-13.

As mentioned previously, IVIG products should originate from large donor pools and contain a natural distribution of IgG subclasses. The products listed in Table 6-13 have been compared in several studies.[85,93,98–100] Specific quantities, values, and relative percentages differ among the studies, perhaps because of differences in manufacturing and purification processes, in the assay procedures used by investigators, and in the donor pools. Until these manufacturing processes and assay procedures are standardized, it will be difficult to directly compare IVIG products reliably. Given these caveats, the following information is generally accepted. Sandoglobulin® has lower levels of IgG1 and higher levels of IgG2 than the WHO standard.[98] Iveegam® has no detectable IgG3, making it unsuitable for replacement therapy. The greatest relative differences between the products were in the levels of IgG4. Gamimune® and Gammagard® had significantly lower levels of IgG4 than the other products. This low level may be caused by an IgA-removing step in the manufacturing process.[98] Low levels of IgA are desirable in products given to patients with IgA deficiency and anti-IgA antibodies. In fact, the low IgA content of Gammagard® makes it the only IVIG product indicated for patients with IgA deficiency.[93] Older IgG products prepared using different methods had no IgG3 and very little IgG4.[92] IgG4 deficiency has been associated with severe pyogenic respiratory infections.[101]

The importance of the variation in subclass distributions in these IVIG products is unknown. Five of the products closely mimic the natural distribution of IgG. These products are preferred in treating agammaglobulinemia because subclass imbalances may result in infectious sequelae.[98] Gammagard® has considerably lower levels of IgG4 than the other products, which may be of concern in treating patients with documented IgG4 deficiency.

IgA Deficiency

IgA deficiency is the most common primary immunodeficiency, although it occurs in only 1 of every 700–23,000 people.[102] Most IgA-deficient patients are prone to frequent infections, especially respiratory tract infections, and they also often have low levels of IgG subclasses, especially the IgG2 subclass (combined IgA and IgG2 deficiency). Administration of IVIG could help correct the IgG2 deficiency. However, the exogenous IgA found in many IVIG products is antigenic, and anti-IgA antibody titers can quickly increase in response. This rapid increase may cause anaphylactic reactions following infusion of any material containing IgA, such as blood, plasma, or IVIG.[103] Therefore, to avoid unnecessary stimulation of the immune system and to decrease the incidence and severity of adverse reactions, only IgA-free or IgA-deficient IVIG products should be administered in this patient population. Increasing antibody titers may indicate an enhanced risk of anaphylaxis.[104,105] Between 10 and 60% of these patients will have measurable titers of anti-IgA antibodies in their blood.[102,103] Patients who have an IgA deficiency and anti-IgA antibodies should not be treated with IVIG; an alternate treatment should be considered. Serum anti-IgA antibody titers should be closely monitored during immunoglobulin replacement therapy.

In conclusion, each IgG subclass plays an important role in the immune system. Clinical deficiency of a subclass may manifest itself as disease, most commonly as a chronic respiratory infection. Development and standardization of technology for quantification has added to our knowledge of IgG subclass deficiencies, especially with the advent of subclass-specific monoclonal antibodies. IVIG products with adequate subclass representation can normalize the plasma of patients with subclass deficiency.

Side Effects

IVIGs cause side effects in approximately 1–10% of patients, but they are generally mild (e.g., chills, nausea,

Table 6-13. Percentage of IgG Subclasses in Licensed IVIG Products[92,94,102]

PRODUCT	IgG1 (%)	IgG2 (%)	IgG3 (%)	IgG4 (%)
WHO reference plasma	60–70	23–29	4–8	2–6
Gamimune® N	59	29	6	5
Gammagard® S/D	69	22	4	5
Gammar®-PIV	69	23	6	2
Iveegam®	64	30	4	1.5
Sandoglobulin®	61	30	7	3
Venoglobulin®-I	61	29	5	4
Venoglobulin®-S	66	25	6	3
Polygam® S/D	57	30	8	5

WHO, World Health Organization.

abdominal pain) and can often be avoided by premedicating the patient or by slowing the rate of infusion.[106] Between October 1993 and June 1994, the CDC received 112 reports associating HCV infection with IVIG administration.[107] In 92% of these cases, IVIG administration was the only risk factor identified. Only one case was reported with Polygam®; the remaining 111 cases were associated with Gammagard® use. Epidemiologic studies suggest that HCV transmission is not related to the administration of any other IVIG or IMIG product. Since May 1994, the manufacturers of these two products have incorporated a solvent/detergent in the manufacturing process that effectively removes any risk of HCV transmission.

Therapeutic Uses

IVIG has many therapeutic uses. The FDA-labeled indications include the treatment of hypogammaglobulinemia (as a primary immunodeficiency), ITP, Kawasaki disease, and hypogammaglobulinemia in patients with chronic lymphocytic leukemia (CLL). However, as can be seen from the partial list of potential uses shown in Table 6-14, IVIG is being studied as a potential treatment for a wide variety of autoimmune and immunodeficiency disease states.

IVIG is the treatment of choice for primary immunodeficiencies, such as hypogammaglobulinemia, because it exerts its therapeutic action through repletion of antibodies.[108] The presence of impaired antibody responses, not IgG subclass deficiencies, is associated with an increased risk of infection and a beneficial response to IVIG.[109] Diseases characterized as "secondary" or "acquired" immunodeficiencies vastly outnumber primary immunodeficiencies. IVIG has been studied as a treatment for a variety of secondary immunodeficiencies, many of which are listed in Table 6-14.

IVIG has also been studied extensively in the treatment of ITP, a bleeding disorder characterized by destruction of platelets and easy bruising. ITP is associated with the presence of antibodies in plasma and on platelets to platelet glycoproteins IIb/IIIa and Ib/IX.[109] The exact mechanism of action of IVIG in treating ITP is unclear. One suggested mechanism is that IVIG saturates Fc receptors on platelets, rendering antibody-coated cells that are less susceptible to Fc-mediated phagocytosis and destruction by the reticuloendothelial system. Although several mechanisms may actually be involved, the important fact is that IVIG is clinically effective in raising platelet counts in adults and children.[109] This increase in platelet counts is especially important before a surgical procedure or when active bleeding is present. In responding patients, the increase in platelet count is usually rapid (within one to five days) but is generally only a transient rise, lasting from several days to a month.[85]

The effectiveness of IVIG in other secondary (acquired) immunodeficiencies is thought to be due to both its immunomodulatory effect and its ability to replace specific antibodies. The infectious complications—bacterial, viral, and fungal—that often accompany these secondary immunodeficiencies can be devastating, especially in transplant patients, cancer patients, and premature infants, among others. It is now known that hypogammaglobulinemia may be an important contributing factor in the development of these infectious complications. Based on this information and placebo-controlled clinical trials, the FDA approved the use of IVIG in the prevention of recurrent bacterial infections in some patients with B-cell chronic CLL.[110] However, there is still some question

Table 6-14. Potential and FDA-Approved Indications for IVIGs

Primary immunodeficiencies
Agammaglobulinemia, hypogammaglobulinemia[a]
Secondary (acquired) immunodeficiencies
Malignancies associated with antibody deficiency
Chronic lymphocytic leukemia (CLL)[a], multiple myeloma
Bacterial infections
Pseudomonas, group B streptococcus
Viral infections
Cytomegalovirus (CMV), herpes simplex
Kidney/heart/bone marrow transplant patients
High-risk premature infants/neonates
AIDS patients, primarily children
Burn patients
Guillain-Barré syndrome
Thrombocytopenias
Autoimmune thrombocytopenia purpura (ATP)
Idiopathic thrombocytopenia purpura (ITP)[a]
Other autoimmune disorders
Collagen vascular diseases
Myasthenia gravis
Kawasaki disease
Autoimmune neutropenia and hemolytic anemia

[a]FDA-approved indications.

whether the use of prophylactic IVIG therapy is cost effective. In a cost analysis of IVIG in treating CLL and hypogammaglobulinemia, it was found that IVIG may not result in an improved quality or length of life in comparison to other, less expensive treatments.[111]

IVIG continues to show promise as a therapy for autoimmune diseases. It has now become standard therapy, in combination with aspirin, for Kawasaki disease.[109,112] IVIG decreases the incidence of coronary artery lesions, a complication of Kawasaki disease. In the treatment of myasthenia gravis, 73% of patients have noted clinical improvement with IVIG therapy.[110] However, no placebo-controlled studies have been performed.

Antigen-specific (hyperimmune) immune globulins have also shown promise in the management of specific infections. For example, the incidence and severity of cytomegalovirus (CMV) infections in transplant patients has been modulated by the administration of CMV-IVIG. CMV-IVIG has received FDA approval as an orphan drug for the attenuation of primary CMV disease associated with renal transplantation.[113] Use of CMV-IVIG is limited to CMV-seronegative patients receiving a kidney from a CMV-seropositive donor.[85] Prospective clinical studies have shown a 50% decrease in primary CMV disease in kidney transplant recipients who received CMV-IVIG versus untreated controls. CMV-IVIG is manufactured by the Massachusetts Public Health Biologics Laboratory and distributed by Connaught Laboratories and MedImmune.[85,113]

In addition to clinical studies in renal transplant recipients, CMV-IVIG has also been evaluated for its ability to decrease CMV pneumonitis and graft-versus-host disease in bone marrow, heart, and liver transplant recipients.[102,114–20] The use of hyperimmune CMV-IVIG to attenuate or prevent CMV infection in transplants other than kidney transplants remains controversial (see chapter 8). The high doses used in the majority of these trials may be prohibitively expensive outside a research setting.[119] In addition, several studies have documented the efficacy of standard IVIG in preventing the CMV complications of bone marrow transplantation. A recent meta-analysis suggested that IVIG was effective in preventing interstitial pneumonia in CMV-seropositive and seronegative recipients and in decreasing the incidence of CMV infection in CMV-seronegative recipients.[120] The future use of antigen-specific hyperimmune IVIGs still remains in question; however, further studies are warranted before a final assessment of therapeutic utility can be made.

Selection Variables

The therapeutic consequences of the differences among the licensed IVIG products have never been evaluated in a controlled trial, but because of their similarity, these products are generally considered to be therapeutic equivalents. Factors that should be considered by the pharmacist when making a product selection include plasma source, IgA content, method of preparation, reconstitution time, storage requirements, available concentrations, available diluents, and cost. Unfortunately, all available IVIG products are quite expensive, especially since fairly substantial doses are commonly used. For example, recommended doses of IVIG used for one of its approved uses, ITP treatment, average 400 mg/kg.[109] This dose, 25–35 g for an average-sized adult, may cost $1000, regardless of the manufacturer. Therefore, indiscriminate use of this product for uses not approved by the FDA should be closely monitored as a part of every institution's ongoing drug utilization evaluation program.

In summary, IVIG has had a substantial therapeutic impact in primary immunodeficiencies and thrombocytopenias. The efficacy of additional uses, such as in secondary immunodeficiencies, autoimmune diseases, and neonatal sepsis, is under investigation.

SUMMARY

The body may be immunized by either active or passive processes. Active immunization exposes the immune system to a relatively harmless form of an antigen to stimulate the body's defenses against a specific disease. Passive immunization facilitates the antigen-antibody response by administering exogenous immunoglobulin from an immune donor to an unprotected individual.

Active immunization with live vaccines poses a risk that the patient will develop the disease rather than only an immune response. Allergic reactions are also possible, most frequently as a result of the culture media. The risk of vaccination must be assessed within the context of the disease and the relative risk of adverse or long-term effects. Adverse reactions to vaccines should be reported to the Vaccine Adverse Effect Reporting System (VAERS).

Vaccines may contain attenuated live organisms (generating long-lasting immunity) or killed organisms. The latter require multiple administrations because they usually do not provide permanent protection with a single dose. Stability is crucial to live vaccines. Vaccines with killed organism may, however, produce more adverse effects because of large quantities of extraneous material in the vaccine.

Biotechnological methods of producing vaccine subunits include cloning antigenic viral peptides (e.g., hepatitis B and malaria vaccines) or creating synthetic antigenic peptides (e.g., influenza and malaria vaccines) to produce large amounts of a critical antigen. Recombinant technology is used to produce attenuated vaccines that are genetically altered to a nonpathogenic state. Through recombinant DNA technology, vaccinia viruses can be altered to express the antigenic peptides of a variety of pathogens, functioning as a carrier organism. Adjuvants and anti-idiotypes are also being studied to enhance immunogenicity.

Passive immunization can be transmitted through animal or human sera. Passive immunization provides more immediate protection than active immunization, but its protection is only temporary. Animal sera may produce a higher incidence of serum sickness than human products. Intramuscular immune globulin vaccines are presently used to treat toxin-induced illnesses and to prevent viral infections. Intravenous immune globulin vaccines are used for many therapeutic purposes, such as immunoglobulin subclass deficiencies. They have several advantages over intramuscular immune globulins but are much more costly. Antigen-specific immune globulins can prevent disease, but their high cost and restricted supply limit their use.

Pharmacists have an important role in the implementation of immunization programs. With a knowledge of the products available and the recommendations for their use, pharmacists can actively assist in the goal of the elimination of vaccine-preventable diseases.

REFERENCES

1. Plotkin SL, Plotkin SA. A short history of vaccines. In: Plotkin SA, Mortimer EA Jr., editors. *Vaccines*. Philadelphia, PA: WB Saunders; 1988.
2. Stites JP, Stobo JD, Fudenberg HH, *et al. Basic and Clinical Immunology*. 5th ed. Los Altos, CA: Lange Medical Publications; 1984.
3. Centers for Disease Control, Advisory Committee on Immunization Practices. Measles prevention: recommendations of the Advisory Committee on Immunization Practices. *MMWR* 1989;38(S9):1–18.
4. Centers for Disease Control. Discontinuation of duck embryo virus for rabies vaccines. *MMWR* 1981;30:407–8.
5. Katz SL, Gelin BG. Measles vaccine: do we need new vaccines or new programs? *Science* 1994;265:1391–2.
6. Pabst HF, Spady DW, Marusyk RG, *et al*. Reduced measles immunity in infants in a well vaccinated population. *Pediatr Infect Dis J*. 1992;11:525–9.
7. Centers for Disease Control. Measles—United States, first 26 weeks, 1994. *MMWR* 1994;43:673–6.
8. Committee on Infectious Diseases of the American Academy of Pediatrics. Recommendations for the use of live, attenuated varicella vaccine. *Pediatrics* 1995;95:791–6.
9. Drawl-Klein LA, O'Donovan CA. Varicella in pediatric patients. *Ann Pharmacother*. 1993;27:938–49.
10. Preblud SR, Orenstein WA, Koplan JP, *et al*. A benefit-cost analysis of a childhood vaccination program. *Postgrad Med J*. 1985;61:17–22.
11. Lieu T, Coch SL, Black SB, *et al*. Cost-effectiveness of a routine varicella vaccination program for United States children. *JAMA* 1994;271:375–81.
12. Gershon AA, Steinberg S, LaRussa P, *et al*. Immunization of healthy adults with live, attenuated varicella vaccine. *J Infect Dis*. 1988;158:132–7.
13. White CJ, Kuter BJ, Ngai A, *et al*. Modified cases of chickenpox after varicella vaccination: correlation of protection with antibody response. *Pediatrics* 1991;87: 604–10.
14. Watson BM, Piercy SA, Plotkin SA, *et al*. Modified chickenpox in children immunized with the Oka/Merck varicella vaccine. *Pediatrics* 1993;91:17–22.
15. Bernstein HH, Rothstein EP, Pennbridge Pediatric Associates, *et al*. Clinical survey of natural varicella compared with breakthrough varicella after immunization with live, attenuated Oka/Merck varicella vaccine. *Pediatrics* 1993;92:833–7.
16. Hardy I, Gerston AA, Steinberg SP, *et al*. The incidence of zoster after immunization with live, attenuated varicella vaccine: a study in children with leukemia. *N Engl J Med*. 1991;325:1545–50.
17. Watson B, Gupta R, Randall T, *et al*. Persistence of cell mediated and humoral immune responses in healthy children immunized with live, varicella vaccine. *J Infect Dis*. 1994;169:197–9.
18. Marks JS, Halpin TJ. Guillain-Barre syndrome in recipients of a New Jersey influenza vaccine. *JAMA* 1980;243:2490–4.
19. Centers for Disease Control. Vaccine Adverse Event Reporting System (VAERS)—United States. *MMWR* 1990;41:730–3.
20. Chen RT, Rastogi SC, Mullen JR, *et al*. The Vaccine Adverse Event Reporting System (VAERS). *Vaccine* 1994;12:542–50.
21. Barret J. *Textbook of Immunology*. 5th ed. St. Louis, MO:

CV Mosby; 1988.
22. Centers for Disease Control. Reported vaccine-preventable diseases—United States 1983 and the Childhood Immunization Initiative. *MMWR* 1994;43:959–60.
22a. Centers for Disease Control. National, state, and urban area vaccination coverage levels among children aged 19–35 months—United States, January–December 1995. *MMWR* 1997;46:176–82.
23. Centers for Disease Control. Recommended childhood immunization schedule—United States, January 1995. *MMWR* 1994;43:959–60.
24. Hinman AR, Orenstein WA, Bart KJ, *et al.* Immunization. In: Mandell GL, Douglas RG Jr., Bennett JE, editors. *Principles and Practice of Infectious Disease.* 3rd ed. New York: Churchill Livingstone; 1990.
25. Ellis RW. New technologies for making vaccines. In: Plotkin SA, Mortimer EA Jr., editors. *Vaccines.* Philadelphia, PA: WB Saunders, 1988.
26. Almond JW, Cann AJ. Attenuation. In: Roitt IM, editor. *Immune Intervention: New Trends in Vaccines.* London: Academic; 1984. p. 13–56.
27. Nkowane BJ, Wassilak SGF, Orenstein WA, *et al.* Vaccine-associated paralytic poliomyelitis. *JAMA* 1987;257: 1335–40.
28. Centers for Disease Control. Monthly immunization table. *MMWR* 1995;43:961.
29. Centers for Disease Control. Lack of evidence for wild poliovirus circulation—United States, 1993. *MMWR* 1995;43:957–9.
31. Nathanson N, Langmuir AD. The Cutter incident. Poliomyelitis following formaldehyde-inactivated poliovirus vaccination in the United States during spring of 1955. I. Background. *Am J Hygiene* 1963;78:16–28.
32. Furesz J, Scheifele DW, Palkonyay L. Safety and effectiveness of the new, inactivated hepatitis A virus vaccine. *Can Med Assoc J.* 1995;152:343–8.
33. Margolis HS, Alter MJ. Will hepatitis A become a vaccine-preventable disease? *Ann Intern Med.* 1995;122: 464–5.
34. Harrison LH, Tajkowski C, Croll J, *et al.* Postlicensure effectiveness of the *Haemophilus influenzae* type b polysaccharide—*Neisseria meningiditis* outer-membrane protein complex conjugate vaccine among Navajo children. *J Pediatr.* 1994;125:571–6.
35. Peltola H, Kayhty H, Virtanen M. Prevention of *H. influenzae* type b bacteremic infections with the capsular polysaccharide vaccine. *N Engl J Med.* 1984;310:1566–9.
36. Kayhty H, Karanko V, Peltola H, *et al.* Serum antibodies after vaccination with *H. influenzae* type b capsular polysaccharide and responses to reimmunization: no evidence of immunologic tolerance or memory. *Pediatrics* 1984;74: 857–65.
37. Insel RA, Anterson P, Pichichero ME, *et al.* Anticapsular antibody to *H. influenzae* type b. In: Sell SH, Wright PF, editors. *Haemophilus influenzae: Epidemiology, Immunology, and Prevention of Disease.* New York: Elsevier; 1982. p. 155–68.
38. Granoff DM, Shackelford PG, Suarex BK, *et al. Haemophilus influenzae* type b disease in children vaccinated with type b polysaccharide vaccine. *N Engl J Med.* 1986;315:1583–90.
39. Shapiro ED. New vaccines against *Haemophilus influenzae* type b. *Pediatr Clin North Am.* 1990;37:567–82.
40. Ward J. Newer *Haemophilus influenzae* type b vaccines and passive prophylaxis. *Pediatr Infect Dis J.* 1987;6:799–803.
41. Eskola J, Petola H, Takala AK, *et al.* Efficacy of *Haemophilus influenzae* type b polysaccharide-diphtheria toxoid conjugate vaccine in infancy. *N Engl J Med.* 1987;317:717–22.
42. Ward J, Brenneman G, Letson GW, *et al.* Limited efficacy of a *Haemophilus influenzae* type b conjugate vaccine in Alaska Native infants. *N Engl J Med.* 1990;323:1393–401.
43. Centers for Disease Control, Advisory Committee on Immunization Practices. *Haemophilus* b conjugate vaccines for prevention of *Haemophilus influenzae* type b disease among infants and children two months of age and older. *MMWR* 1991;40(RR-1):1–7.
44. Black SB, Shinefield HR, Fireman B, *et al.* Efficacy in infancy of oligosaccharide conjugate *Haemophilus influenzae* type B (HbOC) vaccine in a United States population of 61080 children. *Pediatr Infect Dis J.* 1991;10:97–104.
45. [Anonymous]. *H. influenzae* vaccine for infants. *Med Lett.* 1991;33(836):5–7.
46. Singleton RJ, Davidson NM, Desmet IJ, *et al.* Decline of *Haemophilus influenzae* type b disease in a region of high risk: impact of passive and active immunization. *Pediatr Infect Dis J.* 1994;13:362–7.
47. Greenberg DP, Lieberman JM, Marcy SM, *et al.* Enhanced antibody responses in infants given different sequences of heterogenous *Haemophilus influenzae* type b conjugate vaccines. *J Pediatr.* 1995;126:206–11.
48. Greenberg DP, Vadheim CM, Partridge S, *et al.* Immunogenicity of *Haemophilus influenzae* type b tetanus toxoid conjugate vaccine in young infants. *J Infect Dis.* 1994;170:76–81.
49. Murphy TV, Pastor P, Medley F, Osterholm MT, Granoff DM. Decreased *Haemophilus* colonization in children vaccinated with *Haemophilus influenzae* type b conjugate vaccine. *J Pediatr.* 1993;122:517–23.
50. Bureau of Communicable Diseases and Epidemiology, Canada. Canadian Communicable Disease Report. Supplementary statement on newly licensed *Haemophilus influenzae* type b conjugate vaccines in combination with other vaccines recommended for infants. *Can Med Assoc J.* 1995;152:527–9.
51. Gold R, Scheifele D, Barreto L, *et al.* Safety and immunogenicity of *Haemophilus influenzae* vaccine (tetanus toxoid conjugate) administered concurrently or combined with diphtheria and tetanus toxoids, pertussis vaccine and inactivated poliomyelitis vaccine to healthy infants at two, four and six months of age. *Pediatr Infect Dis J.* 1994;13: 348–55.
52. Dagan R, Botujansky C, Watemberg N, *et al.* Safety and immunogenicity in young infants of *Haemophilus* b-tetanus protein conjugated vaccine, mixed in the same syringe with diptheria-tetanus-pertussis-enhanced inactivated polio vaccine. *Pediatr Infect Dis J.* 1994;13:356–61.
53. Committee on Infectious Diseases of the American Academy of Pediatrics. Universal hepatitis B immunization. *Pediatrics* 1992;89:795–800.
54. Centers for Disease Control, Advisory Committee on Immunization Practices. Update of hepatitis B prevention. *MMWR* 1987;36:353–66.

55. Centers for Disease Control, Advisory Committee on Immunization Practices. Protection against viral hepatitis. *MMWR* 1990;39:1–26.
56. Zahradink JM, Couch RB, Gerin JL. Safety and immunogenicity of a purified hepatitis B virus vaccine prepared by using recombinant DNA technology. *J Infect Dis*. 1987;155:903–8.
57. Goudeau A, Denis F, Mounier M, *et al.* Comparative multicentre study of the immunogenicity of different hepatitis B vaccines in health volunteers. *Postgrad Med J.* 1987;63(*Suppl* 2):125–8.
58. Just M, Berger R, Just V. Reactogenicity and immunogenicity of a recombinant hepatitis B vaccine compared with a plasma-derived vaccine in young adults. *Postgrad Med J.* 1987;63(*Suppl* 2):121–3.
59. Zajac BA, West DJ, McAleer WJ, *et al.* Overview of clinical studies with hepatitis B vaccine made by recombinant DNA. *J Infect Dis.*1986;13(*Suppl* A):39–45.
60. Stevens CE, Taylor PE, Tong MJ, *et al.* Yeast-recombinant hepatitis B vaccine: efficacy with hepatitis B immune globulin in prevention of perinatal hepatitis B virus transmission. *JAMA* 1987;257:2612–16.
61. Young JF, Hockmeyer WT, Gross M, *et al.* Expression of *Plasmodium falciparum* circumsporozoite proteins in *Escherichia coli* for potential use in a human malaria vaccine. *Science* 1985;228:958–62.
62. Ballou WR, Sherwood JA, Neva FA, *et al.* Safety and efficacy of a recombinant DNA *Plasmodium falciparum* sporozoite vaccine. *Lancet* 1987;1:1277–81.
63. Lerner RA. Synthetic vaccines. *Sci Am.* 1983;248:66–74.
64. Zavala F, Tam JP, Hollingdale MR, *et al.* Rationale for development of a synthetic vaccine against *Plasmodium falciparum* malaria. *Science* 1985;228:1436–40.
65. Herrington DA, Clyde DF, Losonsky M, *et al.* Safety and immunogenicity in man of a synthetic peptide malaria vaccine against *Plasmodium falciparum* sporozoites. *Nature* 1987;328:257–9.
66. Alonso PL, Smith T, Armstrong-Schellenberg JRM, *et al.* Randomised trial of efficacy of Spf66 vaccine against *Plasmodium falciparum* malaria in children in southern Tanzania. *Lancet* 1994;344:1175–81.
67. White NJ. Tough test for malaria vaccine. *Lancet* 1994;344:1172–3.
68. Nuzzenzweig RS, Long CA. Malaria vaccines: multiple targets. *Science* 1994;265:1381–3.
69. Fields BN, Chanock RB. What biotechnology has to offer vaccine development. *Rev Infect Dis.* 1989;11(*Suppl* 3):S519–S523.
70. Levine MM, Kaper JB, Herrington D, *et al.* Safety, immunogenicity, and efficacy of recombinant live oral cholera vaccines, CVD 103 and CVD 103-HgR. *Lancet* 1988;2: 467–70.
71. Mekalanos JJ, Sadoff JC. Cholera vaccines: fighting an ancient scourge. *Science* 1994;265:1387–9.
72. Levine MM, Herrington D, Murphy JR, *et al.* Safety, infectivity, immunogenicity, and in vivo stability of two attenuated auxotrophic mutant strains of *Salmonella typhi*, 541Ty and 543Ty, live oral vaccines in humans. *J Clin Invest.* 1987;79:888–902.
73. Paoletti E, Perkus ME, Piccini A, *et al.* Vaccinia vectored vaccines. In: Quinnan GV Jr., editor. *Vaccinia Viruses as Vectors for Vaccine Antigens.* New York: Elsevier; 1985. p. 137–51.
74. Karzon DT. Considerations of safety, efficacy and potential applications of vaccinia vectors for immunoprophylaxis: an alternative approach for control of human diseases for which vaccines are available. In: Quinnan GV Jr., editor. *Vaccinia Viruses as Vectors for Vaccine Antigens.* New York: Elsevier; 1985. p. 231–36.
75. Perkus ME, Piccini BR, Lipinskas BR, *et al.* Recombinant vaccinia virus: immunization against multiple pathogens. *Science* 1985;229:981–4.
76. Rabinovich NR, McInnes P, Klein DL, *et al.* Vaccine technologies: view to the future. *Science* 1994;265:1401–4.
77. Arnon R. Synthetic vaccines. In: Roitt IM, editor. *Immune Intervention: New Trends in Vaccines.* London: Academic; 1984. p. 93–116.
78. Adam A, Lederer E. Muramyl dipeptides and analogues. In: Bell R, Torrigiani G, editors. *Progress Towards Better Vaccines.* New York: Oxford University Press [on behalf of the World Health Organization]; 1986. p. 185–203.
79. Lambert PH. Anti-idiotypic vaccines. In: Bell R, Torrigiani G, editors. *Progress Towards Better Vaccines.* New York: Oxford University Press [on behalf of the World Health Organization]; 1986. p. 89–96.
80. Sacks DL, Esser KM, Sher A. Immunization of mice against African Trypanosomiasis using anti-idiotypic antibodies. *J Exp Med.* 1982;155:1108–19.
81. Roitt I. *Essential Immunology.* 6th ed. Oxford, UK: Blackwell Scientific, 1987.
82. Sell S. *Immunology, Immunopathology and Immunity.* 3rd ed. Hagerstown, MD: Harper & Row; 1980.
83. Rose RR, Milgrom F, van Oss CJ, editors. *Principles of Immunology.* 2nd ed. New York: Macmillan; 1979.
84. Dienstag JL. Passive-active immunoprophylaxis after percutaneous exposure to hepatitis B virus. *Hepatology* 1989; 10:385–7.
85. American Hospital Formulary Service. *Drug Information 90.* Bethesda, MD: American Society of Health-System Pharmacists; 1997. p. 2530–36.
86. Centers for Disease Control, Advisory Committee on Immunization Practices. Adult immunization: recommendations of the ACIP. *MMWR* 1989;38:205–14, 219–27.
87. Centers for Disease Control, Advisory Committee on Immunization Practices. Varicella-zoster immune globulin for the prevention of chicken pox: recommendations of the ACIP. *Ann Intern Med.* 1984;100:859–65.
88. Feldman S, Lott L. Varicella in children with cancer; impact of antiviral treatment and prophylaxis. *Pediatrics* 1987;80:465–72.
89. Kastrup EK, editor. *Drug Facts & Comparisons.* St. Louis, MO: JB Lippincott; 1997. p. 445a–448h.
90. Bialecki C, Feder HM. Questions and controversies about varicella-zoster infections. *Hosp Pract.* 1989;24(3A):21–32.
91. Massachusetts Public Health Biologic Labs [MPHBL]. *Product Information: Varicella Zoster Immune Globulin (Human).* Boston, MA: MPHBL; 1997.
92. Skvaril F, Gardi A. Differences among available immunoglobulin preparations for intravenous use. *Pediatr Infect Dis J.* 1988;7(5S):S43–S48.
93. Knapp MJ, Colburn PA. Clinical uses of intravenous im-

mune globulin. *Clin Pharm*. 1990;9:509–29.
94. Gordon DS. Intravenous immunoglobulin: a historical perspective. *Am J Med*. 1987;83(4A):1–2.
95. Hansen LA, Soderstrom R, Avanzini A, *et al*. Immunoglobulin subclass deficiency. *Pediatr Infect Dis J*. 1988;7(5S):S17–21.
96. Aucouturier P, Lacombe C, Bremard C, *et al*. Serum IgG subclass levels in patients with primary immunodeficiency syndromes or abnormal susceptibility to infections. *Clin Immunol Immunopathol*. 1989;51:22–37.
97. Soderstrom T, Soderstrom R, Avanzini A, *et al*. Immunoglobulin G subclass deficiencies. *Int Arch Allergy Appl Immunol*. 1987;82:476–80.
98. Burckhardt JJ, Gardi A, Oxelius V, *et al*. Immunoglobulin G subclass distribution in three human intravenous immunoglobulin preparations. *Vox Sang*. 1989;57:10–14.
99. Lundblad JL, Londeree N, Mitra G. Characterization of various intravenous immunoglobulin preparations. *J Infect Dis*.1987;15(S1):3–12.
100. Eibl MM, Leibl H, Mannhalter JW. IgG subclass distribution in intravenous immunoglobulin preparations [letter]. *J Infect Dis*.1988;17:271–6.
101. Heiner DC. Significance of immunoglobulin (IgG) subclasses. *Am J Med*. 1984;76(3A):1–6.
102. [Anonymous]. *Immunofacts: Vaccines and Immunologic Drugs*. Saint Louis, MO: Facts and Comparisons; 1996. p. 8–16.
103. Klemola T. Deficiency of immunoglobulin A. *Ann Clin Res*. 1987;19:248–57.
104. Burks AW, Sampson HA, Buckley RH. Anaphylactic reactions after gamma globulin administration in patients with hypogammaglobulinemia. *N Engl J Med*. 1986;314:560–4.
105. Bjorkander J, Hammarstrom L, Smith CI, *et al*. Immunoglobulin prophylaxis in patients with antibody deficiency syndrome and anti-IgA antibodies. *J Clin Immunol*. 1987;7:8–15.
106. ASHP Commission on Therapeutics. ASHP therapeutic guidelines for intravenous immunoglobulin. *Clin Pharm*. 1992;11:117–36.
107. Centers for Diseases Control. Outbreak of hepatitis C associated with intravenous immunoglobulin administration—United States, October 1993–June 1994. *MMWR* 1994;43:505–9.
108. So A, Brenner MK, Hill ID, *et al*. Intravenous gamma globulin treatment in patients with hypogammaglobulinemia. *Br Med J*. 1984;289:1171–8.
109. Dwyer JM. Manipulating the immune system with immune globulin. *N Engl J Med*. 1992;326:107–16.
110. Buckley RH, Schiff RI. The use of intravenous immune globulin in immunedeficiency diseases. *N Engl J Med*. 1993;325:110–7.
111. Weeks JC, Tierny MR, Weinstein MC. Cost effectiveness of prophylactic intravenous immunoglobulin in chronic lymphocytic leukemia. *N Engl J Med*. 1991;325:81–6.
112. Arav-Boger R, Assia A, Jurgenson U, Spirer Z. The immunology of Kawasaki disease. *Adv Pediatr Infect Dis*. 1994;41:359–67.
113. [Anonymous]. FDA approves marketing of CMVIG. *Clin Pharm*. 1990;9:493.
114. Winston DJ, Pollard RB, Ho WG, *et al*. Cytomegalovirus immune plasma in bone marrow transplant recipients. *Ann Intern Med*. 1982;97:11–8.
115. Sullivan KM, Kopecky KJ, Jocom J, *et al*. Immunomodulatory and antimicrobial efficacy of IVIG in bone marrow transplantation. *N Engl J Med*. 1990;323:705–12.
116. Weimar W, Metselaar HJ, Balk A, *et al*. Passive immunization to prevent CMV disease after kidney and heart transplantation. *Transplant Proc*. 1990;22:229–32.
117. Snydman DR. CMVIG in the prevention and treatment of CMV disease. *Rev Infect Dis*. 1990;12(S7):S839–48.
118. Meyers JD. Prevention of CMV infection after marrow transplantation. *Rev Infect Dis*. 1989;11(S7):S1691–703.
119. Bailey TC. IVIG to prevent graft-versus-host disease after bone marrow transplantation [letter]. *N Engl J Med*. 1990;324:631–2.
120. Bass Eb, Powe NR, Goodman SN, *et al*. Efficacy of immune globulin in preventing complication of bone marrow transplantation: a meta analysis. *Bone Marrow Transplant*. 1993;12:273–82.

SELF-ASSESSMENT QUESTIONS

1. Which of the following is another term for active immunization?
   a. secondary response
   b. serotherapy
   c. vaccination
   d. variolation

2. The utility of vaccination is based on which of the following principles?
   a. Endogenous antigen will combine with endogenous antibody to prevent disease.
   b. Endogenous antigen will combine with exogenous antibody to prevent disease.
   c. Exogenous antigen will combine with endogenous antibody to prevent disease.
   d. Exogenous antigen will combine with exogenous antibody to prevent disease.

3. Injection of measles virus to prevent measles would best be described as:
   a. attenuation.
   b. passive immunization.
   c. vaccination.
   d. variolation.

4. Possible risks associated with vaccination include all of the following *except*:
   a. allergic reaction.
   b. encephalitis.
   c. excessive antibody production.
   d. possible development of the disease.

5. Which of the following sequelae followed the 1976 swine flu vaccination program?

   a. allergic reactions
   b. cancer
   c. encephalitis
   d. Guillain-Barré syndrome.

6. An example of a currently available attenuated vaccine is:

   a. diphtheria toxoid.
   b. oral polio vaccine.
   c. pertussis vaccine.
   d. pneumococcal vaccine.

7. Characteristics of inactive vaccines include:

   a. a requirement for smaller doses than those necessary with attenuated vaccines.
   b. ability to revert to pathogenic variant.
   c. long-lasting immunity following a single dose.
   d. the need for multiple injections.

8. Methods of attenuation include:

   a. chemical treatment with formalin.
   b. passage at suboptimal temperatures.
   c. purification of toxoids.
   d. all of the above.

9. Which of the following is true regarding the vaccines for *Haemophilus influenzae*?

   a. The surface component for polyribosylribitol phosphate–diphtheria toxoid (PRP-D) is composed of 23 capsular polysaccharides.
   b. All of the conjugated vaccines can be administered to infants.
   c. This conjugated vaccine is more immunogenic than the unconjugated form.
   d. These vaccines are examples of genetically engineered, attenuated vaccines.

10. The recombinant hepatitis B vaccine:

   a. is an attenuated vaccine.
   b. is an example of a subunit vaccine.
   c. is more immunogenic than the plasma vaccine.
   d. may be capable of transmitting HIV infection.

11. Which of the following is not true of malaria vaccines?

   a. Protection against multiple antigens will probably be necessary for an effective vaccine.
   b. Protective antibody has been demonstrated with subunit vaccines.
   c. The circumsporozite (CS) protein has been cloned into vaccinia.
   d. Traditional strategies to develop inactivated vaccines are conducive to malaria vaccine production.

12. Recombinant vaccinia vaccines:

   a. are likely to cause encephalitis.
   b. are not likely to have advantages over traditional vaccination strategies.
   c. are not likely to stimulate an immune reaction in a previously vaccinated host.
   d. may contain more than one foreign antigen.

13. Which of the following is not true of varicella?

   a. Varicella vaccine is associated with higher rates of zoster in leukemic children than natural disease.
   b. Varicella disease is generally more severe in adults and immunocompromised persons.
   c. Breakthrough varicella disease after vaccination is milder.
   d. Children achieve a higher seroconversion rate with varicella vaccine.

14. Which of the following is another term for passive immunization?

   a. secondary response
   b. serotherapy
   c. vaccination
   d. variolation

15. Which of the following agents has a human source?

   a. black widow spider bite
   b. botulism
   c. diphtheria
   d. tetanus

16. Immune globulins for prophylaxis or treatment are available for all of the following viral diseases *except*:

   a. AIDS
   b. measles
   c. rabies
   d. varicella-zoster

17. Intravenous immune globulins (IVIGs) have been used to treat all of the following *except*:

   a. chronic lymphocytic leukemia
   b. diphtheria
   c. hypogammaglobulinemia
   d. idiopathic thrombocytopenic purpura

18. Which of the following is most likely to help in decreasing the incidence of side effects associated with IVIG administration?

    a. increasing the IV infusion rate
    b. premedicating the patient
    c. switching from IgG to IgA administration
    d. switching to another IVIG product

19. Which one of the following statements regarding IgG subclasses is not true?

    a. All IVIG products should closely match the World Health Organization's reference plasma.
    b. IgG subclass distribution in IVIG products should closely resemble that in normal serum.
    c. Older IVIG products caused recurrent infections because of an excess of IgG4.
    d. The functions of IgG2 and IgG4 appear to be closely linked.

CHAPTER 7

Immunology of HIV Infection and AIDS

Bonnie D. Purdy, Pharm.D.
AIDS Clinical Specialist
Albany Medical Center
Albany, NY

Karen I. Plaisance, Pharm.D.
Associate Professor
Department of Pharmacy Practice and Science
University of Maryland School of Pharmacy
Baltimore, MD

HIV Infection ... 117
Etiology ... 117
Viral Replicative Cycle ... 117
Immunopathogenesis ... 119
Transmission ... 121
Sexual Exposure ... 121
Parenteral Exposure ... 122
Intravenous Drug Use ... 122
Blood Transfusion, Organ Exposure, and Artificial Insemination ... 122
Occupational Exposure ... 122
Perinatal Exposure ... 123
Routes Not Associated with HIV Transmission ... 123
Prevention ... 123
Sexual Transmission ... 123
Parenteral Transmission ... 123
Perinatal Transmission ... 124
HIV Testing ... 124
Antibody Testing ... 124
Enzyme-Linked Immunosorbent Assay ... 124
Western Blot ... 125
Other Assays ... 125
p24 Antigen Assay ... 125
HIV Culture ... 125
Polymerase Chain Reaction ... 125
Quantitation of HIV RNA ... 126
Home Testing Kits ... 126
Saliva and Urine Tests ... 126

Spectrum of Disease ... 126
Acute Infection ... 126
Asymptomatic Infection ... 127
Persistent Generalized Lymphadenopathy ... 127
AIDS: CDC Clinical Definition ... 127
Opportunistic Infections ... 128
Pneumocystis carinii Pneumonia ... 128
Cryptococcal Meningitis ... 129
Toxoplasmosis ... 129
Mycobacterium avium Complex and *Mycobacterium tuberculosis* ... 129
Candidiasis ... 129
Herpesvirus ... 129
Neoplasms ... 130
Kaposi's Sarcoma ... 130
Non-Hodgkin's Lymphoma ... 130
Treatment Approaches for HIV Infection ... 130
Antiviral Therapy ... 130
Inhibitors of Viral Binding ... 130
Reverse Transcriptase Inhibitors ... 131
Non-nucleoside Reverse Transcriptase Inhibitors ... 132
Development of Antiretroviral Resistance ... 132
Protease (Proteinase) and Integrase Inhibitors ... 133
Late Stages of Viral Replication ... 133
Combination Therapy ... 133
Immunologic Therapy ... 133
Immune Replacement ... 134
Bone Marrow Transplantation ... 134
Autologous $CD8^+$ T-Cell Transfusions ... 134
Intravenous Immune Globulin and Passive Immunotherapy ... 134
Immune Enhancement ... 134
Therapeutic Immunization ... 135
Cytokines ... 135
Ampligen ... 136
Immune Suppression ... 136
Cyclosporine ... 137
Corticosteroids ... 137
Cytokine Modulation ... 137
Other Host-Directed Therapies ... 137
Vaccine Development ... 138
Developmental Considerations ... 138
Vaccine Approaches ... 139
Human Trials ... 139
Summary ... 139
References ... 140
Self-Assessment Questions ... 147

Since its recognition in 1981, acquired immunodeficiency syndrome (AIDS) has affected a substantial portion of the U.S. population. As of December 1996, over 581,000 cases of AIDS had been reported in the United States alone, largely reflecting infections that occurred during the 1970s and 1980s.[1] Of the cases of AIDS reported to the Centers for Disease Control and Prevention (CDC), over 60% have resulted in death.[1] In January 1993, it was estimated that between 630,000 and 897,000 adults and adolescents in the United States were living with human immunodeficiency virus (HIV) infection.[2] The World Health Organization (WHO) estimates that, as of 1992, 8 to 10 million adults were infected with HIV worldwide and at least 1 million children were born with the infection. The WHO also estimates that, by the year 2000, 30 to 40 million will be infected worldwide, with 90% of infections occurring in developing countries.[3]

As accessible members of the health care profession, pharmacists can play an important role in educating their communities and patients about HIV infection. In practice, pharmacists may be asked to advise individuals about high-risk behaviors, risk-reduction strategies, and the appropriateness of HIV testing. Pharmacists may serve in a different capacity by advising AIDS patients about adverse drug reactions, drug interactions, and the potential of investigational treatment strategies. This chapter will highlight the immunologic aspects of HIV infection and discuss its etiology, pathogenesis, transmission, prevention, clinical manifestations, and treatment. With such a background, pharmacists should be able to provide sound counsel, not only to HIV-infected patients, but to the communities in which they live. After completing this chapter, the reader should be able to:

1. Describe the pathogenesis of HIV infection.
2. Discuss the modes of transmission of HIV.
3. Identify the stages of the viral replicative cycle that have potential for antiviral attack.
4. Discuss the use of immunomodulators in the treatment of HIV infection.
5. Identify various approaches to the development of AIDS vaccines.

HIV INFECTION

The first part of this chapter will review the etiology of HIV infection and AIDS; a discussion of the viral replicative cycle and the immunopathogenesis of HIV infection follows. Finally, the modes of transmission and potential means of prevention of HIV infection will be summarized.

Etiology

HIV was first isolated in 1983 by groups in the United States and France.[4,5] The virus is believed to have been present for several decades in localized areas of central Africa and has since spread extensively throughout both developed and undeveloped countries.

HIV type 1 (HIV-1), the predominant type of HIV in the United States, is related to a group of nontransforming cytopathic retroviruses.[6] It is very closely related to a simian immunodeficiency virus (SIV) that causes a form of simian AIDS with encephalitis.[7] HIV type 2 (HIV-2), relatively uncommon in the United States, causes an immunodeficiency syndrome similar to AIDS.[8] Isolates of HIV-2 appear to be more closely related, both antigenically and genetically, to SIV than to HIV-1.[7,9] There is cross-reactivity between the core proteins of HIV-1 and HIV-2, but the envelope glycoproteins are not cross-reactive.[7,9]

Globally, there are at least three epidemiologic patterns of HIV infection. Both the timing of the introduction of HIV into the population and the relative frequency of various routes of transmission in that population differentiate these patterns.[10]

In the first pattern, prevalent in developed countries with large numbers of AIDS cases (e.g., those in North America and Western Europe), HIV began to spread extensively through the population in the late 1970s and continues to spread through this population even today. Although the majority of cases in this population occur in homosexual or bisexual males and intravenous drug users (IVDUs), heterosexual and perinatal transmission is increasing.

The second pattern occurs primarily in central, eastern, and southern Africa and the Caribbean basin. HIV also began to spread through this population in the late 1970s. However, in contrast to the first pattern, the majority of AIDS cases in this population occur in heterosexuals, and perinatal transmission is frequent. Transmission through intravenous drug use or homosexual activity is virtually absent.

A third pattern of HIV infection is prominent in Eastern Europe and Asia. HIV was introduced into these populations in the early to mid-1980s, presumably through travel to or contact with individuals from countries with one of the other patterns of infection. Only recently has transmission through indigenous homosexual and heterosexual practices and intravenous drug use been documented.

The impact of the AIDS epidemic is partially reflected by the increase in adult mortality. Over 50,000 people with AIDS died in the United States in 1995 alone.[1] In 1993, HIV became a leading cause of death among people between 25 and 44 years old.[11]

More than 80,000 cases of AIDS-related conditions were reported to the CDC in 1994. As shown in Table 7-1, a larger proportion of cases occurred among women, racial and ethnic minorities, and children than in 1993. The largest decline in AIDS-related conditions was reported among homosexual and bisexual men. Of the 1017 cases occurring in children in 1994, 92% were infected through perinatal transmission, and most of the children were black (62%) or Hispanic (23%).[11] Furthermore, it is estimated that 1 in 50 black men between the ages of 18 and 59 are infected with HIV.[2]

Viral Replicative Cycle

As demonstrated in Figure 7-1, infection with HIV begins when the envelope glycoprotein of HIV, gp120, binds to the CD4 receptor of helper T cells and other types of cells (e.g., monocytes and macrophages, glial cells, gut epithelium, and bone marrow progenitors).[12] The virus is then internalized and uncoated. The precise mechanism by which the virus enters the cell has not yet been clearly established; however, the most recent evidence suggests that virus-mediated membrane fusion appears to be the

Table 7-1. Characteristics of Reported AIDS Cases in the United States, 1993–1994[11]

CHARACTERISTIC	1993 (%)	1994 (%)
Sex		
Male	83.8	81.9
Female	16.2	18.1
Race/Ethnicity		
White	45.1	41.1
Black, non-Hispanic	36.1	39.0
Hispanic	17.7	18.7
HIV exposure		
Homosexual/bisexual men	47.3	43.3
History of intravenous drug use		
Women/heterosexual men	28	27
Homosexual/bisexual men	6.2	4.8
Heterosexual contact	9.2	10.3
Transfusion	1.1	1.2
Perinatal	0.8	1.2

AIDS, acquired immunodeficiency syndrome; HIV, human immunodeficiency virus.

dominant pathway of entry.[13,14]

With uncoating of the viral envelope, viral genomic ribonucleic acid (RNA) and the enzyme reverse transcriptase are released into the cytoplasm. The genomic RNA is then transcribed by the viral reverse transcriptase to proviral deoxyribonucleic acid (DNA). The proviral DNA either remains in the cytoplasm in linear or circularized form or integrates into the host's chromosomal DNA. Large amounts of unintegrated viral DNA can accumulate inside the infected cell. If the viral DNA is integrated into the host's chromosomal DNA, restricted gene expression allows the virus to remain in a latent phase until the cell is activated.[15] During clinical latency, the intracellular virus is protected from removal by the host's immune system.[16] However, recent evidence indicates that the virus is not truly latent.[17] Dur-

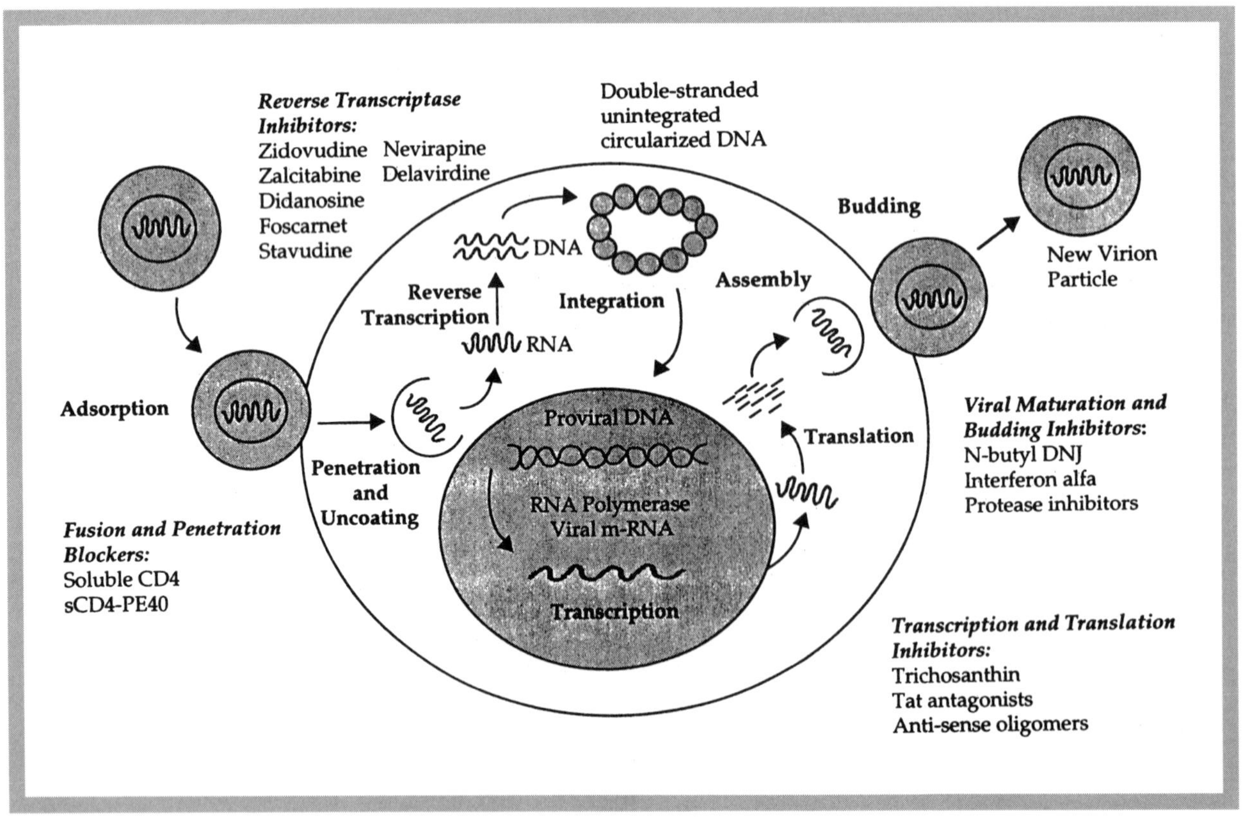

Figure 7-1. Replicative cycle of human immunodeficiency virus (HIV). *N*-butyl DNJ, *N*-butyldeoxynojirimycin.

SOURCE: *©1994, Courtney V. Fletcher. Used with permission.*

ing this time, there is persistent chronic viral replication within the germinal center of the lymph nodes, which eventually leads to depletion of CD4⁺ T lymphocytes and progression of disease.

When the infected cell is activated, the proviral DNA is transcribed into viral genomic RNA and messenger RNA (mRNA). Translation of this mRNA results in the formation of viral proteins. After protein modification and assembly of the viral proteins and genomic RNA, a mature virion is released by budding.[15]

With viral replication and release, the CD4⁺ T lymphocyte is usually killed. This cytopathic effect may result from the accumulation of large amounts of unintegrated DNA, the presence of high levels of viral RNA and aberrant RNAs in the cytoplasm, or the weakening of the cellular membrane during budding of the mature virion.[18] In addition, cell-to-cell fusion and syncytia formation result in the cytolysis of both infected and uninfected cells. These mechanisms may contribute to the disproportionate quantitative deficiency in CD4⁺ T cells relative to the number of cells actually infected.[15] An inappropriate induction of apoptosis (programmed cell death) in CD4⁺ T lymphocytes may also play a role in CD4⁺ T-cell depletion.[17]

Immunopathogenesis

Acute HIV infection is associated with active replication of the virus and, consequently, high levels of plasma viremia. It is during this time that dissemination of the virus to lymphatic tissue and the central nervous system occurs. In addition, the circulating population of CD4⁺ T cells transiently declines. Within the first few weeks to months, both cellular and humoral responses are observed, and the infected patient enters a period of clinical latency. This phase is characterized by a lack of symptoms, a minor reduction in circulating CD4⁺ T cells, and low levels of virus in the blood. It has recently been shown through sensitive molecular and histopathologic methods that the viral burden in lymphatic tissue during this period of clinical latency is high. HIV replicates persistently, even during the asymptomatic phase.[19] These events are depicted in Figure 7-2. These data suggest that high levels of viral burden are present from the start of HIV infection and that both the quantity of virus as well as the intensity of viral replication increase as HIV infection progresses. Although the depletion of CD4⁺ T cells may be attributable in part to indirect effects triggered by the virus, it is clear that active replication within CD4⁺ T cells is the primary force behind CD4⁺ T-cell loss. Mechanisms that may contribute to the quantitative and qualitative dysfunction of CD4⁺ T lymphocytes are summarized in Table 7-2.[19]

By studying the effects of potent inhibitors of viral replication on viral load, as measured by sensitive assays of HIV RNA, an understanding of HIV dynamics has

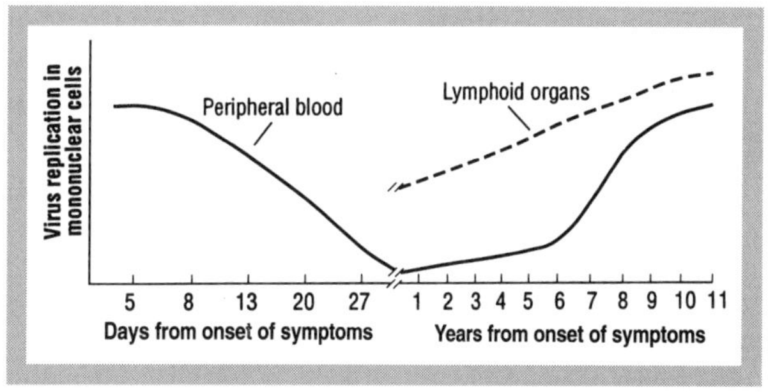

Figure 7-2. HIV replication in peripheral blood and lymph nodes

SOURCE: *Reprinted with permission from Fauci AS. Multifactorial nature of human immunodeficiency virus disease: implications for therapy.* Science *1993;262:1011–8.*

emerged. The life span of plasma virus and virus-producing cells is short, with a half-life of approximately two days. Viral clearance appears to be independent of the stage of disease. Potent antiretroviral drugs may decrease plasma viremia by an average of 98.5–99%.[20,21] The majority of circulating virus must therefore be the result of newly infected cells, not chronically or latently infected cells. Assuming first-order kinetics, to sustain a steady-state viremia of 10^2–10^7 virions/ml, 30% or more of the total plasma viral population must be replaced daily. In patients studied, the rate of CD4⁺ T-cell turnover was approximately 10^9 cells/day.[20,21] The observation that CD4⁺ T-cell counts increase following initiation of antiretrovirals is consistent with a continuous and brisk recruitment of CD4⁺ T cells into a rapidly cleared virus-expressing pool. It is likely that the decline in CD4⁺ T cells over time reflects destruction, not lack of production. This unrelenting cycle of new infection, viral replication, and rapid cell death may be the key dynamic driving HIV pathogenesis.[20,21]

Table 7-2. Potential Mechanisms of CD4⁺ T-Cell Dysfunction[17]

Direct HIV-induced cytolysis
HIV-mediated syncytia formation
Immune response Tc, NK cells, ADCC
Autoimmune mechanisms
Anergy
Superantigen-induced expansion of highly specific T cells followed by anergy
Apoptosis

Tc, cytotoxic T cells; NK, natural killer; ADCC, antibody-dependent cell-mediated cytotoxicity.

Normally, when an infectious pathogen is encountered, the immune response triggers both humoral and cellular factors, the pathogen is eliminated, and the immune system restores itself to its resting state. Because HIV is persistently replicating, the normal return to quiescence is not observed, and the immune system enters a state of chronic activation. Evidence of persistent activation of the various components of the immune system is detailed in Table 7-3.[19]

Chronic stimulation of the immune system contributes to the immunopathogenesis of HIV infection. Although resting $CD4^+$ T cells may be infected with HIV, the processes necessary for the replication of HIV are enhanced within activated cells. In addition, persistent antigenic exposure may cause the immune system to lose adequate response to either the initiating antigen or new antigens. Normal destruction of corrupt cells through apoptosis is closely associated with cell activation. The chronic activation of the immune system caused by HIV may result in inappropriate induction of apoptosis, leading to the destruction of large numbers of uninfected lymphocytes exposed to viral antigens in the lymphoid microenvironment.[19]

There is a progressive diminution over time in the number of circulating $CD4^+$ T cells at a modal rate of approximately 30–50 cells/µl over six months.[22] This loss of $CD4^+$ T cells is accompanied by disruption of nodal architecture and resurgence of plasma viremia. The median time of progression to AIDS is 10 years.[17] On the basis of observational studies, however, it is estimated that 10–17% of HIV-infected individuals will be AIDS-free for as long as 20 years following infection.[22] The contribution of viral attenuation[23] or differential immune responsiveness[24] to nonprogressive infection remains to be determined. It is likely that control of HIV infection is multifactorial. It is unclear whether this control in these long-term survivors will eventually result in clearance of the infection or if the control is transient, albeit prolonged, with infection ultimately progressing to AIDS. Clearance of HIV infection has been reported. An infant perinatally infected with HIV had both culture and HIV DNA evidence of infection at days 19 and 51, but by 12 months of age, however, the infant appeared to have cleared the infection. Numerous attempts at virus isolation by culture and polymerase chain reaction have failed to demonstrate any evidence of HIV infection over four years of follow-up study.[25]

Table 7-3. Evidence for Activation of the Immune System in HIV Infection[19]

Spontaneous hyperactivation of B cells
Spontaneous lymphocyte proliferation
Activation of monocytes
Expression of T-cell activation antigens on $CD4^+$ ($CD25^+$, DR^+) and $CD8^+$ cells
Lymph node hyperplasia
Increased cytokine expression
Elevated neopterin, β_2-microglobulin, acid-labile interferon, IL-2 receptors
Autoimmune manifestations

IL, interleukin.

The hallmark of the immunodeficiency found in patients infected with HIV is a quantitative deficiency of T lymphocytes bearing the CD4 receptor, resulting in an imbalance of the $CD4^+/CD8^+$ (helper-to-suppressor) T-cell ratio.[26] In addition to this quantitative deficiency, functional abnormalities exist, including the inability to respond to soluble antigen (e.g., tetanus toxoid), impaired proliferative responses, and abnormalities in lymphokine production.[27–29] The proliferative responses of lymphocytes not expressing the CD4 marker may also be suppressed.[29] Other functional defects in cellular immunity include impaired natural killer cell and cytomegalovirus (CMV)-specific cytotoxicity responses.[30] As the cellular response is progressively suppressed, the patient becomes increasingly susceptible to the development of opportunistic infections and tumors.

Helper T cells play a critical role in the regulation of the immune system; therefore, even a selective dysfunction of this cell type would be expected to result in impairment of all arms of the immune system. However, although helper T cells are the major target of the virus, monocytes and macrophages can also be infected with HIV.[31,32] Monocytes can engulf the virus, and some monocytes and macrophages express the CD4 receptor and can bind to the gp120 glycoprotein of HIV.[33] Monocytes and macrophages infected with HIV demonstrate defective chemotaxis and altered monokine release.[15,34] Cytokines can promote or inhibit HIV replication, both in vitro and in vivo. B cells from HIV-infected individuals spontaneously secrete large amounts of interleukin 6 (IL-6) and tumor necrosis factor alpha (TNF-α) in vitro. Because these cells are close to latently infected $CD4^+$ T cells in vivo, these cytokines may be involved in the activation of HIV in the lymph nodes.[19] Table 7-4 summarizes the effect of various cytokines on HIV replication. Monocytes and macrophages are not destroyed with replication of the virus and may serve as a reservoir for latent infection;[32] infected monocytes and macrophages probably play a major role in the dissemination of HIV infection.[32]

Dysfunction in the humoral immune system results from helper T-cell dysregulation and destruction of the follicular dendritic cell network within the germinal centers of the lymph nodes. Because this microenvironment is the primary site of antigen-dependent differentiation of B cells, the progressive disruption of its architecture

Table 7-4. Cytokine Regulation of HIV Replication[19]

CYTOKINE	TARGET CELLS	EFFECT
IL-1	T, M	I
IL-2	T	I
IL-3	M	I
IL-4	T, M	I, D
IL-6	M	I
IL-10	M	I, D
IL-13	M	D
TNF-α, -β	T, M	I
GM-CSF	M	I
IFN-α, -β	T, M	D
IFN-γ	M	I, D

T, T lymphocyte; M, monocyte or macrophage; I, increased; D, decreased; TNF, tumor necrosis factor; GM-CSF, granulocyte-macrophage colony-stimulating factor; IFN, interferon.

Table 7-5. Abnormalities in the Immune System Caused by HIV Infection

Cell-mediated abnormalities
- Quantitative decrease in the number of helper T cells
- Inability to recognize and respond to soluble antigen
- Diminished delayed-type hypersensitivity response
- Decreased lymphokine production
- Decreased NK cell activity
- Decreased cytomegalovirus-specific cytotoxicity
- Diminished ability to activate cells dependent on helper T cells

Humoral abnormalities
- Elevated serum levels of nonspecific immunoglobulin (hypergammaglobulinemia)
- Circulating immune complexes
- Inability to produce antibody to new antigens

Abnormalities in monocytes/macrophages
- Defective chemotaxis
- Increased monokine release (IL-1, TNF)
- Decreased in vitro killing of *Giardia lamblia* and *Toxoplasma gondii*

results in the inability to develop effective humoral responses.[19] Infants and children with HIV infection have had little opportunity to develop a protective humoral response against common bacterial pathogens before acquiring HIV infection, so this humoral dysfunction is particularly evident in that population. Adults also show some increased susceptibility to pyogenic infections. Anomalies of the humoral immune system include polyclonal activation, hypergammaglobulinemia, circulating immune complexes, and the formation of autoantibodies.[35] Polyclonal B-cell activation may be induced by Epstein-Barr virus, CMV, or HIV. Table 7-5 reviews the abnormalities in the various components of the immune system that result from HIV infection.

Transmission

HIV can be transmitted through sexual contact with an infected individual, through blood exposure to contaminated needles or infected blood products, or perinatally from an infected mother to her child. The virus has been isolated from essentially all body fluids, including blood, semen, vaginal fluid, tears, breast milk, and saliva.[36–39] However, transmission of the virus to a susceptible host has only been observed through blood, semen, and vaginal secretions.[40]

Sexual Exposure

In the United States, AIDS was first identified in the homosexual population, and homosexual transmission of HIV comprises a majority of the AIDS cases. A number of potential risk factors for the transmission of HIV in this setting have been evaluated. Rectal trauma was most strongly associated with HIV infection.[41] Seropositivity has been associated with both the number of sexual partners and the frequency with which the individual is the receptive partner in anal intercourse.[42,43]

Although uncommon, HIV infection through female-to-female sexual contact has been reported.[44] Trauma resulting from sexual practices may contribute to the transmission of HIV in this population.

Fundamentally, HIV infection should be considered a sexually transmitted disease that can result from either homosexual and heterosexual activity. Heterosexual transmission, first described in early 1983, may well be the predominant route of infection worldwide.[45,46]The frequency of AIDS cases in the United States due to heterosexual transmission is increasing at a faster rate than cases associated with other high-risk behaviors.[11]

Transmission occurs from male to female and, although probably less efficiently, from female to male.[47] Sexual transmission appears to be facilitated by breaks in vaginal or rectal mucosa.[48,49] Ulcerative sexually transmitted diseases, such as genital herpes simplex, chancroid, and syphilis, are significantly correlated with HIV infection, even after adjustment for numbers of sexual partners.[48]

Heterosexual transmission is more common in geographic locations with a high prevalence of intravenous drug use.[46] The reported rate of infection in the female partners of infected male IVDUs is significantly higher (48%) than that in the female partners of other index patients with AIDS (13%).[40] It may be that IVDUs are more efficient transmitters of HIV through sexual intercourse than persons with other high-risk behaviors.[48]

Parenteral Exposure

Transmission of HIV and the development of AIDS have been associated with intravenous drug use, blood and blood product transfusions, and occupational exposure.

Intravenous Drug Use

Transmission of HIV through intravenous drug use is linked to the heterosexual spread of HIV. Eighty-seven percent of heterosexually transmitted cases in New York City have occurred from a drug user to a non-drug-injecting partner.[50] Of the women acquiring HIV infection through heterosexual contact, more than 60% reported having sex with an IVDU.[51]

Infection with HIV in IVDUs appears related to the frequency of injection, the number of days using unsterilized needles, and the median number of injections in shooting galleries.[46,50] Shooting galleries are places where used drug injection equipment is rented, returned after use, and then rented to other IVDUs. Although the amount of blood remaining in any one needle is small, the syringes become contaminated with blood from many individuals.[46] Once contaminated with HIV, this equipment may infect thousands of drug users before being discarded.

Blood Transfusion, Organ Exposure, and Artificial Insemination

Receiving blood from an HIV-seropositive donor is likely to result in infection. Seroconversion was reported in approximately 89% of recipients of HIV-positive transfusions.[52,53] Several studies have found that if a donor has transmitted HIV to one transfusion recipient, all subsequent recipients of that donor's blood also seroconverted.[52,53] Seropositive recipients of HIV-infected blood develop immunologic parameters consistent with active HIV infection.[54] Lack of transmission may be related to the variation in the actual infectivity of the donor. In addition, packed red blood cells appear to have reduced infectivity when stored for more than three weeks. Therefore, the age of the product may also influence transmission.[55]

Blood donations in the United States have been screened for antibodies to HIV since early 1985; however, instances of HIV transmission from antibody-negative donations have been identified. One study investigated 13 HIV-seropositive individuals who had received blood from seven donors screened as negative for antibodies at the time of donation;[53] 12 of the 13 recipients had no identifiable risk behaviors for HIV infection. Retrospectively, the seven donors were found to be infected with HIV. Most of these donors acknowledged a risk behavior associated with HIV infection or reported a mononucleosis-like syndrome in the four months preceding the donation. The authors concluded that there is a small (1 in 40,000) but identifiable risk of acquiring HIV infection through antibody-negative blood. Important modifications in donor and unit exclusion processes occurred around the time of that study and remain in practice today, so this risk may be overstated now. To further minimize this risk, the reasons for deferral of donation need to be communicated more effectively to blood donors who are at high risk, and new assays that detect HIV infection earlier should be evaluated.

Transmission of HIV has been reported to occur among recipients of various organ transplants, including kidney, bone, liver, heart, pancreas, and skin transplants.[56] Currently, the U.S. Public Health Service recommends HIV antibody testing of all potential organ donors. Organs are also screened for the presence of HIV antibodies as part of the procurement process.[56] With careful screening and deferral of individuals with high-risk behaviors, the risk of acquiring HIV infection through transplantation is probably small.

Finally, transmission of HIV has been reported to occur through artificial insemination. In one report, seven cases of HIV infection through artificial insemination were reported to the Los Angeles County Department of Health Services.[57] These women had been identified retrospectively from five clinics performing artificial insemination. All seropositive recipients had undergone artificial insemination prior to 1986. Although the number of reported cases of HIV infection associated with artificial insemination is low, the risk exists, especially for those women who were artificially inseminated before routine HIV screening of semen donors.

Occupational Exposure

Health care workers represent 5.4% of the work force in the United States and 5.5% of AIDS patients. Thus, they do not appear over-represented among individuals with AIDS.[58]

In combining the results from 21 prospective studies, it is estimated that the risk of acquiring HIV infection from a percutaneous exposure is 0.2% per exposure (95% confidence interval, 0.1 to 0.5%).[59,60] Variables that may influence the risk of HIV transmission through percutaneous exposure include the patient's disease stage, volume of blood injected, type and gauge of needle, depth of penetration, and glove use. The risk of HIV infection associated with mucous membrane or cutaneous exposure is much smaller.[59,60]

Postexposure antiretroviral therapy has been recommended in health care workers in an effort to prevent occupationally acquired HIV infection.[61] Some animal models suggest that antiretroviral prophylaxis is effective in this setting.[60,61a] Although failure to prevent HIV infection after using postexposure prophylaxis (PEP) has occurred, a case-controlled study in health care workers suggested that zidovudine PEP decreased the risk of seroconversion after percutaneous exposure to HIV-infected blood by 79%.[61b]

Transmission of hepatitis B virus has been reported to occur from infected health care workers to patients during invasive medical, surgical, and dental procedures. Until recently, no cases of HIV transmission from an HIV-infected health care worker to a patient had been reported. In 1990, the CDC reported the first case consistent with possible transmission of HIV infection from an HIV-infected dentist to a patient during an invasive dental procedure.[62] Since this report, four more of this dentist's patients have been reported to be HIV-infected. Evidence, including the similarity of the strains of HIV isolated from the dentist and these five patients, strongly suggests that these patients were infected with HIV during their dental care.[63] Although the risk of transmission in this setting has not been precisely defined, it is probably very low. However, this case does support the strict adherence to published guidelines for the prevention of transmission of HIV and other blood-borne pathogens in health care settings.[62]

Perinatal Exposure

Transmission of HIV may occur in utero, at birth, or through breast-feeding. Although HIV has been isolated from breast milk and a small number of cases have been identified in which transmission through breast-feeding was likely, transmission is probably less efficient than in utero or during birth. It appears that infection with HIV occurs predominantly in utero.[64] Infants born to mothers with AIDS or low $CD4^+$ T-cell counts during pregnancy may be at an increased risk for perinatal transmission of HIV infection.[65,66] In addition, one study noted that infants born to HIV-seropositive mothers with high viral loads (i.e., maternal plasma HIV-1 RNA >10^5 copies/ml) have an increased risk of HIV transmission.[67]

Studies of transmission and natural history of HIV infection in the newborn are complicated by lack of reliable diagnostic procedures. Infants born to HIV-infected mothers have maternally-acquired antibodies to HIV, which can be detected up to 18 months of age. It is therefore necessary to follow these infants to detect the loss of maternal antibodies and the development of serologic or virologic markers of infection (see section on HIV testing). Larger, prospective studies of HIV-seropositive mothers and their newborns have suggested a perinatal transmission rate of 25–35%.[65] Antiretroviral therapy, initiated during pregnancy and followed by antiretroviral therapy in the infant, appears to significantly reduce the likelihood of perinatal transmission.

Routes Not Associated with HIV Transmission

The lay press has devoted considerable attention to the potential for transmission of HIV by routes other than those described above. Large-scale epidemiologic investigations have repeatedly confirmed the association between transmission and sexual, blood, or perinatal exposure. Studies in family members of individuals with HIV infection have failed to document transmission of HIV through casual contact over periods of extensive and prolonged exposure.[68,69] Likewise, careful study has failed to document transmission of HIV by insect vectors. Finally, donation of blood has not been associated with HIV transmission, although this myth still exists.

Prevention

Currently, there is no vaccine to prevent the spread of HIV infection, so education is the prime tool for containing the dissemination of HIV.

Sexual Transmission

To accomplish a substantial reduction in sexual transmission, fundamental changes in behavior are necessary. Health education should emphasize methods of reducing disease transmission, such as abstinence, monogamy, reduction in number of sexual partners, and correct and consistent use of latex condoms. Latex condoms have been shown to be effective in preventing in vitro passage of herpes simplex, CMV, and HIV.[70] In addition, preliminary epidemiologic surveys suggest that consistent use of condoms will slow the spread of HIV via sexual transmission.[68,71] Nonoxynol 9–containing spermicidal jellies and foams may be a useful adjunct to condoms because this agent had been shown to inactivate HIV and kill lymphocytes.[72] The female condom, Reality™, has been shown to be an effective barrier against HIV, herpes simplex virus, and hepatitis B virus in laboratory studies. However, its effectiveness in pregnancy prevention with consistent and correct use is only approximately 89% in clinical studies. Studies investigating protection against HIV infection or sexually transmitted diseases have not been completed.[73] There is no risk of sexual exposure in individuals who practice sexual abstinence or in those in a mutually monogamous relationship in which neither partner is infected or engages in high-risk behaviors.

Parenteral Transmission

Intravenous drug use is becoming the behavior associated

with the greatest risk of acquiring and transmitting HIV infection. Measures to reduce the transmission of HIV in this setting are urgently needed.

Innovative prevention strategies have been advocated by various groups. The advisability of teaching methods of sterilizing equipment, providing injection equipment, or legalizing recreational drug use has been questioned because of the potential of magnifying our existing drug problem. Other less controversial preventive strategies include large-scale expansion of drug-abuse treatment centers, one-on-one health promotion activities between current and former drug users, empowering individuals to practice safer behaviors (such as safer sex practices and refusing to share equipment). Preliminary data from various programs suggest that facilitating safer injection practices and treating the underlying drug addiction are complementary rather than self-defeating.[74]

Blood-borne transmission of HIV through infected donated blood and blood products has virtually been eliminated in developed countries through self-deferral of high-risk donors, testing of all blood and plasma for HIV antibodies, discarding units that test positive, and use of heat-inactivated factor VIII. The processes by which plasma-derived hepatitis B virus vaccine and immune globulin are manufactured either physically remove or chemically inactivate HIV, making these plasma-derived products safe.[75]

Perinatal Transmission

In the United States, reduction in perinatal transmission is linked to reducing heterosexual spread and transmission through intravenous drug use. Women seeking routine health care should be counseled about family planning and safer sexual practices, especially condom and spermicide use. In the United States, it is generally recommended that HIV-infected mothers avoid breast-feeding.

Antiretroviral therapy may have a major impact on reducing perinatally acquired HIV infection. In a double-blind, placebo-controlled study of pregnant HIV-infected women, zidovudine therapy reduced the risk of perinatally acquired HIV infection by approximately two-thirds.[76] The women enrolled in this study were between 14 and 34 weeks gestation, had $CD4^+$ T-cell counts of greater than 200 cells/µl, and had no prior antiretroviral therapy. The treatment group received oral zidovudine until the time of delivery, at which time they received continuous intravenous infusions of zidovudine. The newborns born in the treatment group received oral zidovudine syrup beginning within 8–12 hours of delivery and continuing for 6 weeks after delivery. At interim analysis, 27.7% of infants born to placebo recipients were HIV infected, compared with 7.9% of infants born to zidovudine recipients.[76] Guidelines have since been published regarding the use of zidovudine in HIV-infected pregnant women.[77] Further studies are needed to see if this benefit extends to women with more advanced disease or who have received previous antiretroviral therapy and to assess the relative benefit provided by specific portions of the therapy (e.g., therapy administered during gestation, during delivery, or after delivery). Furthermore, the long-term effects of gestational and perinatal exposure to zidovudine therapy are unknown.

HIV Testing

Serologic tests for antibodies to HIV are the mainstay in the diagnosis of HIV infection in adults and children older than 18 months. However, after infection with HIV, seroconversion occurs on average six weeks after initial exposure, with 95% of individuals seroconverting within 6 months.[78] An individual infected with HIV may have a negative test for antibodies during this period.

Currently available antibody tests are generally inadequate for diagnosing infection in infants born to HIV-seropositive mothers. Almost all infants will passively acquire maternal antibodies in utero. Maternal antibodies may persist up to 15 to 18 months of age, and serologic antibody tests will detect passively acquired antibodies. True HIV infection of the infant cannot be serologically detected until maternal antibodies have cleared. These tests therefore lack the specificity necessary for detection of infection in infants less than 18 months of age.[79]

This section will briefly summarize the serologic tests currently available for detection of antibodies to HIV and other diagnostic tests that may become useful in diagnosing HIV infection.

Antibody Testing

Enzyme-Linked Immunosorbent Assay

The enzyme-linked immunosorbent assay (ELISA) was first licensed by the U.S. Food and Drug Administration (FDA) in 1985, primarily for the screening of blood and plasma products. Testing by ELISA is now the most useful screening tool for HIV infection. Several commercially available ELISA kits are licensed by the FDA. Under optimal conditions, ELISAs have a sensitivity and specificity of 99.5% and 99.8%, respectively.[80]

Serum samples deemed positive by ELISA must be tested again in duplicate. Only samples tested by ELISA that are repeatedly reactive are considered positive. A positive ELISA is not sufficient to make the diagnosis of HIV infection, especially in low-prevalence populations, and must be followed by a confirmatory test. The Western blot is the most commonly used confirmatory test, although some laboratories have used a radioimmunoprecipitation assay (RIPA).[81] A diagnosis of HIV infection is made when an individual has repeatedly tested positive with ELISA and has a positive confirmatory test.

Table 7-6. Possible Causes of False-Positive ELISA Results

Autoimmune diseases
Liver disease (e.g., alcoholic hepatitis)
Multiple myeloma

Certain infections/immunizations
  HIV-2
  Positive syphilis serology
  Malaria
  Recent influenza vaccination

Multiple blood transfusions
Certain HLA phenotypes

ELISA, enzyme-linked immunosorbent assay; HLA, human leukocyte antigen.

A "window period" of low sensitivity has been noted to occur with ELISA.[82] This is the time between initial infection and the production of antibodies. Seroconversion generally occurs within six weeks. False-negative results may occur during this window period. An individual is still considered infectious during this time despite the absence of antibodies to HIV. In addition, hypogammaglobulinemic children of HIV-seropositive mothers may have false-negative ELISA results because their immune systems cannot produce antibodies to HIV.[83,84] Potential reasons for false-positive ELISAs are listed in Table 7-6.

Western Blot

The Western blot assay is the most commonly used confirmatory test. Controversy exists among various groups as to the interpretation of a positive Western blot.[85] The CDC and the Association of State and Territorial Public Health Laboratory Directors suggest that a positive test should be defined by the presence of at least two of the following HIV protein bands: p24, gp41, or gp120/160.[76] A negative test is the absence of all bands. An indeterminant result is one in which at least one band is present but the bands necessary for a positive test are not. An indeterminant result can be seen in individuals recently infected with HIV with incomplete serologic response and in patients with advanced disease.[85] An indeterminant result in patients whose physical examination and medical history are highly suggestive of HIV infection should be repeated by a second Western blot in six months, which will likely yield a positive result. Conversely, repeat testing of an indeterminant result in individuals at low risk for infection will generally yield the same banding pattern as their previous indeterminant result. These individuals are rarely, if ever, truly infected with HIV.[86]

Other Assays

p24 Antigen Assay

The detection of p24 antigen, one of the HIV core proteins, in the serum of an HIV-infected person is an indicator of active viral replication. Serum p24 antigen can be detected during two different phases of HIV infection: immediately after HIV infection but before the development of antibodies to HIV, and in the late stages of illness.[87–89] The p24 antigen assay is, at present, primarily utilized as a research tool. One of the major disadvantages of this assay is that it cannot detect p24 antigen in the presence of high titers of HIV-specific antibodies because of the formation of antibody-antigen complexes.[79] This assay is valuable in detecting HIV infection during the "window period" before people develop antibodies to HIV and in hypogammaglobulinemic children.[79,90] The assay for p24 antigen has also been used to monitor the progression of disease and the effect of antiviral therapy in patients with advanced disease.[91,92]

Less than 30% of HIV-infected patients have detectable p24 antigen at any given point in the infection, using the standard assay.[93] This assay was recently modified to increase its sensitivity by using an "acid-dissociated method" in which p24 antibody-antigen complexes dissociate, allowing more p24 antigen to be detected by the ELISA. With this modified method, over 50% of HIV-infected patients have detectable p24 antigen.[93,94]

HIV Culture

The use of viral cultures is restricted to research settings. These cultures are costly and labor intensive, often taking up to 28 days or more to complete.[95] Special precautions to prevent exposure of laboratory personnel are required. The significant amount of blood required for viral cultures limits their utility in infants less than 18 months of age.[79] The sensitivity of the virus culture varies among the different laboratories and during the course of the illness. In individuals with AIDS, culture yield may be as high as 100%, compared with 10% in asymptomatic individuals with HIV infection.[96]

Polymerase Chain Reaction

Polymerase chain reaction (PCR) is a method for amplifying the viral DNA a million times or more to increase the probability of detection.[79] This method offers several advantages over other diagnostic tests, including its potential use in detecting virus in infants less than 18 months of age. PCR is not affected by the presence of maternal antibodies.[97] The assay can be completed in one day, making it less labor intensive than an HIV culture.

Because PCR detects viral genetic material, not antibodies, infection with HIV can be detected earlier. Early detection may have favorable prognostic implications because antiretroviral therapy and other medical interventions may be initiated earlier in the course of infection. PCR may also be used to: (1) resolve the infection status of individuals with an indeterminate Western blot, (2) directly detect and quantify HIV DNA and RNA from cells of infected persons, and (3) define the patterns of transmission and evolution of the virus through the population.[98] However, the sensitivity of PCR can vary with the course of HIV illness, and it may be less sensitive during asymptomatic periods and highly sensitive in patients with AIDS.[99]

Quantitation of HIV RNA

Measuring the quantity of HIV RNA (i.e., viral load) in the blood is a relatively new method attracting widespread interest among researchers and practitioners. The ability to quantitate the amount of HIV in the blood will aid in the staging of HIV infection as well as in evaluating the response to antiretroviral therapy. A more rapid progression to AIDS has been observed in patients with a high viral load at the time of seroconversion ($>10^5$ copies/ml) compared with patients with lower viral loads.[100] Viral load testing is becoming standard of care management of HIV infection.

Several assays are commercially available for quantitating viral load. They include Amplicor HIV Monitor Test (Roche Molecular Systems), Nucleic Acid Sequence-Based Amplification (NASBA; Organon Technika), and quantitative branched-chain DNA (bDNA; Chiron).[101] The bDNA assay is a "first-generation test" and has a sensitivity of 10^4 copies/ml.[101,102] Results from these assays are generally available in two to three days. Recent modifications of this assay have increased the sensitivity to as few as 500 copies/ml.[101,102]

Home Testing Kits

There are currently three over-the-counter home HIV testing kits commercially available: Confide® by Johnson and Johnson's Direct Access Diagnostics, and Home Access™ and Home Access Express™ by Home Access Health Corporation.[103,103a] These home HIV testing kits allow people to be tested and counseled regarding their test results in the privacy of their own homes. The user provides a drop of blood on blot paper and sends it to a FDA-licensed laboratory, where both the ELISA and a confirmatory test are performed. After a specified period of time, the user calls for the result and receives appropriate counseling. The entire process is anonymous. Although the concept of home HIV antibody testing kits is controversial, one advantage of home HIV testing kits is that it expands access to testing in those at risk for HIV infection.

Saliva and Urine Tests

Assays for detecting HIV antibodies in saliva have been studied. Earlier studies of these assays demonstrated a specificity and sensitivity ranging from 93 to 100% and from 98.7 to 100%, respectively.[104] In December of 1994, the FDA approved the first saliva-based collection kit for HIV-antibody screening, OraSure HIV-1 test (Epitope; Beaverton, Oregon).[103,105] The sensitivity and specificity were 99.5 and 100% when compared to ELISA assays of the serum but were somewhat lower when compared to Western blot assays. Individuals repeatedly testing positive by this test should then undergo standard testing methods. Assays for detecting antibodies in urine have also been studied.[106,107] In one study using a modified ELISA, 157 (99.4%) of 158 HIV-infected individuals tested positive by this test. Commercially available ELISAs for serum were not accurate enough to use on urine specimens.[106] The potential advantages of these tests are ease of collection, lower cost, and the detection of HIV infection in areas removed from traditional settings, where technical skills may be lacking.

SPECTRUM OF DISEASE

The spectrum of HIV infection ranges from asymptomatic infection to the manifestations of a severely compromised immune system, such as opportunistic infections and tumors, that define AIDS. The interval between initial infection with HIV and the development of AIDS appears to be long and variable. Studies from 1984 of patients who developed AIDS associated with blood transfusions suggested incubation periods of 21 months for children and 31 months for adults.[40] More recent data suggests an incubation period of approximately eight years or more for infection acquired by both transfusion-related and homosexual exposures.[40] Prognostic indicators, such as the decline in antibodies to p24, the appearance or persistent presence of HIV antigenemia, and oral candidiasis, suggest progression of HIV infection to AIDS.[100,108,109] In one study, the mean cumulative survival of individuals with AIDS was approximately 50% at one year and 15% at five years, though sex, race, age, and AIDS-defining illness appeared to contribute to the overall survival of specific subgroups of this population.[110] There also appears to be a small group of individuals infected for more than 10 years with HIV who have not progressed to the development of AIDS.[23,24]

The most severe consequence of advanced HIV infection is AIDS, often resulting in death within two years. The various manifestations of HIV infection will be briefly discussed in this section.

Acute Infection

Acute infection with HIV occurs before seroconversion and may or may not be associated with symptoms.[111] Seroconversion usually occurs in approximately six weeks, with 95% of individuals seroconverting within six months after initial exposure to HIV.[78]

In those experiencing symptoms, a mononucleosis-like illness is most frequently reported. During the acute illness, the individual may have fever, sweats, lethargy, malaise, myalgia, arthralgia, headaches, photophobia, diarrhea, sore throat, lymphadenopathy, and a truncal maculopapular rash. Thrombocytopenia and lymphopenia have also been reported to occur during the first several days, with inversion of the $CD4^+/CD8^+$ T-cell ratio shortly thereafter.[112] Central nervous system abnormalities, such as aseptic meningitis or encephalopathy and peripheral neuropathy, have also been reported during acute infection.[113]

It is unclear what percentage of primarily infected people experience this mononucleosis-like illness or whether the described illness is a reliable and consistent indicator of HIV infection. However, one study investigated the clinical and immunologic manifestations of findings occurring during seroconversion in a group of homosexual men.[112] Approximately 92% of those patients seroconverting experienced signs of acute illness, compared with 40% in the control group of seronegative homosexual men. The mean duration of this acute illness was approximately three weeks. In addition, 50% of seroconverting subjects had an inverted $CD4^+/CD8^+$ T-cell ratio; none of the control subjects did.

Asymptomatic Infection

The guidelines established by the CDC define asymptomatic infection as the absence of clinical signs and symptoms of HIV infection in people with laboratory evidence of antibodies to HIV.[114] Individuals may or may not have hematologic abnormalities often associated with HIV infection, such as lymphopenia, thrombocytopenia, and a decrease in $CD4^+$ T lymphocytes.

Persistent Generalized Lymphadenopathy

Persistent generalized lymphadenopathy is the presence of a palpable lymph node greater than or equal to one centimeter at two or more extrainguinal sites persisting for more than three months with no other illness. Persistent generalized lymphadenopathy indicates progression of HIV infection and may herald the development of an AIDS-defining illness.

AIDS: CDC Clinical Definition

The CDC surveillance definition of AIDS was revised and expanded for adolescents and adults in 1993 and categorizes individuals on the basis of $CD4^+$ T-cell count and clinical conditions associated with HIV infection, such as opportunistic infections and neoplasms. The expanded definition for AIDS now includes HIV-infected individuals with $CD4^+$ T-cell count under 200 cells/µl or a $CD4^+$ T-cell percentage below 14%. The current definition also includes the presence of pulmonary tuberculosis, recurrent pneumonia (more than two episodes per year), and invasive cervical cancer.[115] Conditions included in the CDC definition of AIDS are listed in Table 7-7. This section will discuss the presentations of some selected opportunistic infections and neoplasms.

Many of the opportunistic infections and neoplasms seen in HIV-infected patients are a direct result of a severely impaired cellular immune system. The cell-medi-

Table 7-7. AIDS-Defining Conditions[116]

OPPORTUNISTIC INFECTIONS	OTHER CONDITIONS	NEOPLASMS
Cryptosporidiosis	Lymphoid pneumonia	Kaposi's sarcoma
Cytomegalovirus infection	Progressive multifocal leukoencephalopathy	Lymphoma Cervical dysplasia
Isosporiasis	HIV encephalopathy	
Pneumocystis carinii pneumonia	HIV wasting syndrome	
Toxoplasmosis	Bacterial infections	
Candidiasis	$CD4^+$ T-cell count <200/µl	
Coccidioidomycosis		
Herpes simplex infection		
Histoplasmosis		
Tuberculosis		
Other mycobacterial infections		
Salmonellosis		

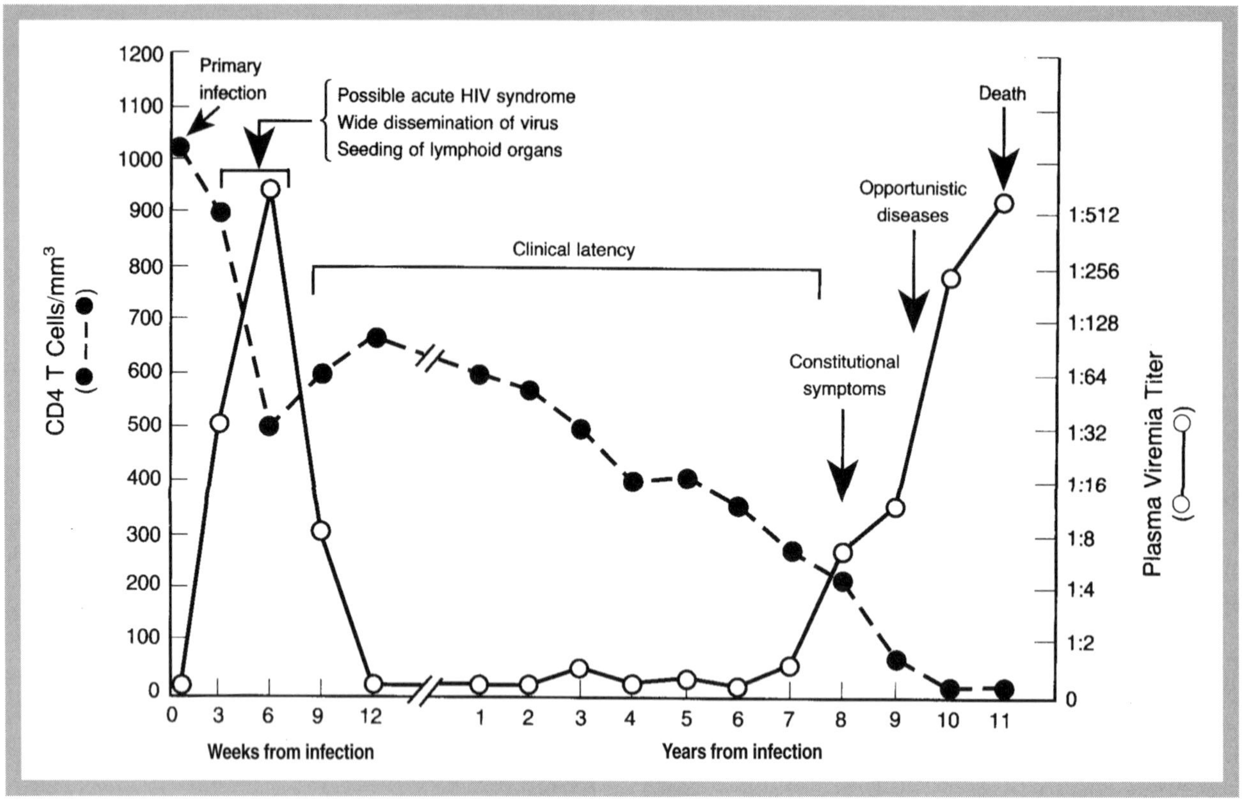

Figure 7-3. Relationship of CD4+ T-cell count and plasma viremia titer to progression of HIV illness

SOURCE: *Reprinted with permission from Pantaleo G, Graziosi C, Fauci AS. The immunopathogenesis of human immunodeficiency virus infection.* N Engl J Med. *1993;328:327–35.*

ated arm of the immune system is responsible for protecting against these infections and neoplasms. The presence of these infections and neoplasms can be correlated with CD4+ T-cell count. In a healthy adult, the normal CD4+ T-cell count is about 1000 cells/µl.[116] This number will progressively decline in an HIV-infected individual, on average, by approximately 40–80 cells/µl or more every year.[116] The first infections usually begin to appear when the CD4+ T-cell count is between 200 and 500 cells/µl. Once the CD4+ T-cell count falls below 200 cells/µl, the more severe, life-threatening infections and neoplasms develop.[116–118] This progression is illustrated in Figure 7-3.

Opportunistic Infections

Because of the profound, irreversible immunodeficiency in AIDS patients, opportunistic infections are generally less responsive to conventional therapy and frequently recur when therapy is discontinued. Life-long suppressive therapy is often required for many of these infections. Opportunistic infections are the leading cause of death in patients with AIDS.

Pneumocystis carinii Pneumonia

Pneumocystis carinii pneumonia (PCP) occurs in up to 80% of AIDS patients not receiving PCP prophylaxis and is the initial opportunistic infection in approximately 60% of AIDS patients. The rate of occurrence in individuals with a CD4+ T-cell count below 200 cells/µl is approximately 8% and 18% after six months and one year, respectively.[119] Since the publication of current guidelines, which recommend prophylaxis for all individuals with CD4+ T-cell counts below 200 cells/µl, the relative incidence of PCP has decreased.[120] As with other infections, PCP may represent reactivation of latent infection.[121] The presentation of PCP in HIV-infected patients is a more subtle, indolent process than that observed in patients whose immunodeficiencies are not caused by HIV. In one study, the median duration of symptoms at the time of diagnosis was 28 days in AIDS patients, compared with 5 days in patients whose immunodeficiencies are not caused by HIV.[122] Clinical manifestations of PCP include fever, shortness of breath, and nonproductive cough, with only subtle changes on chest radiography. Definitive diagnosis is made by identification of the organism in the sputum, by bronchoscopy with bronchoalveolar lavage, or by biopsy.[123,124] Although 80% of patients survive their initial hospitalization, 60% of patients relapse within one year without prophylaxis.[119,125] Survival decreases to 40–60% with recurrent episodes.[125]

Cryptococcal Meningitis

Cryptococcal meningitis occurs in approximately 5–10% of HIV-infected patients. In addition to the central nervous system, cryptococcal infection can occur in the lungs, skin, genitourinary tract, bone marrow, and blood.[126–128] Manifestations of cryptococcal meningitis may be subtle. Fever and headache are the most common symptoms; meningismus, photophobia, mental status changes, and seizures occur less frequently.[126–128] Time from onset of symptoms to diagnosis ranges from a day to four months, with a mean of 31 days.[128] Diagnosis is established by the detection of yeast cells by India ink stain and culture and/or the presence of cryptococcal antigen in the cerebrospinal fluid (CSF).[126–128] Cryptococcal antigen can also be detected in the serum. Even with therapy, cryptococcal antigen titers may remain elevated. Patients who present with altered mental status, high cryptococcal antigen titers in the CSF (>1:1024), and low white-cell count in the CSF (<20 cells/mm^3) are at increased risk of death.[129] Once acute therapy is completed, suppressive therapy is always indicated.

Toxoplasmosis

Toxoplasmosis is the most common cause of focal encephalitis in patients with AIDS.[130] Symptoms include fever, confusion, hemispheric signs (such as hemiparesis and aphasia), meningeal signs, coma, and seizures. The most useful tool in the diagnosis of toxoplasmosis has been the computerized tomography scan, which reveals multiple low-density lesions and/or ring-enhancing lesions.[130,131] Serology has proven of limited value. Definitive diagnosis requires the demonstration of tachyzoites in brain tissue obtained through biopsy. However, brain biopsy is generally reserved for patients who fail to respond to empiric therapy.

Empiric therapy may be considered in patients with positive serology and a clinical and radiologic profile suggestive of toxoplasmosis. An initial response is usually observed after two weeks of therapy.[130,131] Again, as with many of the opportunistic infections, relapse is common when treatment is stopped.

Mycobacterium avium Complex and *Mycobacterium tuberculosis*

Mycobacterium avium complex (MAC) and *Mycobacterium tuberculosis* infection occur frequently in AIDS patients, often as disseminated disease.[132] Before the AIDS epidemic, MAC infection was a rare condition seen only occasionally in patients with chronic pulmonary disease. The diagnosis of MAC infection is usually made in the late stages of HIV illness, and the presence of MAC has been documented in as many as 53% of AIDS patients at autopsy.[132–134] The manifestations of MAC infection range from asymptomatic to a constellation of nonspecific findings including diarrhea, abdominal pain, malabsorption, persistent fevers, anemia, and/or weight loss.[132–134] Quantitative blood cultures and cultures of bone marrow, lymph node, and liver biopsies may be employed to guide in the diagnosis of disseminated infection. In addition, positive cultures from respiratory secretions, urine, and stool have been reported to precede disseminated infection.[132]

Tuberculosis is prevalent among individuals infected with HIV, particularly those in areas endemic for tuberculosis.[132,135] Tuberculosis typically precedes the development of other AIDS-defining opportunistic infections. As in the general population, tuberculosis usually represents reactivation of latent infection acquired earlier in life. However, reinfection has also been observed. Disseminated, extrapulmonary disease is encountered frequently, representing 67% of tuberculosis seen in patients with AIDS.[132,135] Clinical manifestations depend on the site involved. As with MAC, diagnosis is made with the finding of M. *tuberculosis* in the affected tissues or secretions. The CDC has recommended administering tuberculin skin tests to HIV-infected patients. However, because of depressed cellular responses (anergy), a negative reaction does not rule out infection.[136] Therefore, an anergy panel (i.e., candida, mumps) should be used as a control for the purified protein derivative (PPD) test.

Candidiasis

Candidiasis, often presenting as oral thrush and/or esophagitis, is the most common fungal infection in HIV-infected patients.[137] In addition, unexplained oral or vaginal candidiasis in individuals at risk for HIV infection may indicate impending progression of HIV infection. Approximately 60% of these patients will develop an opportunistic infection or Kaposi's sarcoma (KS) within a median of three months after the diagnosis of oral candidiasis.[138] Relapses following antifungal therapy are common, and suppressive therapy is often warranted.

Herpesvirus

Infections with herpesviruses, such as herpes simplex and CMV, are frequently encountered in HIV-infected individuals. Mucocutaneous herpes simplex (oral, genital, or perianal) can be painful, and patients may experience frequent relapses.[139] CMV is particularly common in the homosexual population and is a frequent cause of morbidity and mortality.[140–143] Like other herpesviruses, CMV can cause persistent infection, with viral shedding in a number of body sites.[141,142] Viremia occurs in approximately 50% of AIDS patients, and more than 90% show tissue evidence of CMV at autopsy.[139] Retinitis is the most common manifestation of CMV infection and is a leading cause of blindness in patients with AIDS. In addition to CMV retinitis, other clinical syndromes seen with CMV include colitis, esophagitis, encephalitis, adrenalitis, pneumonitis, sclerosing cholangitis, and hepatitis. Relapse rates are high, especially with CMV retinitis; therefore, long-term suppressive therapy is often necessary.[140–143]

Neoplasms

Severe cellular suppression and polyclonal B-cell activation may contribute to the development of cancers in patients with AIDS. Although both KS and non-Hodgkin's lymphoma (NHL) are relatively rare outside the HIV setting, these tumors occur more frequently and often present atypically in patients with AIDS.

Kaposi's Sarcoma

KS was one of the first described clinical manifestations of AIDS.[144,145] KS occurs in approximately 12% of patients diagnosed with AIDS, with the highest prevalence among homosexual men (19%) and homosexual male IVDUs (15%).[146] KS is more likely to occur in white men than in black men and rarely occurs in women or children infected with HIV.[146] Although the incidence of KS in HIV-infected patients declined from 22% in 1985 to 8% in 1993, a significant number of cases are still reported each year, and this cancer continues to be a major cause of morbidity in these patients.[146] The presence of herpes-like DNA sequences has been detected in the KS lesions of both HIV-infected and non-HIV-infected individuals. This and other epidemiologic data suggest that AIDS-related KS may have an infectious etiology.[147]

Before the AIDS epidemic, KS was a rare tumor occurring predominantly among middle-aged men of Eastern European or Mediterranean extraction. The clinical presentation of KS in AIDS patients is very diverse and differs from the classic, localized presentation. In HIV-infected patients, KS tends to involve the skin, especially the head, neck, and trunk; lymph nodes; mucous membranes; and the entire gastrointestinal tract.[148] More than 50% of patients have visceral lesions, particularly in the gastrointestinal tract, at the time of initial presentation.[149] The rate of progression varies among patients. Most individuals with KS have rapid, progressive disease with multiple organ involvement, particularly the gastrointestinal tract and pulmonary parenchyma. However, a small percentage experience a slow and indolent process similar to that seen in the classic form. Patients with cutaneous KS and no history of opportunistic infections or symptomatic HIV infection have the most favorable prognosis. Patients with gastrointestinal KS have a slightly reduced survival rate, and those with pulmonary KS have the worst prognosis.[149]

Non-Hodgkin's Lymphoma

NHL occurs in approximately 5–10% of patients with AIDS.[150] NHL has been reported in homosexual men, male and female IVDUs, and hemophiliacs.[150–152] Although the reason for the increased incidence of aggressive lymphomas in AIDS patients is unclear, the presence of Epstein-Barr virus, which results in polyclonal B-cell proliferation, may have a permissive effect.[148] AIDS-related lymphomas differ from lymphomas in other populations because they occur in a younger population, are often disseminated, are predominantly high- or intermediate-grade B-cell type, and generally follow a rapidly progressive clinical course.[153,154] Over 70% of these patients have involvement of extranodal sites, especially the brain, bone marrow, and bowel.[155–157] Primary lymphoma of the brain in patients with AIDS carries a poor prognosis and is associated with advanced disease and $CD4^+$ T-cell count below 50 cells/μl.[150] Treatment of patients with AIDS-related NHL is associated with a complete response rate of approximately 50% and high relapse and mortality rates.[158,159] Decisions regarding aggressive chemotherapy are made on an individual basis.

TREATMENT APPROACHES FOR HIV INFECTION

An intensive program has been undertaken to develop strategies aimed at either preventing HIV infection or altering the progression of HIV illness. The purpose of this section is to review both antiviral and immunomodulatory approaches under investigation and to summarize the current efforts at the development of vaccine candidates.

Antiviral Therapy

The stages in the viral replicative cycle that are potentially susceptible to antiviral intervention are summarized in Table 7-8. Potential targets include binding of the virus to the CD4 receptor, viral entry or uncoating, reverse transcriptase, viral transcription, viral protein synthesis and processing, viral assembly, and viral release.[160,161]

Inhibitors of Viral Binding

Although a number of approaches to inhibition of viral binding are being investigated, the greatest amount of interest has centered on the production of soluble, truncated forms of the CD4 molecule. Presenting HIV with excess, non-cell-bound, recombinant CD4 (rCD4) could inhibit the portions of the replicative cycle that require the CD4 receptor, and it may block the cytolysis of uninfected cells induced by syncytia formation.[160,161] Phase I trials suggested that, although rCD4 was nontoxic and had no measurable adverse effect on immune function, only a small antiviral effect was observed at the highest doses.[162,163]

Because of the relatively short half-life (45 minutes) and the suboptimal antiviral effects observed in the phase I trials of rCD4, second-generation versions of rCD4 hybrids are now under study. By linking domains of the rCD4 molecule with the Fc portion of immunoglobulin G

Table 7-8. Potential Targets for Antiretroviral Therapy

MECHANISM	AGENT
Inhibition of viral binding Inhibit gp120-CD4 interaction	 Soluble CD4 Soluble CD4 hybrids
Inhibit membrane fusion	
Inhibit reverse transcriptase	Dideoxynucleosides (AZT [Zdv], ddI, ddC, d4T, 3TC) Non-nucleoside inhibitors
Inhibit integration of provirus	Integrase inhibitors
Inhibit transcription of provirus	*tat* inhibitors
Inhibit translation of viral mRNA	Antisense oligonucleotides
Inhibit post-translational processing	Glycosylation inhibitors Protease inhibitors
Inhibit budding and release	Interferon

AZT (ZdV), zidovudine; ddI, didanosine; ddC, zalcitabine; d4T, stavudine; 3TC, lamivudine.

(rCD4-IgG), the dual goals of extending the half-life and incorporating specific functions of immunoglobulin may be achieved.[164] These immunoadhesins should promote antibody-mediated phagocytic engulfment. One of the potential advantages of immunoadhesins is their ability to cross the placenta and, therefore, possibly play an important role in preventing perinatally acquired HIV infection.[165] Elevations in platelet counts have been noted with high doses of rCD4-IgG in patients with HIV-associated thrombocytopenic purpura.[166] However, the antiviral effects of rCD4-IgG have not been demonstrated clinically;[167] perhaps clinical isolates of HIV are less sensitive to these compounds than laboratory strains of HIV.[168,169]

rCD4 has also been linked to cellular toxins, such as *Pseudomonas* exotoxin A and ricin. These compounds should selectively bind to cells expressing HIV and, through the toxin, kill the infected cells. This may be a particularly attractive approach to targeting cells, such as macrophages, that are relatively resistant to the cytopathic effect of HIV.[160,161]

Reverse Transcriptase Inhibitors

Because reverse transcriptase, which makes DNA from RNA, is an essential and relatively unique feature of HIV, inhibition of this enzyme was recognized early as an important target for antiretroviral therapy. In 1985, it was observed that the dideoxynucleosides had potent in vitro activity against HIV. These compounds must be converted to the active 5′-triphosphate derivative by the biochemical machinery of the cell. This anabolic phosphorylation involves a series of kinases. There are substantial differences in the rates at which human cells phosphorylate these compounds that are reflected in their antiretroviral activity.[160,161,170]

Two mechanisms may contribute to the activity of the dideoxynucleosides. First, as triphosphates, they compete with cellular deoxynucleoside 5′-triphosphates, which are the essential substrates for formation of proviral DNA. In addition, because of the 3′ modification, once reverse transcriptase adds these nucleotides to a growing chain of DNA, no additional nucleotides can be added, and HIV replication is halted.[170]

Reverse transcriptase inhibitors currently available in the United States include zidovudine (AZT or ZdV), didanosine (ddI), zalcitabine (ddC), stavudine (d4T), and lamivudine (3TC). Following a multicenter phase II trial that demonstrated a significant survival advantage in patients receiving zidovudine compared to placebo, zidovudine was approved by the FDA in March 1987 for the treatment of AIDS patients with a history of PCP or with CD4+ T-cell counts below 200 cells/µl. In addition, patients receiving zidovudine had fewer opportunistic infections, gained weight, and had improved overall prognosis.[171]

The efficacy of zidovudine in delaying progression to AIDS was assessed in patients with mildly symptomatic disease. Significant differences in the time to first critical event were apparent in subjects with baseline CD4+ T-cell counts of 200–500 cells/µl but not in those with initial counts of 500–799 cells/µl.[172]

Several studies have suggested that the addition of acyclovir to zidovudine therapy might improve survival.[173,174] An analysis of data from the Multicenter AIDS Cohort Study suggested that concurrent use of acyclovir and zidovudine significantly prolonged survival. This benefit was most pronounced in patients with AIDS and herpesvirus infections who received continuous acyclovir therapy.[175]

Didanosine was originally approved by the FDA for use in adults and children over six months of age with advanced HIV infection who are intolerant to or failing zidovudine therapy.[170] However, in ACTG 175, didanosine monotherapy was as effective as the combinations of zidovudine plus didanosine and zidovudine plus zalcitabine and was superior to zidovudine monotherapy in zidovudine-naive patients. Most of the patients in this trial had asymptomatic disease with CD4+ T-cell counts of 200–500 cells/µl. Similar results were seen in zidovudine-experienced patients. This study expanded the role of didanosine in the management of HIV infection and lends further support to the early initiation of antiretroviral therapy in asymptomatic individuals.[174a] Dose-limiting toxicity, including peripheral neuropathy and pancreatitis, occurred with increased frequency at doses above 12 mg/kg.[175]

Zalcitabine was approved by the FDA for the management of HIV infection and was initially approved for use in combination with zidovudine. Two phase I studies suggested that zalcitabine would reduce viral load as well as produce immunologic improvements. However, painful peripheral neuropathy developed in patients receiving higher doses for long periods of time.[170,176]

Stavudine was approved by the FDA in 1994 for use in adults with advanced HIV infection who are intolerant to or have experienced significant clinical or immunologic deterioration while receiving other therapies with proven clinical benefit. In a recent study,[176a] switching patients from long-term zidovudine therapy (six months or more) to stavudine monotherapy demonstrated a clinically significant benefit in delaying progression of disease in patients will all stages of HIV infection. Studies that examine the use of stavudine in combination with other antiretroviral agents are currently ongoing. Dose-related peripheral neuropathy was the major dose-limiting toxicity. Other adverse effects include macrocytosis without anemia, nausea, and modest liver enzyme elevations.[177]

Lamivudine has been approved by the FDA for use in combination with zidovudine for the management of HIV infection when there is evidence of disease progression.[178] When used as monotherapy, high-level resistance to lamivudine occurs within two to four weeks.[179] However, combination therapy with lamivudine appears to restore susceptibility to zidovudine in patients with zidovudine-resistant isolates.[180] Combinations of lamivudine with other antiretroviral agents are under investigation. Because of the high risk of pancreatitis (15%) noted in the pediatric population, lamivudine should be used with *extreme* caution in children.[178]

Non-nucleoside Reverse Transcriptase Inhibitors

Non-nucleoside reverse transcriptase inhibitors include tetrahydroimidazobenzodiazepinthione (TIBO) compounds, a dipyridodiazepinone analogue (nevirapine), and bis(heteroaryl)piperazines (delavirdine and atevirdine).[181] These non-nucleoside analogues are highly specific, noncompetitive inhibitors of HIV-1 reverse transcriptase. They do not require cellular metabolism to be active and are relatively nontoxic.[181,182] When these agents are used as monotherapy, resistance develops rapidly. Therefore, these agents should be used in combination with other antiretroviral agents. Nevirapine and delavirdine are currently approved in adults for the treatment of HIV infection in combination with other nucleoside analogues. Major adverse effects of these two agents are rash and elevated liver enzymes.

Development of Antiretroviral Resistance

The emergence of resistance to antiretroviral agents was first noted soon after FDA approval of zidovudine for the treatment of HIV infection.[183] Resistance of HIV viral isolates has been detected as early as six months after initiation of zidovudine therapy in patients with advanced HIV infection. Resistance to a variety of other antiretroviral agents has also been observed.[184] Resistance arises from mutations in specific regions of the HIV reverse transcriptase gene. Because of the specificity of these mutations, resistance may or may not extend to other antiretroviral agents. Table 7-9 lists various mutations of the reverse transcriptase gene that confer resistance. The clinical significance of antiretroviral resistance is not com-

Table 7-9. Antiviral Resistance Mediated Through Reverse Transcriptase Mutations

RT CODON MUTATION	EFFECT ON HIV PHENOTYPE
41, 67, 70, 215, 219	Resistance to AZT (ZdV); no cross-resistance to other RT inhibitors
74, 184	Resistance to ddI, cross-resistance to ddC
69	Resistance to ddC; no cross-resistance to AZT (ZdV) or ddI
103	Resistance to nevirapine, TIBO compounds, and pyridinone derivatives; no cross-resistance to nucleoside analogues
181	Resistance to nevirapine, TIBO compounds, and pyridinone derivatives

RT, reverse transcriptase; TIBO, tetrahydroimidazobenzodiazepinthione.

SOURCE: *Reprinted with permission from Erice A, Balfour HH. Resistance of human immunodeficiency virus type I to antiretroviral agents: a review.* Clin Infect Dis. *1994;18:149–56.*

pletely understood. However, current data suggest that the development of resistance correlates with depletion of CD4⁺ T lymphocytes, higher viral burden, more rapid clinical progression, and death.[185–188]

Protease (Proteinase) and Integrase Inhibitors

HIV encodes for enzymes, in addition to reverse transcriptase, that are important in viral replication. The protease enzyme appears to be essential for viral infectivity and the processing of core proteins. Protease cleaves the polyprotein precursors of viral proteins Gag and Pol, creating the mature virion components. Inhibition of this enzyme prevents the formation of mature core proteins and reverse transcriptase and thereby results in the release of a noninfectious virion from the host cell. Inhibition of this target may therefore have an impact at multiple steps in the viral replicative cycle.[160,161]

Protease inhibitors are among the most potent of the antiretrovirals, with activity against zidovudine-resistant isolates. However, some of these agents have poor oral bioavailability and are difficult to formulate because of their poor water solubility. In addition, these compounds are metabolized through the cytochrome P-450 system, and multiple drug interactions have been reported.[188] There are currently four protease inhibitors that have undergone extensive clinical study: saquinavir, ritonavir, indinavir, and nelfinavir. Saquinavir was the first protease inhibitor to receive FDA approval and is indicated for use in combination with nucleoside analogues in the treatment of advanced HIV infection in selected patients. Ritonavir, indinavir, and nelfinavir have also been approved.

A triple regimen of zidovudine, zalcitabine, and saquinavir was compared with zidovudine plus zalcitabine and zalcitabine plus saquinavir in patients with advanced HIV infection and prior zidovudine exposure. The triple combination was associated with enhanced viral suppression and a larger, more sustained increase in CD4⁺ T-cell counts than the other two regimens.[189] The bioavailability of saquinavir is poor, and the drug must be taken within two hours of a full meal for maximum absorption. Saquinavir appears to be well tolerated, and the most common adverse effects include diarrhea, abdominal discomfort, and nausea.

Limited clinical data suggest that ritonavir, indinavir, and nelfinavir have a major impact on both viral load and CD4⁺ T-cell counts.[190–192a] These agents represent an important advance in the antiretroviral armamentarium.

Retroviral integrases are the enzymes that integrate proviral DNA into cellular DNA. Mutants that lack integrase do not appear to be able to replicate in cell culture.[160,161] Thus, inhibition of retroviral integrase may be an important target for antiviral strategies. These agents are in the early stages of clinical development.

Late Stages of Viral Replication

Once the proviral DNA has integrated into the host's DNA, viral proteins, such as Tat, Rev, and Nef, are believed to regulate the expression of a mature virion. Strategies that target these regulatory proteins are being explored.[160,161] Another interesting approach to inhibiting protein synthesis is the use of anti-sense segments of DNA, modified to prevent degradation (phosphorothioate oligodeoxynucleosides). These complementary strands of DNA bind to viral RNA and block the movement of ribosomes along the RNA, preventing protein synthesis.[160,161]

After viral proteins are synthesized, they must be modified for assembly. Sugar residues are added to form glycoproteins; during this process, terminal sugars are cleaved by glucosidases. Glucosidase inhibition results in the production of viral glycoproteins that are less infectious, less able to form syncytia, and of larger molecular weight. Specific analogues, such as *N*-butyldeoxynojirimycin, are now under evaluation.[160,161]

Finally, viral components must assemble at the cell surface and be released from the cell as a mature viral particle. Interferons alpha, beta, and gamma (IFN-α,-β, and -γ) are known to inhibit HIV replication in both acute and chronic infection. The dynamics of HIV susceptibility to interferon therapy is discussed later in this chapter.

Combination Therapy

Monotherapy of HIV infection is of limited benefit, as demonstrated by disease progression, transient elevations of CD4⁺ T-cell counts, incomplete inhibition of viral replication, and resistance emergence. Therefore, combination therapy may reduce the incidence of resistance and more effectively inhibit viral replication. Possible synergy or additive inhibitory activity has been demonstrated with combinations of acyclovir and zidovudine,[173,174] zidovudine and didanosine,[183] and zidovudine and zalcitabine.[182] In addition, positive effects on surrogate markers have been demonstrated when zidovudine or other nucleoside analogues are combined with non-nucleoside reverse transcriptase inhibitors and protease inhibitors.[185,189] Combination therapy with two or more antiretroviral agents has become the standard approach in the management of HIV infection.

Immunologic Therapy

The immunopathogenesis of HIV infection is a consequence of both chronic stimulation from persistent antigenic exposure and the resultant immunosuppression that accumulates over time. Strategies that target the immune

Table 7-10. Strategies Targeted at the Immune Response

Immune replacement therapy
Bone marrow transplantation
Intravenous immune globulin
Passive immunization
Immune enhancement
Therapeutic immunization
Cytokines
Ampligen
Immune suppression
Cyclosporine
Corticosteroids
Cytokine modulation
Other therapies
Intracellular processes
Genetic approaches

system could theoretically include methods to replace or enhance immune response and tactics that suppress the state of chronic activation. Although these two strategies appear diametrically opposed, containment of the destruction rendered by HIV may require each of these approaches to be employed at specific time points in the infection. Finally, immunomodulators may actually modulate the toxicities of other medications. Examples of these approaches are listed in Table 7-10.

Immune Replacement

Bone Marrow Transplantation

Interest in bone marrow transplantation has waned since the early days of the AIDS epidemic. In 1984, the National Institute of Allergy and Infectious Disease (NIAID) attempted to reconstitute the immune system of a patient with AIDS by adoptive transfer of lymphocytes and bone marrow transplantation from a non-HIV-infected identical twin. Although the patient died, immunologic improvement was documented, suggesting the potential utility of this approach.[193] Bone marrow transplantation has been combined with antiviral therapy in patients with AIDS.[194,195] Although viral infection may be eliminated, the failures of this strategy suggest fundamental obstacles. Complete reconstitution of the immune system may be hindered by HIV infection of the transplanted elements. Cytoablative therapy may iatrogenically damage the bone marrow microenvironment, inhibiting hematologic reconstitution.[195] Finally, the lack of an intact thymic microenvironment in the recipient may impede maturation of T-cell progenitors.[19]

Autologous CD8⁺ T-Cell Transfusions

Other attempts to reconstitute the immune system include transfusion of autologous $CD8^+$ T cells that have been expanded and activated in vitro. HIV-specific $CD8^+$ T cells are capable of killing HIV-antigen-expressing cells in both a major histocompatibility complex–restricted and non-restricted fashion. In addition, $CD8^+$ T cells release a cytokine that appears to suppress the replication of HIV in peripheral blood mononuclear cells.[196] These antiviral effects may be important in early containment of HIV infection. Progression of disease has been associated with a loss of cytotoxic $CD8^+$ T cells. A small phase I trial of autologous $CD8^+$ T-cell transfusions suggests that this approach may be feasible, at least in individuals with a $CD4^+$ T-cell count above 150 cells/μl.

Intravenous Immune Globulin and Passive Immunotherapy

The administration of intravenous immune globulin (IVIG) has been used to treat immune-mediated cytopenias, particularly thrombocytopenia, and to prevent pyogenic infections in HIV-infected pediatric patients. Recently, the utility of IVIG in preventing serious bacterial infections was compared to placebo (albumin) in children with symptomatic HIV infection receiving zidovudine. Although the estimated two-year rates of serious bacterial infections were significantly lower in the IVIG recipients, the benefit was confined to those children not receiving trimethoprim–sulfamethoxazole prophylaxis.[197]

A variety of approaches to passive immunotherapy of HIV infection are under development.[198] Clinical trials published to date have used plasma containing high titers of anti-p24 antibodies from HIV-infected donors, and all have shown a diminution in p24 antigenemia in the recipients (Table 7-11).[199–202] The largest of these trials compared passive immunotherapy with placebo sera in 63 individuals with AIDS. Although p24 antigenemia declined in the majority of immunotherapy recipients, there was no effect on $CD4^+$ T-cell count or viremia. In addition, even though trends were suggested, there was no significant improvement in survival or time to new opportunistic infection.[202] Finally, a high titer of neutralizing antibodies in HIV- infected pregnant women appears to confer a protective effect, reducing the likelihood of maternal-fetal transmission. The efficacy of exogenous hyperimmune HIV antibodies in reducing maternal-fetal transmission is under evaluation.[202]

Immune Enhancement

Several strategies to enhance the immune deficiency caused by HIV infection are also under evaluation. HIV-infected individuals have been administered HIV vaccines in an attempt to boost their immune response to the vi-

Table 7-11. Passive Immunotherapy with Anti-p24 Antibody in Patients with AIDS[198]

PREPARATION	PATIENTS TREATED	NUMBER OF TRANSFUSIONS	RESULTS	REFERENCE
Plasma (heat inactivated)	6	7	Decreased OI, p24	199
Plasma (β-propriolactone treated)	10	2–23	Decreased p24	200
Plasma (heat inactivated)	9	7	Decreased OI, p24	201
Plasma (β-propriolactone treated)	31	every 4 wk	No clinical improvement Decreased p24	202

OI, opportunistic infection.

rus. This strategy is referred to as "therapeutic immunizations" to differentiate it from vaccines administered to non-HIV-infected individuals in an attempt to prevent HIV infection. The immune enhancement potential of various cytokines and ampligen (synthetic, double-stranded RNA) are also under evaluation. Hematopoietic growth factors may be able to minimize leukopenia, which occurs either as a consequence of HIV infection or medications.

Therapeutic Immunization

Attempts at potentiating the immune response to HIV by immunizing HIV-infected individuals with a therapeutic vaccine are currently under investigation. A phase I trial conducted in subjects with early HIV infection ($CD4^+$ T-cell count >400 cells/μl) evaluated a recombinant gp160 expressed in a baculovirus system (MicroGeneSys) at three different doses (40, 160, and 640 μg/ml) and two different dosage schedules (three inoculations over four months or six inoculations over six months). Response was defined as a reproducible and selective potentiation of both cellular and humoral responses against specific HIV envelope epitopes associated with the timing of the inoculations. Response was noted in 19 of the 30 vaccine recipients and was associated with both the number of injections and the baseline $CD4^+$ T-cell count. Over a 10-month follow-up period, $CD4^+$ T-cell counts remained stable in the responders whereas the $CD4^+$ T-cell counts in the nonresponders declined by 7.3%. No systemic adverse effects from the vaccine were observed.[203]

The results of a phase II/III efficacy trial conducted in 103 asymptomatic HIV-infected individuals have been reported. The immunogen used in this trial was a gp120-depleted, inactivated HIV-1 presented in incomplete Freund's adjuvant. The control group received the adjuvant alone. Both humoral and cellular immune responses were observed, and both were significantly more pronounced in the immunogen recipients. Antibodies to p24 were maximal at 32 weeks (8 weeks after the last injection). Although a gradual decline was observed during the one-year follow-up period, the titers observed in the group receiving immunogen were still above baseline at the end of the study. Significant differences were also observed in viral burden (viral DNA) and progression of disease ($CD4^+$ T-cell decline) between the immunogen recipients and the controls.[204]

These studies suggest that therapeutic immunization of HIV-infected individuals is safe and does stimulate a specific anti-HIV response. Long-term follow-up study of the subjects is clearly needed to define the role of this strategy in affecting disease progression.

Cytokines

Defects in the production of various cytokines have been reported in patients with HIV infection. Replacement strategies initially focused on the interferons because of the triad of antiviral, immunomodulatory, and antiproliferative effects of these agents. IFN-α has been combined with zidovudine in patients with AIDS-related Kaposi's sarcoma. At a maximum tolerated dose of 600 mg/day of zidovudine and 18 MU/day of IFN-α, tumor regression was observed in 17 of 37 patients.[205] This combination yields higher regression rates than higher doses of IFN-α alone.[206]

The antiviral effects of IFN-α, however, are complex, and the response to therapy is likely to depend on whether the patient has progressed to AIDS. Clinical isolates of HIV have variable susceptibility to IFN-α. Progression to AIDS has been associated with high circulating endogenous levels of IFN-α. It appears that IFN-α–resistant HIV occurs naturally at a low level, and its frequency is probably independent of endogenous IFN-α. However, as disease progresses, the higher levels of endogenous IFN-α select for the IFN-α–resistant phenotype. Thus, patients in the later stages of HIV infection are likely to have a high prevalence of IFN-α–resistant HIV variants.[207] This suggests that the benefits of exogenous IFN-α therapy may be greatest at early stages of infection. In one study of asymptomatic HIV-infected individuals, both an antiviral effect and stabilization in $CD4^+$ T-cell counts were observed in IFN-α recipients. However, even in asymptomatic individuals, exogenous IFN-α was associated with significant toxicity. All the recipients experienced flu-like symptoms, and over half developed granulocytopenia. More than one-third of the recipients withdrew from treatment because of toxicity.[208] These data together suggest that early intervention, perhaps using IFN-α gene therapy directed at HIV target cells, might have potential.[209]

Impaired production of IL-2 has also been described in patients with AIDS. Human $CD4^+$ T cells may be separated into two subsets, TH1 and TH2. TH1 cells secrete the cytokines important for enhancing cell-mediated immunity (IL-2, TNF-β, and IFN-γ), and TH2 cells secrete cytokines that increase antibody production. Impaired production of IL-2 appears to result from a progressive, selective deficiency of TH1 responses and a predominance of TH2 responses (mediated by IL-4, IL-5, IL-6, and IL-10). This defect in TH1 response might be corrected by exogenous administration of IL-2 or IL-12.[19]

Although immunoenhancing effects of IL-2 have been observed in vitro, early results in patients have been disappointing, perhaps because of suboptimal dosing.[209] Recent strategies have focused on intermittent IL-2 therapy (five-day course every eight weeks). A preliminary evaluation in 25 HIV-infected subjects suggested that in some patients administered IL-2, temporary increases in circulating lymphocytes were observed. Specifically, in 6 of the 10 individuals with baseline $CD4^+$ T-cell counts above 200/μl, at least a 50% increase in circulating $CD4^+$ T cells was observed with IL-2 therapy. However, in the remaining patients, whose baseline $CD4^+$ T-cell counts were below 200/μl, IL-2 administration was associated with increased viral replication, toxicity, and little immunologic improvement.[210] IL-2 administration, however, can increase the concentration of circulating HIV particles. This appears to be more sustained in individuals with low $CD4^+$ T-cell counts than in those with high counts. This emphasizes the need for antiretroviral therapy in the setting of IL-2 treatment. The optimal dosing regimen to achieve the most sustained clinical and immunologic benefits from IL-2 remains to be clarified.

Recent studies have also suggested that IL-12 therapy might be useful in the management of HIV infection. Antigenic stimulation of peripheral blood mononuclear cells from subjects with HIV infection yield poor cell-mediated responses in vitro. This can be corrected by stimulating the cultures in the presence of IL-12. This finding suggests that IL-12 administration may be effective in restoring HIV-specific cell-mediated immunity, at least in vitro.[211]

Colony-stimulating factors, glycoprotein hormones that regulate cellular development from hematopoietic progenitors, might be useful in stimulating the production of both erythrocytes and leukocytes. Patients with AIDS who are receiving zidovudine and have low endogenous erythropoietin levels may benefit from epoetin alfa therapy. A reduction in red blood cell transfusion requirements has been observed in patients receiving concomitant therapy with recombinant epoetin alfa.[212,213] A phase I/II trial of granulocyte-macrophage colony-stimulating factor (GM-CSF) was undertaken in 16 patients with AIDS and leukopenia. This study revealed dose-dependent increases in circulating leukocytes. Mature neutrophils, band forms, and eosinophils accounted for the majority of the increase. Circulating monocytes increased two- to fourfold over baseline. Dose-related changes in lymphocyte counts were not observed.[214] The use of GM-CSF may reduce the morbidity associated with either disease-related or therapy-related leukopenia in patients with AIDS. However, the ability of GM-CSF to stimulate HIV replication in monocytes is a cause for concern. Moreover, whether colony-stimulating factors will be able to sustain hematopoiesis in a setting of continued suppression is uncertain. A small study of GM-CSF, used as a single agent followed by an alternating regimen with zidovudine, supports these concerns. In that study, GM-CSF increased both circulating monocyte number and function and increased HIV replication (as measured by increased p24 antigen) in six of nine patients. Furthermore, bone marrow evaluations performed at 14 weeks revealed increased cellularity and increased myeloid precursors in only three of seven patients.[215] Because of the potential for enhancement of viral replication, it is likely that the ultimate role of GM-CSF will be in combination with antiviral therapy. Although neither granulocyte colony-stimulating factor (G-CSF) nor GM-CSF are approved by the FDA for the management of leukopenia in patients with AIDS, G-CSF has become widely used for bone marrow support in this setting.

Ampligen

Ampligen [or poly(I):poly(C_{12}U)] is a synthetic, mismatched, double-stranded RNA molecule that stimulates interferon production. In vitro, this agent has been shown to exhibit both antiviral and immunomodulatory properties. Ampligen appears to be synergistic with zidovudine in both zidovudine-sensitive and zidovudine-resistant isolates without concomitant bone marrow toxicity.[216] A dose escalation study in asymptomatic individuals with $CD4^+$ T-cell counts below 500 cells/μl suggested that immunologic stabilization was dose related. Patients receiving 10 and 40 mg/m^2 twice weekly had a significant decline in $CD4^+$ T-cell counts; those receiving 120 mg/m^2 or more had either stabilized or improved $CD4^+$ T-cell counts. No effect on p24 antigenemia was noted.[217]

Immune Suppression

Recently, investigators have targeted chronic activation of the immune system in an effort to preserve immune function. As reviewed in the discussion of immunopathogenesis above, chronic activation of the immune system enhances viral replication and promotes the destruction of CD4⁺ T cells. Although this approach may be reasonable and preliminary data suggest promise, it is imperative that this strategy target patients unlikely to be harmed by additional immunosuppression.

Cyclosporine

Cyclosporine may be useful in blocking the state of chronic activation of the immune system promoted by HIV. Cyclosporine blocks the transcriptional activation of T lymphocytes by inhibiting nuclear factors, which results in reduced HIV expression.[218] In addition, cyclosporine may disrupt the production of infectious viral particles by interfering with the binding of cellular cyclophilin A and B to the Gag protein of HIV-1.[219] The clinical experience with cyclosporine has been mixed, with one trial suggesting improvement and another suggesting further deterioration of an already compromised immune system.[19] However, one retrospective analysis of transplant recipients infected with HIV at about the time of transplantation suggested that cyclosporine administration soon after infection delayed the progression to AIDS. Of the 13 individuals who did not receive cyclosporine as part of the transplantation regimen, the five-year cumulative risk of AIDS was 90%, compared with 31% in the 40 individuals who received cyclosporine.[220] These data suggest that the optimal time to administer immunosuppressives, such as cyclosporine, would be before the development of HIV-related immunosuppression. In patients who have already developed HIV immune dysfunction, less immunosuppressive analogues of cyclosporine may be of greater benefit.[19,221]

Corticosteroids

Corticosteroids have potent immunosuppressive effects, and concern has arisen over even short courses administered as adjunctive therapy for PCP. Long-term use of corticosteroids has been associated with the reactivation of protozoal, mycobacterial, and fungal infections in patients without HIV infection. Therefore, the theoretical benefit of reducing immune hyperactivation must be balanced against the risk of exacerbating latent infections. Phase I studies conducted in children[222] and adults[223] have addressed the potential of corticosteroid therapy in HIV infection. Pharmacologic doses of prednisolone (0.5 mg/kg for six months, 0.3 mg/kg thereafter) were administered to asymptomatic, HIV-infected adults (CD4⁺ T-cell counts of 200–799 cells/µl) for a period exceeding one year. Evaluations at one year suggested a decrease in activation of both the cellular and humoral components of the immune system (CD25⁺, DR⁺, and CD4⁺ phenotypes; decrease in IgG, IgA, and β_2-microglobulin). Measures of HIV replication remained stable, but the CD4⁺ T-cell counts increased from baseline and remained elevated throughout the period of study in the majority of patients. At one year, the median increase in CD4⁺ T-cell count was 119 cells/µl.[223] Sustained increases in CD4⁺ T-cell counts were more common in those that had baseline CD4⁺ T-cell counts of 500–799 cells/µl than those with 200–499 cells/µl.[224] Clinically, the patients gained weight and had a decrease in lymphadenopathy. No patient developed AIDS. Although the numbers are small, T-cell function did not appear to be compromised, and there did not appear to be an increase in reactivations of viral or fungal infections.[223]

Cytokine Modulation

As described in the discussion of immunopathogenesis above, HIV infection is associated with abnormal release of various cytokines. Many of those cytokines have a direct effect on HIV replication (see Table 7-4). Attempts to modulate cytokine secretion in HIV infection have focused on TNF-α. The production of TNF-α may be inhibited by thalidomide and pentoxifylline. Thalidomide, a drug known for its teratogenicity, has been associated with a reduction in TNF-α–related symptoms in patients with leprosy, and clinical trials in HIV-infected patients are underway.[19]

In addition to inhibiting TNF-α production, pentoxifylline also appears to directly inhibit HIV expression by decreasing the activity of the transcription factor NF-κB.[225,226] Because the effect of pentoxifylline on HIV replication is modest at best,[221,227] it is most likely to be useful as an adjunct to antiretrovirals. Preliminary results from phase I/II trials of pentoxifylline combined with zidovudine suggest the potential of this approach.[226] Other approaches to the inhibition of TNF-α are under development.

Other Host-Directed Therapies

Intracellular processes play an important role in HIV replication. HIV replication is sensitive to the intracellular concentrations of deoxynucleoside triphosphates.[228] The rate of synthesis of HIV DNA is slower in resting lymphocytes than in stimulated cells. Hydroxyurea treatment, in vitro, returns the level of DNA synthesis to that of quiescent lymphocytes.[229] HIV replication may also be inhibited in vitro by mycophenolic acid, which appears to block the incorporation of nucleotides into DNA.[230] Intracellular levels of glutathione, which protects against oxygen free radicals, is depleted in individuals with HIV infection. Glutathione also appears to inhibit NF-κB, an HIV replication inducer. *N*-acetyl-L-cysteine blocks HIV replication by increasing intracellular glutathione concentrations.[231,232] In addition, *N*-acetyl-L-cysteine enhances antibody-dependent cellular cytotoxicity.[233] Phase II clinical trials of *N*-acetyl-L-cysteine are underway.[221]

Finally, genetic approaches that target either the host or the virus are being considered. Targeted ribozymes that cleave HIV RNA,[234,235] introduction of transdominant mutations in critical HIV genes (such as *rev*),[236] and introduction of decoy *tat*- or *rev*-binding antisense RNAs are strategies that successfully inhibit HIV replication in vitro.[221] The application of these approaches to clinical medicine await innovative methods of drug delivery.

Vaccine Development

Although vaccine development is probably crucial to the ultimate containment of HIV, the development of an effective and safe vaccine is a formidable challenge. Optimism has been stimulated by recent advances in the molecular understanding of viral variability and immunologic response to specific epitopes. In addition, meaningful progress in development of a suitable animal model has been achieved with experimental trials of SIV infection. These models enable evaluation of the cross-protection afforded to isolates dissimilar to those contained in the vaccine. Mucosal models of infection are also under development.[237] Although these are important advances in the evolution of a vaccine for HIV, several developmental considerations remain.

Developmental Considerations

Despite the progress made in the development of animal models, HIV is uniquely pathogenic for humans, so an exact animal model in which to study the spectrum of the disease does not exist. The only animal known to be susceptible to HIV infection is the chimpanzee.[238] Once infected, chimpanzees produce antibody profiles similar to those of humans, shed virus, and demonstrate cytopathic changes in $CD4^+$ T cells. Chimpanzees occasionally develop lymphadenopathy and temporary $CD4^+$ T-cell count depression, but they do not develop an AIDS-like illness. The chimpanzee therefore appears to be an adequate model in which to assess the efficacy of a vaccine against primary HIV infection, but this model may not accurately reflect the ability of the vaccine to prevent the development of AIDS in humans. Adding to the problem is the severely limited availability of chimpanzees for research in vaccine development. Given these limitations, a great deal of excitement has been generated by the progress made with the SIV model. However, genetic and biological differences between HIV and SIV may limit the value of this model, particularly with respect to extent of virus variability.[237,239]

HIV is notable for the high degree of antigenic variation among its isolates. The region of greatest variability is the external envelope glycoprotein.[240] The extent of protection conferred by vaccine candidates against divergent isolates must be evaluated. Although HIV-1 and HIV-2 share common core proteins, their envelope proteins differ, and only infection with HIV-2 has been well described. Finally, both phenotypic and genotypic mixing are known to exist, allowing for the possibility that mutations constantly occur in nature. It will be necessary to determine whether an immunogen from a single virus is group-specific or will stimulate the formation of antibodies capable of neutralizing unrelated variants.[241]

The role of antibody protection from HIV infection is not completely understood. Some patients with HIV infection have neutralizing antibodies against HIV. However, in vitro viral neutralization may not reflect in vivo activity. The presence of neutralizing antibodies in the sera of both asymptomatic seropositive persons and in patients with AIDS suggests that these antibodies do not extend adequate protection.[242]

Other retroviral systems suggest that the antigens important for vaccine development are the external envelope glycoproteins. Because the antigens are found on the exterior portion of the virion, they are the first to be exposed to the immune system.[243] However, infected cells may express other gene products from within the virion on their cell surfaces.[241,243] Therefore, antigens defined by genes critical for viral growth and cytopathogenicity, even if not located on the outside of the virus, should be considered as potential immunogens. These genes are listed in Table 7-12.

Strategies for optimizing the presentation of immunogen will need evaluation. The only adjuvant systems approved for human use are aluminum hydroxide and aluminum phosphate. Although alum is effective in some vaccines, a more efficient stimulator of humoral and cellular responses may be necessary for a vaccine effective against HIV. Alternative systems, such as muramyl dipeptides, liposomes, and immune-stimulating complexes, are

Table 7-12. Viral Gene Products for Vaccine Consideration

GENE	MOLECULAR WEIGHT	FUNCTION
env	gp160	External structural proteins
	gp120	Envelope glycoprotein
	gp41	Transmembrane anchor
pol	p66/51/31	Viral enzymes
		Reverse transcriptase
		Integrase
		Protease
gag	p55/24/17	Structural capsid proteins
tat	p14	Viral transactivator
rev	p20	RNA transport/stability factor

Table 7-13. General Approaches to HIV Vaccine Development

Purified natural products
Synthetic peptide or subunit + adjuvant
Subunit in viral vector
Anti-idiotype

under development. The immunogenicity of the preparation may be enhanced by several orders of magnitude if a potent adjuvant system is used.[241]

To test the efficacy of vaccine candidates, phase III studies of seronegative individuals who engage in high-risk behaviors are necessary. Investigators in these studies must balance their ability to obtain HIV vaccine efficacy data with their ethical obligation to inform and educate the subjects about the avoidance of risky behaviors. The implication of these conflicting goals is that the reported efficacy of the vaccine may be clouded by the impact of counseling.

Vaccine Approaches

The two approaches that appear to hold greatest promise for an HIV vaccine are recombinant vaccines and subunit vaccines consisting of cloned, purified, or synthetic HIV proteins (see chapter 6). These subunits may be presented with a suitable adjuvant, or the gene encoding for the desired subunit can be inserted into an attenuated vector. Both these approaches focus on the envelope glycoprotein as the cloned antigen. Finally, anti-idiotype vaccines are in the early stages of human trials. The object of these vaccines is to stimulate the production of antibodies that resemble CD4, potentially interfering with viral binding to CD4 receptors on host cells. The approaches currently under investigation are listed in Table 7-13.

Human Trials

Table 7-14 lists the types of HIV vaccines under evaluation and their current status. The phase III trials of candidate vaccines in the United States have been delayed by the NIAID. There were two principal concerns regarding initiation of these large-scale efficacy trials. First, the markers of successful immunization are unknown. Whether a protective response is engendered by antibodies to the envelope subunit is unclear. Second, potential vaccine recipients may not fully appreciate the possible lack of protection produced by the vaccine. The impact of this second issue was emphasized by the higher than expected rates of new HIV infection in the vaccine recipients enrolled in the phase I and II studies.[3,243]

Efficacy studies are likely to be performed initially in developing countries, where HIV infection is spreading most rapidly. The dynamics of the infection in these regions suggest a public health imperative and indicate that much smaller sample sizes will be necessary to demonstrate the effectiveness (or lack thereof) of the vaccine. It is hoped that these trials will provide more information about the correlates of protection, which will aid in the further quest for an effective vaccine. Phase I and II trials are underway to assess the reproducibility of the U.S. experience in the target countries. Groups of HIV-seronegative, high-risk individuals are currently being assembled for phase III testing in Thailand.[243]

Table 7-14. Status of Recombinant Subunit Protein HIV Vaccines[3]

TYPE OF VACCINE	STATUS
HIV envelope proteins	
gp160-baculovirus vectoralum	Phase II complete
gp160-vaccinia–infected Vero cells	Phase I trials
gp120-CHO cells (IIIB and MN strains) in alum adjuvant	Phase II trials
gp120-CHO cells (SF-2 strain) in MF-59 MTP adjuvant	Phase II trials
gp120-yeast (SF-2 strain) in MF-59 and MF-59 MTP adjuvant	Phase II trials
Fusogenic envelope peptides	Phase I trials
gp120 cocktails	Phase I trials
Modified live-virus vectors	
Vaccinia/gp160 recombinant	Phase II trials
Vaccinia (vac*gagpol*) construct	Phase I trials
Avipoxvirus (gp160)	Phase I trials
Combination	
vac/*env*-gp160 and recombinant gp160 or gp120 boost	Phase I trials

CHO, Chinese hamster ovary; MTP, muramyl tripeptide; MF-59, squalene adjuvant.

SUMMARY

The acquired immunodeficiency syndrome is clearly a disease of both national and global consequence. The long incubation period of the virus and the considerable number of people already infected with HIV ensure that AIDS will continue to have a major impact on our health care system for years to come. As research defining the usefulness of various antiviral and immunomodulating strategies evolve, our approach to the management of patients, potentially combining immunomodulators and multiple antiviral agents directed at specific points in the viral replicative cycle, will change.

Pharmacists can serve an important role in this epidemic by providing up-to-date information and advice for their patients and other health care providers. By participating in community outreach, pharmacists can educate their communities about HIV transmission, risky behaviors, and risk-reduction strategies—especially correct and consistent condom and spermicide use. As an integral member of the medical team, the pharmacist can participate in the management of patients infected with HIV. Pharmacists' specialized knowledge of pharmacology, drug interactions, adverse drug effects, and reimbursement can aid in the provision of optimal health care for patients with HIV infection.

REFERENCES

1. Centers for Disease Control [CDC]. HIV/AIDS Surveillance Report. Year-end Edition. Atlanta, GA: CDC; 1996:1–39.
2. Rosenberg PS. Scope of the AIDS epidemic in the United States. *Science* 1995;270:1372–5.
3. Hoth DR, Bolognesi DP, Corey L, Vermund SH. HIV vaccine development: a progress report. *Ann Intern Med.* 1994;121:603–11.
4. Gallo RC, Salahuddin SZ, Popovic M, *et al.* Frequent detection and isolation of cytopathic retroviruses (HTLV III) from patients with AIDS and at risk for AIDS. *Science* 1984;224:500–3.
5. Barre-Sinoussi F, Chermann JC, Rey F, *et al.* Isolation of a T-lymphotropic retrovirus from a patient at risk for the acquired immune deficiency syndrome (AIDS). *Science* 1983;220:868–71.
6. Clavel F, Guetard D, Brun-Vezinet F, *et al.* Isolation of a new human retrovirus from West African patients with AIDS. *Science* 1986;233:343–6.
7. Franchini G, Gurgo C, Guo H-G, *et al.* Sequence of simian immunodeficiency virus and its relationship to the human immunodeficiency viruses. *Nature* 1987;238:539–43.
8. Clavel F, Mansinho K, Chamaret S, *et al.* Human immunodeficiency virus type 2 infection associated with AIDS in West Africa. *N Engl J Med.* 1987;316:1180–5.
9. Kanki PJ, Barin F, M'Boup S, *et al.* New human T-lymphotropic retrovirus related to simian T-lymphotropic virus type III (STLV-III_{AGM}). *Science* 1986;232:238–43.
10. Piot P, Plummer FA, Mhalu FS, *et al.* AIDS: an international perspective. *Science* 1988;239:573–9.
11. Centers for Disease Control. Update: acquired immunodeficiency syndrome—United States, 1994. *MMWR* 1995;44:64–7.
12. Castro BA, Cheng-Mayer C, Evans LA, Levy JA. HIV heterogeneity and viral pathogenesis. AIDS. 1988;2(*Suppl* 1):S17–S27.
13. Stein BS, Gowda SD, Lifson JD, *et al.* pH-independent HIV entry into CD4-positive T-cells via virus envelope fusion to the plasma membrane. *Cell* 1987;49:659–68.
14. Bedinger P, Moriarty A, von Borstel RC II, *et al.* Internalization of the human immunodeficiency virus does not require the cytoplasmic domain of CD4. *Nature* 1988; 334:162–5.
15. Ho DD, Pomerantz RJ, Kaplan JC. Pathogenesis of infection with human immunodeficiency virus. *N Engl J Med.* 1987;317:278–86.
16. Southern P, Oldstone MBA. Medical consequences of persistent viral infection. *N Engl J Med.* 1986;314:356–67.
17. Pantaleo G, Graziosi C, Fauci AS. The immunopathogenesis of human immunodeficiency virus infection. *N Engl J Med.* 1993;328:327–35.
18. Fauci AS. The human immunodeficiency virus: infectivity and mechanisms of pathogenesis. *Science* 1988;239:617–22.
19. Fauci AS. Multifactorial nature of human immunodeficiency virus disease: implications for therapy. *Science* 1993;262:1011–8.
20. Ho DD, Neumann AU, Perelson AS, *et al.* Rapid turnover of plasma virions and CD4 lymphocytes in HIV-1 infection. *Nature* 1995;373:123–6.
21. Wei X, Ghosh SK, Taylor ME, *et al.* Viral dynamics in human immunodeficiency virus type 1 infection. *Nature* 1995;373:117–22.
22. Phair JP. Variations in the natural history of HIV infection [keynote address]. *AIDS Res Hum Retroviruses* 1994; 10:883–5.
23. Cao Y, Quin L, Zhang L, *et al.* Virologic and immunologic characterization of long-term survivors of human immunodeficiency virus type 1 infection. *N Engl J Med.* 1995; 332:201–8.
24. Pantaleo G, Menzo S, Vaccarezza M, *et al.* Studies in subjects with long-term nonprogressive human immunodeficiency virus infection. *N Engl J Med.* 1995;332:209–16.
25. Bryson YJ, Pang S, Wei LS, *et al.* Clearance of HIV infection in a perinatally infected infant. *N Engl J Med.* 1995; 332:833–8.
26. Klatzmann D, Barre-Sinoussi F, Nugeyre MT, *et al.* Selective tropism of lymphadenopathy associated virus (LAV) for helper-inducer T-lymphocytes. *Science* 1984;225:59–64.
27. Lane HC, Depper JM, Greene WC, *et al.* Qualitative analysis of immune function in patients with the acquired immunodeficiency syndrome: evidence for a selective defect in soluble antigen recognition. *N Engl J Med.* 1985; 313:79–84.
28. Murray HW, Rubin BY, Masur H, *et al.* Impaired production of lymphokines and immune (gamma) interferon in the acquired immunodeficiency syndrome. *N Engl J Med.* 1984;310:883–9.
29. Margolick JB, Volkman DJ, Folks TM, *et al.* Amplification of HTLV-III/LAV infection by antigen-induced activation of T-cells and direct suppression by virus of lymphocyte blastogenic responses. *J Immunol.* 1987;138:1719–23.
30. Rook RH, Masur H, Lane HC, *et al.* Interleukin-2 enhances the depressed natural killer and cytomegalovirus-specific cytotoxic activities of lymphocytes from patients

with the acquired immunodeficiency syndrome. *J Clin Invest*. 1983;72:398–403.
31. Ho DD, Rota TR, Hirsch MS. Infection of monocyte/macrophage by human T lymphotropic virus type III. *J Clin Invest*. 1986;77:1712–5.
32. Gartner S, Markovits P, Markovits DM, *et al*. The role of mononuclear phagocytes in HTLV-III/LAV infection. *Science* 1985;233:215–9.
33. Talle MA, Rao PE, Westberg E, *et al*. Patterns of antigenic expression on human monocytes as defined by monoclonal antibodies. *Cell Immunol*. 1983;78:83–99.
34. Smith PD, Ohura K, Masur H, *et al*. Monocyte function in the acquired immunodeficiency syndrome: defective chemotaxis. *J Clin Invest*. 1984;74:2121–8.
35. Lane HC, Masur H, Edgar LC, *et al*. Abnormalities of B-cell activation and immunoregulation in patients with the acquired immunodeficiency syndrome. *N Engl J Med*. 1983;309:453–8.
36. Ho DD, Schooley TI, Rota TR, *et al*. HTLV-III in semen and blood of a healthy homosexual man. *Science* 1984; 226:451–3.
37. Wofsy CB, Cohen JB, Hauer LB, *et al*. Isolation of AIDS-associated retrovirus from genital secretions of women with antibodies to the virus. *Lancet* 1986;1:527–9.
38. Fujikawa LS, Palestine AG, Nussenblatt RB, *et al*. Isolation of human T-lymphotropic virus type III from the tears of a patient with the acquired immunodeficiency syndrome. *Lancet* 1985;2:529–30.
39. Ho DD, Byington RE, Schooley RT, *et al*. Infrequency of isolation of HTLV-III virus from saliva in AIDS. *N Engl J Med*. 1985;313:1606.
40. Curran JW, Jaffe HW, Hardy AM, *et al*. Epidemiology of HIV infection and AIDS in the United States. *Science* 1988;239:610–6.
41. Chmiel JS, Detels R, Kaslow RA, *et al*. Factors associated with prevalent human immunodeficiency virus (HIV) infection in the multicenter AIDS cohort study. *Am J Epidemiol*. 1987;126:568–77.
42. Darrow WW, Echenberg DF, Jaffe HW, *et al*. Risk factors for human immunodeficiency virus (HIV) infections in homosexual men. *Am J Public Health* 1987;77:479–83.
43. Winkelstein W, Lyman DM, Padian N, *et al*. Sexual practices and risk of infection by the human immunodeficiency virus: The San Francisco Men's Health Study. *JAMA* 1987;257:321–5.
44. Marmar M, Weiss LR, Lyden M, *et al*. Possible female-to-female transmission of human immunodeficiency virus. *Ann Intern Med*. 1986;105:969.
45. Harris C, Butkus C, Klein RS, *et al*. Immunodeficiency in female sexual partners of men with the acquired immunodeficiency syndrome. *N Engl J Med*. 1983;308:1181–4.
46. Friedland GH, Klein RS. Transmission of the human immunodeficiency virus. *N Engl J Med*. 1987;317:1125–35.
47. Al-Nozha M, Ramia S, Al-Frayh A, *et al*. Female to male: an inefficient mode of transmission of human immunodeficiency virus. *J Acquir Immune Defic Syndr*. 1990;3:193–4.
48. Holmberg SD, Horsburgh CR Jr., Ward JW, *et al*. Biologic factors in the sexual transmission of human immunodeficiency virus. *J Infect Dis*. 1989;160:116–25.
49. Padian NS, Shiboski SC, Jewell NP. The effect of number of exposures on the risk of heterosexual HIV transmission. *J Infect Dis*. 1990;161:883–7.
50. Des Jarlais DC, Friedman SR, Stoneburner RL. HIV infection and intravenous drug use: critical issues in transmission dynamics, infection outcomes, and prevention. *Rev Infect Dis*. 1988;10:151–8.
51. Guinan ME, Hardy A. Epidemiology of AIDS in women in the United States: 1981–1986. *JAMA* 1987;257:2039–42.
52. Ward JW, Deppe DA, Samson S, *et al*. Risk of human immunodeficiency virus infection from blood donors who later developed the acquired immunodeficiency syndrome. *Ann Intern Med*. 1987;106:61–2.
53. Ward JW, Holmberg SD, Allen JR, *et al*. Transmission of human immunodeficiency virus (HIV) by blood transfusions screened as negative for HIV antibody. *N Engl J Med*. 1988;318:473–8.
54. Donegan E, Stuart M, Niland JC, *et al*. Infection with human immunodeficiency virus type 1 (HIV-1) among recipients of antibody-positive blood donations. *Ann Intern Med*. 1990;113:733–9.
55. Donegan E, Lenes BA, Tomasulo PA, *et al*. Transmission of HIV-1 by component type and duration of shelf storage before transfusion. *Transfusion* 1990;30:839–40.
56. Rivers EP, Buse SM, Bivins BA, *et al*. Organ and tissue procurement in the acute care setting: principles and practice—part 2. *Ann Emerg Med*. 1990;19:193–200.
57. Araneta MRG, Mascola L, Eller A, *et al*. HIV transmission through donor artificial insemination. *JAMA* 1995;273:854–8.
58. Lifson AR, Castro KG, McCray E, *et al*. National surveillance of AIDS in health care workers. *JAMA* 1986; 256:3231–4.
59. Henderson DK, Fahey BS, Willy M, *et al*. Risk for occupational transmission of human immunodeficiency virus type 1 (HIV-1) associated with exposures. *Ann Intern Med*. 1990;113:740–6.
60. Gerberding JL. Management of occupational exposures to blood-borne viruses. *N Engl J Med*. 1995;332:444–51.
61. Centers for Disease Control. Update: provisional public health service recommendations for chemoprophylaxis after occupational exposure to HIV. *MMWR* 1996;45:468–72.
61a. Niu MT, Stein DS, Schnittmann SM. Primary human immunodeficiency virus type-1 infection: review of pathogenesis and early treatment interventions in humans and animal retrovirus infections. *J Infect Dis*. 1993;168:1490–501.
61b. Centers for Disease Control. Case-control study of HIV seroconversion in health-care workers after percutaneous exposure to HIV-infected blood—France, United Kingdom, and United States, January 1988–August 1994. *MMWR* 1995;44:929–33.
62. Centers for Disease Control. Update: transmission of HIV infection during an invasive dental procedure—Florida. *MMWR* 1991;40:21–7.
63. Ciesielski C, Marianos D, Ou CY, *et al*. Transmission of human immunodeficiency virus in a dental practice. *Ann Intern Med*. 1992;116:798–805.
64. Oxtoby MJ. Perinatally acquired HIV infection. In: Pizzo

PA, Wilfert CM, editors. *Pediatric AIDS: The Challenge of HIV Infection in Infants, Children, and Adolescents*. Baltimore, MD: Williams and Wilkins; 1991. p. 3–21.

65. Puel J, Izopet J, Lheritier D, *et al*. Viral load and mother-to-infant HIV transmission. *Lancet* 1992;340:859.
66. European Collaborative Study. Risk factors for mother-to-child transmission of HIV-1. *Lancet* 1992;339:1007–12.
67. Fang F, Burger H, Grimson R, *et al*. Maternal plasma human immunodeficiency virus type 1 RNA level: a determinant and projected threshold for mother-to-child transmission. *Proc Natl Acad Sci USA* 1995;92:12001–4.
68. Fischl MA, Dickinson GM, Scott GM, *et al*. Evaluation of heterosexual partners, children, and household contacts of adults with AIDS. *JAMA* 1987;257:640–4.
69. Friedland GH, Saltzman BR, Rogers MF, *et al*. Lack of transmission of HTLV-III/LAV infection to household contacts of patients with AIDS or AIDS-related complex with oral candidiasis. *N Engl J Med*. 1986;314:344–9.
70. Rietmeijer CM, Krebs WJ, Feorino PM, *et al*. Condoms as physical and chemical barriers against human immunodeficiency virus. *JAMA* 1988;259:1851–3.
71. Mann J, Quinn TC, Piot P, *et al*. Condom use and HIV infection among prostitutes in Zaire. *N Engl J Med*. 1987; 316:345.
72. Hicks DR, Martin LS, Voeller B, *et al*. Inactivation of LAV/HTLV-III infected cultures of normal human lymphocytes by nonoxynol-9 in vitro. *Lancet* 1985;2:1422–3.
73. Centers for Disease Control. Update: barrier protection against HIV infection and other sexually transmitted diseases. *MMWR* 1993;42:589–90.
74. Brickner, PW, Torres RA, Barnes M, *et al*. Recommendations for control and prevention of human immunodeficiency virus (HIV) infection in intravenous drug users. *Ann Intern Med*. 1989;110:833–7.
75. Centers for Disease Control. Hepatitis B virus vaccine safety: report of an interagency group. *MMWR* 1982;31: 465–7.
76. Connor EM, Sperling RS, Gelber R, *et al*. Reduction of maternal-infant transmission of human immunodeficiency virus type 1 with zidovudine treatment. *N Engl J Med*. 1994;331:1173–80.
77. Centers for Disease Control. Recommendations of the U.S. Public Health Service Task Force on the use of zidovudine to reduce perinatal transmission of human immunodeficiency virus. *MMWR* 1994;43:1–20.
78. Horsburgh CR, Ou CY, Jason J, *et al*. Duration of human immunodeficiency virus infection before detection of antibody. *Lancet* 1989;2:637–40.
79. Rogers MF, Ou CY, Kilbourne B, *et al*. Advances and problems in the diagnosis of HIV infection in infants. In: Pizzo PA, Wilfert CM, editors. *Pediatric AIDS: The Challenge of HIV Infection in Infants, Children and Adolescents*. Baltimore, MD: Williams and Wilkins; 1991. p. 159–74.
80. Centers for Disease Control. Serologic testing for antibody to human immunodeficiency virus. *MMWR* 1987;36:833–45.
81. Centers for Disease Control. Public Health Service guidelines for counseling and antibody testing to prevent HIV infection and AIDS. *MMWR* 1987;36:509–15.
82. Marlink RG, Allan JS, McLane MP, *et al*. Low sensitivity of ELISA testing in early HIV infection. *N Engl J Med*. 1986;315:1549.
83. Parks WP, Scott GB. An overview of pediatric AIDS: approaches to diagnosis and outcome assessment. In: Broder S, editor. *AIDS—Modern Concepts and Therapeutic Challenges*. New York: Marcel Dekker; 1987. p. 245–62.
84. Purdy BD, Plaisance KI. Infection with the human immunodeficiency virus: epidemiology, pathogenesis, transmission, diagnosis, and manifestations. *Am J Hosp Pharm*. 1989;46:1185–209.
85. Steckelberg JM, Cockerill FR. Subspeciality clinics: infectious diseases: serologic testing for human immunodeficiency virus antibodies. *Mayo Clin Proc*. 1988; 63:373–80.
86. Centers for Disease Control. Interpretation and use of the Western blot assay for serodiagnosis of human immunodeficiency virus type 1 infections. *MMWR* 1989;38:S1–S7.
87. Kessler HA, Baauw B, Spear J, *et al*. Diagnosis of human immunodeficiency virus infection in seronegative homosexuals presenting with an acute viral syndrome. *JAMA* 1987;258:1196–9.
88. Wittek AE, Phelan MA, Wells MA, *et al*. Detection of human immunodeficiency virus core protein in plasma by enzyme immunoassay. Association of antigenemia with symptomatic disease and T-helper cell depletion. *Ann Intern Med*. 1987;107:286–92.
89. Allain JP, Laurian Y, Paul DA, *et al*. Long-term evaluation of HIV antigen and antibodies to p24 and gp41 in patients with hemophilia. Potential clinical importance. *N Engl J Med*. 1987;317:1114–21.
90. Borkowksy W, Krasinski K, Paul D, *et al*. Human-immunodeficiency-virus infections in infants negative for anti-HIV by enzyme-linked immunoassay. *Lancet* 1987; 1:1168–71.
91. Chaisson RE, Allain J, Volberding PA. Significant changes in HIV antigen level in the serum of patients treated with azidothymidine. *N Engl J Med*. 1986;315:1610–11.
92. Fahey JL, Taylor JMG, Detels R, *et al*. The prognostic value for cellular and serologic markers in infection with human immunodeficiency virus type 1. *N Engl J Med*. 1990; 322:166–72.
93. Ascher DP, Roberts C, Fowler A. Acidification modified p24 antigen capture assay in HIV seropositives. *J Acquir Immune Defic Syndr*. 1992;5:1080–3.
94. Nishanian P, Huskins KR, Stehn S, *et al*. A simple method for improved assay demonstrates that HIV p24 antigen is present as immune complexes in most sera from HIV-infected individuals. *J Infect Dis*. 1990;162:21–8.
95. Michalski FT. The diagnosis of human immunodeficiency virus infection: progress in less than five years. *Yale J Biol Med*. 1989;62:93–102.
96. Schochetman G, Epstein JS, Zuck TF. Serodiagnosis of infection with the AIDS virus and other human retroviruses. *Ann Rev Microbiol*. 1989;43:629–59.
97. Rogers MF, Ou CY, Rayfield M, *et al*. Use of the polymerase chain reaction for early detection of proviral sequences of human immunodeficiency virus in infants born to seropositive mothers. *N Engl J Med*. 1989;320:1649–54.
98. Schochetman G. Diagnosis of HIV infection. *Clin Chim Acta* 1992;221:1–26.
99. Simmonds P, Balfe P, Peutherer JF, *et al*. Human

immunodeficiency virus-infected individuals contain provirus in small numbers of peripheral mononuclear cells and at low copy numbers. *J Virol.* 1990;64:864–72.
100. Mellors JW, *et al.* Quantitation of HIV-1 RNA in plasma predicts outcome after seroconversion. *Ann Intern Med.* 1995;122:573–9.
101. Caliendo AM. Laboratory Methods for Quantitating HIV RNA. *AIDS Clin Care* 1995;7:89–93.
102. Bartlett JG. Quantitative HIV virology. *Moore News* 1995;4:11–2.
103. Roberts J. US approves HIV "home test." *Brit Med J.* 1996;312:1317.
103a. Frank AP, Wandell MG, Headings MD, *et al.* Anonymous HIV testing using home collection and telemedicine counseling; a multicenter evaluation. *Arch Intern Med.* 1997; 157:309–14.
104. Frerichs R, Eskes N, Htoon M. Validity of three assays for HIV-1 antibodies in saliva. *J Acquir Immune Defic Syndr.* 1994;7:522–5.
105. Soto-Ramirez LE, Hernandez-Gomez L, Sifuentes-Osornio J, *et al.* Detection of specific antibodies in gingival crevicular transudate by enzyme-linked immunosorbent assay for diagnosis of human immunodeficiency virus type 1 infection. *J Clin Microbiol.* 1992;30:2780–83.
106. Connell JA, Parry JV, Mortimer PP, *et al.* Preliminary report: accurate assays for anti-HIV in urine. *Lancet* 1990; 335:1366–69.
107. Cao YZ, Friedman KA, Mirabile M, *et al.* HIV-1 neutralizing antibodies in urine from seropositive individuals. *J Acquir Immune Defic Syndr.* 1990;3:195–9.
108. Rothenberg R, Woelfel M, Stoneburner R, *et al.* Survival with the acquired immunodeficiency syndrome: experience with 5833 cases in New York City. *N Engl J Med.* 1987;317:1297–302.
109. Pederson C, Nielsen CM, Vestergaard BF, *et al.* Temporal relation of antigenemia and loss of antibodies to core antigens to development of clinical disease in HIV infection. *Br Med J. (Clin Res Ed)* 1987;295:567–9.
110. Klein RS, Harris CA, Small CB, *et al.* Oral candidiasis in high-risk patients as the initial manifestation of acquired immunodeficiency syndrome. *N Engl J Med.* 1984;311: 354–8.
111. Nicholson JKA, McDougal S, Jaffe HW, *et al.* Exposure to human T-lymphotropic virus type III/lymphadenopathy-associated virus and immunologic abnormalities in asymptomatic homosexual men. *Ann Intern Med.* 1985;103:37–42.
112. Tindall B, Barker S, Donovan B, *et al.* Characterization of the acute clinical illness associated with human immunodeficiency virus infection. *Arch Intern Med.* 1988;148:945–9.
113. Ho DD, Sarngadharan MG, Resnick L, *et al.* Primary human T-lymphotropic virus type III infection. *Ann Intern Med.* 1985;103:880–3.
114. Centers for Disease Control. Classification system for human T-lymphotropic virus type III/lymphadenopathy-associated virus infections. *Ann Intern Med.* 1986;105: 234–7.
115. Castro KG, Ward JW, Slutsker L, *et al.* 1993 revised classification system for HIV infection and expanded surveillance case definition for AIDS among adolescents and adults. *Clin Infect Dis.* 1993;17:802–10.
116. Crowe S, Stewart K, Carlin J, *et al.* Relationship between opportunistic infections (OI) and malignancy (OM) in HIV patients and CD4 lymphocyte number. Paper presented at the Sixth International Conference on AIDS. San Francisco, CA, June 1990.
117. Mills J, Masur H. AIDS-related infections. *Sci Am.* 1990;263:50–7.
118. Masur H, Ognibene FP, Yarchoan R, *et al.* CD4 counts as predictors of opportunistic pneumonias in human immunodeficiency virus (HIV) infection. *Ann Intern Med.* 1989;111:223–31.
119. Phair T, Munoz A, Detels R, *et al.* The risk of *Pneumocystis carinii* pneumonia among men infected with human immunodeficiency virus type 1. *N Engl J Med.* 1990; 322:161–5.
120. Bozzette SA, Finkelstein DM, Spector SA, *et al.* A randomized trial of three antipneumocystis agents in patients with advanced human immunodeficiency virus infection. *N Engl J Med.* 1995;332:693–9.
121. Hughes WT. *Pneumocystis carinii* pneumonitis. *N Engl J Med.* 1987;317:1021–3.
122. Kovacs JA, Hiemenz JW, Macher AM, *et al.* *Pneumocystis carinii* pneumonia: a comparison between patients with the acquired immunodeficiency syndrome and patients with other immunodeficiencies. *Ann Intern Med.* 1984; 100:663–71.
123. Ognibene FP, Shelhamer J, Gill V, *et al.* The diagnosis of *Pneumocystis carinii* syndrome using subsegmental bronchoalveolar lavage. *Am Rev Resp Dis.* 1986;133:226–9.
124. Bigby TD, Margolskee D, Curtis JL, *et al.* The usefulness of induced sputum in the diagnosis of *Pneumocystis carinii* pneumonia in patients with the acquired immunodeficiency syndrome. *Am Rev Resp Dis.* 1986;133:515–8.
125. Allegra CJ, Chabner BA, Tuazon CU, *et al.* Trimetrexate for the treatment of *Pneumocystis carinii* pneumonia in patients with the acquired immunodeficiency syndrome. *N Engl J Med.* 1987;317:978–85.
126. Powderly WG. Cryptococcal meningitis and AIDS. *Clin Infect Dis.* 1993;17:837–42.
127. Kovacs JA, Kovacs AA, Polis M, *et al.* Cryptococcosis in the acquired immunodeficiency syndrome. *Ann Inter Med.* 1985;103:533–8.
128. Zuger A, Louie E, Holzmann RS, *et al.* Cryptococcal disease in patients with the acquired immunodeficiency syndrome: diagnostic features and outcome of treatment. *Ann Intern Med.* 1986;104:234–40.
129. Saag MS, Powderly WG, Cloud GA, *et al.* Comparison of amphotericin B with fluconazole in the treatment of acute AIDS-associated cryptococcal meningitis. *N Engl J Med.* 1992;326:83–9.
130. Wong B, Gold JWM, Brown AE, *et al.* Central nervous system toxoplasmosis in homosexual men and parenteral drug abusers. *Ann Intern Med.* 1984;100:36–42.
131. Leport C, Raffi F, Matheron S, *et al.* Treatment of central nervous system toxoplasmosis with pyrimethamine/sulfadiazine combination in 35 patients with the acquired immunodeficiency syndrome: efficacy of long-term continuous therapy. *Am J Med.* 1988;84:94–100.
132. Hawkins CC. Managing mycobacterial infections in AIDS patients. *Infect Med.* 1988;5:157–9, 207–8.

133. Hawkins CC, Gold JWM, Whimbey E, *et al*. Mycobacterium avium complex infections in patients with the acquired immunodeficiency syndrome. *Ann Intern Med*. 1986;105:184–8.
134. Young LS. Mycobacterium avium complex infection. *J Infect Dis*. 1988;157:863–67.
135. Chaisson RE, Slutkin G. Tuberculosis and human immunodeficiency virus infection. *J Infect Dis*. 1989;159:96–100.
136. Centers for Disease Control. Diagnosis and management of mycobacterium infections and disease in persons with human immunodeficiency virus infection. *Ann Intern Med*. 1987;106:254–6.
137. Glatt AE, Chirgwin K, Landesman SH. Current concepts: treatment of infections with human immunodeficiency virus. *N Engl J Med*. 1988;318:1439–48.
138. Klein RS, Harris CA, Small CB, *et al*. Oral candidiasis in high-risk patients as the initial manifestation of acquired immunodeficiency syndrome. *N Engl J Med*. 1984;311: 354–8.
139. Quinnan GV Jr, Masur H, Rook AH, *et al*. Herpes virus infections in the acquired immunodeficiency syndrome. *JAMA* 1984;252:72–7.
140. Macher AM, Reichert CM, Straus SE, *et al*. Death in the AIDS patient: role of cytomegalovirus. *N Engl J Med*. 1983;309:1454.
141. Jacobson MA, Mill J. Serious cytomegalovirus disease in the acquired immunodeficiency syndrome (AIDS): clinical findings, diagnosis, and treatment. *Ann Intern Med*. 1988;108:585–94.
142. Drew WL. Cytomegalovirus infection in patients with AIDS. *J Infect Dis*. 1988;158:449–55.
143. Pau AK, Pitrak DL. Management of cytomegalovirus infection in patients with acquired immunodeficiency syndrome. *Clin Pharm*. 1990;9:613–31.
144. Centers for Disease Control. Kaposi's sarcoma and pneumocystis pneumonia among homosexual men—New York City and California. *MMWR* 1981;30:305–8.
145. Hymes KB, Cheung T, Greene JB, *et al*. Kaposi's sarcoma in homosexual men: a report of eight cases. *Lancet* 1981;2:598–600.
146. Denning P, Chu S, Fleming P. Current trends in the epidemiology of Kaposi's sarcoma. Paper presented at the 35th Interscience Conference on Antimicrobial Agents and Chemotherapy, San Francisco, CA, September 1995. (Abstract #I23)
147. Moore PS, Chang Y. Detection of herpesvirus-like DNA sequences in Kaposi's sarcoma in patients with and those without HIV infection. *N Engl J Med*. 1995;332:1181–5.
148. Safai B, Lowenthal DA, Koziner B. Malignant neoplasms associated with the HTLV-III/LAV infection. *Antibiot Chemother Basel* 1987;38:80–98.
149. Groopman JE, Broder S. Cancer in AIDS and other immunodeficiency states. In: Devita VT, Hellman S, Rosenberg SA, editors. *Cancer: Principles and Practice of Oncology*. Vol. 2. Philadelphia, PA: JB Lippincott; 1989. p. 1953–70.
150. Ziegler JL, Beckstead JA, Volberding PA, *et al*. Non-Hodgkin's lymphoma in 90 homosexual men. *N Engl J Med*. 1984;311:565–70.
151. Levine AM, Meyer PR, Begandy MK, *et al*. Development of B-cell lymphoma in homosexual men. *Ann Intern Med*. 1986;104:737.
152. Gill PS, Meyer PR, Pavlova Z, *et al*. B-cell ALL in adults: clinical, morphologic, and immunologic findings. *J Clin Oncol*. 1986;4:747.
153. Kalter SP, Riggs SA, Cabanillas F, *et al*. Aggressive non-Hodgkin's lymphoma in immunocompromised homosexual males. *Blood* 1985;66:655–9.
154. Levine AM. Non-Hodgkin's lymphomas and other malignancies in the acquired immunodeficiency syndrome. *Semin Oncol*. 1987;14(*Suppl* 3):34–8.
155. Bermudez MA, Grant KM, Rodvien R, *et al*. Non-Hodgkin's lymphoma in a population with or at risk for acquired immunodeficiency syndrome. *Am J Med*. 1989;86:71–6.
156. Lamb R, Gonzales R, Myers A, *et al*. Aggressive non-Hodgkin's lymphoma in AIDS: the University of Colorado experience. *Am J Med Sci*. 1990;300:345–9.
157. Kaplan LD, Abrams DI, Feigal E, *et al*. AIDS-associated non-Hodgkin's lymphoma in San Francisco. *JAMA* 1989;261:719–24.
158. Levine AM, Sullivan-Halley J, Pike MC, *et al*. Human immunodeficiency virus-related lymphoma: prognostic factors predictive of survival. *Cancer* 1991;68:2466–72.
159. Kaplan LD, Abrams DI, Feigal E, *et al*. AIDS-associated non-Hodgkin's lymphoma in San Francisco. *JAMA* 1989;261:719–24.
160. Hirsch MS. Chemotherapy of human immunodeficiency virus infections: current practice and future prospects. *J Infect Dis*. 1990;161:845–57.
161. Broder S, Mitsuya H, Yarchoan R, *et al*. Antiretroviral therapy in AIDS. *Ann Intern Med*. 1990;113:604–18.
162. Schooley RT, Merigan TC, Gaut P, *et al*. Recombinant soluble CD4 therapy in patients with the acquired immunodeficiency syndrome (AIDS) and AIDS-related complex. *Ann Intern Med*. 1990;112:247–53.
163. Kahn JO, Allan JD, Hodges TL, *et al*. The safety and pharmacokinetics of recombinant soluble CD4 (rCD4) in subjects with the acquired immunodeficiency syndrome (AIDS) and AIDS-related complex. *Ann Intern Med*. 1990;112:254–61.
164. Capon DJ, Chamow SM, Mordenti J, *et al*. Designing CD4 immunoadhesins for AIDS therapy. *Nature* 1989;337:525–31.
165. Duliege AM, Shearer WT, Hammill H, *et al*. Transplacental transfer of rCDA-IgG given one week and immediately prior to birth: safety and pharmacokinetics in HIV-1 seropositive pregnant women and their newborn infants. Paper presented at Eighth International Conference on AIDS. Amsterdam, Netherlands, July 20, 1992.
166. Kahn J, Hassner A, Arri C, *et al*. A phase I study of recombinant human CD4 immunoglobulin G (rCD4-IgG) in patients with HIV associated immune thrombocytopenia purpura. Seventh International Conference on AIDS. Florence, Italy, 1991. p. 211.
167. Hodges TL, Kahn JO, Kaplan LD, *et al*. Phase I study of recombinant human CD4-immunoglobulin G therapy of patients with AIDS and AIDS-related complex. *Antimicrob Agents Chemother*. 1991;35:2580–6.
168. Daar ES, Li XL, Moudgil T, *et al*. High concentrations of

recombinant soluble CD4 are required to neutralize primary human immunodeficiency virus type 1 isolates. *Proc Natl Acad Sci USA* 1990;87:6574–8.

169. Ashkenazi A, Smith DH, Marsters SA, *et al*. Resistance of primary isolates of human immunodeficiency virus type 1 to soluble CD4 is independent of CD4-rgp120 binding affinity. *Proc Natl Acad Sci USA* 1991;88:7056–60.
170. Yarchoan R, Mitsuya H, Myers C, *et al*. Clinical pharmacology of 3′-azido-2′,3′-dideoxythymidine (zidovudine) and related dideoxynucleosides. *N Engl J Med*. 1989;321: 726–38.
171. Fischl MA, Richman DD, Grieco MH, *et al*. The efficacy of 3′-azido-3′deoxythymidine (azidothymidine) in the treatment of patients with AIDS and AIDS-related complex: a double-blind placebo-controlled trial. *N Engl J Med*. 1987;317:185–91.
172. Fischl MA, Richman DD, Hansen M, *et al*. The safety and efficacy of zidovudine (AZT) in the treatment of subjects with mildly symptomatic human immunodeficiency virus type 1 (HIV) infection. *Ann Intern Med*. 1990; 112:727–37.
173. Cooper DA, Pehrson PO, Pedersen C, *et al*. The efficacy and safety of zidovudine alone or as co-therapy with acyclovir for the treatment of patients with AIDS and AIDS-related complex: a double-blind, randomized trial. *AIDS* 1993;7:197–207.
174. Stein DS, Graham NMH, Park LP, *et al*. The effect of the interaction of acyclovir with zidovudine on progression to AIDS and survival: analysis of data in the Multicenter AIDS Cohort Study. *Ann Intern Med*. 1994;121:100–8.

174a. Hammer SM, Katzenstein DA, Hughes MD, *et al*. A trial comparing monotherapy with combination therapy in HIV-infected adults with CD4 cell counts from 200 to 500 per cubic millimeter. AIDS Clinical Trial Group Study 175 Virology Study Team. *N Engl J Med*. 1996;335:1081–90.

175. Lambert JS, Seidlin M, Reichman RC, *et al*. 2′,3′-Dideoxyinosine (ddI) in patients with the acquired immunodeficiency syndrome or AIDS-related complex. *N Engl J Med*. 1990;322:1333–40.
176. Broder S, Yarchoan R. Dideoxycytidine: current clinical experience and future prospects. *Am J Med*. 1990;88(*Suppl* 5B):31S–33S.

176a. Spruance SL, Pavia AT, Mellors, *et al*. Clinical efficacy of monotherapy with stavudine compared with zidovudine in HIV-infected zidovudine-experienced patients: a randomized, double-blind, controlled trial. *Ann Intern Med*. 1997;126:355–63.

177. Bristol-Myers Squibb. Zerit™ (stavudine) package insert. New York, NY; June 1994.
178. GlaxoWellcome. Epivir™ (lamivudine) package insert. Research Triangle Park, NC; November 1995.
179. [Anonymous]. Guidelines for management of HIV infection. *HIV/AIDS Clin Insight* 1995;5:1–11.
180. Larder BA, Kemp SD, Harrigan PR. Potential mechanism for sustained antiretroviral efficacy of AZT-3TC combination therapy. *Science* 1995;269:696–9.
181. Mitsuya H, Yarchoan R. Development of antiretroviral therapy for AIDS and related disorders. In: Broder S, Merigan TC, Bolognesi D, editors. *Textbook of AIDS Medicine*. Baltimore, MD: Williams and Wilkins; 1994. p. 721–42.
182. Fischl MA. Treatment of HIV infection. In: Sande MA, Volberding PA, editors. *The Medical Management of AIDS*. Philadelphia, PA: WB Saunders; 1995. p. 141–60.
183. Larder BA, Darby G, Richman DD. HIV with reduced sensitivity to zidovudine (AZT) isolated during prolonged therapy. *Science* 1989;243:1731–4.
184. Erice A, Balfour HH. Resistance of human immunodeficiency virus type I to antiretroviral agents: a review. *Clin Infect Dis*. 1994;18:149–56.
185. Ogino MT, Dankner WM, Spector SA. Development and significance of zidovudine resistance in children infected with human immunodeficiency virus. *J Pediatr*. 1993; 123:1–8.
186. D'Aquila RT, Johnson VA, Welles SL, *et al*. Zidovudine resistance and HIV-1 disease progression during antiretroviral therapy. *Ann Intern Med*. 1995;122:401–8.
187. Kozal MJ, Kroodsman K, Winters MA, *et al*. Didanosine resistance in HIV-infected patients switched from zidovudine to didanosine monotherapy. *Ann Intern Med*. 1994;121:263–8.
188. Roche Laboratories. Invirase™ (saquinavir) package insert. Nutley, NJ; December 1995.
189. Collier AC, Coombs RW, Schoenfeld DA, *et al*. Treatment of human immunodeficiency virus infection with saquinavir, zidovudine, and zalcitabine. *N Engl J Med*. 1996;334:1011–7.
190. Danner SA, Carr A, Leonard JM, *et al*. A short-term study of the safety, pharmacokinetics, and efficacy of ritonavir, an inhibitor of HIV-1 protease. *N Engl J Med*. 1995; 333:1528–33.
191. Markowitz M, Saag M, Powderly WG, *et al*. A preliminary study of ritonavir, an inhibitor of HIV-1 protease, to treat HIV-1 infection. *N Engl J Med*.1995;333:1534–9.
192. Massari F, Staszewski S, Berry P, *et al*. A double-blind, randomized trial of indinavir (MK-639) alone or with zidovudine vs. zidovudine alone in zidovudine naive patients. Paper presented at the 35th Interscience Conference on Antimicrobial Agents and Chemotherapy. San Francisco, CA, September 1995. (Abstract # LB–6)

192a. Powderly W, Sension M, Conant M, *et al*. The efficacy of Viracept™ (nelfinavir mesylate, NFV) in pivotal phase II/III double-blind randomized controlled trials as monotherapy and in combination with d4T or AZT/3TC. Paper presented at the 4th Conference on Retroviruses and Opportunistic Infections. Washington DC, January 1997. (Abstract #370)

193. Lane HC, Masur H, Longo DL, *et al*. Partial immune reconstitution in a patient with the acquired immunodeficiency syndrome. *N Engl J Med*. 1984;311:1099–103.
194. Holland HK, Saral R, Rossi JJ, *et al*. Allogeneic bone marrow transplantation, zidovudine, and human immunodeficiency virus type 1 (HIV-1) infection. Studies in a patient with non-Hodgkin lymphoma. *Ann Intern Med*. 1989;111:973–81.
195. Contu L, La Nasa G, Arras M, *et al*. Allogeneic bone marrow transplantation combined with multiple anti-HIV-1 treatment in a case of AIDS. *Bone Marrow Transplant*. 1993:12:669–71.

196. Ho M, Armstrong J, McMahon D, *et al.* A phase 1 study of adoptive transfer of autologous CD8+ T lymphocytes in patients with acquired immunodeficiency syndrome (AIDS)-related complex or AIDS. *Blood* 1993;81:2093–101.
197. Spector SA, Gelber RD, McGrath N, *et al.* A controlled trial of intravenous immune globulin for the prevention of serious bacterial infections in children receiving zidovudine for advanced human immunodeficiency virus infection. *N Engl J Med.* 1994;331:1181–7.
198. Zolla-Pazner S, Gorny MK. Passive immunization for the prevention and treatment of HIV infection. *AIDS* 1992;6:1235–47.
199. Jackson GG, Perkins JT, Rubenis M, *et al.* Passive immunoneutralization of human immunodeficiency virus in patients with advanced AIDS. *Lancet* 1988;2:647–52.
200. Karpas A, Hill F, Youle M, *et al.* Effects of passive immunization in patients with the acquired immunodeficiency syndrome-related complex and acquired immunodeficiency syndrome. *Proc Natl Acad Sci USA* 1988;85:9234–7.
201. Vittecoq D, Mattlinger B, Barre-Sinoussi F, *et al.* Passive immunotherapy in AIDS: a randomized trial of serial human immunodeficiency virus-positive transfusions of plasma rich in p24 antibodies versus transfusions of seronegative plasma. *J Infect Dis.* 1992;165:364–8.
202. Jacobson JM, Colman N, Ostrow NA, *et al.* Passive immunotherapy in the treatment of advanced human immunodeficiency virus infection. *J Infect Dis.* 1993;168:298–305.
203. Redfield RR, Birx DL, Kettler N, *et al.* A phase I evaluation of the safety and immunogenicity of vaccination with recombinant gp160 in patients with early human immunodeficiency virus infection. *N Engl J Med.* 1991;324:1677–84.
204. Trauger RJ, Ferre F, Daigle AE, *et al.* Effect of immunization with inactivated gp120-depleted human immunodeficiency virus type 1 (HIV-1) immunogen on HIV-1 immunity, viral DNA, and percentage of CD4 cells. *J Infect Dis.* 1994;169:1256–64.
205. Krown SE, Gold JWM, Niedzwiecki D, *et al.* Interferon-alfa with zidovudine: safety, tolerance and clinical and virologic effects in patients with Kaposi sarcoma associated with the acquired immunodeficiency syndrome. *Ann Intern Med.* 1990;112:812–21.
206. Krown SE. Approaches to interferon combination therapy in the treatment of AIDS. *Semin Oncol.* 1990;17(*Suppl* 1):11–5.
207. Kunzi MS, Farzadegan H, Margolick JB, *et al.* Identification of human immunodeficiency virus primary isolates resistant to interferon-alpha and correlation of prevalence to disease progression. *J Infect Dis.* 1995;171:822–8.
208. Lane HC, Davey V, Kovacs JA, *et al.* Interferon-alfa in patients with asymptomatic human immunodeficiency virus infection. *Ann Intern Med.* 1990;112:805–11.
209. Lotze MT, Franan LW, Sharrow DO, *et al.* In vivo administration of purified human interleukin 2. I. Half-life and immunologic effects of the Jurkat cell line-derived interleukin 2. *J Immunol.* 1985;134:157–66.
210. Kovacs JA, Baseler M, Dewar RJ, *et al.* Increases in CD4 T lymphocytes with intermittent courses of interleukin-2 in patients with human immunodeficiency virus infection: a preliminary study. *N Engl J Med.* 1995;332:567–75.
211. Clerici M, Lucey DR, Berzofsky JA, *et al.* Restoration of HIV-specific cell-mediated immune responses by interleukin-12 in vitro. *Science* 1993;262:1721–4.
212. Fischl M, Galpin JE, Levine JD, *et al.* Recombinant erythropoietin for patients with AIDS treated with zidovudine. *N Engl J Med.* 1990;322:1488–93.
213. Henry DH, Beall GN, Benson CA, *et al.* Recombinant human erythropoietin in the treatment of anemia associated with human immunodeficiency virus infection and zidovudine therapy: overview of four clinical trials. *Ann Intern Med.* 1992:117:739–48.
214. Groopman JE, Mitsuyasu RT, DeLeo MJ, *et al.* Effect of recombinant human granulocyte-macrophage colony-stimulating factor in the acquired immunodeficiency syndrome. *N Engl J Med.* 1987;317:593–8.
215. Pluda JM, Yarchoan R, Smith PD, *et al.* Subcutaneous recombinant granulocyte-macrophage colony-stimulating factor used as a single agent and in an alternating regimen with azidothymidine in leukopenic patients with severe human immunodeficiency virus infection. *Blood* 1990;76:463–72.
216. Gillespie D, Hubbell HR, Carter WA, *et al.* Synergistic inhibition of AZT-resistant HIV by AZT combined with poly(I):poly(C12U), without synergistic toxicity to bone marrow progenitor cell elements. *In Vivo* 1994;8:375–81.
217. Armstrong JA, McMahon D, Huang XL, *et al.* A phase I study of ampligen in human immunodeficiency virus-infected subjects. *J Infect Dis.* 1992;166:717–22.
218. Fliri H, Baumann G, Enz A, *et al.* Cyclosporins: structure-activity relationships. *Ann NY Acad Sci.* 1993;696:47–53.
219. Luban J, Bossolt KL, Franke EK, *et al.* Human immunodeficiency virus type 1 gag protein binds to cyclophilins A and B. *Cell* 1993;73:1067–78.
220. Schwarz A, Offermann G, Keller F, *et al.* The effect of cyclosporine on the progression of human immunodeficiency virus type 1 infection transmitted by transplantation—data on four cases and review of the literature. *Transplantation* 1993;55:95–103.
221. Lederman MM. Host-directed and immune-based therapies for human immunodeficiency virus infection. *Ann Intern Med.* 1995;122:218–22.
222. Ferdman RM, Church JA. Immunologic and virologic effects of glucocorticoids on human immunodeficiency virus infection in children: a preliminary study. *Pediatr Infect Dis J.* 1994;13:212–6.
223. Andrieu JM, Lu W, Levy R. Sustained increases in CD4 cell counts in asymptomatic human immunodeficiency virus type 1-seropositive patients treated with prednisolone for 1 year. *J Infect Dis.* 1995;171:523–30.
224. Corey L. Reducing T cell activation as a therapy for human immunodeficiency virus infection [editorial]. *J Infect Dis.* 1995;171:521–2.
225. Biswas DK, Dezube BJ, Ahlers CM, Pardee AB. Pentoxifylline inhibits HIV-1 LTR-driven gene expression by blocking NF-kappa B action. *J Acquir Immune Defic Syndr.* 1993;6:778–86.
226. Dezube BJ. Pentoxifylline for the treatment of infection with human immunodeficiency virus. *Clin Infect Dis.*

1994;18:285–7.
227. Luke DR, McCreedy BJ, Sarnoski TP, *et al.* Phase I/II study of pentoxifylline with zidovudine on HIV-1 growth in AIDS patients. *Int J Clin Pharmacol Ther Toxicol.* 1993;31: 343–50.
228. Meyerhans A, Vartanian JP, Hultgren C, *et al.* Restriction and enhancement of human immunodeficiency virus type 1 replication by modulation of intracellular deoxynucleoside triphosphate pools. *J Virol.* 1994;68:535–40.
229. Gao WY, Cara A, Gallo RA, Lori F. Low levels of deoxynucleotides in peripheral blood lymphocytes: a strategy to inhibit human immunodeficiency virus type 1 replication. *Proc Natl Acad Sci USA* 1993;90:8925–8.
230. Levy JA. *HIV and the Pathogenesis of AIDS*. Washington, DC: ASM; 1994. p. 217–36.
231. Lioy J, Ho WZ, Cutilli JR, *et al.* Thiol suppression of human immunodeficiency virus type 1 replication in primary cord blood monocyte-derived macrophages in vitro. *J Clin Invest.* 1993;91:495–8.
232. Roederer M, Stall FJT, Raju PA, *et al.* Cytokine-stimulated human immunodeficiency virus replication is inhibited by *N*-acetyl-L-cysteine. *Proc Natl Acad Sci USA* 1990; 87:4884–8.
233. Roberts RL, Aroda VR, Ank BJ. *N*-acetylcysteine enhances antibody-dependent cellular cytotoxicity in neutrophils and mononuclear cells from healthy adults and human immunodeficiency virus-infected patients. *J Infect Dis.* 1995;172:1492–502.
234. Sioud M, Drlica K. Prevention of human immunodeficiency virus type 1 integrase expression in *Escherichia coli* by a ribozyme. *Proc Natl Acad Sci USA* 1991;88:7303–7.
235. Ojwang JO, Hampel A, Looney DJ, *et al.* Inhibition of human immunodeficiency virus type 1 expression by a hairpin ribozyme. *Proc Natl Acad Sci USA* 1992;89:10802–6.
236. Malim MH, Freimuth WW, Liu J, *et al.* Stable expression of transdominant rev protein in human T cells inhibits human immunodeficiency virus replication. *J Exp Med.* 1992;176:1197–1201.
237. Bolognesi DP. AIDS vaccines: progress and unmet challenges. *Ann Intern Med.* 1991;114:161–2.
238. Goudsmit J, Smit L, Krone WJA, *et al.* IgG response to human immunodeficiency virus in experimentally infected chimpanzees mimics the IgG response in humans. *J Infect Dis.* 1987;155:327–31.
239. Fauci AS, Gallo RC, Koenig S, *et al.* Development and evaluation of a vaccine for human immunodeficiency virus (HIV) infection. *Ann Intern Med.* 1989;110:373–85.
240. Starcich BR, Hahn BH, Shaw GM, *et al.* Identification and characterization of conserved and variable regions in the envelope gene of HTLV-III/LAV, the retrovirus of AIDS. *Cell* 1986;45:637–48.
241. Koff WC, Hoth DF. Development and testing of AIDS vaccines. *Science* 1988;241:426–32.
242. Fischinger PJ, Gallo RC, Bolognesi DP. Toward a vaccine against AIDS: rationale and current progress. *Mt Sinai J Med.* 1986;53:639–47.
243. Cotton P. International disunity on HIV vaccine efficacy trials. *JAMA* 1994;272:1090–1.
244. Acosta EP, Fletcher CV. Agents for treating human immunodeficiency virus infection. *AJHP* 1994;51:2251–67.

SELF-ASSESSMENT QUESTIONS

1. Destruction of $CD4^+$ T lymphocytes is related to:

   a. direct HIV-induced cytolysis.
   b. apoptosis.
   c. cellular response to HIV.
   d. all of the above.

2. Which of the following is the initial event in the HIV replicative cycle?

   a. p24 attaches to reverse transcriptase.
   b. The $CD4^+/CD8^+$ T-cell ratio is inverted.
   c. gp120 binds to the CD4 receptor.
   d. Viral proteins are assembled into a virion.

3. All of the following cytokines stimulate HIV replication *except*:

   a. IL-13.
   b. IL-1.
   c. IL-2.
   d. TNF.

4. Health care workers, as a demographic group, are disproportionally represented among the HIV-infected population in the United States.

   a. true
   b. false

5. The fastest growing numbers of cases of HIV infection are in which of the following demographic groups?

   a. infants
   b. homosexuals
   c. heterosexuals
   d. a and c

6. HIV infection is a leading cause of death among all persons in the United States between 25 and 44 years old.

   a. true
   b. false

7. A newborn who shows two positive ELISAs and a positive Western blot over a six-week period definitely has HIV infection.

   a. true
   b. false

8. PCR is used to detect:

   a. antibodies to HIV in the patient's blood.
   b. HIV proteins in the patient's blood.

c. HIV viral DNA in the patient's blood.
d. replicating virus in culture.

9. According to the 1993 revised classification for HIV infection, which of the following would be considered to have a diagnosis of AIDS?

   a. an asymptomatic patient with a $CD^{+}4$ T-cell count of 550 cells/µl
   b. an asymptomatic patient with a $CD^{+}4$ T-cell count of 150 cells/µl
   c. a patient with oral candidiasis and a $CD^{+}4$ T-cell count of 550 cells/µl
   d. a patient with persistent generalized lymphadenopathy and a $CD^{+}4$ T-cell count of 600 cells/µl

10. During the asymptomatic phase of HIV infection, which of the following statements is true?

    a. The virus is latent and not replicating.
    b. There is an absence of clinical signs and symptoms of HIV infection in people with laboratory evidence of antibodies to HIV.
    c. There is a high level of viremia.
    d. The individual is not infectious to others.

11. Which of the following agents does not inhibit reverse transcriptase?

    a. stavudine
    b. lamivudine
    c. saquinavir
    d. nevirapine

12. An HIV isolate is resistant to zidovudine through a mutation of the reverse transcriptase enzyme gene. Does this mutation inherently confer cross resistance to other dideoxynucleosides?

    a. yes
    b. no

13. Potential immune-based therapies for HIV include all of the following *except*:

    a. therapeutic vaccination.
    b. corticosteroids.
    c. TIBO compounds.
    d. IFN-α.

14. Strategies that either suppress or enhance the immune response to HIV infection are under evaluation.

    a. true
    b. false

15. FDA-approved colony-stimulating factors may be useful in alleviating:

    a. neutropenia.
    b. thrombocytopenia.
    c. anemia.
    d. a and c.

16. Drugs that may modify TNF release include:

    a. thalidomide.
    b. pentoxifylline.
    c. both thalidomide and pentoxifylline.
    d. neither thalidomide nor pentoxifylline.

17. Phase III studies of preventive HIV vaccines have been delayed by:

    a. an unanticipated excess of new HIV infections in phase II vaccine recipients.
    b. a lack of defined markers of a protective response from the vaccine.
    c. both a and b.
    d. neither a nor b.

CHAPTER 8

Solid Organ Transplantation

Kathleen D. Lake, Pharm.D., B.C.P.S.
Program Director, Cardiothoracic Transplantation and Research
Minneapolis Heart Institute Foundation and Abbott Northwestern Hospital
Clinical Associate Professor
College of Pharmacy, University of Minnesota
Minneapolis, MN

Stephen J. Rossi, Pharm.D.
Director, Clinical Program Development
The Transplant Pharmacy™
Sang Stat Medical
Menlo Park, CA

Lawrence Chodoff, Pharm.D.
Associate Director—Clinical Research
Novartis Pharmaceutical Corporation
East Hanover, NJ

PART I. TRANSPLANT IMMUNOLOGY AND IMMUNOTHERAPY

Historical Overview 152
Transplant Immunology 154
Basic Components of the Immune System 154
Major Histocompatibility Complex 154
T-Cell, CD4, and CD8 receptors 154
Cytokine Mediators 154
Adhesion Molecules 155
Pathogenesis of Acute Cellular Rejection 155
Transplant Immunotherapy 155
Corticosteroids 156
Pharmacology and Clinical Uses 156
Dosing and Monitoring 156
Adverse Effects and Toxicity 156
Inhibitors of Early T-Cell Activation 157
Cyclosporine 157
Pharmacology and Clinical Uses 157
Dosing and Monitoring 158
Adverse Effects and Toxicity 159

CsA Analogues . . . 159
Tacrolimus . . . 159
Pharmacology and Clinical Uses . . . 160
Dosing and Monitoring . . . 160
Adverse Effects and Toxicity . . . 161
Inhibitors of Late T-Cell Function . . . 161
Sirolimus . . . 161
Deoxyspergualin (Gusperimus) . . . 162
Leflunomide . . . 162
Inhibitors of Cell Proliferation . . . 162
Azathioprine . . . 162
Pharmacology and Clinical Uses . . . 162
Dosing and Monitoring . . . 162
Adverse Effects and Toxicity . . . 163
Cyclophosphamide . . . 163
Pharmacology and Clinical Uses . . . 163
Dosing and Monitoring . . . 163
Adverse Effects And Toxicity . . . 163
Methotrexate . . . 164
Pharmacology and Clinical Uses . . . 164
Dosing and Monitoring . . . 164
Adverse Effects and Toxicity . . . 164
Mycophenolate Mofetil . . . 164
Pharmacology and Clinical Uses . . . 164
Dosing and Monitoring . . . 164
Adverse Effects and Toxicity . . . 165
Miscellaneous Antiproliferatives . . . 165
Polyclonal Antilymphocyte Antibodies . . . 165
Pharmacology and Clinical Uses . . . 165
Dosing and Monitoring . . . 165
Adverse Effects and Toxicity . . . 166
Monoclonal Antibodies . . . 166
OKT3 . . . 166
Immunologic Effects . . . 166
Dosing . . . 166
Monitoring . . . 167
Lymphocyte Subsets . . . 167
HAMA Formation (Xenosensitization) . . . 167
OKT3 Serum Concentrations . . . 168
Adverse Effects and Toxicity . . . 168
New MoABs . . . 168
Drug Interactions . . . 168
Pharmacokinetic Interactions . . . 169
Pharmacodynamic Interactions . . . 170
Management of Drug Interactions . . . 170
Serious Interactions . . . 171
Moderately Serious Interactions . . . 171
Minor Interactions . . . 171
Other Considerations . . . 171
Nonpharmacologic Means of Immunosuppression . . . 172
Transfusion . . . 173
Splenectomy . . . 173
Irradiation . . . 173
Apheresis . . . 173
Photopheresis . . . 173
Summary . . . 173

PART II. TRANSPLANT PROCEDURES AND COMPLICATIONS

Kidney Transplantation ... 174
- Indications and Candidate Selection ... 174
- Transplantation Technique ... 174
- Immunosuppressive Treatment ... 175
- Postoperative Complications ... 175
- Immunologic Complications ... 175
- De Novo and Recurrent Renal Disease ... 176

Pancreas Transplantation ... 176
- Indications and Candidate Selection ... 176
- Transplantation Technique ... 177
- Immunosuppressive Treatment ... 177
- Postoperative Complications ... 177
- Immunologic Complications ... 177
- Islet Cell Transplantation ... 177

Liver Transplantation ... 178
- Indications and Candidate Selection ... 178
- Organ Allocation ... 179
- Immunology of the Transplanted Liver ... 179
- Immunosuppressive Treatment ... 179
- Postoperative Complications ... 180

Heart Transplantation ... 181
- Indications and Candidate Selection ... 181
- Transplantation Technique ... 182
- Mechanical Bridging ... 182
- Immunosuppressive Treatment ... 183
- Postoperative Complications ... 183
  - Immunologic Complications ... 183
  - Chronic Rejection ... 183

Lung and Heart-Lung Transplantation ... 183
- Indications and Candidate Selection ... 184
- Immunosuppressive Treatment ... 184
- Postoperative Complications ... 184

Small Intestine Transplantation ... 186
- Indications and Candidate Selection ... 186
- Immunosuppressive Treatment ... 186
- Postoperative Complications ... 186

Complications After Solid Organ Transplantation ... 186
- Acute Rejection ... 187
- Chronic Rejection ... 187
- Infectious Complications ... 187
  - Bacterial Infections ... 187
  - Viral Infections ... 188
    - Herpes Group Viruses ... 188
      - Cytomegalovirus ... 188
      - Epstein-Barr Virus ... 189
      - Other Herpes Group Viruses ... 190
    - Hepatotrophic Viruses ... 190
  - Fungal Infections ... 191
  - Opportunistic Infections ... 191
- Hypertension ... 191
- Hyperlipidemia ... 192
- Diabetes Mellitus ... 193
- Bone and Muscle Disorders ... 193
- Malignancy ... 194

Summary 195
References 195
Self-Assessment Questions 209

For many years, scientists were unsuccessful in their attempts to replace diseased and injured organs with donated healthy organs. As discussed in chapter 3, only an organ donated from an identical twin was acceptable to the host's immune system. Organs donated from family members or cadavers were not likely to be sufficiently compatible to avoid rejection.

New drugs, genetic engineering techniques, improved surgical procedures, better organ preservation, major histocompatibility complex (MHC) tissue typing, and an advanced understanding of the mechanisms of the immune system have elevated organ transplantation from an experimental procedure to an accepted treatment for end-stage organ failure. Even though one-year graft survival rates are very good, problems still remain, with immunosuppressive agents adding their own array of complications to patient therapy. Suppressing a patient's immune system reduces the incidence of graft rejection but leaves the patient vulnerable to opportunistic infections and malignant disorders. In addition, immunosuppressive agents have detrimental side effects that increase the patient's risk for other complications. The long-term survival (more than 10 or 20 years) of solid organ recipients is complicated by the development of chronic rejection processes that in most cases can be treated only by retransplantation.

The pharmacist's role in providing pharmaceutical care for the transplant patient is very important. Many opportunities exist, such as optimizing immunosuppressive and other drug therapy, designing nutritional support regimens, developing protocols for preventive and palliative therapy for adverse reactions, monitoring and adjusting drug concentrations, managing drug interactions, providing advice about appropriate investigational agents, and counseling patients to insure compliance. In addition to understanding pharmacokinetic changes that may occur in transplant candidates and recipients,[1] it is important for the pharmacist to have a thorough understanding of the physiologic consequences of organ transplantation.

This chapter begins with an overview of the development of solid organ transplantation and the basic immunology of allograft rejection. Immunosuppressive agents are categorized according to primary mechanism of action. A discussion of the clinical use, dosing, monitoring, and adverse effects of these agents is included. Nonpharmacologic therapies are briefly reviewed.

In part II, solid organ transplant procedures are discussed in the following order: kidney, pancreas and islet cell, islet-thymic, liver, heart, lung, and small intestine. The history, indications, patient selection criteria, immunosuppressive protocols, complications, and postoperative care are discussed briefly for each type of transplant. The discussion of solid organ transplantation concludes with an expanded section about complications and management strategies for preventing and/or treating these common problems.

After completing this chapter, the reader should be able to:

1. Describe the basic immune response involved in an acute rejection episode and identify the sites of action of the various immunosuppressive agents.
2. Discuss the immunosuppressive therapies for solid organ transplant procedures and explain how to monitor for efficacy and toxicity.
3. Compare rescue therapies available for the treatment of acute organ rejection.
4. Describe management strategies for dealing with immunosuppressant drug interactions.
5. Recognize postoperative transplant complications and describe treatment plans for immunotherapy-related adverse effects.

PART I—TRANSPLANT IMMUNOLOGY AND IMMUNOTHERAPY

HISTORICAL OVERVIEW

Although the idea of solid-organ transplantation dates back to ancient times, the first major milestone was the development of the vascular anastomosis technique by Alexis Carrel and Charley Claude Guthrie in 1902.[2] Using this technique, a variety of tissue and organ grafts were performed in various animal species.

The first attempt at kidney transplantation occurred in 1933, although it was not until 1954, in Boston, that the first long-term surviving kidney transplant was performed between identical twins. The first successful attempts at intentionally suppressing the immune system in humans occurred between 1958 and 1962 when Murray in Boston[3] and Hamburger in Paris used varying dosages of total body irradiation to circumvent rejection of transplanted kidneys in nonidentical twins.[4] This was the beginning of immunosuppression, and the advances in transplantation have paralleled those in immunosuppressive therapy.

Subsequent major milestones in organ transplantation occurred in the 1960s with the development of tissue-typing techniques and new immunosuppressive agents. Early work with the antimetabolite 6-mercaptopurine (6-MP) by Schwartz and Dameshek[5] led to the development of an imidazole derivative of this drug, azathioprine (AZA), by Hitchings and Elion.[6] The combination of this agent with corticosteroids demonstrated increased efficacy in preventing rejection.[7] During the next decade, a variety of techniques and agents, including thoracic duct drainage, splenectomy, thymectomy, lymphoid or graft irradiation, cyclophosphamide (CTX), and the polyclonal antilymphocyte and antithymocyte globulins, were used in attempts to suppress the immune response.[4]

The next major milestone occurred in the mid-1970s with the discovery of cyclosporine (CsA). The success demonstrated with heart, liver, pancreas, pancreas-kidney, heart-lung, and lung transplantation during the past decade has been credited to the introduction of CsA (Table 8-1). By the mid-1980s, combinations of two, three, and four drugs were being used to augment immunosuppression while minimizing the toxicity of the individual agents.

The discovery by Kohler and Milstein[8] of the technique to produce monoclonal antibodies (MoAbs) heralded a new era of immunosuppressive therapy for clinical organ transplantation in the 1980s. Their contribution was recognized with the Nobel Prize in 1984. The development of new agents using MoAb technology has been stimulated by the selectivity and specificity of MoAbs against specific immunologic targets.

Despite a dramatic increase in the number of transplants performed each year and the number of centers performing them, the major limitation is the availability of donor organs. The Uniform Anatomical Gift Act of 1968 formalized a consensus definition of brain death and paved the way for legal donation of solid organs. Organ procurement and distribution remained largely the responsibility of the individual centers until the early 1980s. The United Network for Organ Sharing (UNOS) was established in 1972 as a voluntary association, but by the 1980s it was recognized as the only viable organization operating a computerized national registry of all patients awaiting solid organ transplantation. Patients are matched with cadaveric donor organs according to human leukocyte antigen (HLA) compatibility (kidneys), blood type, size, time waiting, and degree of need for transplantation. The

Table 8-1. Success of Organ Transplants Performed in the United States, 1995

ORGAN	NUMBER OF PROGRAMS	NUMBER OF TRANSPLANTS PERFORMED	ONE-YEAR ACTUARIAL SURVIVAL RATE, %	
			GRAFT	PATIENT
Heart	167	2,361	81	82
Heart-Lung	93	68	61	61
Lung	90	871	70	72
Kidney				
CAD		7,683	81	93
LRD		3,209	91	97
Total	246	10,892		
Liver				
CAD		3,881		
LRD		44		
Total	119	3,925	69	79
Kidney-Pancreas				
Kidney-Pancreas		918	72	90
Pancreas alone		110		
Total	124	1,028	72	90

Based on United Network for Organ Sharing (UNOS) Scientific Registry data of April 22, 1996. CAD, cadaveric donor; LRD, living related donor.

Table 8-2. Registrations on the UNOS National Patient Waiting List for Organ Transplants as of April 2, 1997[9]

35,420	for *kidney* transplants
8,037	for *liver* transplants
340	for *pancreas* transplants
1,497	for *kidney-pancreas* transplants
88	for *intestine* transplants
3,797	for *heart* transplants
224	for *heart-lung* transplants
2,378	for *lung* transplants
51,859	**total registrations**

NOTE: *UNOS policies allow patients to be listed with more than one transplant center (multiple listing), and thus the number of registrations may be greater than the actual number of patients.*

most critically ill patients usually receive priority when all other factors are equal. Currently, there are thousands of candidates listed at UNOS awaiting various transplants (Table 8-2).[9] There is a great disparity between the number of patients awaiting transplants and those who actually receive a donor organ. Future efforts need to be directed at maximizing the use of donor organs and developing other therapeutic modalities, such as the use of xenografts or implantable artificial organs, to meet the needs of patients with end-stage organ disease.

TRANSPLANT IMMUNOLOGY

Allograft rejection remains the major barrier to long-term patient and graft survival after solid organ transplantation. The process of rejection is a normal immune response in which the allograft is recognized as foreign, resulting in the activation of cytotoxic responses. Significant advances have been made in understanding the immunologic mechanisms of rejection and how to interrupt these processes with various pharmacologic and immunologic interventions. Experience gained using these agents for the prevention and reversal of the rejection has helped to expand our understanding of the specific molecular processes involved in this complex immune response. However, the development of graft acceptance without immunosuppressive therapy (i.e., tolerance) remains an elusive goal in current clinical transplantation.

Basic Components of the Immune System

Acute rejection episodes are primarily regulated by cell-mediated immunity. The basic components of this arm of the immune system involved in allograft rejection have been discussed in previous chapters. However, to develop appropriate antirejection or tolerance-inducing strategies, an understanding of the specific roles and complex relationships among these components during an acute rejection episode is required.

Major Histocompatibility Complex

The MHC (or HLA) complex is a specific cluster of genes that controls the expression of class I and II HLA proteins, the primary antigens of the immune response pathways.[10] T-cell recognition of foreign antigens is determined by class I and class II HLA molecules. Class I HLAs are cell-surface proteins that serve as primary targets for cytotoxic lymphocytes as well as direct activators of cytotoxic cell responses. These proteins are expressed in varying degrees on the surface of most somatic cells. Conversely, expression of class II HLA proteins is more restricted, and these antigens are found primarily on macrophages, monocytes, B lymphocytes, and dendritic cells. Class I and II HLAs serve as primary activators of the helper T-cell response in initiating the first steps of the immune response to foreign tissue. Both classes of HLA molecules are responsible for the binding, processing, and presentation of key antigens associated with acute rejection response. Other clusters of genes have been associated with the pathogenesis of rejection, but they encode for only minor antigens.[10,11]

T-Cell, CD4, and CD8 Receptors

The specific immune response to allograft tissue is dependent on donor antigens (alloantigens) presented by class I and II HLA molecules to the T-cell receptor (TCR). The TCR is directly associated with the CD3 complex and is clonally restricted in its expression and antigen recognition properties. The TCR is responsible for direct (class I) and indirect (class II) alloantigen recognition.[11] The CD4 marker is expressed exclusively on helper T cells and preferentially interacts with class II HLA molecules. Conversely, the CD8 marker is expressed on the surface of cytotoxic T cells, which react with class I HLA molecules.[11]

Cytokine Mediators

Cytokines, including interleukins (IL), interferons (IFN), colony-stimulating factors, and growth hormones, are the chemical mediators of most immune responses.[12] These cytokines mediate their activity through both self-regulating and direct stimulatory or inhibitory pathways. Increased concentrations of IL-1, IL-2, IL-6, tumor necrosis factor alpha (TNF-α), and IFN-γ are observed within the allografts of patients having a rejection episode. The activating properties of cytokines are exemplified by the upregulation of class I and class II HLA expression on endothelial cells exposed to TNF-α and IFN-γ. Other examples include the roles of IL-1, IL-2, and IL-6 in T-cell postantigenic differentiation, activation, and proliferation. In contrast, other cytokines, such as IL-4, IL-5, and IL-10, are associated with a suppression of T-cell activation and may be clinically relevant in the induction of tolerance.

Adhesion Molecules

Adhesion molecules are specific glycoproteins involved in key receptor-ligand cellular interactions. Three primary families of adhesion molecules (integrin, selectin, and immunoglobulin super) have been identified as having a role in the immune activation of acute rejection episodes. The integrin family is expressed primarily on leukocytes and is involved with initial T-lymphocyte binding to endothelial cells as well as other graft-infiltrating cells.[11,12] Clinically significant integrins, such as lymphocyte function-associated antigen 1 (LFA-1), may also serve as signal transduction molecules necessary for the co-stimulatory signal of antigen-TCR binding.[12] The selectins are also expressed on the majority of lymphocytes and facilitate cellular binding to endothelial sites of activation within the graft. The immunoglobulin super family often serves as counter-receptors to the integrins and selectins and tends to be expressed on both circulating lymphocytes and allograft endothelial cells.[11,12] Increased expression of adhesion molecules is regulated by a variety of activating cytokine mediators, including TNF-α, IL-1β, and IFN-γ.[12]

Pathogenesis of Acute Cellular Rejection

The process of acute allograft rejection involves two distinct phases: (1) recognition and sensitization to donor alloantigens by the host immune system, and (2) deployment of various effector responses, resulting in graft cell injury.[13,14] Sensitization is initiated by the interaction of host antigen-presenting cells (APCs) with donor antigens on the surface of the graft or in peripheral circulation. Additional peripheral sensitization is mediated by donor dendritic cells and donor-derived leukocytes migrating into host lymphoid tissue.[13] Preprogrammed reactive lymphocytes are responsible for the initial step in T-cell activation. Class II HLA antigens are recognized via the binding of APC-processed alloantigens to TCR on $CD4^+$ helper T cells.[13,14] Antigen-TCR binding is further enhanced by adhesion molecule interactions, which result in co-stimulatory transduction of T cell–activating signals.[12,14] A secondary pathway of T-cell activation involves direct binding of MHC class I alloantigens to host $CD8^+$ cytotoxic T cells.[13,14]

Helper T-cell activation requires APC-derived release of IL-1 as well as antigen-binding stimulatory signals. Once activated, these antigenic, differentiated helper T cells upregulate the genes encoding for IL-2 synthesis and IL-2 receptors.[14] Synthesis and secretion of IL-2 stimulates helper T-cell proliferation and recruitment and activation of other proximate helper T cells. Additional cytokine mediators are released by activated helper T cells, including IL-3, IL-4, IL-5, IL-6, and INF-γ,[14] resulting in secondary macrophage and B-cell activation. Several studies support the development of two distinct helper T-cell populations based on functional properties and cytokine release patterns. T-helper 1 cells are the primary mediators of allograft rejection and release activating cytokines (IL-1, IL-6, and TNF-α).[10] T-helper 2 cells are primarily involved with indirect antibody production and release inhibitory cytokines (IL-4, IL-5, and IL-10).[10] Cytotoxic T-cell activation by class I alloantigens stimulates an upregulation of IL-2 receptor expression, which in turn binds IL-2 secreted from the activated helper T cells. Subsequently, antigenic differentiation and clonal proliferation of these cytolytic cells occur.[11]

After T-cell activation, the effector phase of graft rejection is initiated, involving a complex interaction of helper and cytotoxic T cells, alloantigen-specific B-cell antibodies, natural killer cells, and macrophages.[14] Although initial immunologic studies suggested graft injury was completely mediated by cytotoxic T cells, recent evidence points toward both helper and cytotoxic cell-mediated injury.[11] Both cell types release abundant intragraft concentrations of inflammatory cytokines and granular lysozymes, which directly injure the graft cells.[12] Macrophage-mediated cytokine and enzyme release further contributes to graft injury during rejection.[11,14] Although acute rejection is primarily a cell-mediated immune response, the production of antigen-specific antibodies from activated B cells results in complement- and neutrophil-mediated cellular injury.[11]

TRANSPLANT IMMUNOTHERAPY

For almost 20 years, immunosuppression for solid organ transplantation was accomplished with only four drugs—cyclosporine, AZA, corticosteroids, and polyclonal antilymphocyte antibodies (Figure 8-1).[15] In the 1980s, the first MoAb, OKT3, was introduced, and it played a key role in both induction and rejection protocols. In the early 1990s, a number of promising new immunosuppressive agents appeared to be on the horizon. In contrast to the previous three decades, the list of potential new agents seemed almost endless, as many of the major pharmaceutical companies had one (or even several) products in their developmental pipelines. Although two new agents, tacrolimus[16,17] and mycophenolate mofetil,[18,19] and a new microemulsion formulation of CsA[20–22] made it to market in the mid-1990s, an equal number of other agents (cyclosporine G [OG 37-235],[23,24] brequinar,[15] and leflunomide[25,26]) have been abandoned, at least temporarily.

The following discussion of immunosuppressive

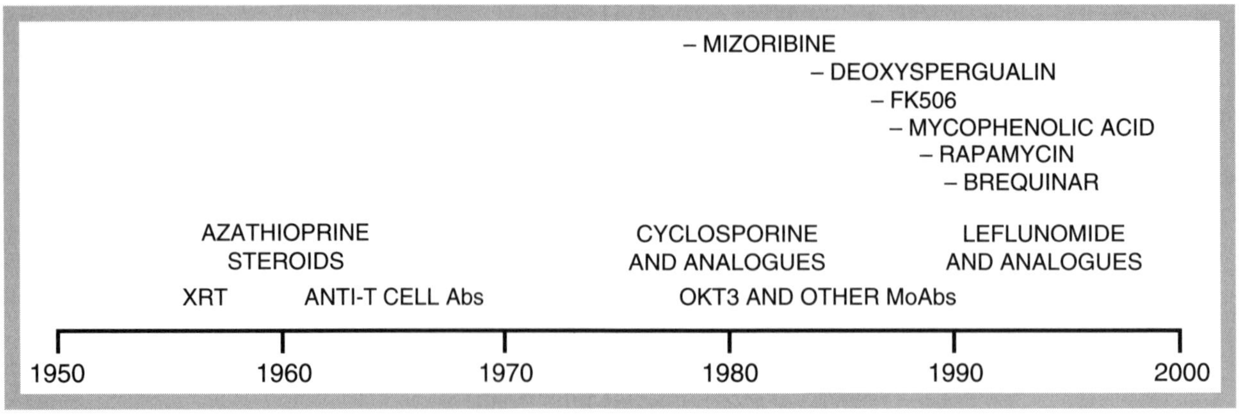

Figure 8-1. Four decades of immunosuppressive drug discovery and development in transplantation. Abs, antibodies; MoAbs, monoclonal Abs.

SOURCE: *Reprinted with permission from Morris RE. New small molecule immunosuppressants for transplantation: reveiw of essential concepts [review].* J Heart Lung Transplant. *1993;12(6 Pt 2):5275–86.*

agents provides information about the pharmacology, pharmacokinetics, and toxicology of these drugs and practical guidelines for their therapeutic use; specific organ transplants and their complications and management strategies are discussed later in this chapter.

Corticosteroids

Pharmacology and Clinical Uses

The usefulness of corticosteroids in solid organ transplantation results from three of their pharmacologic effects: (1) a direct effect on circulating lymphocytes, (2) modulation of specific cellular immune functions, and (3) a nonspecific anti-inflammatory effect.

Corticosteroids cause a rapid and profound drop in circulating T lymphocytes, not as a result of direct destruction of lymphocytes but, rather, from sequestration of lymphocytes in the bone marrow. Besides decreasing the number of circulating monocytes and lymphocytes (particularly $CD4^+$ T lymphocytes) and increasing the number of circulating neutrophils, corticosteroids have major effects on the function of these cells. Corticosteroids bind to an intracytosolic steroid receptor and are transported to the nucleus, where they alter DNA and RNA synthesis. They also potently inhibit phosphodiesterase, leading to accumulation of intracellular cyclic adenosine monophosphate and inhibition of lymphocyte activation. Inhibition of IL-1 secretion from macrophages and IL-2 secretion from T lymphocytes inhibits the generation of cytotoxic T lymphocytes. The nonspecific, potent anti-inflammatory effect is a result of the inhibition of arachidonic acid release and suppression of macrophage phagocytosis.

Dosing and Monitoring

Corticosteroids have a broad spectrum of use in clinical transplantation. They are used in preventing and treating graft rejection. High-dose methylprednisolone is routinely used as part of induction immunosuppression in virtually all organ transplant settings; methylprednisolone or hydrocortisone IV 250–1000 mg is administered preoperatively or intraoperatively immediately before revascularization of the newly placed allograft. Thereafter, a rapid taper of methylprednisolone is accomplished over the first three to seven days following the transplant, at which time the patient is switched to oral prednisone. In general, initial prophylactic doses in solid organ transplantation are in the range of 1–2 mg/kg per day and are tapered over months to 0.1–0.3 mg/kg per day. Dosing requirements are consistently higher in pediatric recipients and may vary among races.[27] Similar high-dose regimens are used for the treatment of episodes of acute rejection. Pulses of 250–1000 mg of methylprednisolone once daily for two to four days, followed by a rapid taper back to the patient's baseline maintenance dose of prednisone over three to five days, successfully aborts 60–80% of acute rejections. Large doses of oral prednisone (100–200 mg) have also been used for "pulse" treatment of rejection.[27,28]

Adverse Effects and Toxicities

The wide array of acute and chronic side effects associated with corticosteroids stems from the presence of steroid receptors on nearly every cell in the body. Because of the significant toxicities associated with long-term corticosteroid use, there has been more aggressive use of steroid-sparing drugs, such as CsA and tacrolimus, so that lower doses of steroids can be given.[29] Table 8-3 lists some of the side effects associated with corticosteroid therapy.

Recent efforts to reduce the short- and long-term consequences of corticosteroid administration have focused on the use of newer agents with less potential for adrenal suppression and metabolic effects and attempts at programmed steroid withdrawal during long-term main-

Table 8-3. Selected Side Effects of Corticosteroid Therapy

Central nervous system
Euphoria
Depression
Adrenal axis suppression
Hypertension
Sodium and water retention
Myopathy
Avascular necrosis
Infection
Impaired wound healing
Increased appetite and weight gain
Osteoporosis
Cataracts
Hyperglycemia
Hyperlipidemia
Impaired growth and sexual maturation

tenance immunosuppression. Deflazacort is a new synthetic glucocorticoid that has been shown to be well-tolerated in a number of organ transplant settings, both as primary therapy at induction and as a substitute for prednisone during maintenance treatment.[30,31] One study of 26 heart transplant recipients demonstrated that switching from prednisone to deflazacort maintenance therapy was associated with significantly improved glycemic control and reductions in total cholesterol and low-density lipoprotein (LDL) cholesterol without an increase in frequency or severity of rejection.[32] Deflazacort has not been approved by the Food and Drug Administration (FDA) for use in the United States.

The elimination of corticosteroids as part of maintenance immunosuppression holds great appeal in minimizing the consequences of chronic steroid treatment, with particular significance among pediatric recipients, in whom chronic steroid administration can interfere with normal growth and sexual maturation. Steroids have been successfully withdrawn 3–12 months after the transplant with widely varying rates of success in heart, liver, and kidney transplantation.[33–38] Although the results of these evaluations are variable, up to 80% of patients in some series can be successfully withdrawn from maintenance steroids. These attempts are not without risk, however; episodes of acute rejection can be precipitated by steroid withdrawal in an otherwise stable patient. Unfortunately, none of the series published to date has adequately identified predictors of successful steroid withdrawal. Suggested predictors of successful withdrawal include prior low maintenance steroid doses, stable graft function, no episodes of rejection within 6–12 months, and selective HLA matching. Rejection episodes that occur during steroid withdrawal may require the temporary or permanent reintroduction of higher doses of maintenance steroids. In addition, increases in cyclosporine or tacrolimus doses may be necessary to compensate for the reduction in immunosuppression. Finally, there remains concern that steroid withdrawal may increase the risk of chronic rejection.

Inhibitors of Early T-Cell Activation

Cyclosporine

CsA is an 11–amino acid cyclic peptide with reversible immunosuppressive activity. This agent is a naturally occurring metabolic product of the soil fungus *Tolypocladium inflatum gams*, first isolated in the early 1970s and introduced into human use in transplantation in 1978. Since 1982, it has formed the basis for the development of a new era in the history of organ transplantation, resulting in a dramatic improvement in renal allograft survival and allowing the widespread growth of extrarenal transplantation. The discovery and development of CsA as an immunosuppressive agent brought with it new insights into the mechanisms of alloimmunity and opened a floodgate of investigation into further innovations in drug development.

Pharmacology and Clinical Uses

The mechanism of action of CsA is unique. CsA binds to cyclophilin, a cytosolic binding protein that is key in signal transmission for de novo IL-2 production. The CsA-cyclophilin complex binds competitively to and inhibits calcineurin, a phosphatase whose activity is dependent on its being bound to calcium and calmodulin. Inhibition of calcineurin is believed to mediate the immunosuppressive activity of both CsA and tacrolimus. Calcineurin activity results in activation of the promoter region for the gene encoding IL-2, which leads to transcription. Inhibition of calcineurin activity by CsA inhibits transcription. Thus CsA interferes with the transcription of the genes encoding for the enzyme peptidyl-prolyl-*cis-trans* isomerase, thereby blocking signal transduction for lymphokine synthesis from the cytoplasm to the nucleus. The production of IL-2 from $CD4^+$ T cells is inhibited, with no apparent direct effect on $CD8^+$ T cells, B cells, macrophages, or granulocytes. Clonal expansion of allosensitized T cells is also reduced by inhibiting expression of IL-2 surface receptors. Because CsA selectively inhibits the synthesis of other lymphokines, including IFN-γ, the lymphokine that provides an amplification signal activating macrophages and monocytes, preformed cytotoxic ($CD8^+$) T lymphocytes are not affected by CsA.

Hyperacute rejection and other humorally mediated processes are also not affected.[39,40]

CsA exhibits wide inter- and intrapatient variation in its pharmacokinetic profile. Oral absorption, which occurs primarily in the duodenum, is slow and incomplete (mean bioavailability 30%), in part due to presystemic metabolism by cytochrome P-450 (CYP450) in the gut wall. Absorption is influenced by biliary diversion (see the discussion on bile duct anastomosis after liver transplantation below), cholestasis, delayed gastric emptying, dietary fat content, increased gastrointestinal motility, and reduced pancreatic exocrine secretions. After administration, CsA is widely distributed, with more than 90% of total drug bound to serum lipoproteins and erythrocytes (volume of distribution reported between 3.5 and 13 L/kg). Biotransformation of the parent compound occurs via the hepatic and gut microsomal mixed function oxidase enzyme system (CYP450-3A4) and results in the formation of at least 21 metabolites. The mean terminal half-life is 10–27 hours, and varies widely owing to differences in patient age and liver function and the effects of interacting drugs that induce or inhibit the CYP450 system. The pharmacokinetics of CsA are not influenced by hemodialysis, peritoneal dialysis, or continuous venovenous hemofiltration.

Dosing and Monitoring

CsA pharmacokinetics are complex and vary among transplant populations.[40,41] Red blood cells (RBCs) bind CsA; thus, because of its low to intermediate extraction ratio, clearance increases with decreased binding. CsA pharmacokinetics may therefore be altered in patients with low hematocrit. Age also seems to be an important factor in the disposition of CsA; pediatric patients have higher clearance values than older patients. One study has suggested that this age-related difference in clearance may result from lower serum lipoprotein concentrations and CsA binding in younger patients.[42] In addition, many drugs are capable of altering the clearance of CsA (Table 8-4).[43–45]

Cyclosporine absorption and disposition from the commercially available oral formulations are markedly variable, which complicates dosing and monitoring strategies with respect to maintenance of desired target blood concentrations and avoidance of toxicity. A microemulsion concentrate of CsA (Neoral®, Novartis) has been developed that demonstrates an increased rate and extent of drug absorption with lower intra- and interindividual pharmacokinetic variability when compared with the original formulation (Sandimmune®). Initial studies in normal volunteers and in renal transplant recipients have demonstrated that Neoral® is well-tolerated and exhibits greater relative bioavailability (faster time to peak [T_{max}] and maximum concentration [C_{max}]), greater area under the plasma drug concentration vs. time curve (AUC), and less intra- and interindividual variability than Sandimmune®.[20–22] Prospective comparative trials in primary cadaveric renal and liver transplantation are under way.

Table 8-4. Representative Drug Interactions with Cyclosporine[45]

INCREASE CsA CONCENTRATIONS	DECREASE CsA CONCENTRATIONS	ALTER CsA NEPHROTOXICITY
Increase CsA's absorption	**Decrease CsA's absorption**	**Increase nephrotoxicity**
Erythromycin	Phenytoin	Aminoglycosides
Metoclopramide	Rifampin	Amphotericin B
Grapefruit juice	Cholestyramine (?)	Nonsteroidal anti-inflammatory agents
Cisapride	Octreotide	Tacrolimus
	Probucol	
Decrease CsA's metabolism[a]	**Increase CsA's metabolism[a]**	**Decrease nephrotoxicity**
Diltiazem, nicardipine, verapamil	Nafcillin	Diltiazem, verapamil
Ketoconazole, itraconazole, fluconazole	Phenytoin	
Erythromycin, josamycin, clarithromycin	Phenobarbital	
Oral contraceptives	Carbamazepine	
Danazol	Primidone	
Tacrolimus	Rifampin, isoniazid	
	Sulfadimidine	

[a]*Many of the interactions reported to affect the hepatic metabolism of cyclosporine (CsA) may also alter CsA's absorption by either inhibiting or enhancing its intestinal (presystemic) metabolism.*

The use of therapeutic drug monitoring to reduce the risk of nephrotoxicity and maintain adequate immunosuppression associated with CsA remains controversial. A number of studies have demonstrated an association between elevated CsA concentrations and renal dysfunction, but a therapeutic range has not been identified. Despite more than a decade of widespread use, a clear correlation between the maintenance of defined cyclosporine blood concentrations and either efficacy or toxicity has not been defined.[46] The therapeutic drug monitoring of CsA is complicated by important assay and biologic fluid considerations.[47] One of the difficulties in assessing CsA concentrations comes from the fact that many of the early studies used a polyclonal radioimmunoassay (RIA) that is no longer available. The current polyclonal assay using a fluorescence polarization immunoassay (FPIA) has different metabolite-binding affinities and demonstrates about 1.6 times higher concentrations in plasma than the polyclonal RIA. In whole blood, the FPIA and RIA give about the same value.[48] Whether a specific (i.e., high-performance liquid chromatography [HPLC]) or nonspecific (i.e., FPIA) assay should be used is still controversial. More complete studies have been performed using nonspecific assays and have shown the most convincing positive correlation between concentration and effect.[49]

In most investigations of the relationship between CsA concentrations and efficacy or toxicity, serum or plasma concentrations have been measured. The issue of the use of whole blood versus serum or plasma remains controversial. CsA is highly bound to RBCs, and the binding is temperature dependent. As the temperature of blood is lowered from body temperature to room temperature, the CsA increasingly partitions into the RBCs, resulting in serum or plasma concentration variations. Because of this temperature-dependent effect, it may be advantageous to assay whole blood if the samples cannot be handled with consistent temperature restriction. However, with appropriate sample handling—which means that one consistent temperature is used to separate serum or plasma, such as a two-hour equilibration at room temperature—consistent results can be obtained. Until more is known about the activity of the metabolites, it is difficult to recommend one assay method or biologic matrix over another; it may be reasonable to use the assay and matrix that is most convenient for the given institution.[50] Most recently, routine use of a monoclonal whole blood FPIA specific for parent CsA (TDx®, Abbott) has gained widespread popularity because of its ease of performance, reproducibility, rapid turnaround time, and low cost.

Adverse Effects and Toxicity

CsA has a number of important toxicities (Table 8-5), the most common and clinically relevant of which is renal dysfunction. CsA nephrotoxicity can manifest as an acute renal failure or as chronic nephrotoxicity. The acute renal dysfunction associated with CsA is characterized by decreased glomerular filtration within days of starting the drug. A number of drugs have also been reported to produce additive nephrotoxicity with CsA (see Table 8-4).[43–47] Despite the high frequency of CsA-associated nephrotoxicity, the long-term efficacy and safety of this agent has been documented, and chronic CsA toxicity rarely results in graft loss.[51]

A number of renal protectants have been investigated to decrease the acute renal failure syndrome: misoprostol,[52] clonidine,[53] and pentoxifylline.[54] Patients on amphotericin and CsA who received pentoxifylline were able to receive significantly higher CsA doses with lower serum creatinine values than patients not receiving pentoxifylline.[54] Calcium antagonists have also been evaluated for their renal protective effects.[55,56]

In addition to nephrotoxicity, CsA can cause liver dysfunction, neurotoxicity, hirsutism, gingival hyperplasia, and infusion-related reactions characterized by burning of the soles and palms.[57] Hypertension occurs as a result of CsA administration in 50–90% of transplant patients. The requirement for effective treatment of hypertension cannot be overemphasized, for uncontrolled blood pressure will result in premature loss of allograft function. Calcium-channel blockers, particularly those of the dihydropyridine class, are preferred antihypertensive agents owing to their favorable effects on renal blood flow and serum lipid profile.[58] Angiotensin-converting enzyme-inhibitors are also effective, but they can compromise renal blood flow and exacerbate the hyperkalemia associated with CsA.

CsA Analogues

The frequent and often severe side effects associated with CsA have prompted research into the use of analogues that may preserve or enhance its efficacy as an immunosuppressive agent while reducing or eliminating its toxicities, particularly nephrotoxicity.[59] Cyclosporin G (OG-37-325, Sandoz) has undergone the most extensive evaluation in renal transplant recipients.[23] Cyclosporin G differs from CsA structurally by one amino acid substitution. Although initial studies demonstrated a reduction in nephrotoxicity, recent large multicenter analyses demonstrated equivalent patient and graft survival. In addition, there was a significant incidence of elevation of liver enzymes and hepatotoxicity, which appears to be dose and concentration dependent and responsive to dosage reduction.[24] Because no significant improvement in outcomes accompanied the increased hepatotoxicity, the agent was recently removed from further clinical investigation.

Tacrolimus

Tacrolimus (FK506) is a naturally occurring macrolide product of the soil fungus *Streptomyces tsukubaensis* and has immunosuppressive ability similar to that of CsA.

Table 8-5. Incidence of Adverse Events with Tacrolimus and Cyclosporine[a]

ADVERSE EVENT[b]	TACROLIMUS (*n* = 263)	CYCLOSPORINE (*n* = 266)	(*P* VALUE)
Alopecia	20	6	<0.001
Anemia	47	38	0.047
Anorexia	34	24	0.01
Diarrhea	72	47	<0.001
Fever	48	56	0.089
Headache	64	60	0.408
Hirsutism	7	31	<0.001
Hyperglycemia	47	38	0.07
Hyperkalemia	45	26	<0.001
Hypertension	47	56	0.06
Nausea	46	37	0.046
Paresthesia	40	30	0.039
Pruritus	36	20	<0.001
Rash	24	19	0.101
Tremor	56	46	0.032
Vomiting	27	15	0.001

[a]Values are the percentages of patients reporting the first occurrence of any treatment-related event on the basis of history, physical examination, or laboratory examination or diagnostic tests during the one-year follow-up.

[b]Hypertension was defined as elevated blood pressure (regardless of the specific value) that was being treated with at least one medication. Anemia, hyperglycemia, and hyperkalemia were defined at each study site on the basis of accepted laboratory values at that institution.

SOURCE: *Reprinted from U.S. Multicenter FK506 Liver Study Group,* N Engl J Med. *1994;331(17):1110–5.*

Tacrolimus shares a mechanism of action similar to that of CsA but binds to a specific cytoplasmic immunophilin (FK binding protein) different from the calcineurin binding site of CsA. Both agents inhibit calcium-dependent signal transduction pathways in T cells, thereby blocking the secretion of IL-2 and other lymphokines.[68–70] Their pharmacokinetic profiles are also similar. Reported clinical pharmacokinetic parameters for tacrolimus include a half-life of 8.7 hours (range, 5.5–16.6 hours), mean volume of distribution of 19.4 L/kg, and mean clearance of 143 L/hr (range, 88–269 L/hr). After oral administration, tacrolimus is poorly, erratically, and incompletely absorbed. The mean bioavailability is 27%; wide interpatient variability is observed, particularly among pediatric patients.[71] Unlike CsA, it does not require bile to ensure adequate absorption.[72] The newer Neoral® formulation of CsA is less dependent on the presence of bile for absorption, similar to tacrolimus. After an oral dose of 0.15 mg/kg, peak plasma concentrations of 0.4–3.7 ng/ml were achieved. The time to peak varied from one to four hours. Tacrolimus is metabolized by the CYP450 enzyme system, as is CsA,[72] which accounts for the similar drug interactions (e.g., ketoconazole, erythromycin, and phenytoin) that have been reported.[72–74] Metabolism is significantly impaired in the presence of poor hepatic function, requiring close attention to blood concentration monitoring and careful dosage adjustment.

Pharmacology and Clinical Uses

Clinical use of tacrolimus began in February 1989 at the University of Pittsburgh. Multicenter, randomized, prospective clinical trials comparing a tacrolimus-based regimen with CsA-based regimens in liver transplantation began in the fall of 1990, resulting in FDA approval for this indication in April 1994.[60,61] Tacrolimus has also been shown to be an effective agent for the prevention of allograft rejection in noncomparative trials in primary renal,[62,63] lung,[64] and cardiac[65] transplantation and as rescue therapy for patients experiencing persistent allograft rejection during primary immunosuppression with CsA.[66,67] Reviews of its extensive clinical use are presented elsewhere.[16,17]

Dosing and Monitoring

Therapy is initiated with a dose of 0.05–0.1 mg/kg administered orally twice daily.[75] Tacrolimus is adequately absorbed in the immediate post-transplant period, and routine parenteral administration is neither required nor desirable, because of the potentially greater neurotoxicity and nephrotoxicity associated with the intravenous dosage form. However, for those patients who cannot receive oral medication, tacrolimus may be administered at initial doses of 0.05–0.075 mg/kg per day as a continuous intravenous infusion over 24 hours. Therapy is adjusted based on whole blood or plasma trough concentrations as measured by enzyme-linked immunosorbent assay (ELISA) or by microparticle enzyme immunoassay (IMX).[76,77] Typical whole blood trough concentrations range from 5 to 20 ng/ml, and plasma concentrations from 0.5 to 2.0 ng/ml. As for CsA, the optimal target blood concentrations for tacrolimus have not been determined.

Adverse Effects and Toxicity

Table 8-5 compares the adverse effects of tacrolimus with those of CsA. Tacrolimus may have a lesser incidence of certain side effects (e.g., hypertension, hypercholesterolemia, hirsutism, and gingival hyperplasia) than CsA.[78] The propensity of tacrolimus to cause nephrotoxicity and diabetes and predispose patients to opportunistic infections is similar to that of CsA.[79–81] A variety of neurotoxic effects has been reported, including akinetic mutism, expressive aphasia, seizures, confusion, psychosis, encephalopathy, coma, tremors, headache, and sleep disturbances.[16] Gastrointestinal toxicity may be manifest as nausea or severe anorexia with weight loss. Many patients will respond to dosage reductions, but in other cases neurotoxicity and/or gastrointestinal toxicity may necessitate withdrawal of this agent and conversion to CsA.[82–84]

Inhibitors of Late T-Cell Function

Sirolimus

Sirolimus (Rapamycin; Wyeth-Ayerst) was discovered in the mid-1970s during a screening program intended to identify novel antifungal agents. However, further development was not pursued at that time. When the structure of tacrolimus was elucidated, sirolimus was found to be structurally similar (Figure 8-2), and investigations into its use as an antirejection agent were initiated. The immunosuppressive activity of sirolimus appears to be mediated through a mechanism distinct from that of tacrolimus or CsA. Unlike the latter two agents, which inhibit T-cell stimulation through a mechanism involving reduction of IL-2 production and IL-2 receptor expression, sirolimus has little or no effect on these immunologic events. Instead, sirolimus markedly suppresses IL-2– and IL-4–driven T-cell proliferation, thus acting at a later phase of the cell cycle (G_1) than tacrolimus or CsA. Sirolimus inhibits the response to activating cytokines IL-2 and IL-6, rather than the direct synthesis and secretion of these mediators. This agent is also inhibitory to IL-6–supported proliferation and IFN-α and IFN-β activity.[85,86] Sirolimus has been shown to compete for binding to the same intra-

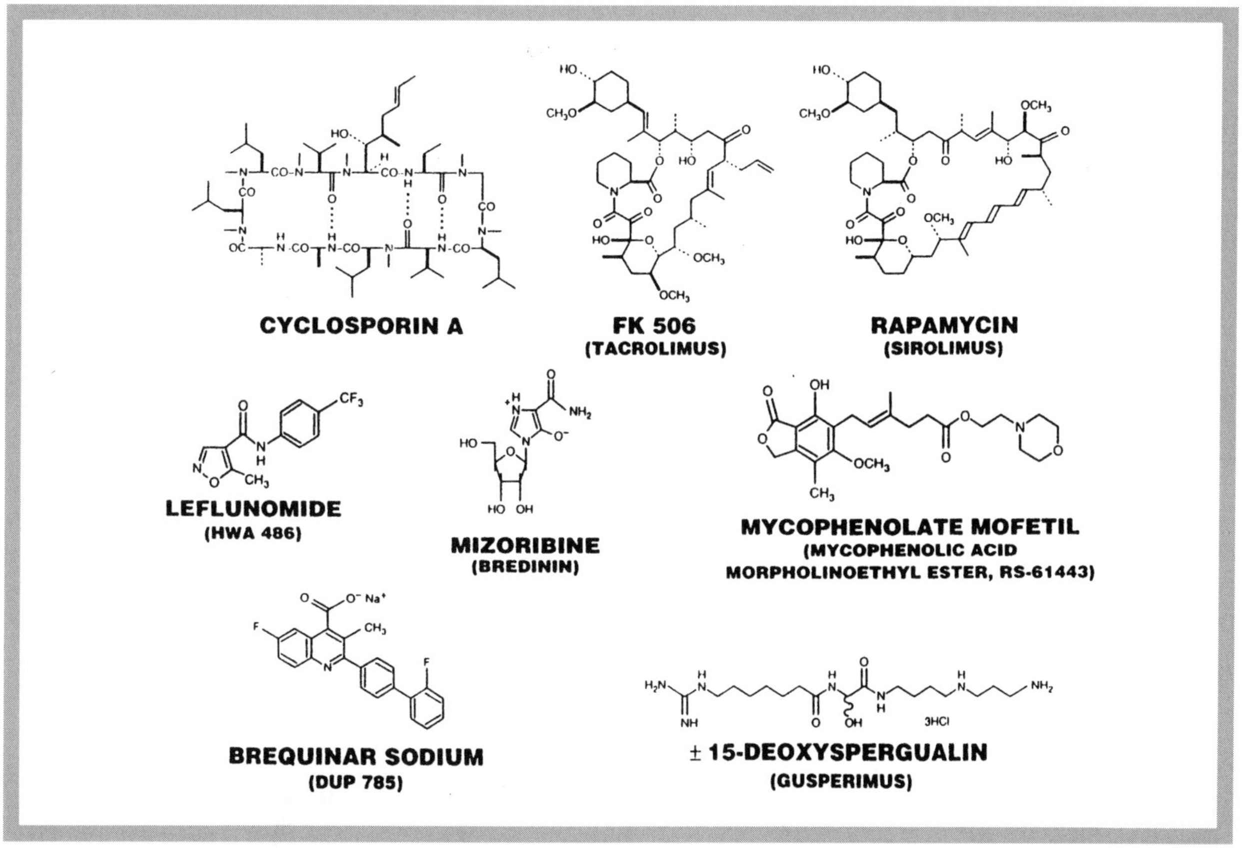

Figure 8-2. Structures of new immunosuppressive drugs

SOURCE: *Reprinted with permission from Morris RE. New small molecule immunosuppressants for transplantation: reveiw of essential concepts [review].* J Heart Lung Transplant. *1993;12(6 Pt 2):5275–86.*

cellular site as tacrolimus, suggesting these agents cannot be used in combination. In contrast, the potency of sirolimus is markedly augmented by combination with CsA, permitting at least threefold reduction of the dose of each agent.[87] Human and animal trials are under way to clarify sirolimus's dose-response relationship, toxicology profile, and potential for drug interactions.[88,89]

Deoxyspergualin (Gusperimus)

Deoxyspergualin (15-DSG; Bristol-Myers) entered phase I and II clinical trials for kidney transplantation in 1991. This guanidine derivative has been found to exert a powerful immunosuppressive effect in animal models. Because 15-DSG must be given parenterally, its clinical potential lies in induction of immunosuppression at the time of transplantation and in the management of acute rejection. Its mechanism of action has not been completely elucidated. In vitro, 15-DSG preferentially suppresses the generation of effector cytotoxic T cells from antigen-stimulated precursor T cells. It does not modulate IL-2 production like CsA and tacrolimus, nor does it block TCR recognition. Early trials in the United States and Japan have shown that it is effective in the prevention and treatment of acute renal transplant rejection, with a variety of tolerable side effects, including headache, fatigue, facial and peroral numbness, mild leukopenia, thrombocytopenia, and gastrointestinal discomfort.[90–95]

Leflunomide

Leflunomide (HWA 486, Hoechst) is an isoxazol derivative that has shown promise as an immunosuppressive agent in a number of animal models of organ transplantation.[25] After oral absorption, it undergoes metabolism in the liver to the active compound A77-1726, which constitutes more than 90% of the parent and its derivatives. Its mechanism of action is poorly defined, but it has been shown to interfere with both B- and T-lymphocyte responsiveness to multiple stimuli, acting at a point later in the cell cycle than CsA. Although no human studies have been reported, leflunomide has shown considerable activity alone and in combination with subtherapeutic concentrations of CsA in prolonging allograft survival in animals without evidence of organ toxicity.[26] Leflunomide is an investigational agent not yet approved by the FDA.

Inhibitors of Cell Proliferation

Azathioprine

Azathioprine (AZA) is a purine analogue that has been used as a component of immunosuppressive regimens since 1961.[4] Its popularity has waned through the decades as new immunosuppressive agents have been introduced, but it has played a major role in the evolution of clinical transplantation.

Pharmacology and Clinical Uses

AZA is an imidazolyl derivative of 6-MP and is readily converted to this active metabolite.[96] It acts by incorporating into cellular DNA, and inhibiting purine synthesis; purines are required for both DNA and RNA synthesis. AZA is most toxic to rapidly proliferating cells that are making new DNA. It inhibits humoral and cellular immunity during the initial stages of lymphoid differentiation. Thus, it is useful in the prevention but not the treatment of acute rejection. AZA may also reduce neutrophil production and macrophage function, thereby reducing the nonspecific inflammatory aspect of the immune reaction.[97]

Dosing and Monitoring

Even though AZA has been used for more than 30 years, its pharmacokinetics have not been fully characterized. The development of more sensitive and specific assays has allowed for a better understanding of the pharmacokinetics of AZA and its metabolites.[98–102] The absorption of orally administered AZA is rapid but incomplete. It is rapidly converted by glutathione to 6-MP in the liver and RBCs.[98–100,103,104] Both AZA and 6-MP have short half-lives—12.5 ± 3.0 and 50.4 ± 36.6 minutes, respectively. Bioavailability of 6-MP after administration of AZA has been estimated to be 41–44%.[105] Based on these findings, it has been suggested that the dose of AZA be reduced by 50% when converting from the oral to the intravenous route of administration.[96] However, because the immunologic activity is actually conveyed by its metabolites, it is unclear whether dosage adjustments of the prodrug (i.e., AZA) are necessary. 6-MP is either transformed intracellularly to thioinosinic acid and 6-thioguanine nucleotides (TGNs) or further broken down to 6-thiouric acid, an inactive end product primarily eliminated by the kidneys.[103] Thioinosinic acid is an inhibitor of purine synthesis. The TGNs incorporate into DNA and probably are toxic to dividing cells. The half-life of RBC TGN appears to be quite long (i.e., approximately 13 days), allowing for once-daily dosing of AZA[103] but also contributing to delayed reversal of toxicity. The concentration of TGN in the tissues may be the more clinically relevant level to be measured, but at this time therapeutic drug monitoring is only investigational. The clearance of AZA is not affected by renal impairment, but its metabolite 6-thioguanine may accumulate, with renal impairment contributing to enhanced toxicity.[100] Dosing guidelines for renal impairment are not available.

AZA has been used extensively in double- (also known as "conventional therapy"), triple-, and quadruple-drug regimens for organ transplantation. Clinical studies using AZA are reviewed elsewhere.[96] An initial, one-time dose of 3–5 mg/kg per day of AZA is administered preoperatively. Immediately after transplantation, the dose is usually tapered to a maintenance dose of 1–3 mg/kg per day or titrated to patient tolerance as determined by a desired white blood cell (WBC) count of 3500–6000 cells/mm^3.[96] WBC counts below 3000 usually necessitate temporary discontinuation of the drug and/or subsequent dosage reduction (e.g., 25 mg/day). Infectious complications (e.g., cytomegalovirus [CMV]) and other medications commonly used in transplant patients (e.g., trimethoprim–sulfamethoxazole, ganciclovir, etc.) may further confound the differential diagnosis of leukopenia observed in patients treated with AZA.

A reduction of 75–80% of the AZA dose is necessary in patients receiving the xanthine-oxidase inhibitor allopurinol, which blocks the metabolism of AZA's metabolites.[106–108] This interaction can cause life-threatening pancytopenia, which may not become clinically apparent until after one month of concomitant therapy. Administration of granulocyte colony-stimulating factor may be necessary to decrease the risk of infection and other complications associated with profound marrow suppression. AZA has been associated with increased requirements of the nondepolarizing muscle relaxant pancuronium, but it potentiates the activity of succinylcholine, a depolarizing muscle relaxant.[109,110] Increased warfarin requirements have been reported for patients receiving 6-MP and may be expected with AZA.[111]

Adverse Effects and Toxicity

The primary toxicity of AZA is its dose-related bone marrow suppression, appearing 7–14 days after initiation of therapy.[112] The myelosuppression is characterized by leukopenia,[113,114] thrombocytopenia, macrocytic anemia, pure red cell aplasia, and reticulocytopenia.[115] Other adverse effects include increased predisposition to infections (viral, bacterial, and fungal),[116] hepatic dysfunction and jaundice,[117,118] alopecia, stomatitis,[119] acute pancreatitis,[120] and increased risk of malignancy.[121] The adverse effects of AZA are reviewed in greater detail elsewhere.[96]

Cyclophosphamide

Pharmacology and Clinical Uses

Cyclophosphamide (CTX) is used occasionally in solid organ transplantation because it suppresses both humoral and cell-mediated immunity.[122,123] In low doses it is toxic to precursors of suppressor T cells, and it enhances natural killer cell activity and macrophage activation.[124,125] Infrequently, it may be used as a substitute agent in organ transplantation (1.5–2.0 mg/kg per day) when AZA has to be withdrawn because of hepatotoxicity or leukopenia.[126,127] CTX has been used in transplant recipients with severe, prolonged, and uncontrollable rejection that has failed to respond to standard therapy.[128] It has also been suggested as a useful entity in humorally (B-cell) mediated rejection and to decrease OKT3 sensitization because CTX inhibits antibody production.[129] CTX has also been utilized as part of immunosuppressive protocols for ABO-incompatible liver transplantation.[130] However, the use of CTX will likely decrease with FDA approval of mycophenolate mofetil.

Classified as an alkylating agent, CTX is metabolically activated in the liver by phosphoamidases to active alkylating metabolites. Its primary active metabolite, phosphoramide mustard, inhibits the cross-linking of DNA and causes cell death. Unlike AZA, which only acts on proliferating cells, CTX is toxic to both resting and dividing cells. CTX has a greater effect on B-lymphocyte activity than does AZA.

With regard to drug interactions, allopurinol and cimetidine, but not ranitidine, have been reported to increase CTX concentrations and effect, respectively; ranitidine does not interact.[131] Like AZA, the neuromuscular blocking effect of succinylcholine can be prolonged significantly by a decrease in plasma pseudocholinesterase activity during CTX therapy.[132]

Dosing and Monitoring

After oral administration, CTX is well absorbed (90% bioavailability), and maximal plasma concentrations are achieved after one hour. The volume of distribution is 0.64 L/kg. Most of the drug is metabolized by the liver, and only 20% or less is excreted as unchanged drug.[124] Both the parent drug and its metabolites are eliminated primarily via the kidneys. The half-life of CTX after intravenous administration ranges from 4 to 7 hours; however, CTX or its metabolites or both may be detected in the plasma for up to 72 hours. Allopurinol has been found to prolong CTX's half-life substantially by affecting its metabolism.[124] Neither impaired renal function nor liver failure requires dosage adjustments; however, supplementation may be necessary following dialysis, because 72% of CTX in the bloodstream may be removed following a six-hour treatment.[133] Renal impairment also prolongs plasma-alkylating activity. Microsomal enzyme-inducing drugs seem to alter the half-life without modifying the overall toxicity.[124]

Doses of CTX up to 3–4 mg/kg per day for four days followed by a reduction to 1 mg/kg per day have been used to treat graft rejection.[128,130] Doses of 1–2 mg/kg are standard for use in maintenance therapy in AZA-intolerant patients. The nadir in WBC count usually occurs within one to two weeks, and the dosage needs to be titrated to maintain the WBC count between 4000 and 6000/mm^3.[128,130]

Adverse Effects and Toxicity

The toxicity of CTX differs from that of other antineoplastic agents in that significant thrombocytopenia is much less common than leukopenia but alopecia occurs very frequently. It is believed that the toxic metabolites phosphoramide mustard and acrolein account for the cytotoxic properties of the parent drug. Nausea and vomiting are common when CTX is administered at higher doses. Other rare side effects include syndrome of inappropriate antidiuretic hormone, chronic pulmonary fibrosis, bone marrow suppression, and acute myocardial necrosis.[134]

Methotrexate

Pharmacology and Clinical Uses

Methotrexate (MTX) is an antimetabolic folic acid analogue that inhibits DNA synthesis in cell division and suppresses both cellular and humoral immunity. MTX prevents dihydrofolic acid from converting to tetrahydrofolic acid by inhibiting the enzyme dihydrofolate reductase. This inhibition ultimately interferes with DNA and protein synthesis.

Dosing and Monitoring

MTX is minimally metabolized, and only small amounts are excreted via the bile.[135] Elimination occurs primarily by renal excretion via glomerular filtration, absorption in the proximal tubule (which can be blocked by probenecid), and active tubular secretion in the distal tubule (which can be blocked by salicylates). This agent has had limited use in solid organ transplantation and has been primarily used for recalcitrant rejection in heart and heart-lung recipients.[136–138] Lower doses of 7.5–22.5 mg/week (2.5–7.5 mg every 12 hours for three doses weekly) have been used as an adjunct in the treatment of persistent mild cardiac rejection,[137] whereas higher doses (15–50 mg weekly for one to three weeks) have been necessary for recalcitrant rejection.[136] Toxicity is dose dependent and doses greater than 30 mg/week may be too toxic to bone marrow transplant recipients.

Adverse Effects and Toxicity

The toxicity of MTX may depend more on the duration of exposure than on the peak concentration. Because of MTX's action on rapidly proliferating cells, such as those in the bone marrow, intestine, and mouth, it produces side effects such as myelosuppression, diarrhea, and mucositis. Because MTX is partially bound to plasma proteins, other highly protein-bound drugs (e.g., salicylates and sulfonamides) may exacerbate its toxicity.

Mycophenolate Mofetil

Pharmacology and Clinical Uses

Mycophenolate mofetil (CellCept®, Roche Labs) is a semisynthetic agent derived from the fermentation of several *Penicillum* species. The compound is the morpholino-ethyl ester of mycophenolic acid, the active form of the drug, and is rapidly hydrolyzed to this compound in vivo.[18] Mycophenolic acid selectively blocks human B- and T-lymphocyte proliferative responses via inhibition of de novo pathways of purine biosynthesis. This results in decreased intracellular pools of guanosine ribonucleotides and dGTP, which are key for the regulation of DNA polymerase activity and subsequent lymphocyte proliferation. De novo purine synthesis is specific to lymphocytes, and therefore the antiproliferative effects on other cell types are significantly lower with mycophenolic acid than with other agents. Secondary immunologic effects include decreased B-lymphocyte antibody production and reduced expression of selective adhesion molecules responsible for key cellular interactions. Unlike CsA and tacrolimus, mycophenolic acid does not affect IL-1 and IL-2 production, the key cytokines associated with early T-cell signal transduction. In vitro, mycophenolic acid inhibits human arterial smooth muscle, fibroblast, and endothelial cell proliferation, which may prove key in preventing the development and progression of chronic rejection.[19]

Mycophenolic acid undergoes hepatic conjugation to the inactive metabolite mycophenolic acid glucuronide (MPAG).[18,19] However, this compound undergoes enterohepatic recirculation and can be hydrolyzed back to mycophenolic acid by intestinal and cellular β-glucuronidase enzymes. Pharmacokinetic studies after oral administration demonstrated 94% bioavailability, T_{max} of 1.0 hour, a dose-dependent C_{max} of 2.0–18.7 μg/ml, and a plasma half-life of 15.8 hours.[19] The agent undergoes extensive metabolism and enterohepatic recirculation, with more than 90% of mycophenolic acid excreted in the urine. The apparent lack of effect on human CYP450 activity is supported by the absence of a pharmacokinetic drug interaction with CsA.[18,19]

Initially evaluated as an immunosuppressant in the late 1970s for several autoimmune indications, clinical investigations with mycophenolate mofetil in solid organ transplant recipients were not initiated until 1991.[19] Subsequently, mycophenolate mofetil, combined with CsA and prednisone, has undergone extensive phase I–III trials for the prevention of rejection after kidney,[19,139,140] liver,[141] and heart[142] transplantation and was approved by the FDA in the summer of 1995 for this indication in renal allograft recipients. In addition, mycophenolate mofetil appears effective in reversing acute rejection episodes refractory to steroid and antibody therapy.[140,141] Preliminary clinical evaluations are under way to explore the CsA-sparing properties and preventive effects on chronic rejection associated with this unique compound.

Dosing and Monitoring

The immunosuppressive activity of mycophenolate mofetil, as well as adverse effects, appear to be dose dependent, with doses ranging from 100 to 3500 mg/day evaluated in various clinical settings.[139] Doses of 2000 mg/day appear necessary for the prevention of rejection in kidney transplant recipients and provide optimal immunosuppression with minimal adverse effects.[139,143,144] The agent can be administered orally twice a day and is generally adjusted based on adverse effects or intolerance to the agent. Studies evaluating the intravenous form for optimal dosing in extrarenal allograft recipients and for rescue therapy are currently under way. There are several drug-drug interactions documented with mycophenolate mofetil.[145] Acyclovir and probenecid appear to compete for renal tubular secretion with MPAG, increasing the AUC of theses agents and MPAG. Cholestyramine and aluminum- or magnesium-based antacids significantly reduce the bioavailability of mycophenolate mofetil, and these agents should not be administered concomitantly. Although there are no formal dosing guidelines for renal insufficiency, patients with significant acute or chronic failure should be monitored closely for toxicity. Preliminary studies have demonstrated that cirrhosis has no effect on the metabolism of mycophenolate mofetil.

Adverse Effects and Toxicity

Mycophenolate mofetil is generally well tolerated, with fewer dose-limiting effects than other antiproliferative agents.[19,139–144] Gastrointestinal effects, such as gastritis, nausea, anorexia, and abdominal cramping, are most frequently reported at standard doses (2–3 g/day).[139,143–145] Rare cases of gastrointestinal ulceration and bleeding have been reported with larger doses (above 3.5 g/day). Hematologic toxicities, including neutropenia, thrombocytopenia, and anemia, occur at similar or less frequent rates than with standard AZA therapy. The incidence of viral infections is at least equivalent to AZA, with several studies demonstrating an increase in CMV disease in mycophenolate mofetil–treated patients. The incidence of Epstein-Barr virus (EBV)–related lymphoma and malignancy appears similar to that of AZA when combined with CsA and prednisone.[19,139–146] Currently, the safety profile of mycophenolate mofetil is only established in combination with CsA, prednisone, and with or without antithymocyte globulin (Atgam®) induction.[145] It is unclear what effect other immunosuppressive combinations will have on clinical outcomes as well as the adverse effect, infection, and malignancy rates observed with mycophenolate mofetil.

Miscellaneous Antiproliferatives

Other investigational inhibitors of purine and pyrimidine biosynthesis include mizoribine (MZ, also known as bredinin) and brequinar, respectively.[15] Unlike mycophenolate mofetil, MZ inhibits purine synthesis by competitively inhibiting inosine monophosphate dehydrogenase (IMPDH). The drug has antiproliferative effects on lymphocytes and antagonizes the formation of cytotoxic cells but does not affect the function of previously formed cytotoxic cells. MZ has been used extensively in Japan as a substitute for AZA in triple-drug regimens, but large-scale clinical trials have not been completed in the United States. MZ is eliminated via the kidneys (85% of a dose is excreted unchanged in the urine), and dosage adjustments are necessary with renal impairment. The half-life varies from two to eight hours, with creatinine clearances of 22–93 ml/min, respectively. The dosage of MZ ranges from 50 to 300 mg/day and is administered once daily. The drug has considerably less myelotoxicity and hepatotoxicity than AZA.[147]

Brequinar is an antimetabolite that inhibits the de novo synthesis of pyrimidines by inhibiting the enzyme dihydroorotate dehydrogenase. Dose-limiting side effects include headache, thrombocytopenia, leukopenia, stomatitis, and a severe desquamative dermatitis. Because of the inter- and intrapatient pharmacokinetic variability, plasma concentration monitoring is necessary to adjust the dosage. This agent has been in phase II clinical trials in kidney and liver transplant patients, but investigations have been put on hold by the manufacturer because of a high incidence of life-threatening thrombocytopenia.[148]

Polyclonal Antilymphocyte Antibodies

The immunosuppressive qualities of antilymphocyte serum were first described by Woodruff in 1963.[149] Antilymphocyte antibodies were the first form of selective immunosuppression to be used as anti-T-cell therapy. Polyclonal antilymphocyte antibodies have since been used, both alone and in combination with other immunosuppressive agents, to prevent and treat rejection episodes in organ transplantation.[150–158] In addition, these agents have been most recently used in "sequential" regimens in which monoclonal or polyclonal agents are administered in the early phase following renal transplantation in lieu of more nephrotoxic agents, such as CsA or tacrolimus. Once renal function has recovered, CsA or tacrolimus are initiated and the antibody therapy is stopped.[159]

Pharmacology and Clinical Uses

Antilymphocyte globulin (ALG) and antithymocyte globulin (ATG) are produced by first injecting a series of human spleen cells (ALG) or thymocytes (ATG) into various animals (e.g., horse, goat, or rabbit). Antibodies are then isolated from the animal sera.[160,161] Their potency lies primarily in the immunoglobulin G (IgG) antibody fraction. Their action is directed not only against T cells but also against B cells, causing marked lymphocytopenia. Additional binding to nonlymphoid cells (i.e., platelets, RBCs, and WBCs) can also occur, resulting in various blood dyscrasias. ALG acts by binding to surface antigens on host T or B lymphocytes, causing (1) opsonization and removal by the reticuloendothelial system, or (2) direct, complement-assisted lysing of lymphocytes.

Dosing and Monitoring

The pharmacokinetics of ATGs have not been fully elucidated. The plasma half-life of equine IgG averages 6 days (range, 1.5–12 days). The plasma concentrations and half-life of IgG vary, depending on the patient's ability to catabolize foreign IgG. Concentrations of ATG have been detected up to 30 days after administration. Approximately 1% of a dose of ATG is excreted in urine as unchanged equine IgG. The distribution and selective binding to different binding sites vary from product to product.[162]

Antilymphocyte antibodies are produced for investigational use by various institutions around the world. Atgam® (equine) is the only commercially available product in the United States; Frensenius ATG (rabbit) is available in Europe. The equine antilymphoblast globulin (MALG) produced by the University of Minnesota, which was previously used by many transplant centers, is no longer available. The recommended dose for equine preparations is usually 10–20 mg/kg per day for up to 14 days but varies according to institutional protocol and type of transplant. The required dose should be diluted in saline at a maximum concentration of 4 mg/ml and administered through a central line over four to eight hours.[163] The dose of rabbit preparations varies from 1.5 to 3.0 mg/kg per day and is administered either intravenously or intramuscularly. One ATG (Thymoglobulin, Institute Merieux/Sangstat) is currently in phase III trials in the United States.[164]

For all of these agents, efficacy can be monitored by measuring the T-cell count. Controversy exists as to the most appropriate lymphocyte population to monitor the efficacy of polyclonal antibodies. Each preparation has a different binding specificity for CD2, CD3, CD4, CD8, and other specific epitopes.[165] Several studies have used variable dosing of polyclonal antibodies based on reduction in $CD2^+$ or $CD3^+$ T-cell counts during sequential induction.[165] Other centers have utilized reduction in total lymphocyte counts as a marker of response.[166] In general, a 90% reduction in $CD2^+$ or $CD3^+$ T cells from baseline correlates with an adequate response.[164]

Adverse Effects and Toxicity

ALGs and antilymphocyte sera are composed of antibodies directed against multiple-surface antigens. This nonspecificity predisposes the patient to significant side effects from the products' cross-reactivity with nonlymphocytic blood cells and other human tissues.[167,168] Side effects seen with these agents include fever, chills, erythema, pruritus, leukopenia, thrombocytopenia, arthralgias, myalgias, and (rarely) allergic reactions, such as anaphylaxis and serum sickness. Premedication with acetaminophen, antihistamines, and steroids decreases the incidence of adverse reactions. Switching to a different source (e.g., goat or rabbit) or to OKT3 may be necessary if the reactions are severe. Doses are reduced by 50% if the platelet count falls below 50,000–70,000 per microliter and are often held for severe thrombocytopenia. Like other immunosuppressants, these agents have also been associated with increased incidence of infections and neoplasms.[169]

The major limitations associated with the polyclonal antilymphocyte antibodies relate to their (1) batch-to-batch variability in potency and purity, (2) variable immunosuppressive efficacy among different preparations, (3) contamination with other globulins, which can result in substantial side effects, and (4) derivation from animal sources, which incurs the risk of potentially serious allergic reactions and efficacy-reducing xenosensitization.

Monoclonal Antibodies

OKT3

Immunologic Effects

Muromonab OKT3 is a murine MoAb of the IgG2a isotype that binds to the CD3 receptor found on mature circulating T cells and medullary thymocytes.[170,171] The CD3 receptor complex is situated next to the T-cell antigen-recognition site. By binding to the CD3 receptor, OKT3 blocks the ability of cells to become stimulated by foreign antigens, thus inhibiting both the generation and function of cytotoxic T cells responsible for graft rejection. After the initial dose of OKT3, T cells virtually disappear from the circulation within minutes to hours. During treatment with OKT3, T cells bearing the usual array of surface markers (CD2, CD4, CD8) reappear but are devoid of the OKT3 target, the CD3 receptor.[172–174] However, within 48 hours of discontinuing therapy, the normal array of surface markers, including CD3, reappears on T cells. Proposed mechanisms for OKT3's action include opsonization of circulating T cells and subsequent removal by the reticuloendothelial system;[175] modulation (internalization) of the T-lymphocyte antigen receptor–CD3 complex, which would render the T cell nonfunctional;[176] and coating of the TCR, which would inhibit T-lymphocyte antigen recognition for the duration of the therapy.[177,178] The therapeutic effectiveness of OKT3 in reversing acute allograft rejection is related to its ability to block the action of cytotoxic T lymphocytes against the allograft. Potential causes for failure of OKT3 or subsequent need for higher OKT3 doses include immune clearance of the agent as a result of human antimurine antibody (HAMA) production, increased consumption from high antigen production rates, an abnormally high clearance rate of mouse immunoglobulin, and lack of T-cell functional dependence on the CD3 antigen.[174]

Dosing

The clinical efficacy of OKT3 is well established for the first-line treatment of rejection, steroid-resistant rejection, and rejection prophylaxis (induction) in most solid organ transplant populations.[179] The usual dosage regimen for OKT3 is 5 mg intravenously daily for 10–14 days for rejection and 7–10 days for induction. Before administration, OKT3 must be filtered through a 0.20- to 0.22-micron low-protein-binding filter to remove particulate matter. After filtering, OKT3 should be administered as an intravenous bolus via either peripheral or central access. Lower doses have proved equally effective in some patients for rejection prophylaxis.[180] The manufacturer recommends a dose of 2.5 mg be administered daily in children who weigh less than 30 kg, but it has been observed that children may actually require larger doses (5–7.5 mg daily) to achieve similar immunosuppressive efficacy. [181–183]

Monitoring

Immunologic monitoring should be performed during and after OKT3 therapy to monitor the efficacy of treatment and to assess whether retreatment with OKT3 is possible. It is particularly important that immune monitoring be performed during retreatment with OKT3 so that appropriate dose adjustments can be made.[184] The efficacy of OKT3 therapy can be monitored by measuring peripheral lymphocyte subsets ($CD3^+$ T cells), serum OKT3 concentrations, and the production of HAMAs.[185]

Lymphocyte Subsets—Based on the alterations of CD3 expression during OKT3 therapy, lymphocyte subset populations have been the mainstay of monitoring immunologic response to OKT3. The absolute number and percentage of peripheral $CD3^+$ T cells/mm^3 have been correlated with effective immunosuppression. Absolute $CD3^+$ T cell counts below 10–50 cells/mm^3 or percentages of total lymphocyte below 3–5% indicate adequate immunosuppression.[186–189] A consistent increase in $CD3^+$ T cells during treatment reflects therapeutic failure. Although monitoring peripheral circulating $CD3^+$ T cells does not detect lymphocytes infiltrating the allograft or lymphoid tissue, most courses of OKT3 are successfully monitored using this method in conjunction with other biochemical or clinical parameters. In general, the current guidelines for monitoring lymphocyte subsets include trough sample measurement, target number of absolute cell counts below 10–50 cells/mm^3 or percentages of total lymphocyte below 3–5% of $CD3^+$ T cells, and utilization of the Ortho OKT3-FITC staining antibody until better clinical correlations are established with the other products. Frequency of optimal monitoring may be based on indication for OKT3 use (induction vs. rejection) and specific risk factors for possible therapeutic failure (retransplant, pediatric patients, black race, highly sensitized to donor antigens (i.e., multiple blood transfusions, multiparous females), poor HLA match, low anti-OKT3 antibody titer, or previous OKT3 therapy). Dosage adjustments should be made in conjunction with clinical response and based on trends over several consecutive days.

HAMA Formation (Xenosensitization)—HAMA may develop against OKT3 and potentially neutralize the immunosuppressive effects of this agent. Primary exposure to OKT3 can result in the development of anti-OKT3 antibodies as early as 7–10 days into therapy if proper preventive measures are not implemented.[190] Early studies demonstrated general anti-OKT3 antibody formation as high as 80–100% before advances in monitoring and prevention of this response.[190] The formation of anti-idiotypic antibodies is responsible for blocking T-lymphocyte binding of OKT3. Anti-OKT3 antibody titers greater than 1:1000 are associated with a significant reduction in the immunosuppressive effects of OKT3. The HAMA response to OKT3 is oligoclonal, resulting in a highly specific neutralizing effect only against murine IgG2a antibodies. Peak anti-idiotypic antibody response generally occurs four to six weeks after primary exposure, depending on specific risk factors. Although the titer may decrease over a period of time, re-exposure results in a memory response and a rapid increase in blocking antibody. Therefore, detection of peak antibody titer is imperative in determining which patients can receive longer initial courses or retreatment with OKT3.

The primary factor influencing the rate and timing of antibody formation is concomitant immunosuppression. Early studies with OKT3 alone demonstrated HAMA formation rates near 100%, with peak titers developing as early as 7–10 days into therapy.[190] The addition of AZA and prednisone decreased the formation rate to 80%, with higher doses of AZA (3 mg/kg per day) reducing rates to 40–50% and delaying peak antibody time to two to four weeks after initial exposure.[188,191] Recent studies demonstrated reduced xenosensitization with CTX versus AZA during OKT3 induction in heart transplant recipients.[192] However, the concomitant use of CsA has the greatest impact on reducing anti-OKT3 antibodies, with an observed overall antibody formation rate of 11% and no high-titer formation in patients maintained at half their standard CsA doses during OKT3 rejection therapy.[192] Other investigators have demonstrated a reduced antibody response after OKT3 induction when therapeutic CsA concentrations are achieved as early as possible. In general, the concomitant administration of CsA, AZA, and steroids have reduced the risk of high-titer antibody formation to 5–10%.[193,194] The impact of mycophenolate mofetil or tacrolimus on antibody formation has yet to be evaluated but is expected to further reduce the currently observed rates. General guidelines for monitoring anti-OKT3 antibody formation include sampling at baseline prior to the first course of OKT3, approximately four weeks after each course of OKT3, and before initiation of any secondary course of OKT3 to determine possible retreatment success. Patients with high titer (above 1:1000) should receive an alternative agent. In general, concomitant maintenance immunosuppression with CsA and AZA or CTX should be continued, without adjustment if possible, during OKT3 therapy.

OKT3 Serum Concentrations—In vitro, OKT3 concentrations above 800 ng/ml were associated with an inhibition of T-cell effector function.[186] Early reports of the pharmacokinetics of OKT3 showed a rapid decrease in antibody concentrations and short half-life, reflecting the initial CD3 binding and depletion. Subsequent doses were associated with higher trough concentrations and a longer half-life (16–20 hours), reflecting clearance of OKT3 via CD3/TCR modulation.[191] More recently, OKT3 demonstrated linear pharmacokinetics with the initial doses until saturation of CD3 receptors, whereas subsequent doses appear to exhibit nonlinear Michaelis-Menten kinetics.[180] Initial studies with OKT3 induction preliminarily established a clinical correlation between increased rejection rates and low OKT3 serum concentrations, suggesting high trough concentrations were necessary for treatment success.[188,194] More recent evaluations comparing standard versus low-dose induction have demonstrated that the presence of any excess drug may be more critical than the high target trough concentration cited in many early clinical studies.[180] Patients generally achieve relatively steady trough concentrations two to three days into induction and three to four days during rejection therapy.[180,186] A precipitous drop in OKT3 serum concentration often precedes a rise in $CD3^+$ T cells by 24–72 hours and is often associated with xenosensitization and subsequent failed therapy.[188,194] Several recent analyses have suggested appropriate dosage adjustments of OKT3 induction course are better determined with OKT3 serum concentrations versus lymphocyte subset determination.[180,195,196] Based on current clinical evaluations, serum concentration monitoring should be performed in conjunction with lymphocyte subset determinations. There is no clear evidence of a specific therapeutic trough concentration, and each patient should serve as his or her own control to determine steady-state trends and alterations in response. Serial monitoring may provide a better early indicator of inadequate dosing during induction or rejection. Single samples may be obtained to determine therapeutic failure in conjunction with other clinical and laboratory data.

Adverse Effects and Toxicity

Most patients experience a mild to severe flu-like syndrome with the first several doses of OKT3. Symptoms include fever, chills, headache, nausea, vomiting, diarrhea, and myalgias. This reaction is related to the activation of T cells and monocytes by OKT3, which results in the release of cytokines such as IL-2, IL-6, IFN-γ, and TNF.[197–199] With subsequent doses, the severity of the reaction is lessened or the syndrome disappears because of the substantial reduction in the number of circulating $CD3^+$ T cells, the amount of cytokines released, and the depletion of cytokine receptors. Less frequent side effects include pulmonary edema in fluid-overloaded patients (more than 3% over dry weight),[197–200] marked hypotension,[201] aseptic meningitis,[202–204] and seizures.[205] An acute decline in glomerular filtration rate, causing a reversible rise in serum creatinine during the first one to three days of OKT3 therapy, may be the result of cytokine-induced renal toxicity.[206] Initial attempts to prevent these cytokine-mediated toxicities with acetaminophen, antihistamines, and low doses of corticosteroids proved relatively ineffective.[207,208] High doses of corticosteroids given one hour before the administration of OKT3 significantly reduce cytokine release and subsequent side effects in both murine and human models.[209] Current guidelines recommend administering 500–1000 mg of methylprednisolone intravenously in combination with acetaminophen and diphenhydramine one hour before the first two doses of OKT3 for optimal management of cytokine release syndrome. A recent study demonstrated dividing the steroids into two doses and administering them at six and one hour prior to OKT3 may further reduce clinical symptoms.[210] Other adjunctive agents, such as pentoxifylline, indomethacin, and anti-TNF MoAbs, have demonstrated variable clinical effects.[211–213]

As with other antilymphocyte agents, a higher incidence of viral infections and malignancy has been observed after OKT3 therapy.[214] This finding is most likely related to the degree and duration of the overall concentration of immunosuppression that predisposes patients to viral reactivation and compromises the T cell–mediated immunity necessary for combating viral pathogens. Currently, antiviral prophylaxis with ganciclovir and/or acyclovir may reduce the incidence and severity of these secondary viral complications.

New MoAbs

Numerous new MoAbs are currently at various stages of clinical investigation. New targets for antibody immunotherapy include the α/β TCR, specific lymphocyte populations ($CD4^+$ T cells), cytokine (IL-2) receptors, and various adhesion ligands. Several new agents have focused on circumventing several of the complications associated with OKT3 therapy. Chimeric and humanized antibodies have been developed to reduce the incidence of xenosensitization. Nonactivating antibodies are currently under development to reduce the significant side effects associated with the cytokine release after CD3-mediated immunotherapy. Table 8-6 summarizes some of these new MoAbs and their potential sites of action.[215] (See chapter 11 for a more complete discussion of MoAbs.)

Drug Interactions

The pharmacist plays an important role on the transplant team by serving as the drug expert who provides pharmaceutical care to the solid organ transplant recipients. One component of this service is to monitor and manage drug interactions. Contrary to the traditional notion that drug

Table 8-6. New Monoclonal Antibodies in Development

ANTIBODY	SPECIFIC BINDING SITE
HuLy-1	CD2
OKT3* (humanized, non-activating), WT32	CD3
T10B9, BMA 031	T-cell receptor
OKT4a, BL4, MT412	CD4
Anti-T12	CD6
RFT2, CHH380	CD7
Leu 2a	CD8
CHI 621, Anti-TAC, Campath 6	CD25
Campath 1	CDw52
BIRR-1	CD54 (ICAM-1)
25.3	LFA-1

CD, cluster of differentiation; LFA-1, lymphocyte function-associated antigen 1; ICAM-1, intercellular adhesion molecule 1.

interactions are bad and should be avoided if at all possible, drug interactions in the transplant patient are very common and must be dealt with on a daily basis. In fact, some investigators have suggested exploiting drug interactions in the interest of cost containment (e.g., CsA and ketoconazole or diltiazem) for the transplant patient.[216–223] In transplant patients, the inherent possibility of a drug interaction is magnified not only by the multitude of drugs prescribed for these patients but also by the unintended side effects of these medications that require additional drug therapy. It is important to remember that in addition to drug-drug interactions, medications can interact with food or alcohol and that a drug's pharmacokinetics can be altered by the effects of various coexisting disease states seen in transplant patients.[1]

Because it is impossible to be familiar with all potential interactions, it is important for the practitioner to have a thorough understanding of the fundamental mechanisms of these interactions. Anticipation of potential problems allows for early detection and/or avoidance of troublesome regimens whenever possible. Providing advice about which drugs interact and how to manage drug interactions is one of the most important functions of the pharmacist on the transplant team. In addition, pharmacists should use their knowledge and understanding of substantiated drug interactions to predict the interactive potential of many new compounds.

All immunosuppressive drugs are known to interact with at least a few compounds.[45,46] The consequences of drug interactions in the transplant patient can vary from minor inconveniences, such as more frequent drug concentration monitoring and/or dosage adjustments, to more life-threatening complications, such as graft rejection, nephrotoxicity, or infection.[224–226] The best-documented interactions in the transplant patient are typically pharmacokinetic in origin (based on alterations in the absorption, distribution, metabolism, or excretion of the immunosuppressant, resulting in an alteration in the drug concentration); however, pharmacodynamic interactions (i.e., those resulting in altered physiologic or toxicologic effects of the drug) may also occur.

Pharmacokinetic Interactions

The majority of the drugs reported to interact with CsA (and presumably tacrolimus) are inducers, inhibitors, or substrates of the same enzymes in the CYP450-3A gene family.[227–229] When considering CsA's pharmacokinetic interactions, the clinically significant interactions are usually due to changes in its absorption and metabolism rather than distribution and excretion.

The liver is the predominant site of both CsA's and tacrolimus's metabolism, although human intestinal mucosa also contains high concentrations of these enzymes.[230–232] Presystemic metabolism of these compounds in the small intestine is most likely responsible for the poor bioavailability of these compounds (CsA 30%, tacrolimus 26%).[39,231–233] Thus, CYP450 inducers (e.g., phenytoin[234] and rifampin[235–237]) and inhibitors (e.g., erythromycin)[238–240] first alter the absorption of the compound from the gut and then alter its metabolism by affecting similar enzymes in the liver. Interactions with these compounds are less problematic when either of these agents is administered intravenously, again providing evidence that the interactions occur at sites other than just the liver.[240,241]

Grapefruit juice has been shown to facilitate the absorption of CsA and that of other drugs, presumably by inhibiting its gut metabolism.[242–244] Grapefruit juice does not affect systemic clearance when CsA is administered intravenously.[245] The exact mechanism is not known, but flavanoids (particularly naringin) in grapefruit juice may inhibit CYP450-3A4.[242] Another consideration is that interactions involving absorption (i.e., altered CYP450 activity in the small intestine) are more problematic when two interacting agents are administered simultaneously rather than at different dosing intervals.[246,247] This may also account for some of the intra- and interpatient variability seen when patients alter the timing of medication administration to accommodate lifestyle changes.

Other interactions, such as those between AZA and

concomitant allopurinol, also occur predominantly in the small intestine; allopurinol blocks xanthine oxidase function in the gut, causing a three- to fourfold increase in AZA's absorption. This interaction is also far less significant when AZA is administered intravenously.[248,249]

Pharmacodynamic Interactions

Nephrotoxicity is the primary side effect observed in all patients maintained on CsA[49,51] and tacrolimus.[80] Theoretically, any drug capable of causing nephrotoxicity may exacerbate CsA's and tacrolimus's nephrotoxicity. Whether the effects of administering two or more nephrotoxic agents is additive or synergistic remains to be elucidated.

Several drugs, including the aminoglycosides, amphotericin B, acyclovir, ganciclovir, diclofenac, ibuprofen, indomethacin, sulindac, melphalan, and others, have been reported to increase CsA's nephrotoxicity.[46,47]

Acute CsA nephrotoxicity is concentration dependent and is usually reversible following dosage reduction. Chronic nephrotoxicity is irreversible and may be a consequence of persistent renal vasoconstriction and mesangial cell proliferation with resultant glomerulosclerosis. The vasoconstriction appears to be mediated by an increased production of thromboxane A_2 and endothelin. A number of agents, including captopril, enisoprostil, misoprostil,[52] pentoxifylline,[54] cilastatin, urodilatin, and others,[46] have been studied for their potentially beneficial renal protective effects. However, the calcium-channel antagonists (e.g., verapamil, diltiazem, felodipine, nifedipine, nicardipine, and isradipine) appear to be most promising.[55,56] These agents may block the endothelin-induced constriction of smooth muscle cells that is dependent on the influx of calcium.[250] This mechanism may also explain, at least in part, the efficacy of calcium antagonists for the treatment of CsA-induced hypertension.

It is important to remember that increased serum creatinine concentrations may occur in patients treated with trimethoprim, disopyramide, and cimetidine without an apparent change in renal function or CsA concentration. Trimethoprim and cimetidine have been reported to competitively inhibit renal tubular secretion of creatinine.[46]

In addition to observing a decrease in glomerular filtration rate and an increase in serum creatinine and blood urea nitrogen, other CsA-induced laboratory abnormalities include hypomagnesemia, hyperkalemia, and hyperuricemia. Patients treated with CsA commonly require aggressive magnesium supplementation to maintain serum magnesium concentrations at the lower end of the normal range. In addition, a number of other medications used concomitantly in CsA-treated patients may exacerbate these fluid and electrolyte derangements (e.g., diuretics may cause hyperuricemia and gout, hypomagnesemia, or enhanced nephrotoxicity with volume depletion). Potassium-sparing diuretics (e.g., spironolactone, amiloride, and triamterene), β-blockers, and angiotensin-converting enzyme inhibitors may exacerbate hyperkalemia.

Other complications of CsA that are difficult to manage include hypertension and hyperlipidemia. Again, both of these conditions can be complicated by the administration of other drugs capable of exacerbating hypertension (e.g., corticosteroids) and hyperlipidemia (e.g., diuretics, β-blockers) in CsA-treated patients. These disorders require aggressive strategies, including dietary modifications, multidrug regimens, and, if necessary, reduction of CsA concentration or discontinuation of therapy. CsA has also been associated with a number of benign but troublesome dose-related side effects, such as hirsutism, neurotoxicity, and gingival hyperplasia. Gingival hyperplasia has been reported as an adverse effect of certain drugs (e.g., phenytoin, CsA, nifedipine, and the other calcium-channel blockers).[228–240] Concomitant administration of nifedipine and CsA results in an increased rate of this condition (51%) compared with that for CsA alone (8%).[251,252] The mechanism by which these drugs cause this disorder may be related to calcium-channel inhibition; however, a direct local effect may also occur with the liquid but not with capsules.[253] Based on these observations, concurrent administration of drugs capable of inducing gingival hyperplasia should be avoided whenever possible. Plaque control and removal of local irritants have been of some benefit, and a recent four-patient case report suggests that metronidazole therapy may be useful.[254] Surgery and discontinuation of CsA may be necessary in patients who do not respond to these modalities.

Other pharmacodynamic interactions with immunosuppressive agents include enhanced bone marrow toxicity observed with the antiproliferative agents and drugs known to suppress the bone marrow (e.g., trimethoprim–sulfamethoxazole and ganciclovir) that are also commonly used in transplant recipients. Minoxidil and other drugs may exacerbate the hypertrichosis and hirsutism seen with CsA and steroids.

Management of Drug Interactions

Management of confirmed immunosuppressant drug interactions requires proactive measures, such as altering the dose of the affected drug on either initiation or discontinuation of the interacting agent; measuring drug concentrations and, when available, those of the offending agents; and monitoring renal function tests, creatinine phosphokinase concentrations, and any other tests indicative of pharmacologic or toxic response.

Because of the number of drug interactions reported with CsA (and anticipated with tacrolimus), it is useful to categorize the interactions based on severity to assist the pharmacist in making therapeutic decisions.

Serious Interactions

Serious interactions are those that cause the serum concentrations of the object drug to increase at least three- to fourfold, which usually correspond to a significantly increased risk of toxicity. The most serious interactions require immediate intervention on initiation of the concomitant interactant. One such interactant is ketoconazole, which inhibits the metabolism of CsA and is assumed to have a similar effect on tacrolimus. Of the azole antifungals, ketoconazole is the most potent inhibitor of the CYP450 system, and, as expected, CsA dosage reductions of up to 80% are necessary during concomitant therapy.[255,256] Unless the CsA dose is reduced at the outset of concomitant therapy, CsA concentrations rise dramatically within 24–48 hours, placing the patient at unnecessary risk for nephrotoxicity.

Dosage adjustment guidelines for tacrolimus are not yet available, but the need for a similar magnitude of adjustment should be anticipated. Tacrolimus concentrations have been reported to rise with fluconazole[257,258] and clotrimazole,[259] so suspicion should be high for all of the azole antifungals, just as it is with CsA.[255] Because tacrolimus has such a narrow therapeutic index (i.e., therapeutic plasma concentrations of 0.5–2.0 ng/ml or whole blood 5–20 ng/ml), it may be even more susceptible to potentially deleterious interactions. With tacrolimus (as well as with CsA), a doubling of the drug concentration may cause serious consequences in a patient with a higher therapeutic concentration.

Enzyme inducers, such as phenytoin, phenobarbital, and rifampin, can also cause serious interactions with CsA[260,261] and presumably with tacrolimus.[258] Before these drug interactions were well recognized, a number of patients experienced acute rejection episodes and lost their grafts when their CsA concentrations were found to be undetectable.[224–226] In contrast to the concomitant administration of enzyme inhibitors, during which the CsA dosage must be reduced dramatically to counterbalance decreased metabolism, with concurrent enzyme inducer therapy the CsA dosage must be increased at least two- to threefold to maintain therapeutic drug concentrations.

The other important point to remember about these interactions is that when the enzyme inducer is discontinued, the effect may persist up to two to three weeks, thus necessitating more frequent drug concentration monitoring not only when initiating therapy but also after discontinuing the interacting drug. The time frame for reversal of enzyme inhibition depends on whether it is due to actual inhibition of enzyme function or competition for the same sites of metabolism; the latter will reverse upon elimination of the competing drug from the metabolism sites.

Another serious interaction occurs between AZA and allopurinol.[96] The dosage of AZA needs to be reduced by 75% when allopurinol is added to the regimen. The serious consequences of this interaction (e.g., profound pancytopenia) are not usually clinically evident for four to six weeks because of the prolonged half-life of the TGNs and delayed impact on marrow production. However, unlike CsA or tacrolimus, serum concentration monitoring of AZA is not routinely available, so the only markers of toxicity (WBCs, RBCs, and platelets) do not respond acutely to changes in AZA serum concentrations. Certainly, toxicity can be detected by frequent complete blood count monitoring, but again it is better to prevent the consequences of profound marrow suppression than to deal with them after they occur.

Because of the potentially serious consequences of these interactions, the need to alter the dosage of the object drug (e.g., CsA, tacrolimus, or AZA) must be taken into consideration when initiating concomitant therapy.

Moderately Serious Interactions

Moderately problematic interactions include those capable of causing a twofold rise in drug concentrations of the object drug. Some of the drugs that have this effect with CsA, presumably by competing for the same CYP450 substrate, include erythromycin [238–240] and some of the calcium-channel blockers. Diltiazem, verapamil, and nicardipine inhibit CsA's metabolism; diltiazem is the most potent.[262–268] Dosage reductions of approximately 50% can be anticipated with diltiazem, and smaller reductions are necessary with the other drugs. With moderately problematic drug interactions, the time to alter the dosage of the drug may actually depend on the initial drug concentrations. For instance, when adding diltiazem therapy to a patient who has a low therapeutic CsA concentration, it may be better to alter the CsA dosage once the concentrations begin to rise rather than at the outset of therapy. This increases the inconvenience for the patient, but the risks of rejection must be weighed against the benefits of more frequent monitoring.

Minor Interactions

These interactions occur when an increase in CsA concentration of less than 50% is observed during concomitant therapy. In this situation, awareness of the interaction is important and must be considered in light of the clinical status of the patient. Unless the patient has very labile renal function or high therapeutic levels, dosage adjustments of CsA or tacrolimus can usually be made once the concentrations begin to rise, rather than at the outset of therapy.

Other Considerations

When selecting agents to treat the various medical problems of transplant patients, it is important to consider whether the treatment is for an acute (requiring less than two to three weeks of therapy) or a chronic medical condition. In the acute setting, it is preferable to avoid drug interactions because of the inconvenience associated with dosage adjustments and more frequent monitoring. The use of alternative (noninteracting) agents is usually preferable in the short-term setting (e.g., 7–14 days) when equally effective agents are available. Obviously, if therapeutically equivalent products are not available, then it is most appropriate to use the drug of choice for the condition and deal with the drug interaction as needed. Short-term erythromycin therapy (e.g., a 10- to 14-day course) is usually discouraged because it is inconvenient to adjust the CsA dosage for a short period of time and then readjust it. However, in the case of endocarditis prophylaxis in a penicillin-allergic patient, it may be appropriate to administer the standard two doses of erythromycin if the patient's CsA concentration is moderately low. The increased absorption and inhibited metabolism of CsA following one or two doses of erythromycin should not have a major effect on the patient's kidney function unless renal dysfunction is already present. In the case of enzyme inducers, if chronic anticonvulsant drug therapy is necessary in a transplant patient, then it is best to use the agent of choice for the seizure type and deal with the drug interaction to insure optimal immunosuppressive and anticonvulsant efficacy.

The impact on the patient's quality of life should also be considered when dealing with drug interactions. Additional monitoring, more frequent clinic visits, and dosage adjustments may cause an unnecessary burden in a long-term patient who returns to the clinic on an infrequent basis. Because calcium-channel blockers are often used in transplant patients and a number of calcium-channel blockers are available, it seems prudent to consider what impact the drug interaction will have on the patient's quality of life. The initiation of interacting agents (e.g., diltiazem or nicardipine) is most easily accomplished soon after transplantation, when patients generally require more frequent monitoring. Conversely, several years after a transplant, when a patient has returned to work or school, the increased frequency of monitoring and corresponding dosage adjustments may be inconvenient. In this situation it may be preferable to initiate a noninteracting calcium-channel blocker, such as nifedipine, isradipine, or felodipine.[46]

Finally, patient compliance must be considered, especially when dealing with serious interactions. Utmost compliance is necessary when a drug interaction results in a significant dosage reduction of the immunosuppressive agent. The most dramatic impact would be seen in a patient on concomitant CsA and ketoconazole in whom the CsA dosage has been reduced to 20% of the previous steady-state dose. Many of these patients are maintained on only 1 mg/kg per day, so if the patient either stops taking ketoconazole or takes it sporadically, the CsA concentration may drop precipitously, predisposing the patient to a rejection episode. Similar problems can occur even if the CsA dosage has only been reduced by 50% (e.g., by interaction with diltiazem), especially if the patient is running borderline low concentrations. Compliance is a critical factor for transplant patients, so consideration must be given when adding drugs that interact and mandate dosage alterations of the immunosuppressant. Compliance is equally important in a patient on an enzyme inducer (e.g., phenytoin) in whom the CsA dose has been tripled to achieve therapeutic concentrations. At these high doses, the cost of therapy may become prohibitive and patients cannot afford prolonged concomitant therapy.

When making recommendations about drug interactions, pharmacists need to be familiar with the available drug interaction literature and must have a thorough understanding of pharmacokinetic and pharmacodynamic principles of drug interactions. Besides these factors, pharmacists need to rely on their expertise and practical experience when trying to predict whether a drug interaction may occur with a new drug. Anticipating drug interactions promotes the development of a monitoring strategy for the patient when it is not known whether new compounds interact with immunosuppressive drugs. Being aware of some of the problematic therapeutic classes (e.g., azole antifungals, calcium-channel blockers, and nephrotoxic drugs) is useful when considering the likelihood of an interaction. In addition, even though it is difficult to predict a priori the extent of an interaction in an individual patient, being aware of whether the drug is metabolized via the same CYP450 enzymes as the immunosuppressive agent at least raises the level of suspicion and allows the pharmacist to develop a monitoring strategy for the transplant patient. As both CsA and tacrolimus are metabolized by the CYP450-3A enzymes, it is assumed that the interaction profile for tacrolimus will be very similar, if not identical, to CsA. It is possible that, because of tacrolimus's potency, narrow therapeutic index, and strong binding avidity, it may have even more interactions than CsA. Evidence for this premise comes from the observation that clotrimazole interacts with tacrolimus but not with CsA.[259] In addition, tacrolimus is metabolized by the CYP450-1A system, which could raise the potential for other macrolide-like interactions with compounds such as theophylline, caffeine, etc.[269]

NONPHARMACOLOGIC MEANS OF IMMUNOSUPPRESSION

A number of nonpharmacologic methods have been used to prevent and treat graft rejection over the years, including total body and local graft irradiation, total lymphoid irradiation, plasmapheresis, and a variety of methods that decrease the severity of rejection by causing lymphoid depletion, such as splenectomy, leukapheresis, and thoracic duct drainage. Alternatives to the use of immunosuppression include the development of techniques or agents that can be used in the short term to induce permanent tolerance to the grafted organ (i.e., eliminating the need for maintenance immunosuppression) or the development of procedures such as cardiomyoplasty or permanent artificial devices that can be used in lieu of solid organ transplantation.

Transfusion

Blood transfusions have become the most widely used form of pretransplant immunosuppression. Ample evidence exists that pretransplant blood transfusions improve survival rates of cadaveric donor kidney allografts.[270] In addition, donor-specific transfusions may be obtained from the living related donor. AZA and CsA may be started at the time of pretransplant transfusions to reduce the incidence of sensitization associated with donor-specific transfusions. Possible mechanisms for the transfusion immunosuppressant effect are the generation of suppressor T lymphocytes, the action of anti-idiotypic antibodies, and clonal depletion.[270] About half of the total immunosuppressive effect seems to be conferred by 1 transfusion,[271] and the peak effect occurs with about 14 transfusions. The optimal number of pretransplant transfusions remains debatable.[270]

Splenectomy

Pretransplant splenectomy was found to have a beneficial effect for at least the first two years after kidney transplantation, with no decrease in patient survival.[272] However, long-term follow-up showed no significant difference in graft survival between splenectomized and nonsplenectomized recipients, and the incidence of death from sepsis was higher among splenectomized recipients. Therefore, routine pretransplant splenectomy is currently not recommended. However, splenectomy has been used to prevent rejection in ABO-incompatible liver transplants. Appropriate antibiotic prophylaxis with penicillin is necessary in splenectomized patients.

Irradiation

In the late 1950s, whole body irradiation was abandoned and replaced with total lymphoid irradiation, a technique directed at the small fraction of the entire lymphocyte pool that is responsible for the rejection reaction toward a transplanted organ.[273] Targeting irradiation (up to 2000 rads using standard inverted Y-mantle fields) limits toxicity and allows for reduction in post-transplant immunosuppression.

As a mode of immunosuppression, total lymphoid irradiation has been a major therapeutic advance in the treatment of Hodgkin's disease, in which it was found to produce a selective and prolonged reduction in the number and function of circulating helper T cells and certain subsets of B cells.[274]

The dose used in organ transplantation is considerably lower than that used in Hodgkin's disease. Patients awaiting transplants are treated with a course of total lymphoid irradiation and monitored for suppression of their T cells. Thereafter, patients can receive transplants with markedly reduced immunosuppressive requirements.[275] Recent reports have shown the technique to be a useful adjunct for the intermediate-term control of early or recurrent acute cardiac rejection.[276] It has also been used as salvage therapy for cardiac allograft rejection that does not respond to conventional therapy.[277,278]

Apheresis

Therapeutic plasma exchange has been suggested as a useful adjunct to remove a variety of antibodies in the treatment of vascular (e.g., B cell–mediated) rejection and to allow transplantation in highly sensitized individuals.[279]

Photopheresis

Photopheresis is a investigational technique using ultraviolet A light and 8-methoxypsoralens to alter the function of mononuclear cells to enhance suppressor mechanisms, possibly by altering APC activity. The procedure is rather tedious; patients ingest the 8-methoxypsoralens and then undergo leukapheresis. The cells are then treated with ultraviolet light and reinfused. The technique has been used to reverse cardiac rejection,[280,281] and clinical trials evaluating its efficacy are under way.

SUMMARY

Recent advances in solid organ transplantation can be attributed to a number of factors, the foremost of which is immunosuppressive therapy. The introduction of cyclosporine in the late 1970s allowed the successful transplantation of many previously untransplantable organs. For the past decade, the mainstay of most immunosuppressive protocols has been triple-drug regimens consisting of cyclosporine, azathioprine, and prednisone, with or without the use of antilymphocyte preparations. Small intestine transplantation and lung transplantation have still been fraught with less than desirable results. The recent introduction of more potent immunosuppressive agents, including tacrolimus and mycophenolate mofetil, has offered new options for the transplant patient. Combinations of these agents will allow greater flexibility when individualizing patient therapy. Pharmacists play a key role on the transplant team by serving as the drug experts and providing pharmaceutical care to patients.

PART II—TRANSPLANT PROCEDURES AND COMPLICATIONS

KIDNEY TRANSPLANTATION

Dramatic strides have been made in renal transplantation and transplant immunotherapy in the past 35 years. One-year graft and patient survival rates in recipients of a kidney from a living related donor (an HLA-identical sibling) are 91 and 96%, respectively, whereas graft and patient survival rates are 81 and 92% for recipients of cadaveric donor kidneys, respectively.[282,283] In addition to improved survival, the economic ramifications of kidney transplantation have also been recognized, since transplantation is more cost effective than chronic hemodialysis.[284,285] Transplantation also significantly improves patient rehabilitation and quality of life when compared with hemodialysis.[283]

Indications and Candidate Selection

Most patients presenting with end-stage renal disease are considered potential transplant recipients. The etiologic conditions responsible for end-stage renal disease leading to transplantation include progressive chronic diseases, congenital abnormalities, genetic diseases, metabolic disorders, and localized neoplasms. Chronic diseases, such as diabetic nephropathy, glomerulonephritis, nephrotic syndrome, and hypertension, account for the majority of patients considered for renal transplant evaluation. Definitive and relative contraindications to renal transplantation are listed in Table 8-7.[264]

Kidney allografts are acquired from either living or cadaveric sources. Living donors (related and unrelated) are preferred for transplantation because of improved survival rates attributable to the increased degree of histocompatibility matching, the elective nature of the surgery, the ability to optimize the recipient's medical condition, and short organ preservation time.[286,287] However, the majority of transplanted kidneys are from cadaveric donors.[288] Cadaver kidneys are tissue typed by six HLA loci (*A*, *B*, *C*, *DQ*, *DP*, and *DR*) and are transported nationwide to be optimally matched with a recipient of similar HLA type.[288] This process evolved from studies indicating that recipients of kidneys from donors with a six-antigen match and recipients of kidneys from HLA-identical siblings are comparable in allograft survival. Cadaver kidneys that match less than six HLA loci are allocated by UNOS on the basis of points scored for HLA matching, panel reactive antibody, waiting time on transplant list, medical urgency, and logistic or locational factors.[289] Once a cadaveric donor has been matched with an appropriate recipient, the kidney is transported rapidly to the recipient transplant center. Current standard preservation techniques with University of Wisconsin solution (Viaspan®) allow kidney storage for up to 72 hours. However, preservation times of less than 16 hours are preferred and are associated with a significant reduction in delayed graft function and improved graft survival.

Table 8-7. Contraindications to Renal Transplantation

DEFINITIVE	RELATIVE
Immunologic incompatibility	Age >65 years
Active infection	Stable cardiovascular disease
Unstable cardiovascular disease	Hepatic disease
Metastatic symptomatic malignancy	Pulmonary disease
Active connective tissue disorder	Emotional psychiatric disorder
Primary hyperoxalosis	Technical abnormalities
Active gastrointestinal bleeding	Severe bone disease
	Subacute infection

Transplantation Technique

The immunologic evaluation of the donor and recipient includes ABO blood group compatibility and HLA determination before organ allocation, recipient panel reactivity antibody assessment (pretransplant peak and at the time of transplant), and donor-recipient B- and T-lymphocyte cross-match after the organ has been allocated to a specific transplant center. Preoperative management of the kidney transplant recipient includes insertion of a central venous pressure monitoring line, instillation of antibiotic solution into the bladder via a Foley catheter, and administration of immunosuppressive medications and prophylactic antibiotics. Since its inception in the 1950s, the retroperitoneal iliac approach has become the standard technique for kidney transplantation in adults.[3] The transplanted kidney is usually placed in the contralateral iliac fossa of the recipient to keep the ureter and collecting system medial. Vascularization is performed as quickly as possible to minimize ischemic time to the kidney. Urinary continuity is established through attachment of the donor ureter to the recipient bladder via a ureteroneocystostomy. Before the kidneys are unclamped and revascularized, the patient is fluid-resuscitated to maintain a systolic blood pressure of 140 mmHg and central venous pressure of 10–15 mmHg. The patient's vital signs and hemodynamic status are monitored closely, with fluids and electrolytes replaced as needed. Patients are closely monitored for appropriate urine output and decrease in serum creatinine relative to baseline as early indicators of allograft function.

Immunosuppressive Treatment

Prophylactic immunosuppressive regimens for renal transplantation are usually based on triple-drug therapy (i.e., CsA, AZA, and prednisone) for cadaveric and mismatched living related grafts;[290–292] alternative regimens may be used for living related HLA-identical siblings.[293] Some centers use induction therapy with OKT3 (5 mg per day) or ATG (15 mg/kg) for seven days to delay the administration of CsA until renal function is well established.[294–297] Initial doses of CsA (8–10 mg/kg per day orally or 1–2 mg/kg per day intravenously) are adjusted according to CsA drug concentrations. In living related recipients, CsA may actually be administered 48 hours before transplantation. AZA (4–5 mg/kg) is given preoperatively and adjusted postoperatively to keep the WBC count above 4000 cells/mm^3. Prednisone (0.5–2 mg/kg per day) is used initially and then tapered to 0.1–0.2 mg/kg per day by 12 months.[289–292]

The treatment of acute rejection episodes is usually initiated with steroid "pulse" therapy (e.g., 500–1000 mg of methylprednisolone intravenously every day for three days) and a prednisone taper, which is effective in treating 60–70% of first rejections. If the patient does not respond, ATG (15 mg/kg per day) or OKT3 (5 mg per day) for 7–10 days can be used. Alternatively, mild rejection in patients who are ambulatory and in whom CsA toxicity is unlikely can be treated with a minipulse of prednisone (100 mg orally each day for three days).[289]

Postoperative Complications

Early postoperative complications in renal transplant recipients include delayed graft function secondary to mechanical causes (ureteral, arterial, or venous occlusions or thrombosis, renal artery stenosis, or fluid collections) and nonmechanical causes (e.g., hypovolemia and acute tubular necrosis, CsA nephrotoxicity, or rejection).[283] Various laboratory tests have been used to evaluate renal compromise in the transplanted kidneys, but most of them are nonspecific, expensive, and impractical for routine bedside monitoring.[298] In a patient with acute oliguric renal failure, an iodine-131 hippuran renogram can identify other causes of graft dysfunction, such as renal artery thrombosis, ureteral necrosis with urine leak, or an obstruction along the urinary tract. A renal perfusion scan can be used to determine the adequacy of blood flow to the graft. Ultrasound shows dilation of the pelvicalyceal system if the patient has an obstructive uropathy and reveals perirenal fluid collections that might compress the kidney or the ureter. On the basis of these test findings, an antegrade pyelography may be used to delineate the level and nature of obstruction, or a renal arteriogram may be used to confirm a thromboembolic event.[298] Other early postoperative complications include infection, lymphocele, hematoma, and seroma formation.

Immunologic Complications

Although the success rates following renal transplantation have improved in the past two decades, allograft rejection continues to be a major problem and is the leading cause of graft loss in renal transplant recipients.[298] Despite the use of multidrug immunosuppressive regimens, most patients experience one or two clinically evident rejection episodes during the first year after transplantation. Renal allograft rejection episodes are of five types, based on time of onset, clinical criteria, histologic findings, and response to antirejection (Table 8-8).

Hyperacute rejection occurs within minutes to a few hours of renal transplantation, before the patient has left the operating room.[298] This type of rejection is fairly uncommon and is generally prevented when the patient and donor are ABO and HLA compatible. The clinical findings include acute anuria, hypertension, hyperkalemia, metabolic acidosis, pulmonary edema, and possible disseminated intravascular coagulation. Hyperacute rejection must be distinguished from other causes of anuria, such as obstruction of the urinary tract, renal pelvic necrosis, ureteral necrosis with urine leak, ischemic acute tubular necrosis, and severe intravascular volume depletion. Once the diagnosis of hyperacute rejection is confirmed, the graft is generally immediately removed. Advances in tissue typing and immunosuppression have made hyperacute rejection an uncommon phenomenon.

Accelerated rejection usually occurs within six days of transplantation.[298] Initial renal function can progress to acute oliguric renal failure due to previous sensitization to minor donor antigens through blood transfusions, multiple pregnancies, or a previous transplant. Most patients who experience accelerated acute rejection do not respond to antirejection therapy and require nephrectomy, but OKT3 or high-dose steroids are occasionally effective.

Acute cellular rejection is the most common manifestation of immunologic incompatibility in transplant recipients and usually presents within one week to three months following the transplant, depending on the induction immunosuppression regimen.[298] Clinical manifestations may vary from an asymptomatic mild reduction in renal function to acute oliguric renal failure, hypertension, and pulmonary edema. Other clinical events associated with acute cellular rejection include fever, malaise, anorexia, myalgia, oliguria, weight gain, edema, and congestive heart failure. Clinically, it is difficult to differentiate acute rejection from CsA-induced nephrotoxicity. The differentiation can be made by noting that patients with CsA nephrotoxicity are usually afebrile, demonstrate only

Table 8-8. Types of Renal Allograft Rejection

TYPE	TIME OF DAMAGE	EFFECTOR MECHANISM	CAUSE
Hyperacute	Minutes to hours	Ab	Preformed cytotoxic antibodies directed against donor antigens
Accelerated	2–5 days	CMI (± Ab)	Previous sensitization to donor
Acute	7–21 days	CMI (± Ab)	Development of allogenic reaction to donor antigens
Chronic	>3 months	CMI (± Ab)	Disturbance of host's and/or graft's tolerance
Immunopathologic	>3 months		New organ damaged by immunopathologic events related to those that necessitated the transplant

Ab, antibody-mediated (humoral) immunity; CMI, cell-mediated immunity; ±, with or without.

mild oliguria, have increased ratios of blood urea nitrogen to creatinine, and sometimes have elevated CsA concentrations. A renal biopsy is helpful for differentiating between rejection and CsA nephrotoxicity. Biopsies are usually performed when the initial presentation of oligoanuria occurs 7–14 days after transplantation, when renal function deteriorates acutely or gradually without obvious cause, or when the serum creatinine does not return to baseline after treatment of a rejection episode. Histologically, the renal biopsy specimen shows a perivascular mononuclear cell infiltration with acute graft rejection.

Chronic rejection can occur months to years after transplantation and is the predominant cause of graft loss in the late post-transplant period (after one year).[298] Chronic rejection is characterized by the classic triad of hypertension, proteinuria, and progressive decline in renal function. Histologically, obliterative arteriopathy, glomerulosclerosis, interstitial fibrosis, and alterations in the basement membrane are all characteristic of chronic rejection. Because there is no effective treatment for chronic rejection other than retransplantation, therapy is based on delaying the progression of chronic renal failure (i.e., controlling hypertension, adopting a low-protein diet, correcting acidosis, and initiating dialysis when the creatinine clearance approaches 15 ml/min). Lower one-year graft survival rates of 70% or less have been reported after multiple transplants.[288]

De Novo and Recurrent Renal Disease

Immunopathologic destruction of the kidney graft can occur any time after three months and is related to the immunologic process that damaged the original organ.[299] Occasionally, these disorders can occur in patients with no previous history of the disorder. Immunologic diseases that can recur after transplantation include membranoproliferative glomerulonephritis, focal glomerulosclerosis, and lupus nephropathy. Immunosuppressive therapy with AZA, CTX, or mycophenolate mofetil may slow the progression of these diseases; however, the specific role of each agent remains unclear.

PANCREAS TRANSPLANTATION

The first pancreas transplant was performed in 1966,[300] and poor results were seen until the late 1970s (graft and recipient survival rates of 3 and 39%). ABO-identical blood group and HLA-DR matching have also improved allograft survival after cadaveric pancreas transplantation.[301,302] During the past five years, graft function and patient survival rates of 63 and 89%, respectively, have been reported by the International Pancreas Transplant Registry. Functional survival for pancreas grafts (defined as insulin independence and normoglycemia) is more than 74% at one year for recipients of simultaneous cadaveric donor kidney transplant.[303]

Indications and Candidate Selection

Pancreas transplantation is indicated for patients who already have or are likely to develop complications of diabetes that are more serious than the adverse effects associated with immunosuppressive therapy.[303] It is also indicated in nonuremic diabetic patients with other complications (e.g., retinopathy, albuminuria, or diabetic nephropathy) and in those who have extreme difficulty with diabetic control.[304] The intent of pancreas transplantation is to establish an insulin-independent normoglycemic state in type I (insulin-dependent) diabetic patients and to prevent the onset or halt the progression of secondary complications of diabetes.[305] After successful pancreas transplantation, exogenous insulin can be discontinued and the patient's quality of life improved. Contraindications include incapacitating neuropathy, severe cardiovascular disease, severe gastropathy, concurrent malignancy or infection, and extensive psychiatric or emotional instability.

Transplantation Technique

In general, pancreas transplantation is performed simultaneously with a kidney allograft, with the pancreas allograft placed first. Transplantation of the pancreas mandates diverting the pancreatic exocrine secretions into the recipient's intestine or bladder. The latter is preferable because it allows rejection to be monitored by measuring the decrease in urine amylase activity that precedes deterioration of endocrine function.[306] Postoperative management includes close monitoring of fluid and electrolytes, pancreatic function, renal function, and evidence of infection. Plasma glucose should be maintained at concentrations less than 150 mg/dl because chronic hyperglycemia is detrimental to beta cells. Increased exocrine secretions, combined with improved renal function, often result in a metabolic acidosis and dehydration, requiring fluid and sodium bicarbonate supplementation. Uncomplicated pancreas transplant recipients are usually discharged from the hospital during the third postoperative week.[305]

Immunosuppressive Treatment

The immunosuppressive management of pancreas transplant recipients is the same as that for recipients of other solid organ allografts, but pancreas recipients require a higher level of immunosuppression.[307] Regimens usually include OKT3 (5 mg/day) for 14 days, CsA targeted to maintain HPLC-measured whole blood concentrations at 200 ng/ml, AZA (2.5 mg/kg per day) to maintain WBC count at or above 4000 cells/mm^3, and prednisone (1–2 mg/kg per day tapered to 0.5 mg/kg per day by one to two months and then tapered to a long-term maintenance dose of 0.2 mg/kg per day or less by one year).[307]

Rejection is routinely treated with OKT3 (5 mg/day) for seven days along with a rapid prednisone taper of 2 mg/kg per day for two days, 1.5 mg/kg per day for two days, 1.0 mg/kg per day for two days, 0.75 mg/kg per day for two days, 0.5 mg/kg per day for two days, and then back to baseline.[305,307] Attempts are made to limit the amount of OKT3 to 21 doses during the first four months to reduce the risk of malignancy. If there is a second rejection episode in this interval, high-dose steroids (1.0 g/day for three days) are used.

Postoperative Complications

The most common early post-transplant complications include pancreatitis, peripancreatic fluid collection, anastomotic leaks, dehydration, metabolic acidosis, abdominal or pancreatic abscesses, arterial or venous graft thrombosis, and pancreatic fistula. New surgical techniques, improved anti-infective prophylaxis, and better preservation solutions have lowered the incidence of many postoperative complications.

Immunologic Complications

Rejection remains the most common cause of pancreatic graft loss, primarily because of the difficulty in making an early and appropriate diagnosis. In general, obtaining tissue for evaluation is difficult, with a questionable correlation between clinical rejection and histopathology.[308] Acute cellular rejection is generally hallmarked by acinar endothelialitis, lymphocytic transmigration across the acinar lumen, endophlebitis, and occasional visible injury to the small pancreatic ductules. Chronic rejection is characterized by acinar loss and severe interstitial fibrosis, with occasional evidence of pancreatic obliterative arteriopathy. Rejection is frequently difficult to distinguish from infection or graft pancreatitis, but it often presents with a greater than 25% decrease in urine amylase activity (to less than 10,000 IU/L), a drop in serum amylase, or hyperglycemia. Other tests being evaluated as markers of rejection include measurement of C peptide, serum IL-2 receptors, pancreas-specific protein, urinary pH, insulin, trypsin, and pancreatic juice volume and cytology.[309–313] However, the most frequent method of diagnosing pancreas rejection is via diagnosis of rejection in the simultaneously placed kidney allograft; isolated pancreas rejection is a rare event.

Islet Cell Transplantation

Although islet cell transplantation is currently under investigation, successful long-term engraftment to allow withdrawal of insulin has not yet been achieved.[314] This procedure may be an alternative to whole or partial pancreas transplantation as endocrine replacement therapy in type I diabetic patients.[315] It has been proposed that islet cells can be transplanted into the liver, spleen, brain, testes, peritoneal cavity, kidney, muscle beds, and subcutaneous spaces.[316] Limitations to successful islet cell transplantation at this time include the ineffectiveness of current immunosuppressive regimens, the inability to diagnose early graft rejection, and determination of beta cell mass is necessary to restore normal glucose utilization. Pancreatic islet cells have been successfully transplanted into the thymus gland of type I diabetic patients. In the thymus, thymocytes mature and are educated to respond to certain foreign antigens. When the islet cells (antigens) are transplanted into this area, the maturing lymphocytes accept foreign tissue as being part of the self.[317] Another promising method, immunoisolation, is being investigated. This method involves encapsulating islet cells in a membrane that keeps them out of reach of the body's immune cells but still allows insulin to diffuse outward.[315,318] Advances in this procedure may allow transplantation of animal islet cells into humans, potentially reducing the donor shortage problem.[315]

LIVER TRANSPLANTATION

The initial work that led to the current success with liver transplantation occurred more than thirty years ago. Unlike renal transplantation techniques, the surgical techniques for liver transplantation are relatively complex; early work centered on the technical aspects of the surgery itself.[319] Surgical complications were the cause of death in the few patients who received transplants in the early 1960s. The technical problems associated with liver transplant surgery were overcome relatively rapidly, at which point it became apparent that other problems, such as organ availability, preservation of organs, and graft rejection, would be more difficult to solve. One-year patient survival rates throughout the 1960s and nearly all of the 1970s hovered around 20 or 30%. With the availability of CsA at the end of 1979, one-year actuarial graft survival increased to 70%. With the development of University of Wisconsin solution for organ preservation and CsA for immunosuppression, the modern era of liver transplantation had arrived;[320] one-year patient and graft survival now routinely exceed 80%, and five-year patient survival exceeds 70%.

Table 8-9. Native Liver Disease in 400 Pediatric and 858 Adult Recipients of Liver Transplants at the University of Pittsburgh, 1981–1988[351]

DISEASE		NUMBER OF CASES
Parenchymal		**522**
Postnecrotic cirrhosis	348	
Alcoholic cirrhosis	76	
Acute liver failure	54	
Budd-Chiari syndrome	18	
Congenital hepatic fibrosis	9	
Cystic fibrosis	6	
Neonatal hepatitis	8	
Hepatic trauma	3	
Cholestatic		**544**
Biliary atresia	217	
Primary biliary cirrhosis	186	
Sclerosing cholangitis	100	
Secondary biliary cirrhosis	25	
Familial cholestasis	16	
Inborn errors of metabolism		**114**
Tumors		**78**
Benign	10	
Primary malignant	60	
Metastatic	8	
Total		**1258**

Indications and Candidate Selection

Table 8-9 lists the diseases for which liver transplantation is a major treatment modality and reflects the Pittsburgh experience in more than 1200 adult and pediatric patients who received transplants between 1981 and 1988.[321] There is currently no upper age limit for patients undergoing liver transplantation. Patients more than 70 years old and newborns have undergone transplants successfully.

Controversy persists regarding which patients should undergo liver transplantation. This controversy results partly from having too few organs for the number of transplant candidates. Transplants for patients with liver carcinoma are very controversial because of the high incidence of nonhepatic tumor involvement and tumor relapse. Less controversial are transplants for patients with the hepatitis B virus (HBV) or alcoholic liver disease. Recent data indicate that the use of passive immunoprophylaxis with hepatitis B immune globulin can decrease two-year actuarial reinfection rates from the historical 80–90% to about 30%.[322,323]

The use of liver transplantation for fulminant hepatitis (sudden onset of liver failure) is well established. Common causes include type A, B, and C hepatitis and various forms of toxic hepatitis induced by drug and nondrug chemicals. It is important to recognize when to perform transplants in these patients. Conditions that predict rapid progression to death include grade III and IV hepatic encephalopathy, metabolic acidosis, severe irreversible coagulopathy, sepsis, and cardiovascular compromise. It is also important to confirm that liver dysfunction is irreversible before considering transplantation. Therefore, most patients who are at the point of receiving transplants have some or all of these complications. Despite the severely compromised condition of these patients, an impressive 50–80% of patients survive after liver transplantation. In comparison, only about 20% are long-term survivors with medical management alone.[319] In addition to liver transplantation, other options for the management of acute liver failure are under development. Extracorporeal liver assistance devices composed of human or porcine hepatocytes in a hollow fiber cartridge similar to those used for continuous venovenous hemofiltration (CVVH) can be used as a temporary treatment for the effects of acute liver failure or as a bridge to transplantation when a suitable cadaveric donor is not available.[319,324] An auxiliary heterograft may be used as a temporary bridge to allografting. This approach may also be used when the liver has suffered an acute injury (e.g., drug overdose or other toxic exposure) to allow time for the damaged liver to recover; the heterograft may then be removed, freeing the patient from the requirement for lifelong immunosuppression and its sequelae.

Liver transplantation is also indicated for treating end-stage chronic liver disease. The decision to transplant is often more subtle than in the case of acute liver failure and involves issues of worsening dementia, frequent hospital admissions, and, in children, mental and physical growth retardation. Not all patients have the typical jaundiced appearance. When hepatocellular disease is involved, patients often appear minimally jaundiced, but profound hypoalbuminemia and coagulopathy are always present. In comparison, cholestatic disease (biliary atresia and primary biliary cirrhosis) always presents with jaundice.[319] Severe and intractable pruritus is a hallmark of end-stage cholestatic disease.

One of the major predictors for a successful outcome is the pretransplant performance status of the patient. For example, patients without severe complications before transplant have an 80% two-year survival rate; the rate is 55% in patients with a major complication. The difference between these groups is the high perioperative mortality.[319]

Organ Allocation

The allocation of scarce donor organs is made in accordance with rules established and enforced by UNOS. Patients on the waiting list for a liver allograft are prioritized according to the extent of progression of their disease and the acuity of their health status. UNOS status I patients are those who are critically ill and currently maintained on life-support systems; status II are those who require hospitalization for the management of some manifestation of end-stage liver disease; status III are those who suffer from end-stage liver disease but who can be maintained at home without need for acute care; status IV are those patients with liver disease whose condition has not yet progressed to the stage requiring transplantation.[325]

Organs are further allocated according to ABO blood compatibility and size matching. The requirement for size matching puts pediatric recipients at particular disadvantage with respect to organ allocation. The scarcity of suitable pediatric donors causes pediatric patients to wait longer for a cadaveric allograft, with consequent excess mortality while waiting. In response to this need, some centers are dividing adult cadaveric donor livers into two smaller allografts or removing one lobe of living donor livers (partial hepatectomy). Excellent results have been achieved with this approach. There has been no mortality reported among donors, and despite the technical challenges of such a procedure, the survival of pediatric patients receiving such grafts approaches that of similar patients who receive whole cadaveric allografts.[326]

Immunology of the Transplanted Liver

Hyperacute rejection is a result of lymphocytotoxic antibodies directed against lymphocytes in the donor organ. It is not well understood why the liver is relatively resistant to this form of rejection even though it affects heart and kidney transplants. Certain anatomic characteristics of the liver may protect it from immune injury. For example, the dual blood supply of the hepatic artery and portal vein provides protection against ischemia. In addition, much of the vasculature of the liver has endothelium that is different from other vascular beds and that may make the liver relatively resistant to immune complex–mediated injury. A very interesting observation is that lymphocytotoxic antibodies disappear from the circulation shortly after liver transplantation. Consequently, a transplanted liver can actually protect other transplanted solid organs from undergoing hyperacute rejection.

Evidence that the immunology of rejection associated with liver transplantation is different from other solid organs is suggested by the lack of correlation between HLA matching and the incidence of rejection. A number of studies have actually demonstrated an inverse relationship between the degree of HLA matching and graft survival. At the present time, HLA matching is not used for the allocation of cadaveric hepatic allografts.[319]

The role of endotoxemia and TNF in primary nonfunction of the liver is being actively investigated. Endotoxin stimulates the production of various inflammatory cytokines, including TNF and IL-1. These cytokines can cause direct endothelial damage, and their activation of coagulation pathways can lead to vascular congestion and ischemia of the graft. The normal liver serves as a protective organ against endotoxemia, but this ability may be impaired after transplant, exposing the graft to damage from released cytokines.[321]

Chronic rejection is distinctly different from acute rejection. Chronic rejection develops slowly and is not effectively treated by intensifying immunosuppressive therapy with current agents. Chronic rejection frequently presents as obstructive jaundice without other major liver abnormalities.

Immunosuppressive Treatment

Drug combinations currently used to prevent graft rejection in liver transplantation usually include CsA and corticosteroids with or without AZA, or a combination of tacrolimus and corticosteroids. The addition of AZA may allow a reduction in CsA dose to minimize nephrotoxicity. Two randomized prospective studies indicated that patient and graft survival were not different with either a CsA- or a tacrolimus-based regimen.[60,61] OKT3 or ATG can also be used for rejection prophylaxis, although its major role continues to be in treating allograft rejection along with agents such as ATG and corticosteroids.

One method of induction used in adults involves administering one gram of methylprednisolone at the time of transplant, and then later switching to 200 mg/day in four equal doses every six hours, tapered by 40 mg/day. The dose is stabilized at 20 mg/day of prednisone by the end of the first week. In addition, CsA is used, starting at a dose of 4–6 mg/kg per day intravenously; subsequent doses are based on whole blood concentrations. Once the patient's digestive tract begins functioning normally, the patient is converted to oral CsA at about 8.5 mg/kg twice daily. When CsA is being instituted, part of the daily dose continues to be given intravenously and slowly tapered until the entire dose is administered orally.[320] Alternatively, tacrolimus can be administered at 0.05 mg/kg by the oral route twice daily, without routine parenteral administration.[327]

Because of the high variability of CsA or tacrolimus absorption and metabolism in liver transplant patients, the development of assays that measure concentrations in the blood was very important in the appropriate use of these drugs. The dose is adjusted to maintain whole blood trough concentrations at 350–400 ng/ml for CsA, as measured by a MoAb assay specific for parent cyclosporin A. Whole blood tacrolimus concentrations are usually maintained around 10–20 ng/ml. One key difference between these drugs is that CsA requires the presence of bile in the duodenum for adequate absorption to occur. The type of biliary anastomosis employed in each case is key to the proper use of oral CsA. Some patients have a different type of anastomosis, a choledochojejunostomy (or "Roux-en-Y") in which no T tube is employed. End-to-end anastomosis of the donor bile duct to the recipient bile duct, with T-tube diversion of bile to bedside drainage, will necessitate administration of intravenous CsA until such time that the T tube is clamped and bile is allowed to flow into the duodenum. At this point, oral CsA can be introduced, while intravenous administration is maintained. Once target blood concentrations have been achieved, intravenous CsA can be discontinued and the patient can be maintained on oral CsA alone. In the event that the T tube is opened once again, the absorption of oral CsA will be compromised and intravenous administration may be required. Early experience indicates that CsA is well absorbed after administration of Neoral® even when the T tube is opened.[328]

In contrast, the absorption of tacrolimus does not depend on bile. Thus the type of biliary anastomosis employed and the presence and status of a T tube will not influence the bioavailability of tacrolimus.

The diagnosis of acute rejection is made by careful monitoring of the trends in liver function tests. A presumptive diagnosis of rejection can be made in the presence of rising liver enzymes and/or bilirubin in the absence of evidence of obstruction of the bile ducts or major vessels on sonography. However, definitive diagnosis can only be made by percutaneous liver biopsy. Rejection episodes are often treated with high-dose "pulse" steroid therapy (one gram of methylprednisolone); the steroids are then cycled in a manner similar to induction after surgery. In patients for whom high-dose steroids are ineffective, a 10- to 14-day course of OKT3 (5 mg/day) or ATG (10–20 mg/kg) may be used. For those patients maintained on a CSA-based regimen who experience rejection resistant to these treatments, conversion to tacrolimus has been successful in rescuing the allograft in the majority of cases,[17] and conversion to tacrolimus may be the preferred treatment in cases of late acute rejection.

Postoperative Complications

Post-transplant complications that increase the risk of early graft loss (or primary nonfunction) include ischemic injury to the liver and acute rejection. Ischemia is the main cause of graft loss during the early post-transplant period. Ischemia can occur to the organ after the death of the donor or after transplantation in the recipient. The University of Wisconsin solution (ViaSpan®, DuPont), which allows the liver to be refrigerated for up to 24 hours, has significantly decreased the incidence of primary nonfunction of the liver. Despite careful evaluation of the donor before organ harvest and proper handling during cold preservation, 8–10% of newly placed allografts will display primary nonfunction or delayed function that can threaten the recipient in the first hours or days after transplantation. Primary nonfunction of the hepatic allograft is characterized by persistent or worsening hypoprothrombinemia, hyperkalemia, and poor bile production. Primary nonfunction follows an unpredictable course; outcome may be improved by administration of alprostadil by continuous infusion.[329]

Although hyperacute rejection of the transplanted kidney or heart is well recognized clinically, it is not so in liver transplantation. However, some of the primary nonfunction seen in liver transplantation is likely a result of hyperacute rejection of the liver, particularly in cases of ABO mismatch.

The most frequent complications faced by the hepatic allograft recipient in the first days to weeks following transplantation are thrombosis, infection, and acute renal insufficiency. Thrombosis of the hepatic artery and/or portal vein secondary to intimal injury occurs in 5–10% of cases and is more frequent in pediatric recipients because of the small size of the vessels involved. The value of prophylaxis with low-dose heparin or aspirin is uncertain. Once detected by sonography, thrombosis can sometimes be corrected surgically by thrombectomy, but in other cases, nonfunction of the allograft results in requiring retransplantation.

Infection is a major complication after liver transplantation.[330,331] Extensive abdominal surgery, malnutrition, and impaired host immunity are all risk factors; poor early allograft function that compromises the liver's normal function as a bacterial sieve encourages or allows bacterial translocation from the small bowel. Bleeding into the peritoneal cavity is a risk factor for the development of bacterial or fungal peritonitis, with gram-negative enteric flora and *Candida albicans* predominating. Several strategies have been proposed for prevention of these infections, including selective bowel decontamination with nonabsorbable antimicrobials[332,333] or systemic prophylaxis with fluconazole. Identification of the optimal approach requires further study.

Acute renal insufficiency occurs after liver transplantation in up to 40% of recipients. Preexisting renal insufficiency, poor early allograft function, and administration of nephrotoxic drugs (including CsA or tacrolimus) in the immediate post-transplant period are contributing risks. Careful attention must be paid to the selection and management of drug therapy in response to changing renal function; an excellent review of pharmacokinetic and therapeutic considerations for drug dosage during renal replacement with hemodialysis or CVVH is available.[334]

Persistent viremia and reinfection of the graft is a common complication for patients undergoing transplantation for the treatment of end-stage liver disease resulting from infection with HBV or hepatitis C virus (HCV). Reinfection may lead to progressive liver failure in the absence of effective prophylaxis. Treatment of recurrent disease after transplantation with IFN-α is poorly tolerated and rarely effective.[335] Anecdotal reports of treatment with ganciclovir, famciclovir, lamivudine, and ribavirin suggest mixed results.[336] Important progress has been made in the prevention of recurrent HBV using long-term immunoprophylaxis with hepatitis B immune globulin.[322] Intravenous administration of large doses (10,000 IU) during the anhepatic phase of transplant surgery, followed by additional high-dose intravenous or intramuscular administration on a monthly basis to maintain antibody to HBV surface antigen (HBsAb) titers above 100 IU/ml, has been successful in preventing reinfection and has resulted in impressive long-term patient survival.[322,337] The preparations of hepatitis B immune globulin available in the U.S. have not been approved by the FDA for intravenous administration. These are preserved with thimerosal, a mercury-containing compound. Because of the long half-life of mercury and the need to give monthly booster doses, methylmercury may accumulate. Signs and symptoms of chronic methylmercury poisoning include paresthesia and sensory loss in the digits, encephalopathy, and renal insufficiency.[338]

Less progress has been made in the prevention of recurrent HCV infection. Persistent viremia can be detected in 95% of patients transplanted for hepatitis C cirrhosis, and reinfection of the allograft occurs in up to 50% of patients; some of these will progress to recurrent end-stage liver disease, often within the first year. Risk factors for recurrence include the requirement for chronic immunosuppression, the presence of a high concentration of HCV RNA (detectable by PCR), and the requirement for augmented immunosuppression for the treatment of acute rejection early in the post-transplant period.[339] Effective prophylactic or therapeutic strategies have not been defined.

HEART TRANSPLANTATION

The era of human cardiac transplantation was initiated in 1964 by Dr. James Hardy[340] at the University of Mississippi, who used a chimpanzee as the organ donor. In 1967, Dr. Christian Barnard[341] of South Africa performed the first human-to-human cardiac transplant. The initial success of this procedure produced a brief flurry of activity, but the clinical results were disappointing because of the high incidence of complications and low survival rates. By 1978 fewer than 15 cardiac transplantation programs were operating worldwide.

The widespread clinical adoption of CsA-based immunosuppressive regimens by 1983 resulted in dramatic improvement in survival and reduction in the incidence of complications after cardiac transplantation.[342] Other factors, including improvements in organ preservation allowing for distant procurement,[343] introduction of the endomyocardial biopsy for diagnosis of rejection,[344] and advances in the prevention and treatment of opportunistic infections, also contributed to the improved survival rates.[345]

Indications and Candidate Selection

Potential cardiac transplant recipients are patients with end-stage cardiac failure who have New York Heart Association class III or IV symptoms refractory to maximal medical management (e.g., angiotensin-converting enzyme inhibitors, diuretics, inotropes, etc.) and no coexisting conditions that might preclude a successful clinical outcome. The overall annual mortality rate of class IV congestive heart failure continues to be 30–40%.[346–348] In comparison, in-hospital mortality following transplantation is less than 5%, and one- and five-year actuarial survival rates are approaching 85 and 75%, respectively.[349,350] Patient selection criteria are listed in Table 8-10.[351] The excellent results that have been achieved have prompted a dramatic increase in the number of candidates listed for transplantation, resulting in prolonged waiting times, which may exceed one year. Ideally, organs should be allocated to those patients at greatest risk of dying in the near future. Thus, more objective means (i.e., oxygen consumption) other than clinical criteria (e.g., class III or IV congestive heart failure) are advocated to stratify the risk

Table 8-10. Selection and Exclusion Criteria for Heart Transplant Recipients[319]

Indications
- Age, newborn to 60 years old
- Irremediable cardiac disease, class IV New York Heart Association
- Normal function or irreversible dysfunction of liver, kidneys, lungs, or central nervous system
- Pulmonary vascular resistance <6–8 Wood units or pharmacologically irreversible

Contraindications
- Active malignancy or infection
- Recent pulmonary infarction
- Active peptic ulcer disease
- Severe peripheral or cerebrovascular disease
- Insulin-dependent diabetes mellitus, unless under excellent medical control and without renal and neurological dysfunction

for these patients to allow better allocation of a scarce resource.[352,353]

The most common causes of heart failure in potential recipients are idiopathic dilated cardiomyopathy in 50% of patients and ischemic heart disease in 41%.[349] Other causes include congenital, valvular, postpartum, viral, and drug-induced (e.g., ethanol) cardiomyopathies. Absolute contraindications to orthotopic cardiac transplantation are (1) the presence of severe, irreversible pulmonary hypertension that may result in right-sided allograft failure after transplantation, (2) preformed antibodies against the donor organ, and (3) the presence of multiorgan failure or other diseases (infection, malignancy) that may limit survival.[351] Patients with elevated pulmonary vascular resistances can be considered candidates for heart-lung or single-lung transplantation.

Transplantation Technique

The diseased heart is removed and replaced with a donor heart while the patient is on cardiopulmonary bypass. Once the cross-clamp is removed and rewarming is under way, the heart often enters sinus rhythm spontaneously. The heart is subjected to numerous insults during the transplant process, including cold cardioplegia, surgical trauma, and anoxia. The total ischemic time for the donor organ should be limited to four hours to minimize these insults. Lidocaine is used to treat any arrhythmias that may arise after the procedure. Because cardiac output is depressed immediately after transplantation, isoproterenol is titrated to maintain a heart rate of approximately 110 beats per minute for up to seven days after surgery. A limited number of patients, including those who received amiodarone preoperatively, may require temporary or permanent atrial pacing during the postoperative period.[354]

Excision of the donor heart results in severing the afferent and efferent nerves, which are not reconnected following transplantation in the recipient. Afferent nerve interruption impairs renin-angiotensin-aldosterone regulation and impedes the normal vasoregulatory response to changes in cardiac filling pressure.[355] Most important, the loss of afferent nerve signaling eliminates the subjective sensation of angina pectoris experienced during ischemia. The cardiac efferent nerves mediate sympathetic and parasympathetic nervous system effects on the heart. Efferent denervation removes the cholinergic influence provided by the autonomic nervous system, resulting in a higher-than-normal resting heart rate. Thus, those interventions that depend on vagal signaling (e.g., atropine, carotid sinus pressure, and the Valsalva maneuver) have no effect on the donor heart rate.[356] It is important to remember that adrenergic receptors remain intact and respond normally to catecholamines, β-blockers, and glucagon.[357] Because the denervated heart relies on enhancement of ventricular performance through catecholamine-induced stimulation of β-receptors, administration of β-blockers is detrimental during periods of stress and also can impair exercise performance.[355] Reinnervation of the heart may occur long after transplantation, resulting in more normal physiologic and pharmacologic responses. However, the pattern of reinnervation is extremely variable,[358] so heart transplant patients should not be told to ignore pain that resembles angina pectoris.

Mechanical Bridging

In addition to using intravenous inotropic support and intra-aortic balloon pumps, critically ill heart failure patients may require long-term mechanical support and "bridging" to transplantation to allow time to find a suitable donor. A number of devices have been used to bridge patients, including the Symbion-7 (Jarvik-7) Total Artificial Heart, the Penn State Heart, and various temporary ventricular assistance devices;[359,360] however, most were plagued by clotting problems and other complications. Most recently, the HeartMate left ventricular assistance device was FDA approved as a bridge to transplant[361–363] and the Novacor wearable left ventricular assistance system has been in use in Europe since 1994.[364,365] Both devices allow for patient discharge from the hospital and, in general, enable the patient to be in much better physical condition at the time of transplant rather than confined to a critical care unit on a UNOS status I classification (i.e., critically ill patient on multiple intravenous inotropic medications and/or requiring mechanical assistance) for a prolonged waiting period of 30 or more days. Because of the disparity between organ supply (2500 heart transplants per year in the United States) and demand (each year 40,000 people under age 65 die who could possibly benefit from heart transplantation),[366] the obvious goal is to develop a totally implantable permanent artificial heart or assistance device to resolve this supply and demand inequity.

Immunosuppressive Treatment

Current preoperative immunosuppressive regimens consist primarily of varying dosages of CsA (0–10 mg/kg) administered orally within four to six hours of surgery and AZA (2–4 mg/kg orally or intravenously). All patients receive 500 mg of methylprednisolone immediately after the cardiopulmonary bypass is discontinued and for the first 36 hours after surgery (125 mg intravenously every 12 hours).[367–371] A number of heart transplant centers are currently involved in clinical trials evaluating tacrolimus or mycophenolate mofetil as substitutes for CsA and AZA, respectively.[142]

Postoperative care of the uncomplicated transplant recipient is similar to that provided for other cardiac surgical patients in that time to extubation, duration of stay in the intensive care unit, and length of total hospitalization are comparable. CsA is either initiated on day 1 or delayed until day 3 or 4 to decrease potential nephrotoxicity in the immediate postoperative period. For that reason, the postoperative dosage of CsA varies from center to center (4–12 mg/kg per day); however, it is usually titrated to achieve CsA whole blood concentrations as assayed by HPLC in the range of 175–250 ng/ml or whole blood concentrations by FPIA of 350–400 ng/ml. Intravenous CsA (0.5–4 mg/kg per day) may be used in patients with absorption problems.[372–374] However, controversy exists about what steady-state concentrations are desirable. AZA is initiated at 2 mg/kg per day and is adjusted to maintain a peripheral WBC count of 3500–7000 cells/mm^3. Prednisone is tapered from an initial dose of 1.5 mg/kg per day to 0.2 mg/kg per day by the end of 3 months and then to approximately 0.1 mg/kg per day by 6–12 months.[367–370]

Some centers use cytolytic agents—for example, OKT3 5 mg/day, ATG 10–15 mg/kg per day, or rabbit ATG 1–3 mg/kg per day—as induction therapy during the first 7–14 postoperative days to minimize the adverse side effects (e.g., CsA nephrotoxicity) observed with the other agents.[375–386] To date, pooled data series show no clear-cut survival improvements with induction therapy, although it appears that a higher percentage of patients may be weaned from prednisone, thereby reducing the incidence of long-term steroid-associated complications.[380,383,387–389] These protocols usually result in the discontinuation of prednisone by three to six months after transplantation. Controversy exists about whether prophylactic therapy with these antilymphocyte antibodies confers any added benefits.[390–392]

Postoperative Complications

Immunologic Complications

Rejection and infection remain the major causes of morbidity and mortality in the early postoperative period.[393] Endomyocardial biopsies are performed frequently after transplantation to monitor for acute rejection. Histologic features consistent with rejection include diffuse mononuclear infiltrate with cellular necrosis.[394] Depending on the severity of the rejection, the patient may be asymptomatic or manifest a variety of clinical signs and symptoms (e.g., fever, lethargy, weakness, dyspnea, hypotension, S3 gallop, or arrhythmias). Initial treatment of rejection usually consists of a steroid pulse (methylprednisolone 1.0 g/day for three days) or a prednisone taper or both.[395,396] OKT3 or ATG is used to treat refractory rejection episodes.[397–399] Tacrolimus and mycophenolate mofetil have also demonstrated efficacy as rescue agents in patients not responding to steroid pulses and/or antilymphocytic therapy.[400]

Eighty percent of all infections in heart transplantation recipients occur within the first three months after transplantation and after episodes of augmented immunosuppression during rejection episodes.[401] The increased risk lasts for three months after treatment and is highest when combinations of high-dose steroids and other agents (e.g., ATG) are used.[402] Since the introduction of CsA and triple drug regimens, the overall incidence and severity of bacterial infection have decreased,[401] whereas the incidence of viral infections has increased.

Chronic Rejection

The major cause of late morbidity and mortality in the cardiac transplant recipient is the development of transplant coronary artery disease (chronic rejection), which is characterized by a diffuse and often rapidly progressive form of occlusive coronary artery disease. Because the transplanted heart is denervated, patients are usually asymptomatic (i.e., do not sense anginal pain) until sufficient myocardial damage has occurred to cause congestive heart failure. This process may be caused by chronic rejection, but CMV infection has also been identified as a risk factor.[403,404] Because percutaneous transluminal coronary angiography and coronary bypass surgery are not useful for treating diffuse coronary artery disease, retransplantation remains the only viable option. The prognosis after retransplantation is suboptimal; the one-year actuarial survival rate is 49%.[405]

LUNG AND HEART-LUNG TRANSPLANTATION

The first human lung transplant was attempted by Hardy in 1963. For 20 years, experimental lung transplantation was plagued by a variety of complications, including respiratory insufficiency caused by denervation of the lung, dehiscence of the bronchial or tracheal anastomosis associated with high-dose steroid therapy,[406] and the difficulty of diagnosing rejection.[407] The first successful heart-lung transplant was performed in 1981 at Stanford,[408] and the first single-lung transplant was performed at Toronto in 1983.[409]

Further refinements in surgical techniques,[410] new immunosuppressive protocols, and management of complications will permit lung transplantation to achieve long-term survival rates similar to those of the other solid organs.[411]

Indications and Candidate Selection

Lung transplantation has been successfully extended to a variety of advanced lung diseases, including pulmonary fibrosis, chronic obstructive lung disease, cystic fibrosis, primary pulmonary hypertension, and selected forms of Eisenmenger's syndrome. Current selection criteria for lung transplantation are listed in Table 8-11.[410] The most common procedure performed today is the single-lung procedure, which has even been successful in previously contraindicated conditions, including emphysema, cor-pulmonale, and primary pulmonary hypertension. The primary indications for bilateral single-lung transplants are cystic fibrosis, emphysema, and bronchiectasis. These procedures allow more patients to benefit from a given organ donor, as a heart-lung block can be used for two or three recipients instead of just one. A few patients with coexisting severe heart and lung disease (e.g., Eisenmenger's syndrome or congenital defects) will still require heart-lung transplantation (Table 8-12).

Table 8-11. Medical and Psychosocial Selection Criteria for Lung Transplantation[399]

Medical criteria

- Life expectancy from progressive pulmonary disease <18 months
- Age <60 years
- Absence of systemic disease with significant end-organ damage, especially liver and kidney damage
- Absence of significant coronary artery disease
- Absence of extensive mediastinal radiation
- No previous major abdominal surgery *if* an omental wrap is to be employed
- Not on high-dose corticosteroids
- Adequate nutrition
- Ambulatory
- No surgical violation of the pleural space *if* cardiopulmonary bypass is required

Psychosocial criteria

- Demonstrates compliance with medical regimens
- Psychologically stable; no history of alcohol or drug abuse or psychosis
- Able to move to transplant center and maintain self plus support person for 3–6 months

Immunosuppressive Treatment

The lung is one of the largest transplantable organs and has an extensive intrinsic immune apparatus. The lung may be more susceptible to rejection because of its large population of T lymphocytes and macrophages, its constant contact with external antigens, and its extensive vascular bed. Immunosuppressive therapy for lung transplantation has been patterned after earlier experience with other solid organs but modified to take into consideration the unique problems associated with lung transplantation.[412] Preoperative immunosuppression in the lung transplant recipient usually consists of varying dosages of CsA (4–8 mg/kg) or tacrolimus (0.1–0.2 mg/kg per day), AZA (2–4 mg/kg orally or intravenously), and methylprednisolone (500 mg administered during surgery, followed by 0.5–4 mg/kg per day tapered over the next three to four days).[413,414] During the initial years of successful lung transplantation, corticosteroids were avoided during the first one to three weeks in an effort to improve tracheal or bronchial anastomotic healing; however, with improved surgical techniques, steroids are now administered early in the postoperative course. Some centers also use induction regimens including ALGs or antilymphocyte sera (dose varies according to product), ATG (10–15 mg/kg per day), or OKT3 (5 mg/day) to provide an initial steroid-sparing effect.[415] These agents are usually used for a minimum of 7–14 days, at which point CsA (or tacrolimus) concentrations are predictably in the therapeutic range. Most recently, some centers have abandoned the use of antilymphocyte agents in lieu of corticosteroids.[407,416,417]

CsA is initiated after surgery, either orally (6–8 mg/kg per day or more, especially in patients with cystic fibrosis) or intravenously (2–4 mg/hr), and adjusted to achieve therapeutic concentrations. CsA concentrations are maintained in the high therapeutic range unless renal function declines. The AZA dose is adjusted to maintain the WBC count between 3500 and 6000 cells/mm^3. Prednisone (1.5 mg/kg per day) is usually initiated within the first week and tapered to a maintenance dose of 0.1–0.2 mg/kg per day.[407,410] Investigations are under way using tacrolimus and mycophenolate mofetil in lung transplantation.[413,414,418]

Postoperative Complications

Lung transplant recipients undergo considerable intraop-

Table 8-12. Indications for Lung Transplant Procedures[410]

Single-lung transplant
End-stage fibrotic lung disease
COPD[a]
Pulmonary hypertension (selected cases)
Double-lung transplant
Cystic fibrosis
Pulmonary sepsis
Diffuse pulmonary diseases associated with pleural effusion, pneumothorax, etc. (e.g., **eosinophilic granuloma** and **lymphangioleiomyomatosis**)
Pulmonary hypertension (selected cases)
COPD (selected cases)
Heart-lung transplant
Pulmonary parenchymal disease with separate cardiac dysfunction
Chronic pulmonary emoli (if thromboendarterectomy is not feasible)
Pulmonary hypertension, primary and secondary (selected areas)

Lung conditions in ***bold*** *are listed under transplantation procedure of choice.*

[a]*Chronic obstructive pulmonary disease (COPD) includes alpha-1-antitrypsin deficiency.*

erative trauma and are at high risk for early postoperative complications, including bleeding and the pulmonary reimplantation response, which is a form of noncardiogenic pulmonary edema that has its onset within 48 hours following the procedure. Other early complications, including fluid overload, left ventricular failure, rejection, infection, and atelectasis, can confound the differential diagnosis.[410] Management includes aggressive fluid restrictions, concentration of intravenous solutions, and administration of diuretic therapy to facilitate fluid removal. Most lung transplant recipients are cachectic before transplantation because of hypermetabolism and long-standing pulmonary disease. Postoperative nutritional replacement is often necessary but may be complicated by fluid restrictions, hypermetabolism, malabsorption, or a prolonged postoperative ileus (i.e., in patients in whom a laparotomy was performed to mobilize the omentum). Gastric atony or outlet obstruction may also occur if the vagus nerve is severed or damaged during surgical manipulation.[419] Postoperative nutritional support provided by intravenous alimentation or a feeding jejunostomy and oral supplementation is often useful to facilitate weaning from the respirator, promote tissue healing, and prevent subsequent infections.

Lung transplant recipients are predisposed to the same long-term complications as other immunosuppressed transplant patients (e.g., hypertension, hyperlipidemia, obesity, rejection, infection, and malignancy). In the past, acute lung rejection was very common in the first three weeks following transplantation, and this may have been related to the intentional avoidance of corticosteroids during the early postoperative period. Differentiating rejection from infection still remains a challenging dilemma.[407] There is no reliable marker for rejection, except for a rapid response to a bolus of steroids (methylprednisolone 1000 mg). Patients usually respond within 12 hours with resolution of hypoxemia and pulmonary infiltrates. Such a clinical response warrants continuation of high-dose corticosteroids for the next two days. A poor response warrants immediate bronchoscopy, bronchoalveolar lavage, and transbronchial lung biopsy, which have become useful adjuncts for differentiating infection from rejection.[407,420]

Infectious complications in the lung transplant recipient are a major cause of death. Bacterial, viral, and fungal pathogens may cause infections both early and throughout the life span of the lung recipient. The most common type of infection in the lung transplant patient is pneumonia, which can be very problematic, especially in the early postoperative period. The lung is a very susceptible site for infection because the transplanted lung is denervated and there is no cough reflex beyond the bronchial anastamosis. Donor-acquired and nosocomial infections can occur, with gram-negative pathogens being the primary culprits. *Staphylococcus aureus* and *Streptococcus pneumoniae* account for most of the other bacterial pathogens.[420]

CMV pneumonia is the second most common cause of pneumonia in lung transplant patients after bacterial pneumonia. Because CMV can be life threatening in a lung transplant patient, most centers use various prophylactic regimens consisting of intravenous immune globulin (e.g., 500 mg/kg on days 0, 1, 2, and 7, and then weekly for three months) or CMV hyperimmune globulin (100–150 mg/kg weekly to monthly for eight doses),[421] and ganciclovir (5 mg/kg every 12 hours for two weeks or 5 mg/kg every 24 hours while hospitalized, then Monday through Friday for three months) in CMV-negative recipients of CMV-positive organs.[419,420] Other protocols include ganciclovir administered from day 7 to day 90 after transplantation or from day 7 to day 28 followed by high-dose acyclovir.[422] The efficacy of one protocol over another has not been confirmed, but randomized trials are under way. The role of oral ganciclovir has not yet been elucidated.

Pneumocystis carinii pneumonia (PCP) has also been very problematic in lung transplant recipients, but the institution of routine trimethoprim–sulfamethoxazole prophylaxis has decreased the incidence dramatically.[423] Various regimens (e.g., one double-strength tablet three times weekly or therapy for the first seven days of each month) have been used in an attempt to reduce side effects, such as loss of appetite, nausea, or vomiting, observed with this drug in lung recipients.

The most devastating complication and threat to long-term survival after lung transplantation is the development of obstructive airway disease as a result of obliterative bronchiolitis (OB).[423–425] OB is an inflammatory disorder of the small airways characterized clinically by a relatively rapid and progressive form of obstructive airway disease that is frequently fatal. Early detection through the use of serial measurements of pulmonary function, serial transbronchial lung biopsies, and a trial of augmented immunosuppression may slow the progression of the disease.[423] Therapy for OB has included high-dose steroids, ATG, and OKT3, none of which has emerged as superior to the others. Trials are under way to evaluate the efficacy of MTX, which has been used for treating recalcitrant cardiac rejection.[136,137]

SMALL INTESTINE TRANSPLANTATION

Small intestine transplantation was first attempted in 1901 by Carrel and was developed successfully in dogs in 1959 by Lillehei. This work was extended by Starzl in 1983 and by Williams in 1989 in performing multivisceral ("cluster") transplantation (liver, stomach, pancreas, small bowel, and colon).[426] Recent major improvements in surgical techniques and the routine use of tacrolimus-based immunosuppression have resulted in successful long-term patient and allograft survival (i.e., greater than one year).[426,427] Despite these advances, transplantation of the small bowel or multivisceral transplantation must still be considered experimental, and much work will be required before these procedures can become routine.

Indications and Candidate Selection

Transplantation of the small intestine has been proposed as a means of increasing intestinal absorption in patients who have undergone extensive small-bowel resection and become dependent on total parenteral nutrition (TPN). Indications for small intestine transplantation include failure of home parenteral nutrition to sustain a patient with short-bowel syndrome (e.g., Crohn's disease or radiation enteritis), congenital causes of small bowel failure (e.g., microvillus atrophy), and extensive traumatic injury to the small bowel requiring radical resection.

Immunosuppressive Treatment

The use of CsA-based regimens for small intestine transplantation has been disappointing; rejection and graft-versus-host disease (GVHD) were not adequately prevented, and patient survival was unacceptable. Initial immunosuppression is presently accomplished with a combination of intravenous tacrolimus 0.1 mg/kg per day, corticosteroids, and prostaglandin E_1. Later, oral tacrolimus 0.3 mg/kg per day and prednisone are administered for maintenance.[427] Combined small bowel and liver transplantation appears to reduce the risk of intestinal rejection. Graft monitoring after clinical small intestine transplantation includes daily to weekly biopsies during the early postoperative course and less frequent biopsies thereafter. Frequent biopsies are facilitated by a surgical technique that includes the creation of dual enterostomies.[427]

Postoperative Complications

Two major problems were identified early and continue to plague small intestine transplantation. First is the complex immunologic response that occurs after small bowel transplantation, which includes both classic cell-mediated graft rejection by the recipient and GVHD, in which graft lymphocytes within lymphoid tissues in the gut wall attack the recipient.[428] GVHD can be reduced or even abolished if the lymphoid tissue in the graft is reduced by irradiation before transplantation or by resection of mesenteric lymph nodes.[428,429] Second, the physiologic functions of the graft are severely disturbed by the process of transplantation, and further immunologic damage not only hampers recovery but also destroys the barrier functions vital to recipient survival.[430] If the patient survives the perioperative period, the next major obstacle is surviving infection. Rejection of the small bowel may increase intestinal permeability and result in bacterial translocation and sepsis.[430] For this reason, selective decontamination of the gastrointestinal tract is continued for the first four to six weeks.

Following the transplant procedure, parenteral nutrition is continued until adequate graft function is established. Close attention to fluid and electrolyte supplementation is critical, and slow stepwise introduction of enteral feeding is required.

An inevitable consequence of small bowel transplantation is graft denervation. This is important because salt and water absorption is under neurologic control by the autonomic nervous system. Motor function is also disturbed by denervation.[428]

Additional challenges for successful small bowel transplantation include (1) the technical aspects of small vessel anastomoses, (2) the risk of infections related to complications due to routine colonization of the small intestine with microorganisms, (3) the lack of uniform approach to small intestine preservation, and (4) the lack of a consistent method of identifying rejection.[428]

COMPLICATIONS AFTER SOLID ORGAN TRANSPLANTATION

During the past decade, dramatic increases in graft and patient survival following solid organ transplantation have occurred. These increases are due to a variety of factors: identification of better patient selection parameters; improvements in tissue-typing techniques; development of more specific immunosuppressive regimens; improvements in organ preservation; refinement of surgical technique; improvements in the recognition, distinction, and treatment of allograft rejection; and introduction of effective agents for both the prophylaxis and treatment of all types of opportunistic infections. Despite the improved survival rates, the development of complications continues to plague long-term survival after solid organ transplantation.[393,419,431–435] The major complications arise from an imbalance in the recipient's overall level of immunosuppression. Preventing rejection increases the risk of infection and malignancy. The ultimate goal of immunosuppressive therapy is to develop tolerance to the graft while leaving intact the host's defenses against microbial pathogens and tumors.

Acute Rejection

Despite dramatic strides in the advancement of organ transplantation, acute rejection is one of the leading causes of morbidity and mortality. The immune response to an allograft almost invariably results in rejection if not prevented by appropriate treatment. Not only are grafts lost in the early weeks or months after transplantation, but in surviving grafts the lesions may lead to permanent damage and to a gradual deterioration of function months to years later. The accurate diagnosis and effective treatment of allograft rejection remains one of the most critical determinants of both short- and long-term survival. Development of noninvasive means of detecting early rejection is desired.

Chronic Rejection

Although survival rates after transplantation continue to improve, long-term survival in all types of organ transplantation is limited by the development of chronic rejection. Regardless of organ type, chronic rejection is the common denominator that eventually causes graft failure, with resultant ischemia and fibrosis secondary to progressive effects on the arterial and arteriolar circulation. This progressive process is the main cause of long-term kidney graft failure, graft atherosclerosis of transplanted hearts, bile duct obliteration in liver transplants, and OB in lung grafts. Until this process is better understood and can be controlled, indefinite graft survival will remain unattainable in most cases.

Infectious Complications

The clinical approach to infectious complications after solid organ transplant involves a careful analysis of clinical presentation, diagnostic tests and procedures, specific risk factors, and preventive strategies employed. The epidemiology of post-transplant infections is represented in Table 8-13. Risk factor analysis is key in determining the likely pathogen as well as appropriate clinical interventions and anti-infective treatments. The use of various anti-infective agents in transplant recipients is generally classified into three treatment strategies: (1) prophylaxis, (2) preemptive therapy, and (3) treatment. *Prophylaxis* refers to the administration of preventive agents to all individuals and implies a low-toxicity regimen for a high-risk group. *Preemptive* therapy is the selective administration of preventive agents based on specific indicators of high risk for infection. *Treatment* indicates therapeutic intervention with curative agents for an established infection. Pharmacologic, pharmacoeconomic, and anti-infective resistance considerations have pressured the transplant clinician to evolve from generalized prophylaxis to selective preemptive therapy.

Bacterial Infections

The most common bacterial pathogens associated with various sites of infection are represented in Table 8-14. Strategies for both prevention and treatment should focus on the most common pathogens at the suspected or potential site of infection in conjunction with the specific risk factors associated with the type of organ transplant and/or the intended procedure. Table 8-13 displays the most common risk factors for the development of bacterial infections in this population. Although immuno-

Table 8-13. Epidemiology of Post-transplant Infectious Complications

	BACTERIAL (%)	CMV (%)	FUNGAL (%)	INFECTION/PT	COMMON SITE
Kidney	5	8	1–2	0.86	Urinary tract
Liver	19	22	16	1.86	Abdomen/GI tract
Heart	13	16	8	1.36	Respiratory tract

%, percentage of total patient population who will have this type of infection; CMV, cytomegalovirus; pt, patient; GI, gastrointestinal.

Table 8-14. Common Bacterial Pathogens and Sites of Infection

URINE	ABDOMEN	LUNG	BLOOD	CNS	WOUND
E. coli	GNR	PSA/GNR	Staph sp.	Pneumococci	Staph sp.
Enterococci	Enterococci	Staph sp.	GNR	*H. influenza*	PSA
Other GNR		Pneumococci[a] *H. influenza*[a] Nocardia[a] Legionella[a]		Meningococci Listeria	Other GNR

GNR, gram-negative rod; PSA, Pseudomonas aeruginosa.
[a]*Late pathogen.*

suppression compromises the host's ability to fight active infections, specific agents have not been linked to an increased risk of bacterial infections.

The prevention of post-transplant infection should focus on discriminate pre- and post-transplant antibiotic therapy. Unnecessary use of long courses of therapy and broad spectrum antibiotics can result in significant resistance and predispose patients to other pathogenic organisms. Increasing reports of enterococcal and gram-negative rod bacterial resistance in transplant recipients are most likely due to indiscriminate and prolonged antibiotic therapy in this population. Other preventive strategies have focused on specific populations of transplant patients. Selective bowel decontamination with nonabsorbable antibiotics has demonstrated a significant reduction in gram-negative bacterial infections after liver and small bowel transplantation. Urinary tract sterilization with trimethoprim–sulfamethoxazole or fluoroquinolones reduces the frequency of recurrent urinary tract infections in renal transplant recipients. Prophylaxis against viral pathogens and other opportunistic infections appears to contribute to a lower incidence of concurrent bacterial infections.

Viral Infections

Post-transplant viral infections are generally divided into three broad classifications: the herpes group viruses, hepatotrophic viruses, and rare viral pathogens.[436] The most common pathogens in each classification are listed in Table 8-15. These viral pathogens have a significant clinical impact on patient and graft survival, causing clinical infection and disease, increased susceptibility to other bacterial or fungal pathogens due to secondary immunosuppression, indirect and direct allograft injury, and increased risk of malignancy.[436,437] Furthermore, there is growing evidence of the relationship between CMV infection and the subsequent development of acute and chronic rejection.[438] Therefore, preventive strategies against common viral pathogens are a key focus of clinical practice and research in solid organ transplant recipients.

Herpes Group Viruses

Cytomegalovirus—CMV remains the most prevalent viral pathogen in transplant recipients, causing symptomatic infection in up to 60% of this population.[439] CMV presents either latently, without viral replication, or as active infection, with subsequent viral shedding and immune activation.[439] CMV infection is often classified on the basis of donor and recipient CMV IgG antibody status at the time of transplant, the highest risk being the CMV-positive donor/CMV-negative recipient patient (Table 8-16).[439,440] Symptomatic CMV infection gener-

Table 8-15. Viral Infections in Transplant Recipients

Herpes Group Viruses
- Cytomegalovirus
- Epstein-Barr virus
- Herpes simplex viruses
- Human herpes 6
- Varicella-zoster virus

Hepatotrophic Viruses
- Hepatitis A virus
- Hepatitis B virus
- Hepatitis C virus
- Rare hepatotrophic viruses (hepatitis delta virus, hepatitis E and G viruses)

Rare pathogens
- Adenovirus
- HIV
- HTLV
- Papillomavirus
- Rotavirus

HIV, human immunodeficiency virus; HTLV, human T-cell lymphotropic virus.

Table 8-16. Epidemiology of CMV Infection[439,440]

	PRIMARY INFECTION	REACTIVATION	SUPERINFECTION
Serology	D^+/R^-	D^- or D^+/R^+	D^+/R^- or R^+
Incidence of symptoms	60–90%	<20%	40–50%

D, donor; R, recipient; +, positive; –, negative.

ally presents as a flu-like syndrome, often in combination with leukopenia. CMV disease is the progression to invasive infection with biochemical, histopathologic, or radiographic evidence of organ involvement.

The greatest risk for symptomatic CMV infection is during the first two to three months following the transplant.[439] In addition to donor and recipient serology, other risk factors for CMV infection include net immunosuppression, type of organ transplanted, blood product exposure, recipient age, HLA phenotyping, cadaveric transplants, and retransplants.[439–441] The specific role of immunosuppression depends on the ability of the agent to either stimulate reactivation or amplify viral replication.[440] Antilymphocyte antibody preparations (OKT3, ATG, and antithymocyte sera) are associated with a high risk of CMV reactivation from latency, whereas steroids, AZA, mycophenolic acid, CsA, tacrolimus, and sirolimus are associated with a low to moderate risk of viral reactivation.[440] Conversely, cyclosporine, tacrolimus, and sirolimus potently amplify viral replication after reactivation has occurred. Therefore, the sequence and duration of specific immunotherapeutic agents are key to the subsequent development of CMV disease.

General strategies for the prevention of CMV infection have focused on the avoidance of viral exposure, the use of preemptive indicators to predict high-risk patients, and immunologic and pharmacologic inhibition of viral reactivation and replication. Strategies for avoiding viral exposure include donor/recipient serologic matching as well as serologic screening and/or leukocyte filtration of blood products.[440] Immunologic strategies have focused on both active immunization (Towne vaccine) and passive immunization (standard or hyperimmune globulin).[330] However, primary attention has been directed at the use of various antiviral agents, such as acyclovir and ganciclovir, either alone or in combination (i.e., intravenous ganciclovir followed by oral acyclovir).

High-dose oral acyclovir (3200 mg per day) initially demonstrated protection against CMV in renal transplant recipients.[442] However, subsequent studies failed to demonstrate efficacy in high-risk recipients, and the role of this regimen appears to be primarily as an adjunctive suppressive agent.[443,444] Prophylaxis with intravenous ganciclovir demonstrated significant efficacy in preventing reactivation, but not primary infection, in heart transplant recipients.[445] Selective (preemptive) use of ganciclovir 2.5–5.0 mg/kg per day during OKT3 therapy significantly reduced the incidence of subsequent CMV infection and further established the preventive role of this agent.[446] Numerous studies have supported ganciclovir as a key component of most antiviral preventive strategies.[330,447,448] Passive immunization with immune globulin preparations (standard or hyperimmune), although it decreases the severity of infection in kidney and liver recipients, has had variable effects as monotherapy and is best utilized in combination with other antiviral agents.[449–453]

Despite a reduction in the incidence and severity of CMV infection, single-drug therapy does not provide optimal prevention in the high-risk transplant patient.[448] The development of effective preventive strategies should take into account the specific immunosuppressive protocol, the organ transplanted, potential adverse effects, and pharmacoeconomic considerations. Current guidelines suggest that high-risk patients (positive donor/negative recipient, OKT3/ATG-treated, or nonrenal abdominal and lung transplant patients) should receive combination therapy for two to three months. Successful protocols generally utilize intravenous ganciclovir 5–10 mg/kg per day for one to two weeks followed by long-term suppressive therapy with high-dose acyclovir and/or immune globulin preparations for the remaining 8–12 weeks.[299,448–450] The low-risk recipient is sufficiently protected by suppressive therapy with high-dose acyclovir or delayed initiation of treatment with ganciclovir based on clinical and/or laboratory preemptive indicators of CMV infection.[450] New agents, such as oral ganciclovir, valacyclovir, famciclovir, and lobucavir, may provide improved alternatives for initial and suppressive therapy.

Established CMV disease is generally treated with therapeutic doses of intravenous ganciclovir (5 mg/kg twice daily) for 14–28 days, depending on the severity of illness. In cases of life-threatening disease, adjunctive therapy with immune globulin preparations is recommended. Foscarnet has been used for cases of resistant CMV infection, but the general use of this agent in transplantation is limited by its significant nephrotoxicity.[451] In addition, suppressive therapy with acyclovir or immunoglobulin is probably warranted for one to two months following infection to establish viral latency.

Epstein-Barr Virus—Epstein-Barr virus (EBV), a member of the herpes family of viruses, infects B lymphocytes and squamous epithelial cells and has been linked to the development of post-transplant lymphoproliferative disease (PTLD).[454] After acute EBV infection, immunocompetent patients develop an asymptomatic persistent infection in which cytotoxic T cells suppress the acute infection into a latent state. However, in transplant recipients, immunosuppression results in loss of this immune control, which can lead to uncontrolled B-cell proliferation and eventual lymphoma formation.[455] The clinical presentation of PTLD can vary widely from a mild viral illness to fulminant, rapidly fatal disease. The mild form may present with fever, malaise, and lymphadenopathy. Tumors in the gastrointestinal tract often present as acute abdominal pain with subsequent perforation, obstruction, or bleeding.[456,457] PTLD also commonly presents as tumors in the central nervous system or the allograft.

The two primary factors contributing to EBV-related PTLD are pretransplant immune status to the virus and the net level of immunosuppression.[458] Transplant patients naive to the virus are at a greater risk for primary infection and progression to PTLD secondary to personal contact, exposure to blood products, or infection by the transplanted organ. In patients previously infected with EBV, reactivation of the latent virus appears to be directly related to the immunosuppressive regimen administered. The incidence of lymphoma appears to closely correlate with the overall intensity of immunosuppression. This is reflected by higher lymphoma rates in cardiac and liver transplant recipients, who receive more intense immunosuppression than do renal transplant patients.[459] The introduction of CsA significantly increased the incidence of PTLD compared to traditional therapy with prednisone and AZA or CTX.[460] There appears to be a higher risk with tacrolimus than with CsA, especially in pediatric patients, due to its greater immunosuppressive potency. As with CMV, antilymphocyte agents appear to be associated with significant reactivation of EBV and resultant PTLD. Initial reports suggested OKT3 was associated with a greater risk than polyclonal preparations, but subsequent analyses have established equivalent risk with monoclonal and polyclonal antibody therapy.[391,461–463] More important, the duration of therapy and the proximity of multiple courses of antilymphocyte preparations appear to be the primary risk factors, not the total dose.

The current strategies for treating PTLD include reduction or cessation of immunosuppression, antiviral therapy, adjuvant chemotherapy and/or radiotherapy, and surgical resection of the tumors.[458,464] Once a patient is diagnosed with PTLD, it is important to establish the clonality of the lesions to help guide treatment.[454] Polyclonal B-cell proliferation alone carries the best prognosis and should be treated with either discontinuation or reduction of immunosuppression and acyclovir (10 mg/kg intravenously every 8 hours or 800 mg by mouth four times daily) or ganciclovir (5 mg/kg intravenously every 12 hours) therapy for three to four weeks.[465] Long-term maintenance therapy with high-dose acyclovir for 6 months is probably justified, given the potential for reactivation. Hyperimmune globulin contains high titers against EBV and may provide additional adjunctive therapy. Patients with monoclonal, malignant-appearing tumors are generally treated with aggressive measures, such as surgery, adjuvant chemotherapy or radiotherapy, and discontinuance of immunosuppression. Recent studies suggest implementation of appropriate CMV prophylaxis (ganciclovir followed by high-dose oral acyclovir) may also affect the incidence of EBV infection and subsequent PTLD.[458,465]

Other Herpes Group Viruses—Infection with herpes simplex virus (HSV-1, -2) is generally confined to latent infections reactivated by immunosuppression or other stress factors.[466] Most infections are confined to mucocutaneous sites, but occasional rare invasive infections can occur. Prevention and/or treatment with standard doses of acyclovir (oral or intravenous) is generally effective. A significant decrease in HSV infections is a secondary result of implementation of CMV preventive strategies.[330]

Varicella-zoster virus (VZV) infections present as a primary infection (chicken pox) or as reactivation (shingles).[467] VZV will occasionally present as severe hepatitis, pneumonitis, or encephalitis. New advances in the prevention of primary VZV infection include the varicella-zoster vaccine and VZV hyperimmune globulin. Both products are approved for use and appear promising, but further data are needed in transplant recipients. Treatment of established infections with high-dose acyclovir offers variable results with chicken pox but appears to attenuate the duration and severity of other VZV infections. Adjunctive therapy with VZV immune globulin may be warranted in severe systemic infections.

Hepatotrophic Viruses

Liver disease after organ transplantation can result from multiple causes, including drug toxicity, metabolic disturbances, or viral infection. Infection with HBV or HCV is the most common cause of liver disease. Pretransplant screening for the presence of HBV and administration of recombinant HBV vaccine when indicated can prevent the development of HBV hepatitis.

Before donated blood was routinely screened for the presence of HCV, the virus was the most common cause of transfusion-related viral illness. Transmission of HCV by organ transplantation has been documented,[468] and chronic liver disease among renal and heart allograft recipients is frequent among those who were HCV positive before transplantation as well as among those who acquire the virus as a result of transplantation. HCV cirrhosis occurs more frequently among allograft recipients than among the normal population (six- to sevenfold higher) because of the requirement for maintenance immunosuppression. Testing for HCV RNA is important because immunosuppressive medications may interfere with the patient's ability to produce anti-HCV antibodies.[469] These findings have prompted debate about the wisdom of using organs from HCV-positive donors for transplantation,[470] as well as an ethical dilemma about the allocation of those organs (i.e., preferential allocation to HCV-positive candidates). Treatment strategies that include IFN-α or ribavirin have met with mixed results.

Fungal Infection

Fungal infections following solid organ transplantation remain a major cause of morbidity and mortality. *Candida* and *Aspergillus* species continue to account for the majority of these infections, although the attack rate is higher among recipients of organs other than kidneys because those patients receive more immunosuppressive therapy.[471] Attack rates range from 5% among kidney allograft recipients to 40% among liver graft recipients. Risk factors among the latter group that predispose to fungal infection include renal insufficiency, length of the transplant operation, and the need for re-exploration or retransplantation.[472] *Aspergillus* infection in these patients is characterized by pulmonary localization with subsequent dissemination, whereas infection with *Candida albicans* is most often disseminated but rarely involves the lungs. *Aspergillus* infection of the lungs is associated with high mortality despite aggressive treatment with amphotericin B. Superficial infections may also occur in the oropharynx with *Candida* species, or on the skin or nail beds with dermatophytes. The latter may be particularly resistant to treatment and can be a cause of considerable discomfort and concern to patients.

Although amphotericin B remains the drug of choice for treatment of invasive aspergillosis, its toxicity profile limits its widespread use. Liposomal formulations of amphotericin B have shown promise in ameliorating the toxicity associated with amphotericin B deoxycholate and may be preferred for transplant recipients.[473] Recent experience suggests that fluconazole may be a safe and effective alternative for the treatment of fungal infections caused by *Candida* species or *Cryptococcus neoformans*. Prevention of fungal infections remains one of the most important goals in the field of transplantation. New approaches, such as the use of prophylactic or preemptive therapy for patients at greatest risk of developing infection, may assist in attainment of this goal.[330,331] A multicenter randomized blinded trial of fluconazole versus placebo, administered for 10 weeks after liver transplantation, has been completed but results have not been reported to date.

Either nystatin (administered as swish-and-swallow suspension or pastille) or clotrimazole troches (three times daily for six months) are used to prevent fungal colonization and infection.

Opportunistic Infections

Opportunistic infections after organ transplantation may occur with *Pneumocystis carinii* or *Toxoplasma gondii*. The incidence of *P. carinii* pneumonia in organ transplant patients receiving no antimicrobial prophylaxis is approximately 5–10%.[330] Effective prophylaxis for *P. carinii* infection may be accomplished by administration of trimethoprim–sulfamethoxazole once daily (or three times per week) or by monthly administration of inhaled pentamidine.[474,475] In the special case of the heart transplant patient who is seronegative for *T. gondii* prior to transplantation and receives an allograft from a *T. gondii*–seropositive donor (and thus is at high risk for disseminated toxoplasmosis), the combination of sulfadiazine plus pyrimethamine administered for the first three months following transplant provides effective prophylaxis against both pneumocystosis and toxoplasmosis.[330]

Hypertension

Hypertension in the solid organ transplant recipient is worrisome because it is a significant risk factor for the development of morbidity and mortality in the general population. Cardiovascular disease remains the primary cause of death in patients with functioning renal allografts. The contributory role of hypertension to the development of transplant coronary artery disease in the heart transplant recipient is less clear. In addition to the issues associated with increased morbidity and mortality caused by hypertension, treatment of hypertension usually mandates the use of multiple drugs, many of which interact with immunosuppressive therapy, further increasing the risk of drug-related complications and noncompliance.

The pathogenesis of hypertension in solid organ recipients is multifactorial and includes immunosuppressive therapy (e.g., CsA, steroids, tacrolimus), renal disease (including CsA or tacrolimus-induced nephrotoxicity), recurrent essential hypertension, or other causes of secondary hypertension. Renal transplant recipients may become hypertensive with chronic rejection or recurrence of their diabetic nephropathy.

Although there are many potential causes, CsA- and tacrolimus-induced hypertension are probably the primary cause in most solid organ recipients. The incidence of hypertension following solid organ transplantation has increased dramatically since the routine incorporation of CsA into immunosuppressive regimens.[476–478] Corticosteroids may also exacerbate hypertension by causing sodium and water retention after transplantation, but the incidence of hypertension with regimens based on the combination of AZA and prednisone is one-third that of the CsA era. CsA-associated hypertension (CAH) occurs in 50–100% of transplant recipients; both the incidence and severity are more pronounced in heart, lung, bone marrow, and liver transplant recipients.[479–481] Its development is independent of race, sex, age, and prior history of hypertension.[476,480] The onset of CAH is evident within four to six weeks after transplantation. Heart transplant recipients typically require antihypertensive therapy indefinitely,[478,479] whereas the percentage of renal transplant patients requiring treatment has been reported to decrease over time.[481]

Various mechanisms for CAH have been proposed, including enhanced sympathetic activity, altered renin activity, enhanced vasoconstrictor prostaglandins, and hypomagnesemia.[482] CsA decreases renal blood flow and glomerular filtration rate and causes an increase in mean arterial pressure and renal vasculature. The vasoconstrictive effects of CsA on the afferent arteriole result in a volume-dependent hypertension that may be mediated by catecholamines,[483] prostaglandins,[484] endothelin,[485] or the renin-angiotensin system.[486,487]

Treatment of CAH frequently requires the use of multiple agents.[488–490] Calcium antagonists appear to be the most effective.[491] Variable efficacy has been observed with diuretics, vasodilators, and β-blockers.[492] β-blockers are less desirable in cardiac transplant recipients than the other drugs; they impair exercise tolerance, because the denervated heart is dependent on circulating catecholamines. Further research is needed to clarify CsA's role in the development of this form of hypertension and to identify the most effective treatment strategies.

The incidence of hypertension appears to be less with tacrolimus; however, this finding needs to be confirmed with more widespread use in solid organ transplant recipients. Considering its propensity to cause nephrotoxicity, tacrolimus is assumed to be a likely culprit for this disease.[80] However, because it may be more steroid-sparing than CsA, the lower incidence of hypertension reported with this agent may actually be related to steroid discontinuation than to tacrolimus itself. More evidence is needed before deciding to empirically switch all hypertensive transplant patients from CsA to tacrolimus.

Hyperlipidemia

Hyperlipidemia and obesity occur in the majority of solid organ recipients following transplantation.[493–498] Many renal and cardiac transplant recipients have pre-existing hyperlipidemia, which may have contributed to their end-stage organ disease, and transplantation of the corresponding organ does not correct their hyperlipidemia, unlike a new liver. Following transplantation, these patients receive numerous medications that may further exacerbate their hyperlipidemia and inability to control their weight.

The major concern is the increased risk associated with these factors, especially the risk of developing coronary artery disease and the subsequent need for coronary artery bypass surgery in a transplant recipient. In contrast to recipients of other organs, it is not clear whether hyperlipidemia and obesity are the primary causes of transplant coronary artery disease (TCAD) in cardiac transplant recipients or just the adverse milieu in which it thrives.[493] It is also unclear whether improved control of plasma lipids and obesity can prevent chronic graft rejection in heart transplant recipients and coronary artery disease in other organ recipients to the same extent observed in nontransplant patients.

Elevation of plasma lipids has been associated with both corticosteroid and CsA use.[499] Several studies have demonstrated that prednisone is the primary culprit[500–502] and that prednisone withdrawal lowers cholesterol levels,[503,504] but conflicting reports also exist.[505–508] CsA has also been implicated as the causative factor in the development of hyperlipidemia after transplantation. One possible mechanism may be a direct toxic effect imposed by CsA on the hepatocyte that results in impaired cellular clearance of low-density lipoprotein by the liver.[467] Withdrawing CsA after converting to AZA-based regimens has resulted in significant decreases in total cholesterol and triglycerides.[509] The finding that withdrawal of either CsA or prednisone produces a decline in lipid concentrations may actually reflect an additive or synergistic hyperlipidemic response produced by this combination of drugs. If necessary, the use of alternate-day steroids or the discontinuation of prednisone[503,504] or CsA[509] may be considered, but the efficacy of these methods has not been fully evaluated in all types of organ transplants. Preliminary data suggest a much lower incidence of hyperlipidemia with tacrolimus. However, the majority of these studies were conducted in liver transplant recipients, who generally have a lower incidence of hyperlipidemia.[81] The salutary effect of tacrolimus on the incidence of hyperlipidemia may be related to its potency and associated steroid-sparing effects.

Treatment of hyperlipidemia in transplant patients is similar to that of other patients. Before drug therapy is implemented, a low-fat diet in combination with a weight reduction and exercise program should be instituted.[510] In most transplant patients, drug therapy needs to be added to these basic interventions. Because many of these patients receive treatment for hyperlipidemia before transplantation, a thorough drug history can reveal which drugs were most effective. However, because of the problematic drug interactions between CsA and many lipid-lowering drugs, additional caution is necessary following transplantation. The rapidly progressive nature of TCAD in heart transplant patients may require that therapy be started even before the lipid values reach concentrations necessitating drug therapy, according to the National Cholesterol Education Program (NCEP) II guidelines.[493]

Drug treatment of hyperlipidemia has varied; there have been few controlled, randomized trials evaluating the efficacy of the available agents in transplant recipients.[511,512] Cholestyramine is a useful agent but should not be administered within two hours of CsA, as it may alter the absorption of CsA.[513] Cholestyramine should not be administered to patients taking MMF, because the bioavailability of MMF is reduced by at least 40% by concurrent cholestyramine therapy. More important, that cholestyramine can also impair the absorption of other drugs should be taken into consideration, especially in those patients on other life-sustaining medications (e.g., amiodarone, digoxin, or diuretics). Niacin is useful, provided the dosage is titrated slowly. However, it should not be used in transplant patients with diabetes or hyperuricemia or in combination with multiple drugs metabolized by CYP450, because of the increased potential for drug interactions. Newer agents (e.g., pravastatin, simvastatin, and fluvastatin) appear to be the drugs of choice for treatment of hyperlipidemia in CsA-treated patients. Lovastatin is also safe and effective, provided the daily dose does not exceed 20 mg.[511] The major concern is that CsA inhibits the metabolism of lovastatin, resulting in elevated serum concentrations of lovastatin and its metabolites. This drug combination has been associated with elevated creatinine phosphokinase concentrations, rhabdomyolysis, and acute renal failure.[512–515] Because these drugs are metabolized at the CYP450 site, concomitant administration of other inhibitors or competitors (e.g., gemfibrozil, erythromycin, or calcium antagonists) should be undertaken cautiously. In preliminary studies, these agents have been reported to have immunosuppressive properties that result in a lower incidence of rejection.[516] Whether this finding is due to an inherent immunologic effect or to an enhanced pharmacodynamic effect of CsA remains to be proven.

Diabetes Mellitus

The incidence of native diabetes mellitus in solid organ recipients varies with the type of organ transplanted. Diabetes is a common indication for kidney and/or pancreas transplantation, whereas until recently it was an absolute contraindication for heart and/or lung transplantation. Now many patients with cystic fibrosis who undergo lung transplantation also have diabetes. With the availability of more steroid-sparing immunosuppressive agents, a number of these patients with pre-existing diabetes are now considered eligible for lifesaving transplant procedures.

The significance of post-transplant diabetes mellitus (PTDM) is the development of diabetic micro- and macrovascular complications (e.g., coronary heart disease, stroke, retinopathy, nephropathy, or neuropathy) and the higher incidence of infections, all of which can increase morbidity and mortality in the transplant recipient. These findings are especially worrisome because it appears that many of the immunosuppressive agents pose a triple threat by causing hyperlipidemia, hypertension, and hyperglycemia, increasing the risk of death by coronary disease or stroke.[517]

Many patients have a predisposition for diabetes that does not manifest itself until after transplantation, when the patient is treated with corticosteroids or other drugs (e.g., CsA or tacrolimus) known to cause glucose intolerance. The development of de novo PTDM occurs in up to 40% of transplant recipients.[518] Corticosteroids have been reported to decrease insulin receptor number and affinity, impair peripheral glucose uptake in the muscle, impair suppression of endogenous glucose production, impair activation of glucose/fatty acid cycle,[519] and induce insulin resistance.[517] Because it is apparent that reducing steroid dosages has a beneficial effect on PTDM, some centers have advocated the use of steroid-weaning protocols in their diabetic patients; this must be weighed against the risks of both acute and chronic rejection.

Both CsA and tacrolimus are diabetogenic. An increased incidence of PTDM (11–14%) was seen following the introduction of CsA-based regimens, despite a reduction in steroid dosage. CsA may inhibit the clearance of steroids, thus potentiating their diabetogenic effects;[520] however, studies have shown that CsA also affects glycemic control in patients not receiving steroids.[521] CsA has been shown to directly inhibit pancreatic islet cell function and insulin release.[522] Initially, because of tacrolimus's steroid-sparing effects, it was assumed that PTDM would be less problematic with this agent. In fact, the incidence appears to be similar or higher than with CsA-based regimens.[523] Long-term studies are needed to determine what impact tacrolimus's steroid-sparing properties will have on PTDM and its associated complications. These agents may impair insulin secretion, increase insulin resistance, or be directly toxic to beta cells in the pancreas.

The other currently available immunosuppressive agents (AZA, mycophenolate mofetil, and the various antilymphocyte preparations) do not impair glucose tolerance; the use of these agents in addition to much lower doses of steroids and CsA or tacrolimus may be preferable in diabetic patients. The effects of the other investigational agents on glucose tolerance is reviewed elsewhere.[517]

Finally, it is important to remember that, in addition to the primary immunosuppressive agents, many transplant patients may receive other drugs known to exacerbate glycemic control, including thiazide diuretics and β-blockers. Pharmacists can play an important role by identifying drug therapy that can impair glucose tolerance and providing recommendations for alternative agents in these patients. Treatment of diabetes in the transplant patient is similar to that for other diabetic patients; meticulous diabetic control should be the goal in these patients, and a thorough understanding of the added risks and complications is necessary to insure comparable survival to that of nondiabetic organ transplant recipients.

Bone and Muscle Disorders

Musculoskeletal problems are a well-recognized entity following transplantation. As more patients undergo transplantation and survive longer, these complications become even more problematic. In addition, many of the patients have pre-existing bone abnormalities because of older age, postmenopausal status of female recipients, and lower bone mass before transplantation. Cardiac transplant recipients are at risk for a lower pretransplant bone mass because of low cardiac output, prolonged use of loop diuretics, physical inactivity, cardiac cachexia, cigarette smoking, and heparin administration.[524] Many renal transplant recipients have renal osteodystrophy (e.g., osteoporosis, osteomalacia, hyperparathyroidism with osteitis fibrosa, or aluminum-associated bone disease) at the time of transplantation from long-standing renal failure and uremia.[518] Liver transplant patients with cholestatic processes may have low concentrations of 25-hydroxy(vitamin D) due to decreased hepatic production and poor absorption of fat-soluble vitamins, predisposing them to osteomalacia and osteoporosis.[525] Based on a number of clinical studies reviewed elsewhere,[525] most transplant patients appear to be at risk for bone abnormalities going into the transplant procedure. Some of the problems will be corrected (e.g., vitamin D metabolism abnormalities following kidney or liver transplantation), but others will only be further exacerbated by the effects of immunosuppression or subsequent development of renal complications.

Following transplantation, drug-induced bone and muscle complications are common. Corticosteroids are the primary culprit. However, CsA and other immunosuppressants may also contribute to these complications. Corticosteroid complications include osteoporosis, osteopenia, avascular necrosis, and growth retardation. Postulated mechanisms for steroid-related bone complications include direct effects on bone formation and resorption as well as alterations in the secretion of sex hormones, intestinal calcium absorption, the vitamin D system, and renal excretion of calcium and phosphate.[526]

Growth retardation is an especially problematic complication in infants and children undergoing transplantation. Patients on high-dose corticosteroids demonstrate both a delay in bone maturation and lower growth rates, leading to growth retardation.[527]

As the steroid-related bone disturbances appear to be both dose- and duration-dependent, combination therapy with steroid-sparing agents (e.g., CsA or tacrolimus) has been suggested to be beneficial in this regard. A lower incidence of complications, such as avascular necrosis, has been reported,[528,529] but conflicting data are also present. CsA and tacrolimus have both been reported to be deleterious to bone metabolism. AZA and MTX may also have adverse effects on bone turnover.[530] Because most transplant patients receive some combination of immunosuppressive agents, it is difficult to implicate just one unless well-controlled clinical trials are conducted.

Management of bone-related complications in the transplant patient should be based on prevention, including regular exercise and calcium and vitamin D supplementation. Calcitonin, bisphosphonates, and bone-sparing corticosteroids (e.g., deflazacort) may all have a role; however, there are no comprehensive published studies examining the post-transplant effects of these agents.

Because CsA decreases the glomerular filtration rate and the renal handling of urate, it may cause hyperuricemia and gout in the transplant patient.[518] This can be further exacerbated by other drugs, such as diuretics. Treatment of gout is challenging because most of the effective agents can cause other complications in the transplant patient. Uricosuric therapy with probenecid is most effective in patients with a glomerular filtration rate above 50 ml/min and should be used cautiously in the patients with lesser degrees of renal function. Probenecid may also impair the excretion of MTX and mycophenolate mofetil, resulting in increased serum concentrations of these drugs. Allopurinol is very effective, but reductions in AZA dosage are mandatory at the outset of therapy to avoid life-threatening pancytopenia. The use of colchicine may be limited by its propensity to cause gastrointestinal and bone marrow toxicity, exacerbating the known side effects of AZA and mycophenolate mofetil. The nonsteroidal anti-inflammatory drugs are effective for treating gout but may also exacerbate CSA's renal toxicity secondary to prostaglandin inhibition.

Malignancy

Successful maintenance of allograft function requires continuous therapy with potent immunosuppressive agents that interfere with normal immune surveillance and function. The biologic activity of these agents may cause diminished immune surveillance, direct carcinogenic or mutagenic action, chronic antigenic stimulation, or activation of oncogenic viruses, resulting in increased potential for tumor development.[525] Malignant neoplasms are an unfortunate consequence of chronic immunosuppression and may be an unavoidable complication of modifying the normal immune process.[531] Cancers that occur most frequently in the general population (e.g., carcinomas of the lung, prostate, breast, and colon and invasive carcinomas of the uterine cervix) are not increased among transplant recipients. However, various cancers that are uncommon in the general population are often more prevalent in transplant recipients: lymphomas, squamous cell carcinomas of the lip and skin, Kaposi's sarcoma, other sarcomas, carcinomas of the vulva and perineum, carcinomas of the kidney, and hepatobiliary tumors.[532]

The incidence of lymphoma appears to correlate with the intensity of immunosuppression. The use of more intensive immunosuppression in extrarenal transplant recipients is particularly common and is reflected in a higher incidence of lymphomas in cardiac recipients than in renal recipients.[532] The incidence, time to occurrence, and features of the tumors appear to vary with use of various immunosuppressive agents. AZA-based immunosuppressive regimens have been associated with a high incidence of cutaneous malignancies. One possible mechanism to explain this unusually high incidence of skin cancer involves AZA's metabolite nitroimidazole, which causes significant photosensitivity, resulting in subsequent skin cancer.[533,534] One study found that with the introduction of CsA, the incidence of non-Hodgkin's lymphoma or PTLD increased to 29%, in contrast to 11% with regimens based on AZA or CTX.[532] Among patients treated with OKT3 and other MoAbs, lymphomas account for 64% of all tumors. PTLD and its management was discussed earlier under EBV.

SUMMARY

The number of successful heart, lung, liver, kidney, pancreas, and islet cell transplants has increased during the past 15 years as improvements have been made in the effectiveness of immunomodulating agents, surgical techniques, organ donor programs, and preservation fluids for organ transportation.

Postoperative complications following solid organ transplantation can include acute or chronic rejection, infections, hypertension, hyperlipidemia, diabetes, bone disease, or malignancies. Acute rejection is frequently treated with an intravenous steroid pulse with or without a prednisone taper. Chronic rejection may require retransplantation.

REFERENCES

1. Venkataramanan R, Habucky K, Burckart GJ, *et al.* Clinical pharmacokinetics in organ transplant patients. *Clin Pharmacokin.* 1989;116(3):134–61.
2. Carrel A, Guthrie CC. The transplantation of veins and organs. *Am J Med.* 1905;10:1101–2.
3. Murray JE, Merrill JP, Dammin GJ, *et al.* Studies on transplantation immunity after total body irradiation: clinical and experimental investigations. *Surgery* 1960;48:272–84.
4. Flye MW. History of transplantation. In: *Principles of Organ Transplantation.* Philadelphia, PA: WB Saunders; 1989. p. 1–17.
5. Schwartz R, Dameschek W. Drug-induced immunological tolerance. *Nature* 1959;183:1682.
6. Hitchings GH, Elion BG, Falco EA, *et al.* Antagonists of nucleic acid derivatives. I. The lactobacillus case model. *J Bio Chem.* 1950;183:1.
7. Starzl TE, Marchioro TL, Waddell WR. The reversal of rejection in human renal homografts with subsequent development of homograft tolerance. *Surg Gynecol Obstet.* 1963;117:385–95.
8. Kohler G, Milstein C. Continuous cultures of fused cells secreting antibody of predefined specificity. *Nature* 1975; 256:495–7.
9. United Network for Organ Sharing. Personal communication to K. Lake, 1997.
10. Bach FH, Sachs DH. Transplant immunology. *N Engl J Med.* 1987;317:482–92.
11. Halloran PF, Broski AP, Batiuk TD, *et al.* The molecular immunology of acute rejection: an overview. *Transplant Immunol.* 1993;1(1):3–27.
12. Krams SM, Ascher NL, Martinez OM. New immunologic insights into mechanisms of allograft rejection. *Gastroenterol Clin North Am.* 1993;22(2)381–400.
13. Strom TB. Molecular immunology and immunopharmacology of allograft rejection. *Kidney Int.* 1992;42 (*Suppl* 38):S182–7.
14. Krensky AM, Weiss A, Crabtree G, *et al.* T-lymphocyte-antigens interactions in transplant rejection. *N Engl J Med.* 1990;322(8):510–7.
15. Morris RE. New immunosuppressive drugs. In: Busuttil RW, Klintmalm GB, editors. *Transplantation of the Liver.* Philadelphia, PA: Saunders; 1996. p. 760–86.
16. Peters DH, Fitton A, Plosker GL, *et al.* Tacrolimus: a review of its pharmacology, and therapeutic potential in hepatic and renal transplantation. *Drugs* 1993;46(4):746–94.
17. Klintmalm G. A review of FK506: a new immunosuppressant agent for the prevention and rescue of graft rejection. *Transplant Rev.* 1994;8(2):53–62.
18. Allison AC, Eugui EM. The design and development of an immunosuppressive drug, mycophenolate mofetil. *Springer Semin Immunopathol.* 1993;14(4):353–80.
19. Allison AC, Eugui EM, Sollinger HW. Mycophenolate mofetil: mechanisms of action and effects in transplantation. *Transplant Rev.* 1993;7(3):129–39.
20. Kahan BD, Dunn J, Fitts C, *et al.* Reduced inter- and intrasubject variability in cyclosporine pharmacokinetics in renal transplant recipients treated with a microemulsion formulation in conjunction with fasting, low-fat meals, or high-fat meals. *Transplantation* 1995;59(4):505–11.
21. Kovarik JM, Mueller EA, van Bree JB, *et al.* Cyclosporine pharmacokinetics and variability from a microemulsion formulation—a multicenter investigation in kidney transplant patients. *Transplantation* 1994;58(6):658–63.
22. Mueller EA, Kovarik JM, van Bree JB, *et al.* Pharmacokinetics and tolerability of a microemulsion formulation of cyclosporine in renal allograft recipients—a concentration-controlled comparison with the commercial formulation. *Transplantation* 1994;57(8):1178–82.
23. Huser B, Thiel G, Oberholzer M, *et al.* The efficacy and tolerability of cyclosporine G in human kidney transplant recipients. *Transplantation* 1992;54:65–9.
24. Henry ML, Tesi RJ, Elkhammas EA, *et al.* A randomized, prospective, double-blinded trial of cyclosporine vs. OG37-325 in cadaveric renal transplantation—a preliminary report. *Transplantation* 1993;55(4):748–51.
25. Xiao F, Chong AS, Foster P, *et al.* Leflunomide controls rejection in hamster to rat cardiac xenografts. *Transplantation* 1994;58(7):828–34.
26. McChesney LP, Xiao F, Sankary HN, *et al.* An evaluation of leflunomide in the canine renal transplantation model. *Transplantation* 1994;57(12):1717–22.
27. Tornatore KM, Reed KA, Venuto RC. Racial differences in the pharmacokinetics of methylprednisolone in black and white renal transplant patients. *Pharmacotherapy* 1993; 13(5):481–6.
28. Kobashigawa JA, Stevenson LW, Moriguchi JD, *et al.* Is intravenous glucocorticoid therapy better than an oral regimen for asymptomatic cardiac rejection? A randomized trial. *J Am Coll Cardiol.* 1993;21(5):1142–4.
29. Fryer JP, Granger DK, Leventhal JR, *et al.* Steroid-related complications in the cyclosporine era. *Clin Transplant.*

1994;8:224–9.
30. Arizon JM, Anguita M, Valles F, *et al.* A randomized study comparing deflazacort and prednisone in heart transplant patients. *J Heart Lung Transplant.* 1993;12(5):864–8.
31. Elli A, Rivolta R, Di Palo FQ, *et al.* A randomized trial of deflazacort versus 6-methylprednisolone in renal transplantation—immunosuppressive activity and side effects. *Transplantation* 1993;55(1):209–12.
32. Arizon JM, Anguita M, Valles F, *et al.* Preliminary experience with deflazacort, a new synthetic steroid with fewer undesirable side effects, in heart transplant patients. *J Heart Lung Transplant.* 1993;12(3):445–9.
33. O'Connell PJ, d'Apice AJF, Walker RG, *et al.* Results of steroid withdrawal in renal allograft recipients on low-dose cyclosporine A, azathioprine and prednisone. *Clin Transplant.* 1988;2:102–6.
34. Hricik DE, Alamawi WY, Strom TB. Trends in the use of glucocorticoids in renal transplantation. *Transplantation* 1994;57(7):979–89.
35. Opelz G. Effect of the maintenance immunosuppressive drug regimen on kidney transplant outcome. *Transplantation* 1994;58(4):443–6.
36. Romani F, Belli LS, De Carlis L, *et al.* Cyclosporin monotherapy (after 3 months) in liver transplant patients: a prospective randomized trial. *Transplant Proc.* 1994;26(5): 2683–5.
37. Schulak JA, Mayes JT, Moritz CE, *et al.* A prospective randomized trial of prednisone versus no prednisone maintenance therapy in cyclosporine-treated and azathioprine-treated renal transplant patients. *Transplantation* 1990;49 (2):327–32.
38. Au J, Gregory JW, Colquhoun IW, *et al.* Paediatric cardiac transplantation with steroid-sparing maintenance immunosuppression. *Arch Dis Child.* 1992;67(10):1262–6.
39. Schreiber SL, Crabtree GR. The mechanism of action of cyclosporin A and FK506. *Immunol Today* 1992;13:136–42.
40. Kahan BD. Cyclosporine. *N Engl J Med.* 1989;321(25): 1725–38.
41. Canafax DM. Minimizing cyclosporine concentration variability to optimize transplant outcome. *Clin Transplant.* 1995;9(1):1–13.
42. Yee GC, McGuire TR, Gmur DJ, *et al.* Blood cyclosporine pharmacokinetics in patients undergoing marrow transplantation. *Transplantation* 1988;46:399–402.
43. Lake KD. Update and management of CsA drug interactions. *Pharmacotherapy* 1991;11(5):110S–118S.
44. Lake, K.D. Drug interactions in transplant patients. In: Emery RW, and Miller LW, editors. *Handbook of Cardiac Transplantation.* Philadelphia, PA: Hanley & Belfus; 1995. p. 147–64.
45. Yee GC, McGuire TR, *et al.* Pharmacokinetic interactions with cyclosporine. Parts I and II. *Clin Pharmacokin.* 1990; 19:319–32.
46. Cantarovich M, Fitchett D, Latter DA. Cyclosporine trough levels, acute rejection, and renal dysfunction after heart transplantation. *Transplantation* 1995;59(3):444–7.
47. Beutler D, Molteni S, Zeugin T, *et al.* Evaluation of instrumental, nonisotopic immunoassays (fluorescence polarization immunoassay and enzyme-multiplied immunoassay technique) for cyclosporine monitoring in whole blood after kidney and liver transplantation. *Ther Drug Monit.* 1992;14:424–32.
48. Alvarez JS, Sacristan JA, Alsar MJ. Comparison of a monoclonal antibody fluorescent polarization immunoassay with monoclonal antibody radioimmunoassay for cyclosporin determination in whole blood. *Ther Drug Monit.* 1992;14: 78–80.
49. Yee GC, Self SG, McGuire TR, *et al.* Serum cyclosporine concentrations and risk of acute GVHD after allogeneic marrow transplantation. *N Engl J Med.* 1988;319:65–70.
50. Oellerich M, Armstrong VW, Kahan B, *et al.* Lake Louise Consensus Conference on cyclosporin monitoring in organ transplantation: report of the consensus panel [review]. *Ther Drug Monit.* 1995;17(6):642–54.
51. Burke JF, Pirsch JD, Ramos EF, *et al.* Long-term efficacy and safety of cyclosporine in renal-transplant recipients. *N Engl J Med.* 1994;331(6):358–63.
52. Moran M, Mozes MF, Maddux MS, *et al.* Prevention of acute graft rejection by the prostaglandin E_1 analogue misoprostol in renal-transplant recipients treated with cyclosporine and prednisone. *N Engl J Med.* 1990;322(17): 1183–8.
53. Luke J, Luke DR, Williams LA, *et al.* Prevention of cyclosporine-induced nephrotoxicity with transdermal clonidine. *Clin Pharm.* 1990;9:4953.
54. Bianco JA, Almgren, J, Kern DE, *et al.* Evidence that oral pentoxifylline reverses acute renal dysfunction in bone marrow transplant recipients receiving amphotericin B and cyclosporine. *Transplantation* 1991;51:925–7.
55. Dawidson I, Rooth P, Fry WR, *et al.* Prevention of acute cyclosporine-induced renal blood flow inhibition and improved immunosuppression with verapamil. *Transplantation* 1989;48(4):575–80.
56. Morales JM, Andres A, Alvarez C, *et al.* Calcium channel blockers and early cyclosporine nephrotoxicity after renal transplantation: a prospective randomized study. *Transplant Proc.* 1990;22(4):1733–5.
57. Scott JP, Higenbottam TW. Adverse reactions and interactions of cyclosporin. *Med Toxicol.* 1988;3:107–27.
58. Bunke M, Ganzel B. Effect of calcium channel antagonists on renal function in hypertensive heart transplant recipients. *J Heart Lung Transplant.* 1992;11(6):1194–9.
59. Watson CJ, Metcalfe SM, St. John Collier DG, *et al.* A comparative study of cyclosporine and its derivative SDZ IMM-125 in canine renal allografts. *Transplantation* 1993; 56(5):1248–50.
60. U.S. Multicenter FK506 Liver Study Group. A comparison of tacrolimus (FK 506) and cyclosporine for immunosuppression in liver transplantation. *N Engl Med.* 1994; 331(17):1110–5.
61. European FK506 Multicentre Liver Study Group. Randomized trial comparing tacrolimus (FK506) and cyclosporin in prevention of liver allograft rejection. *Lancet* 1994;344: 423–8.
62. Shapiro R, Jordan M, Scantlebury V, *et al.* A prospective, randomized trial of FK-506 in renal transplantation—a comparison between double- and triple-drug therapy. *Clin Transplant.* 1994;8:508–15.
63. Shapiro R, Jordan ML, Scantlebury, *et al.* A prospective randomized trial of FK506-based immunosuppression after renal transplantation. *Transplantation* 1995;59(4):485–90.

64. Griffith BP, Bando K, Hardesty RL, *et al.* A prospective randomized trial of FK506 versus cyclosporine after human pulmonary transplantation. *Transplantation* 1994;57 (6):848–51.
65. Armitage JM, Kormos RL, Morita S, *et al.* Clinical trial of FK 506 immunosuppression in adult cardiac transplantation. *Ann Thorac Surg.* 1992;54:205–11.
66. Egawa H, Esquivel CO, So SK, *et al.* FK506 conversion therapy in pediatric liver transplantation. *Transplantation* 1994;57(8):1169–73.
67. Jordan ML, Shapiro R, Vivas CA, *et al.* FK506 "rescue" for resistant rejection of renal allografts under primary cyclosporine immunosuppression. *Transplantation* 1994;57 (6):860–5.
68. Kino T, Hatanaka H, Miyata S, *et al.* FK-506, a novel immunosuppressant isolated from a streptomyces. II. Immunosuppressive effect of FK-506 in vitro. *J Antibiot.* 1987; 40:1256–65.
69. Sawada S, Suzuki G, Kawase Y, *et al.* Novel immunosuppressive agent, FK506 in vitro effects on the cloned T-cell activation. *J Immunol.* 1987;139:1797–803.
70. Zeevi A, Duquesnoy R, Eiras G, *et al.* Immunosuppressive effect on FK-506 on in vitro lymphocyte alloactivation: synergism with cyclosporine A. *Transplant Proc.* 1987;19 (*Suppl* 6):40–4.
71. McDiarmid SV, Colonna JO, Shaked A, *et al.* Differences in oral FK506 dose requirements between adult and pediatric liver transplant patients. *Transplantation* 1993;55(6): 1328–32.
72. Venkataramanan R, Jain A, Cadoff E, *et al.* Pharmacokinetics of FK506 preclinical and clinical studies. *Transplant Proc.* 1990;22(1):52–6.
73. Starzl TE, Todo S, Fung JJ, *et al.* FK-506 for liver, kidney and pancreas transplantation. *Lancet* 1989;2:1000–4.
74. Burke MD, Omar G, Thomson AW, *et al.* Inhibition of the metabolism of cyclosporine by human liver microsomes by FK506. *Transplantation* 1990;50(5):901–2.
75. Newhaus P, Blumhardt G, Bechstein WO, *et al.* Comparison of FK506- and cyclosporine-based immunosuppression in primary orthotopic liver transplantation. *Transplantation* 1995;59:31–40.
76. Tamura K, Kobayashi M, Hashimoto K, *et al.* A highly sensitive method to assay FK-506 levels in plasma. *Transplant Proc.* 1987;5(*Suppl* 6):23–9.
77. Backman L, Nicar M, Leve M, *et al.* FK506 trough levels in whole blood and plasma in liver transplant recipients: correlation with clinical events and side effects. *Transplantation* 1994;57(4):519–25.
78. Starzl TE, Abu-Elmagd K, Tzakis A, *et al.* Selected topics on FK506, with special references to rescue of extrahepatic whole organs grafts, transplantation of "forbidden organs," side effects, mechanisms and practical pharmacokinetics. *Transplant Proc.* 1991;23(1):914–9.
79. Alessiani M, Kusne S, Martin M, *et al.* Infection in adult liver transplantation under FK-506 immunosuppression. *Transplant Proc.* 1991;23(1):1501–3.
80. McDiarmid SV, Colonna JO, Shaked A, *et al.* A comparison of renal function in cyclosporine- and FK506-treated patients after primary orthotopic liver transplantation. *Transplantation* 1993;56(4):847–53.
81. Steinmuller TM, Graf K, Schleicher J, *et al.* The effect of FK506 versus cyclosporine on glucose and lipid metabolism—a randomized trial. *Transplantation* 1994;58(6):669–74.
82. Reyes J, Gayoiski T, Fung JJ, *et al.* Expressive dysphasia possibly related to FK506 in two liver transplant recipients. *Transplantation* 1990;50(6):1043–4.
83. Abu-Elmagd K, Fung JJ, Alessiani M, *et al.* The effect of graft function on FK-506 plasma levels, doses and renal function with particular reference to the liver. *Transplantation* 1991;52:81–7.
84. Mor E, Sheiner PA, Schwartz ME, *et al.* Reversal of severe FK506 side effects by conversion to cyclosporine-based immunosuppression. *Transplantation* 1994;58(3):380–2.
85. Taylor-Fishwick DA, Kahan M, Hiestand P, *et al.* Evidence that rapamycin has differential effects on IL-4 function. Multiple IL-4 signaling pathways and implications for in vivo use. *Transplantation* 1993;56(2):368–74.
86. Morris RE, Wu J, Shorthouse R, *et al.* A study of the contrasting effects of cyclosporine, FK506, and rapamycin on the suppression of allograft rejection. *Transplant Proc.* 1990; 22(4):1638–41.
87. Wood RP, Katz SM, Kahan BD. New immunosuppressive agents. *Transplant Sci.* 1991;1(1):34–46.
88. Morris RE, Meiser BM, Wu J, *et al.* Use of rapamycin for the suppression of alloimmune reactions in vivo: schedule dependence, tolerance induction, synergy with cyclosporine and FK506, and effect on host-versus-graft and graft-versus-host reactions. *Transplant Proc.* 1991;23(1): 521–4.
89. Almond PS, Moss A, Nakhleh RE, *et al.* Rapamycin: immunosuppression, hyporesponsiveness, and side effects in a porcine renal allograft model. *Transplantation* 1993;56(2): 275–81.
90. Amemiya H, Suzuki S, Ota K, *et al.* A novel rescue drug, 15-deoxyspergualin. First clinical trials for recurrent graft rejection in renal recipients. *Transplantation* 1990;49(2): 337–43.
91. Takahashi K, Ota K, Tanabe K, *et al.* Effect of a novel immunosuppressive agent, deoxyspergualin on rejection in kidney transplant recipients. *Transplant Proc.* 1990;22 (4):1606–12.
92. Groth CG, Ohlman S, Ericson BG, *et al.* Deoxyspergualin for liver graft rejection [letter]. *Lancet* 1990;336(8715):626.
93. Okazaki H, Sato T, Jimbo M, *et al.* Prophylactic use of deoxyspergualin in living related renal transplantation. *Transplant Proc.* 1991;23:1094–5.
94. Koyama I, Amemiya H, Taguchi Y, *et al.* Prophylactic use of deoxyspergualin in a quadruple immunosuppressive protocol in renal transplantation. *Transplant Proc.* 1991;23: 1096–8.
95. Matas AJ, Kelley SL, Bielefield-Skrokov M, *et al.* Pilot evaluation of 15-deoxyspergualin for refractory acute renal transplant rejection. *Clin Transplant.* 1994;8:116–9.
96. Chan GL, Canafax DM, Johnson CA. The therapeutic use of azathioprine in renal transplantation. *Pharmacotherapy* 1987;7(5):165–77.
97. Van Scoik KG, Johnson CA, Porter WR. The pharmacology and metabolism of the thiopurine drugs 6-mercaptopurine and azathioprine. *Drug Metab Rev.* 1985;16(1&2): 157–74.
98. Odlind B, Grefberg N, Hartvig P, *et al.* Pharmacokinetics

of azathioprine and 6-mercaptopurine: methodological aspects and preliminary results in uremic patients. *Scand J Urol Nephrol*. 1981;64(*Suppl*):213–9.

99. Odlind B, Hartvig P, Lindstrom B, *et al.* Serum azathioprine and 6-mercaptopurine levels and immunosuppression activity after azathioprine in uremic patients. *Int J Immunopharmacol*. 1986;8:1–11.
100. Lin SN, Jessup K, Floyd M, *et al.* Quantitation of plasma azathioprine and 6-mercaptopurine levels in renal transplant patients. *Transplantation* 1980;29:290–4.
101. Maddocks JL. Clinical pharmacological observations on azathioprine in kidney transplant patients [abstract]. *Clin Sci Mol Med*. 1978;55:20P.
102. Chan GL, Erdmann GR, Gruber SA, *et al.* Pharmacokinetics of 6-thiouric acid and 6-mercaptopurine in renal allograft recipients after oral administration of azathioprine. *Eur J Clin Pharmacol*. 1989;36(3):265–71.
103. Chan GL, Gruber SA, Skjei KL, *et al.* Principles of immunosuppression. *Crit Care Clin*. 1990;6(4):841–92.
104. Ding TL, Benet LZ. Determination of 6-mercaptopurine and azathioprine in plasma by high-performance liquid chromatography. *J Chromatogr*. 1979;163:281–8.
105. Ding TL, Gamberatoglio JG, Amend WJC, *et al.* Azathioprine (AZA) bioavailability and pharmacokinetics in kidney transplant patients [abstract]. *Clin Pharmacol Ther*. 1980;27(2):250.
106. Watts GF, Corston R. Hypersensitivity to azathioprine in myasthenia gravis. *Postgrad Med J*. 1984;60:362–3.
107. Brooks RJ, Dorr RT, Durie BGM. Interaction of allopurinol with 6-mercaptopurine and azathioprine. *Biomedicine* 1982;36:217–22.
108. Coffey JJ, White CA, Lesk AB, *et al.* Effect of allopurinol on the pharmacokinetics of 6-mercaptopurine (MSC 775) in cancer patients. *Cancer Res*. 1972;32:1283–9.
109. Vetten KB. Immunosuppressive therapy and anesthesia. *South African Med J*. 1973;47:767–70.
110. Dretchen KL, Morgenroth VH III, Standaert FG, *et al.* Azathioprine: effects on neuromuscular transmission. *Anesthesiology* 1976;45:604–9.
111. Spiers ASD, Mibashan PS. Increased warfarin requirement during mercaptopurine therapy: a new drug interaction. *Lancet* 1974;2:221–2.
112. Winklestein A. The effects of azathioprine and 6MP on immunity. *J Immunopharmacol*. 1979;1:429–54.
113. Maddocks JL, Lennard L, Amess J, *et al.* Azathioprine and severe bone marrow depression [letter]. *Lancet* 1986;1:156.
114. Lennard L, Murphy MF, Maddocks JL, *et al.* Severe megaloblastic anaemia associated with abnormal azathioprine metabolism. *Br J Clin Pharmacol*. 1984;17:171–2.
115. Old CW, Flannery EP, Grogan TM, *et al.* Azathioprine-induced pure red blood cell aplasia. *JAMA* 1978;240:552–4.
116. Rosman M, Bertino JR. Azathioprine. *Ann Intern Med*. 1973;79:694–700.
117. Berne TV, Chatterjee SN, Craig JR, *et al.* Hepatic dysfunction in recipients of renal allografts. *Surg Gynecol Obstet*. 1975;141:171–5.
118. Zarday Z, Veith FJ, Gliedman ML, *et al.* Irreversible liver damage after azathioprine. *JAMA* 1972;222:690–1.
119. McCormack JJ, Johns DG. Purine antimetabolites. In: Chabner B, editor. *Pharmacologic Principles of Cancer Treatment*. Philadelphia, PA: WB Saunders; 1982. p. 213–8.
120. Nakashima Y, Howard JM. Drug-induced acute pancreatitis. *Surg Gynecol Obstet*. 1977;145:105–9.
121. Penn I. Cancer is a complication of severe immunosuppression. *Surg Gynecol Obstet*. 1986;162:603–10.
122. Kaufmann SHE, Han H, Diamanstein T. Relative susceptibilities of T-cell subsets involved in delayed type hypersensitivity to sheep red cells to the in vitro action of 4-hydroperoxycyclophosphamide. *J Immunol*. 1980;125:1304–8.
123. Ozer H, Cowens JW, Colvin M, *et al.* In vitro effects of 4-hydroperoxycyclophosphamide on human immunoregulatory T subset function. *J Exp Med*. 1982;155:276–90.
124. Hengst JCD, Kempf RA. Immunomodulation by cyclophosphamide. *Clin Immunol Allergy* 1984;4(2):199–216.
125. Connors TA. Alkylating drugs, nitrosourea and dialkyl triazenes. In: Pinedo HM, editor. *Cancer Chemotherapy*. Amsterdam: Elsevier-North Holland; 1979. p. 25–55.
126. Starzl TE, Halgrimson CG, Penn I. Cyclosphophamide and human organ transplantation. *Lancet* 1971;2:70–4.
127. Yadav RVS, Indudhara R, Kumar P, *et al.* Cyclophosphamide in renal transplantation. *Transplantation* 1988;45(2):421–4.
128. Evrard HM, Miller C, Schwartz M, *et al.* Resistant hepatic allograft rejection successfully treated with cyclophosphamide and plasmapheresis. *Transplantation* 1990;50(4):702–20.
129. Taylor DO, Bristow MR, O'Connell JB, *et al.* A prospective, randomized comparison of cyclophosphamide and azathioprine for early rejection prophylaxis after cardiac transplantation-decreased sensitization to OKT3. *Transplantation* 1994;58(6):645–9.
130. Hanto DW, Eastman J, Park SI, *et al.* Plasmapheresis, cytoxan, splenectomy and quadruple therapy to reduce the risk of antibody-mediated rejection in ABO incompatible liver transplantation [abstract]. Second Congress of the International Liver Transplantation Society; Oct. 6, 1993; Toronto, Ontario.
131. Ahmed AR, Hombal SM. Cyclophosphamide (Cytoxan). A review on relevant pharmacology and clinical uses. *J Am Acad Dermatol*. 1984;11:1115–26.
132. Moore MJ. Clinical pharmacokinetics of cyclophosphamide. *Clin Pharmacokinet*. 1991;20:194–208.
133. Cunningham D, Cummings J, Blackie RB, *et al.* The pharmacokinetics of high dose cyclophosphamide and high dose etoposide. *Med Oncol Tumor Pharmacother*. 1988;5:117–23.
134. Steinherz IJ, Steinherz PG. Cyclophosphamide cardiotoxicity. *Cancer Bull*. 1985;37:231–4.
135. Chabner BA, Myers CE. Clinical pharmacology of cancer chemotherapy. In: DeVita VT Jr., Hellman S, Rosenberg SA, editors. *Cancer: Principles and Practice of Oncology*. Philadelphia, PA: JB Lippincott; 1989. p. 349–95.
136. Costanzo-Nordin MR, Grusk BB, Silver MA, *et al.* Reversal of recalcitrant cardiac allograft rejection with methotrexate. *Circulation* 1988;78(*Suppl* 3):47–57.
137. Olsen SL, O'Connell JB, Bristow MR, *et al.* Methotrexate as an adjunct in the treatment of persistent mild cardiac allograft rejection. *Transplantation* 1990;50(5):773–5.
138. Chan GL, Weinstein SS, Vijayanagar RR, *et al.* Treatment of recalcitrant cardiac allograft rejection with methotrex-

ate. *Clin Transplant*. 1995;9(2):106–14.

139. Sollinger HW, Deierhoi MH, Belzer FO, *et al.* RS-61443 (mycophenolate mofetil)—a phase I clinical study and pilot rescue trial. *Transplantation* 1992;53:428–32.
140. Sollinger HW, Belzer FO, Deierhoi MH, *et al.* RS-61443 (mycophenolate mofetil)—a multicenter study for refractory kidney transplant rejection. *Ann Surg*. 1992;216:513–9.
141. Klintmalm GB, Ascher NL, Busutill RW, *et al.* RS-61443 for the treatment of resistant human liver rejection. *Transplant Proc*. 1993;25(1 *Pt* 1):697.
142. Taylor DO, Ensley RD, Olsen SL, *et al.* Mycophenolate mofetil (RS-61443): preclinical, clinical and three year experience in heart transplantation. *J Heart Lung Transplant*. 1994;13:571–82.
143. Sollinger HW. Mycophenolate mofetil for the prevention of acute rejection in primary cadaveric renal allograft recipients. U.S. Renal Transplant Mycophenolate Mofetil Study Group. *Transplantation* 1995;60(3):225–32.
144. European Mycophenolate Mofetil Cooperative Study Group. Placebo-controlled study of mycophenolate mofetil combined with cyclosporin and corticosteroids for prevention of acute rejection. *Lancet* 1995;345(8961):1321–5.
145. CellCept® (Mycophenolate Mofetil) Package Insert. Roche Laboratories, Nutley, NJ.
146. Alfieri C, Kieff E, Allison AC. Effect of mycophenolic acid on Epstein-Barr virus infection on human B lymphocytes. *Antimicrob Agents Chemother*. 1994;38:126–9.
147. Morris RE. Mechanisms of action of new immunosuppressive drugs [review]. *Ther Drug Monit*. 1995;17(6):564–9.
148. Cramer DV. Brequinar sodium [review]. *Pediatr Nephrol*. 1995;9(*Suppl*):S52–5.
149. Woodruff MFA, Anderson NF. Effect of lymphocyte depletion by thoracic duct fistula and administration of antilymphocyte serum on the survival of skin homografts in rats. *Nature* 1963;200:702–4.
150. Delmonico FL, Auchincloss H, Rubin RH, *et al.* The selective use of antilymphocyte serum for cyclosporine treated patients with renal allograft dysfunction. *Ann Surg*. 1987;206:649–54.
151. Fassbinder W, Scheuermann EH, Stutte HJ, *et al.* Improved graft prognosis by treatment of steroid-resistant rejections with ATG and plasmapheresis. *Proc Eur Dialysis Transplant Assn*. 1983;20:362–7.
152. Hardy MA, Nowygrod R, Elberg A, *et al.* Use of ATG in treatment of steroid-resistant rejection. *Transplantation* 1980;29:162–4.
153. Kreis H, Mansoum R, Descamps JM, *et al.* Antithymocyte globulin in cadaver kidney transplantation: a randomized trial based on T-cell monitoring. *Kidney Int*. 1981;19:438–44.
154. Nelson PW, Cosimi AB, Delmonico FL, *et al.* Antithymocyte globulin as the primary treatment for renal allograft rejection. *Transplantation* 1983;36:587–9.
155. Sheil GR, Mears D, Kelly GE, *et al.* A controlled trial of antilymphocyte globulin therapy (ALG) in man. *Transplant Proc*. 1972;4:501–5.
156. Shield CF, Cosimi AB, Tolkoff-Rubin N, *et al.* Use of antithymocyte globulin for reversal of acute allograft rejection. *Transplantation* 1979;28:461–9.
157. Starzl TE, Marchioro TL, Porter KKA, *et al.* The use of heterologous antilymphoid agents in canine renal and liver homotransplantation and human renal homotransplantation. *Surg Gynecol Obstet*. 1967;124(2):301–8.
158. Fries D, Hiesse C, Lantz O, *et al.* Optimization of antilymphocytes globulin in renal transplantation. *Transplant Proc*. 1990;22(4):1793–4.
159. Stratta RJ, D'Alessandro AM, Armbrust MIJ, *et al.* Sequential antilymphoctye globulin/cyclosporine immunosuppression in cadaveric renal transplantation. *Transplantation* 1989;47(1):96–102.
160. Cosimi AB. Antilymphocyte globulin: a final (?) look. In: Morris PJ, Tilney NL, editors. *Progress in Transplantation*. Edinburgh: Churchill Livingstone; 1985:167–88.
161. Cosimi AB, Delmonico FL. Anti-lymphocyte antibody immunosuppressive therapy. In: Williams GM, Burdick JF, Solez K, editors. *Kidney Transplant Rejection*. New York: Marcel Dekker; 1986. p. 335–40.
162. Macdonald PS, Mundy J. Keogh AM, *et al.* A prospective randomized study of prophylactic OKT3 versus equine antithymocyte globulin after heart transplantation—increased morbidity with OKT3. *Transplantation* 1993;55 (1):110–6.
163. Atgam Package Insert. The Upjohn Company; Kalamazoo, MI.
164. Clark KR, Forsythe JLR, Shenton BK, *et al.* Flow-cytometric monitoring of ATG therapy for steroid-resistant rejection. *Transplant Proc*. 1992;24(1):315.
165. Cerilli G, Brastle L, Clarke J, *et al.* Correlation of cell reaction patterns and in vitro immunosuppression capabilities of six ATG products used clinically. *Transplant Proc*. 1985;17:2760.
166. Clark KR, Forsythe JLR, Shenton BK, *et al.* Administration of ATG according to the absolute T-lymphocyte count during therapy for steroid-resistant rejection. *Transpl Int*. 1993;6:18–21.
167. Lawley TJ, Bielory L, Gascon P, *et al.* A prospective clinical and immunologic analysis of patients with serum sickness. *N Engl J Med*. 1984;311:1407–13.
168. Vermnier I, Giraud P, Eche JP, *et al.* Hematologic side effects of antilymphocyte globulins: prevalence and impact on therapeutic protocol. *Transplant Proc*. 1985;17:2765–6.
169. Melosky B, Karim M, Chui A, *et al.* Lymphoproliferative disorders after renal transplantation in patients receiving triple or quadruple immunosuppression [review]. *J Am Soc Nephrol*. 1992;2(*Suppl* 12):S290–4.
170. Chang TW, Kung PC, Gingras SP, *et al.* Does OKT3 monoclonal antibody react with an antigen-recognition structure on human T-cells? *Proc Natl Acad Sci USA* 1981;78 (3):1805–8.
171. Reinherz EL, Meuer S, Fitzgerald KA, *et al.* Antigen recognition by human T-lymphocytes is linked to surface expression of the T-3 molecular complex. *Cell* 1982;30:735–43.
172. Chatenoud L, Bandrihaye MF, Krefs H, *et al.* Human in vivo antigenic modulation induced by the anti-T-cell OKT3 monoclonal antibody. *Eur J Immunol*. 1982;12:979–82.
173. Delmonico FL, Cosimi AB. Monoclonal antibody treatment of human allograft recipients. *Surg Gynecol Obstet*. 1988;166(1):89–98.

174. Shield CF, Norman DJ. Immunologic monitoring during and after OKT3 therapy. *Am J Kidney Dis*. 1988;11:112–9.
175. Miller RA, Maloney DG, McKillop J, *et al*. In vivo effects of murine hybridoma monoclonal antibody in a patient with T-cell leukemia. *Blood* 1981;58:78–86.
176. Rinnooy Kan EA, Wright SD, Welte K, *et al*. Fc receptors on monocytes cause OKT3-treated lymphocytes to internalize T3 and to secrete IL-2. *Cell Immunol*. 1986;98:181.
177. Carreno M, Miller J, Fuller NL. Are OKT3 binding sites on T-cells modulated or merely converted (blind-folded) by OKT3 during therapy? *Transplant Proc*. 1989;21(1):987–8.
178. Gedel H, Lebeck LL, Jensik FC. Discordant expression of CD3 and T-cell receptor antigen on lymphocytes from patients treated with OKT3. *Transplant Proc*. 1989;21(1):1745–6.
179. Kreis H, Legendre C, Chatenoud L. OKT3 in organ transplantation. *Transplant Rev*. 1991;5:181–99.
180. Alloway R, Kotb M, Hathaway D, *et al*. The pharmacokinetic profile of standard and low-dose OKT3 induction immunosuppression in renal transplant recipients. *Transplantation* 1994;58(2):249–53.
181. Leone MR, Barry JM, Alexander SR, *et al*. Monoclonal antibody OKT3 therapy in pediatric kidney transplant patients. *J Pediatr*. 1990;116(*Suppl* 5):S86–91.
182. Schroeder TJ, Ryckman FC, Hurtubise PE, *et al*. Immunological monitoring during and following OKT3 therapy in children. *Clin Transplant*. 1991;5:191–6.
183. Ryckman FC, Schroeder TJ, Pedersen SH, *et al*. Use of monoclonal antibody immunosuppressive therapy in pediatric renal and liver transplantation. *Clin Transplant*. 1991;5:186–90.
184. Schroeder TJ, First MR, Hurtubise PE, *et al*. Immunologic monitoring with orthoclone OKT3 therapy. *J Heart Transplant*. 1989;8:371–80.
185. Chatenoud L. Immunologic monitoring during OKT3 therapy. *Clin Transplant*. 1993;7:422–30.
186. Colvin RB, Preffer FI. Laboratory monitoring of therapy with OKT3 and other murine monoclonal antibodies. *Clin Lab Med*. 1991;11(3):693–714.
187. Henell KR, Norman DJ. Monitoring OKT3 treatment: pharmacodynamic and pharmacokinetic measures. *Transplant Proc*. 1993;25(*Suppl* 1):83–5.
188. Thistlethwaite JR, Stuart JK, Mayes JT, *et al*. Complications and monitoring of OKT3 therapy. *Am J Kid Dis*. 1988;11:112–9.
189. Shield CF, Norman DJ. Immunologic monitoring during and after OKT3 therapy. *Am J Kid Dis*. 1988;11:120–4.
190. Chattenoud L. Humoral immune response against OKT3. *Transplant Proc*. 1993;25(2 *Suppl* 1):68–73.
191. Goldstein G, Fuccello AJ, Norman DJ, *et al*. OKT3 monoclonal antibody plasma levels during therapy and the subsequent development of host antibodies to OKT3. *Transplantation* 1986;42:507–11.
192. Hricik DE, Mayes JT, Schulak JA. Inhibition of anti-OKT3 antibody generation by cyclosporine-results of a prospective randomized trial. *Transplantation* 1990;50(2):237–40.
193. Schroeder TJ, Hariharan, First MR. Antibody response to OKT3 and methods for monitoring. *Transplant Proc*. 1993;25(2 *Suppl*. 1):77–80.
194. McDiarmid SV, Millis M, Terashita G, *et al*. Low serum OKT3 levels correlate with failure to prevent rejection in orthotopic liver transplant patients. *Transplant Proc*. 1990; 22:1774–6.
195. Abramowicz D, Goldman M, Mat O, *et al*. OKT3 serum levels as a guide for prophylactic therapy: a pilot study in kidney transplant recipients. *Transpl Int*. 1994;7:258–63.
196. Rossi SJ, Schroeder TJ, Schlueter KT, Hanto DW. Pharmacokinetics of OKT3 in liver transplant patients during sequential induction immunosuppression. *Clin Pharmacol Ther*. 1994;55(2):149.
197. Cosimi AB. Clinical development of orthoclone OKT3. *Transplant Proc*. 1987;19(*Suppl* 1):7–16.
198. Chatenoud L, Ferran C, Legendre C, *et al*. In vivo cell activation following OKT3 administration. Systemic cytokine release and modulation by corticosteroids. *Transplantation* 1990;49(4):697–702.
199. Abramowicz D, Schandene L, Goldman M, *et al*. Release of tumor necrosis factor, interleukin-2, and gamma-interferon in serum after injection of OKT3 monoclonal antibody in kidney transplant recipients. *Transplantation* 1989; 47:606–8.
200. Rowe PA, Rocker GM, Morgan AG, *et al*. OKT3 and pulmonary capillary permeability. *Br Med J*. 1987;255:1099.
201. Hosenpud JD, Norman DJ, Pantley GA, *et al*. OKT3-induced hypotension in cardiac allograft recipients treated for resistant rejection. *J Heart Transplant*. 1989;8:159–66.
202. Emmons C, Smith J, Flanigan M. Cerebrospinal fluid inflammation during OKT3 therapy [letter]. *Lancet* 1986; 2:510.
203. Martin MA, Massanaari RM, Nghiem DD, *et al*. Nosocomial aseptic meningitis associated with administration of OKT3. *JAMA* 1988;259:2002–5.
204. Thomas DM, Nicholls AJ, Feest TG, *et al*. OKT3 and cerebral oedema. *Br Med J*. 1987;295:1486.
205. Thistlethwaite JR, Gaber AO, Haag BW, *et al*. OKT3 treatment of steroid resistant renal allograft rejection. *Transplantation* 1987;43(2):176–84.
206. Norman W, Shield CF, Barry J, *et al*. A U.S. clinical study of orthoclone OKT3 in renal transplantation. *Transplant Proc*. 1987;19(*Suppl* 1):21–7.
207. Todd PA, Brogden RN. Muromonab CD3: a review of its pharmacology and therapeutic potential. *Drugs* 1989;37: 871–99.
208. Ortho Multicenter Transplant Study Group. A randomized clinical trial of OKT3 monoclonal antibody for acute rejection of cadaveric renal transplants. *N Engl J Med*. 1985;313:337–42.
209. Chatenoud L, Legendre C, Ferran C, *et al*. Corticosteroid inhibition of the OKT3-induced cytokine-related syndrome—dosage and kinetics prerequisites. *Transplantation* 1991;51(2):334–8.
210. Bemelman FJ, Buysman S, Surachno J, *et al*. Pretreatment with divided doses of steroids strongly decreases the side-effects of OKT3. *Kidney Int*. 1994;46:1674–9.
211. Alegre M, Gastaldello K, Abramowicz D, *et al*. Evidence that pentoxifylline reduces anti-CD3 monoclonal antibody-induced cytokine release syndrome. *Transplantation* 1991;52:674–9.
212. Chatenoud L. OKT3-induced cytokine-release syndrome: prevention effect of anti-tumor necrosis factor monoclonal antibody [review]. *Transplant Proc*. 1993;25(2 *Suppl* 1):47–51.

213. First MR, Schroeder T, Hariharan S, *et al.* The effect of indomethacin on the febrile response following OKT3 therapy. *Transplantation* 1992;53:91–4.
214. Kreis H. Adverse events associated with OKT3 immunosuppression in the prevention of allograft rejection. *Clin Transplant.* 1993;7:431–46.
215. Parlevliet KJ, Schellekens PT. Monoclonal antibodies in renal transplantation: a review. *Transpl Int.* 1992;5:234–46.
216. Butman SM, Wild JC, Nolan PE, *et al.* Prospective study of the safety and financial benefit of ketoconazole as adjunctive therapy to cyclosporine after heart transplantation. *J Heart Lung Transplant.* 1991;10(3):351–8.
217. Albengres E, Tillement JP. Cyclosporin and ketoconazole, drug interaction or therapeutic association? *Int J Clin Pharmacol Ther Toxicol.* 1992;30(12):555–70.
218. Gueco IP, Tan-Torres T, Baniga U, *et al.* Ketoconazole in posttransplant triple therapy: comparison of costs and outcomes. *Transplant Proc.* 1992;24(5):1709–14.
219. Bourge RC, Kirklin JK, Naftel DC, *et al.* Diltiazem-cyclosporine interaction in cardiac transplant recipients: impact on cyclosporine dose and medication costs. *Am J Med.* 1991;90(3):402–4.
220. Neumayer HH, Wagner K. Diltiazem and economic use of cyclosporine. *Lancet* 1986;2:523.
221. Valantine H, Keogh A, McIntosh N, *et al.* Cost containment: coadministration of diltiazem with cyclosporine after heart transplantation. *J Heart Lung Transplant.* 1992; 11:1–8.
222. Patton PR, Brunson ME, Pfaff WW, *et al.* A preliminary report of diltiazem and ketoconazole. *Transplantation* 1994; 57:889–92.
223. Randall T. Cyclosporine-ketoconazole combination offers promise in reducing antirejection therapy costs. *JAMA* 1990;264(4):430–1.
224. Modry DL, Stinson EB, Oyer PE, *et al.* Acute rejection and massive cyclosporine requirements in heart transplant recipients treated with rifampin. *Transplantation* 1985; 39:313–4.
225. Offermann G, Keller F, Molzahn M. Low cyclosporine A blood levels and acute graft rejection in a renal transplant recipient during rifampin treatment. *Am J Nephrol.* 1985; 5:385–7.
226. Wassner SJ, Pennisi AJ, Malekzadeh MH, *et al.* The adverse effect of anticonvulsant therapy on renal allograft survival. *J Pediatr.* 1976;88(1):134–7.
227. Nelson DR, Kamataki T, Waxman DJ, *et al.* The P450 superfamily: update on new sequences, gene mapping, accession numbers, early trivial names of enzymes, and nomenclature. *DNA Cell Biol.* 1993;112(1):1–51.
228. Kronbach T, Fischer V, Meyer UA. Cyclosporine metabolism in human liver: identification of a cytochrome P-450III gene family as the major cyclosporine-metabolizing enzyme with other drugs. *Clin Pharmacol Ther.* 1988;43: 630–5.
229. Vincent SH, Karanam BV, Painter SK, *et al.* In vitro metabolism of FK-506 in rat, rabbit, and human liver microsomes; identification of a major metabolite and of cytochrome P450 3A as the major enzymes responsible for its metabolism. *Arch Biochem Biophys.* 1992;294:454–60.
230. Kaminsky LS, Fasco MJ. Small intestinal cytochromes P450 [review]. *Crit Rev Toxicol.* 1991;21(6);407–22.
231. Kolars JC, Schmiedlin-Ren P, Schuetz JD, *et al.* Identification of rifampin-inducible P450IIIA4 (CYP3A4) in human small bowel enterocytes. *J Clin Invest.* 1992;90(5): 1871–8.
232. Watkins PB, Wrighton SA, Schuetz EG, *et al.* Identification of glucocorticoid-inducible cytochromes P-450 in the intestinal mucosa of rats and man. *J Clin Invest.* 1987;80(4): 1029–36.
233. Jain AB, Venkataramanan R, Fung J, *et al.* Pharmacokinetics of cyclosporine and nephrotoxicity in orthotopic liver transplant patients rescued with FK506. *Transplant Proc.* 1991;23(6):2777–9.
234. Rowland M, Gupta SK. Cyclosporine-phenytoin interaction: re-evaluation using metabolite data. *Br J Clin Pharmacol.* 1987;24:329–34.
235. Hebert MF, Roberts JP, Preuksaritanont T, *et al.* Pharmacokinetics and drug disposition: bioavailability of cyclosporine with concomitant rifampin administration is markedly less than predicted by hepatic enzyme induction. *Clin Pharmacol Ther.* 1992;52:453–57.
236. Van Buren D, Wideman CA, Ried M, *et al.* The antagonistic effect of rifampin upon cyclosporine bioavailability. *Transplant Proc.* 1984;16:1642–5.
237. McAllister WAC, Thompson PJ, Al-Habet SM, *et al.* Rifampicin reduces effectiveness and bioavailability of prednisolone. *Br Med J.* 1983;286(6369):923–5.
238. Wadhwa NK, Schroeder TJ, O'Flaherty E, *et al.* Pharmacokinetics and drug interactions of cyclosporine and erythromycin. *Clin Res.* 1986;34:638A.
239. Wadhwa NK, Schroeder TJ, O'Flaherty E, *et al.* Interaction between erythromycin and cyclosporine in a kidney and pancreas allograft recipient. *Ther Drug Monit.* 1987;9 (1):123–5.
240. Gupta SK, Bakran A, Johnson RWG, *et al.* Cyclosporine-erythromycin interaction in renal transplant patients. *Br J Clin Pharmacol.* 1989;27:475–81.
241. Cakaloglu Y, Tredger JM, Devlin J, *et al.* Importance of cytochrome P-450IIIA activity in determining dosage and blood levels of FK506 and cyclosporine in liver transplant recipients. *Hepatology* 1994;20(2);309–16.
242. Bailey DG, Arnold JMO, Spence JD. Grapefruit juice and drugs: how significant is the interaction? *Clin Pharmacokinet.* 1994;26:91–8.
243. Ducharme MP, Provenzano R, Dehoorne-Smith M, *et al.* Trough concentrations of cyclosporine in blood following administration with grapefruit juice. *Br J Clin Pharmacol.* 1993;36:457–9.
244. Yee GC, Stanley DL, Pessa LJ, *et al.* Effect of grapefruit juice on blood cyclosporin concentration. *Lancet* 1995; 345:955–6.
245. Ducharme PM, Warbasse LH, Edwards DJ. Disposition of intravenous and oral cyclosporine after administration with grapefruit juice. *Clin Pharmacol Ther.* 1995;57(5):485–91.
246. Doble N, Hykin P, Shaw R, *et al.* Pulmonary mycobacterium tuberculosis in acquired immune deficiency. *Br Med J.* 1985;291:849–50.
247. Watkins PB. Drug metabolism by cytochromes P450 in the liver and small bowel. *Gastroenterol Clin North Am.* 1992;21(3):511–26.
248. Ding TL, Gamberatoglio JG, Amend WJC, *et al.* Azathio-

prine (AZA) bioavailability and pharmacokinetics in kidney transplant patients. *Clin Pharmacol Ther.* 1980;27 (2):250.
249. Chan GL, Canafax DM, Johnson CA. The therapeutic use of azathioprine in renal transplantation. *Pharmacotherapy* 1987;7(5):165.
250. Watschinger B, Ulrich W, Vychytil A, *et al.* Cyclosporine A toxicity is associated with reduced endothelin immunoreactivity in renal endothelium. *Transplant Proc.* 1992;24 (6):2618–9.
251. DeCamargo PM. Cyclosporin- and nifedipine-induced gigival enlargement: an overview. *J West Soc Periodontol Periodontal Abstr.* 1989;37(2):57–64.
252. Slavin J, Taylor J. Cyclosporine, nifedipine, and gingival hyperplasia. *Lancet* 1987;2:739.
253. Modeer T, Wondimu B, Larsson E, *et al.* Levels of cyclosporin-A (CsA) in saliva in children after oral administration of the drug in mixture or in capsule form. *Scand J Dent Res.* 1992;100(6):366–70.
254. Wong W, Hodge MG, Lewis A, *et al.* Resolution of cyclosporin-induced gingival hypertrophy with metronidazole. *Lancet* 1994;343(8903):986.
255. Horton CM, Freeman CD, Nolan PE Jr., *et al.* Cyclosporine interactions with miconazole and other azole-antimycotics: a case report and review of the literature. *J Heart Lung Transplant.* 1992;11(6):1127–32.
256. First MR, Schroeder TJ, Weiskittel P, *et al.* Concomitant administration of cyclosporine and ketoconazole in renal transplant patients. *Lancet* 1989;2(8673):1198–201.
257. Nanez R, Martin M, Venkataramanan R, *et al.* Fluconazole therapy in transplant recipients receiving FK506. *Transplantation* 1994;57(10):1521–3.
258. Venkataramanan R, Jain A, Warty VS, *et al.* Pharmacokinetics of FK506 in transplant patients. *Transplant Proc.* 1991;23(6):2736–40.
259. Mieles L, Venkataramanan R, Yokoyama I, *et al.* Interaction between FK506 and clotrimazole in a liver transplant recipient. *Transplantation* 1991;52(6):1086–7.
260. Freeman DJ, Laupacis A, Keown PA, *et al.* Evaluation of cyclosporine-phenytoin interaction with observations on cyclosporine metabolites. *Br J Clin Pharmacol.* 1984;18: 887–93.
261. Keown PA, Laupacis A, Carruthers G, *et al.* Interaction between phenytoin and cyclosporine following organ transplantation. *Transplantation* 1984;38(3):304–6.
262. Brockmoller J, Neumayer HH, Wagner K, *et al.* Pharmacokinetic interaction between cyclosporin and diltiazem. *Eur J Clin Pharmacol.* 1990;38(3):237–42.
263. Grino JM, Sebate I, Castelao AM, *et al.* Influence of diltiazem on cyclosporine clearance. *Lancet* 1986;1:1387.
264. Kohlhaw K, Wonigeit K, Frei U, *et al.* Effect of the calcium channel blocker diltiazem on cyclosporine A blood levels and dose requirements. *Transplant Proc.* 1988;20: 572–4.
265. Renton KW. Inhibition of hepatic microsomal drug metabolism by the calcium channel blockers diltiazem and verapamil. *Biochem Pharmacol.* 1985;34:2549–53.
266. Bourbigot B, Guiserix J, Airiau J, *et al.* Nicardipine increases cyclosporine blood levels. *Lancet* 1986;1:1447.
267. Cantarovich M, Hiesse C, Lockiec F, *et al.* Confirmation of the interaction between cyclosporine and the calcium channel blocker nicardipine in renal transplant patients. *Clin Nephrol.* 1987;28:190–3.
268. McNally P, Mistry N, Idle J, *et al.* Calcium channel blockers and cyclosporine metabolism. *Transplantation* 1989;48: 1071.
269. Ludden TM. Pharmacokinetic interactions of the macrolide antibiotics. *Clin Pharmacokinet.* 1985;10(1):63–79.
270. Fine RN, Terasaki PI, Ettenger RB, *et al.* Renal transplantation update. *Ann Intern Med.* 1984;100:246–57.
271. Opelz G, Graver B, Terasaki PI. Induction of high kidney graft survival rate by multiple transfusion. *Lancet* 1981; 1:223–5.
272. Sutherland DER, Fryd DS, So SKS, *et al.* Long-term effect of splenectomy versus no splenectomy in renal transplant patients. *Transplantation* 1984;38(6):619–24.
273. Flye MW. Immunosuppressive therapy. In: Flye MW, editor. *Principles of Organ Transplantation.* Philadelphia, PA: WB Saunders; 1989. p.155–75.
274. Struber S. Total lymphoid irradiation in alloimmunity and autoimmunity. Part II. *J Pediatr.* 1987;3(6):1051–5.
275. Monaco AP. Development of clinical immunosuppressants for organ transplantation. *Jpn J Surg.* 1988;18(2):119–30.
276. Salter M, Bourge R, Kirklin JK, *et al.* Total lymphoid irradiation as therapy for recurrent allograft rejection [abstract]. *J Heart Transplant.* 1991;10:176.
277. Hunt SA, Strober S, Hoppe RT, *et al.* Total lymphoid irradiation for treatment of intractable cardiac allograft rejection. *Heart Transplant.* 1991;10:211–6.
278. Evans MA, Schombert PJ, Rodeheffer RJ, *et al.* Total lymphoid irradiation: novel therapy for treatment of cardiac allograft rejection. *Mayo Clin Proc.* 1992;67:785–90.
279. Costanzo-Nordin MR, Cooper DKC, Jessup M, *et al.* Task Force 6: future developments. *J Am Coll Cardiol.* 1993; 22(1):54–64.
280. Costanzo-Nordin MR, Hubbell EA, O'Sullivan EJ, *et al.* Successful treatment of heart transplant rejection with photopheresis. *Transplantation* 1992;53:808–15.
281. Wieland M, Randeis MJ, Strauss RG, *et al.* Photopheresis: a promising therapy for intractable cardiac allograft rejection. *J Clin Apheresis.* 1992;7:42–3.
282. Tilney NL. Renal transplantation between identical twins: a review. *World J Surg.* 1986;10:381–8.
283. Tilney NL. Renal transplantation. *Curr Prob Surg.* 1989;26 (9):607–69.
284. Blagg CR. Dialysis or transplantation? JAMA 1983; 250(8):1072–3.
285. Terasaki PI, Takemoto S, Mickey MR. A report of 123 six-antigen matched cadaver kidney transplants. *Clin Transplant.* 1989;3:301.
286. Levinsky NG, Rettig RA. The Medicare end-stage renal disease program. *N Engl J Med.* 1991;324(16):1143–8.
287. Evans RW, Manninen DL, Garrison LP, *et al.* The quality of life of patients with end-stage renal failure. *N Engl J Med.* 1985;312:553–9.
288. Terasaki PI, Cecka Y, Cho S, *et al.* A report from the UNOS Scientific Renal Transplant Registry. *Transplant Proc.* 1991; 23(1):53–4.
289. Frey W, Matas AJ. Renal transplantation. *Crit Care Clin.* 1990;6(4):899–910.
290. Henry ML, Sommer BG, Ferguson RM. Triple drug therapy: an alternative regimen in renal transplantation. *Transplant*

Proc. 1987;19(1):1920–1.
291. Landsberg D, Rae A, Chiu A, *et al*. The effect of triple therapy on cyclosporine nephrotoxicity and hypertension in renal transplantation. *Transplant Proc*. 1989;21(2):3323–4.
292. Landsberg DN, Rae A, Chiu A, *et al*. The use of triple therapy to minimize cyclosporine (CsA) nephrotoxicity in renal transplantation. *Transplant Proc*. 1989;21(1):1550–1.
293. Hodge E, Banowsky L, Novick A, *et al*. Alternative immunosuppressive strategies in the management of recipients of living related renal transplants. *Transplant Proc*. 1989;21(1):1609–14.
294. Michael HJ, Francos GC, Burke JF, *et al*. A comparison of the effects of cyclosporine versus antilymphocyte globulin on delayed graft function in cadaver renal transplant recipients. *Transplantation* 1989;48(5):805–8.
295. Benvenisty AL, Cohen D, Stegall MD, *et al*. Improved results using OKT3 as induction immunosuppression in renal allograft recipients with delayed graft function. *Transplantation* 1990;49(2):321–7.
296. Matas AJ, Tellis VA, Quinn TA, *et al*. Individualization of immediate posttransplant immunosuppression: the value of antilymphocyte globulin in patients with delayed graft function. *Transplantation* 1988;45(2):406–9.
297. Novick AC, Ho-Hsieh H, Steinmuller D, *et al*. Detrimental effect of cyclosporine on initial function of cadaver renal allografts following extended preservation: results of a randomized prospective study. *Transplantation* 1986;42 (2):154–8.
298. Rao KV. Mechanism, pathophysiology, diagnosis, and management of renal transplant rejection. *Med Clin North Am*. 1990;74(4):1039–57.
299. Mathew TH. Recurrent disease after renal transplantation. *Transplant Rev*. 1991;5:31–42.
300. Kelly WD, Lillehei RC, Merkel FK, *et al*. Allotransplantation of the pancreas and duodenum along with the kidney in diabetic nephropathy. *Surgery* 1967;67:827–37.
301. Squifflet JP, Moudry K, Sutherland DER. Is HLA matching relevant in pancreas transplantation? A registry analysis. *Transpl Int*. 1988;1:26–9.
302. Sutherland DER, Gillingham KJ, Moudry-Munns KC. Registry report on clinical pancreas transplantation. *Transplant Proc*. 1991;23(1):55–7.
303. Sutherland DER. Who should get a pancreas transplant? *Diabetes Care* 1988;11:681–5.
304. Grundfest-Broniatowski S. Pancreas transplantation: state of the art. *Cleve Clin J Med*. 1990;57(6):564–70.
305. Sutherland DER, Gruber SA. Pancreas transplantation. *Crit Care Clin*. 1990;6(4):947–53.
306. Prieto M, Sutherland DER, Fernandez-Cruz I, *et al*. Experimental and clinical experience with urine amylase monitoring for early diagnosis of rejection in pancreas transplantation. *Transplantation* 1987;34:71–9.
307. Stratta RJ. Pancreas transplantation. *Ren Fail*. 1995;17(4): 323–37.
308. Allen RDM, Wilson TG, Grierson JM, *et al*. Percutaneous pancreas transplant, fine needle aspiration, and needle core biopsies are useful and safe. *Transplant Proc*. 1990;22: 663–4.
309. Esmatjes E, Fernandez-Cruz L, Ricart MJ, *et al*. Urinary C-peptide excretion in pancreas transplantation with urinary drainage. *Transplant Proc*. 1990;22(4):1598–9.
310. Perkins JD, Munn SR, Barr D, *et al*. Evidence that the soluble interleukin-2 receptor level may determine the optimal time for cystoscopically directed biopsy in pancreaticoduodenal allograft recipients. *Transplantation* 1990;49:363–6.
311. Tyden O, Reinholt F, Bohman S-O, *et al*. Diagnosis of pancreatic graft rejection by pancreatic juice cytology. *Transplant Proc*. 1989;21:2780–1.
312. Fernstad R, Tyden G, Brattstrom C, *et al*. Pancreas-specific protein: new serum marker for graft rejection in pancreas-transplant recipients. *Diabetes* 1989;38(*Suppl* 1):55–6.
313. Teule OJJ, Leunissen KML, Halders SGEA, *et al*. Serial radionuclide determinations of graft perfusion in pancreas transplantation. *Transplant Proc*. 1989;21:2795–6.
314. Gray DWR, Morris PJ. Transplantation of isolated pancreatic islets. In: Groth CG, editor. *Pancreatic Transplantation*. Philadelphia, PA: WB Saunders; 1988. p. 363–83.
315. Skolnick A. Advances in islet cell transplantation: is science closer to a diabetes cure? *JAMA* 1990;264(4):427–8.
316. Weir GC, Bonner-Weir S, Leahy JL. Islet mass and function in diabetes and transplantation. *Diabetes* 1990;39:401–5.
317. Skerrett PJ. New transplant method evades immune attack. *Science* 1990;249:1248.
318. Morris PJ, Gray DW, Sutton R. Pancreatic islet transplantation. *Br Med Bull*. 1989;456(1):224–41.
319. Starzl TE, Demetris AJ, Van Thiel DV. Liver transplantation. *N Engl J Med*. 1989;321:1014–222, 1092–9.
320. Shaw BW, Starzl TE, Iwatsuki S, *et al*. An overview of orthotopic transplantation of the liver. In: Flye ME, editor. *Principles of Organ Transplantation*. Philadelphia, PA: WB Saunders; 1989. p. 347–63.
321. Starzl TE, Demetris AJ. Liver transplantation: a 31 year perspective. *Curr Prob Surg*. 1990;17:55–116, 123–78.
322. Samuel D, Muller R, Alexander G, *et al*. Liver transplantation in European patients with the hepatitis B surface antigen. *N Engl J Med*. 1993;329(25):1842–7.
323. Konig V, Hopf U, Neuhaus P, *et al*. Long-term follow-up of hepatitis B virus-infected recipients after orthotopic liver transplantation. *Transplantation* 1994;58(5):553–9.
324. Sussman NL, Gislason GT, Kelly JH. Extracorporeal liver support. Application to fulminant hepatic failure. *J Clin Gastroenterol*. 1994;18(4):320–4.
325. United Network for Organ Sharing. By-Laws and Policies. Richmond, Virginia; amended November 3, 1995. Section 3, p. 18–9.
326. Broelsch DE, Burdelski M, Rogiers X, *et al*. Living donor for liver transplantation. *Hepatology* 1994;20(1 *Pt* 2):49S–55S.
327. Inomata Y, Tanaka K, Egawa H, *et al*. The evolution of immunosuppression with FK506 in pediatric living-related liver transplantation. *Transplantation* 1996;61:247–52.
328. Levy G, Rochon J, Freeman D, *et al*. Cyclosporine Neoral in liver transplant recipients. *Transplant Proc*. 1994;26: 2949–52.
329. Grieg PD, Woolf GM, Sinclair SB, *et al*. Treatment of primary liver graft nonfunction with prostaglandin E_1. *Transplantation* 1989;48(3):447–53.

330. Rubin RH, Tolkoff-Rubin NE. Antimicrobial strategies in the care of organ transplant recipients. *Antimicrob Agents Chemother.* 1993;37(4):619–24.
331. Paya CV. Fungal infections in solid organ transplantation. *Clin Infec Dis.* 1993;16:677–88.
332. Weisner RH, Hermans PE, Rakela J, *et al.* Selective bowel decontamination to decrease gram-negative aerobic bacterial and candida colonization and prevent infection after orthotopic liver transplantation. *Transplantation* 1988;45(3):570–4.
333. Steffen R, Reinhartz O, Blumhardt G, *et al.* Bacterial and fungal colonization and infections using oral selective bowel decontamination in orthotopic liver transplantations. *Transpl Int.* 1994;7:101–8.
334. Reetze-Bonorden P, Bohler J, Keller E. Drug dosage in patients during continuous renal replacement therapy: pharmacokinetic and therapeutic considerations. *Clin Pharmacokinet.* 1993;24(5):32–79.
335. Wright TL, Donegan E, Hsu HH, *et al.* Recurrent and acquired hepatitic C viral infection in liver transplant recipients. *Gastroenterol.* 1992;103:317–22.
336. Rezieg I, Traif A, Roach C, *et al.* Treatment of chronic hepatitis C viral infection (HCV) in the transplanted patient. *Hepatology* 1993;18(3):739.
337. Guy SR, Post J, Chodoff L, *et al.* Long-term immunoprophylaxis with hepatitis B immune globulin prevents recurrence of hepatitis B after first liver transplant [abstract]. American Society of Transplant Surgeons' 20th Annual Meeting, 1995. Abstract H-4.
338. Annau Z, Eccles CU. Sensory deficits caused by exposure to methyl mercury. In: *The Toxicities of Methyl Mercury.* Baltimore, MD: Johns Hopkins; 1987. p. 102–13.
339. Sheiner PA, Schwartz ME, Mor E, *et al.* Severe or multiple rejection episodes are associated with early recurrence of hepatitis C after orthotopic liver transplantation. *Hepatology* 1995;21(1):30–4.
340. Hardy JD, Chavez CM, Kurrus FD, *et al.* Heart transplantation in man: developmental studies and report of a case. *JAMA* 1964;188:1132–40.
341. Barnard CN. The operation. *South African Med J.* 1967; 41:1271–4.
342. Gorensek MJ, Stewart RW, Keys TF, *et al.* Decreased infections in cardiac transplant recipients on cyclosporine with reduced corticosteroid use. *Cleve Clin J Med.* 1989;56 (7):690–5.
343. Thomas FT, Szentpetery SS, Mammana RE, *et al.* Long distance transportation of human hearts for transplantation. *Ann Thorac Surg.* 1978;26:344–50.
344. Caves PK, Billingham ME, Stinson EB, *et al.* Diagnosis of human cardiac allograft rejection by serial cardiac biopsy. *J Thorac Cardiovasc Surg.* 1973;66:461–6.
345. Dunn DL, Mayoral JL, Gillingham KJ, *et al.* Treatment of invasive cytomegalovirus disease in solid organ transplant patients with ganciclovir. *Transplantation* 1991;51(1):98–106.
346. Cohn JN, Johnson G, Ziesche S, *et al.* A comparison of enalapril with hydralazine-isosorbide dinitrate in the treatment of chronic congestive heart failure. *N Engl J Med.* 1991;325:303–10.
347. The SOLVD Investigators. Effect of enalapril on survival in patients with reduced left ventricular ejection fractions and congestive heart failure. *N Engl J Med.* 1991;325:293–302.
348. The CONSENSUS Trial Study Group. Effects of enalapril on mortality in severe congestive heart failure. Results of the Cooperative North Scandinavian Enalapril Survival Study (CONSENSUS) *N Engl J Med.* 1987;316:1429–35.
349. Hosenpud JK, Novick RJ, Breen TJ, *et al.* The Registry of the International Society for Heart and Lung Transplantation: eleventh official report—1994. *J Heart Lung Transplant.* 1994;July/August:561–70.
350. Young JB, Winters WL, Bourge R, *et al.* Task Force 4: function of the heart transplant recipient. *J Am Coll Cardiol.* 1993;22(1):31–41.
351. Burdine J, Fischel RJ, Bolman RM III. Cardiac transplantation. *Crit Care Clin.* 1990;6(4):927–45.
352. Mudge GH, Goldstein S, Addonizio LJ, *et al.* Task Force 3: recipient guidelines/prioritization. *J Am Coll Cardiol.* 1993;22(1):21–31.
353. Mancini DM, Wong KL, Simson MB. Prognostic value of an abnormal signal-averaged electrocardiograms in patients with nonischemic congestive cardiomyopathy. *Circulation* 1993;87:1083–92.
354. Macdonald P, Hackworthy R, Keogh A, *et al.* The effect of chronic amiodarone therapy before transplantation on early cardiac allograft function. *J Heart Lung Transplant.* 1991;10(5 *Pt* 1):743–8.
355. Schuler S, Thomas D, Thebken M, *et al.* Endocrine response to exercise in cardiac transplant patients. *Transplant Proc.* 1987;19:2506–9.
356. Stinson EB, Schroeder JS, Griepp RB, *et al.* Observations on the behavior of recipient atria after cardiac transplantation in man. *Am J Cardiol.* 1972;30:615–22.
357. Stinson EB, Griepp RB, Schroeder JS, *et al.* Hemodynamic observations one and two years after cardiac transplantation in man. *Circulation* 1972;45:1183–94.
358. Wilson RF, Christensen BV, Olivari MT, *et al.* Evidence for structural sympathetic reinnervation after orthotopic cardiac transplantation in humans. *Circulation* 1991; 83:1210–20.
359. Pennington DG, McBride LR, Kanter KR, *et al.* Bridging to heart transplantation with circulatory support devices. *J Heart Transplant.* 1989;8:116–23.
360. Reedy JE, Swartz MT, Termuhlen DF, *et al.* Bridge to heart transplantation: importance of patient selection. *J Heart Transplant.* 1990;9:473–81.
361. McCarthy PM. HeartMate implantable left ventricular assist device: bridge cotransplantation and future applications [review]. *Ann Thorac Surg.* 1995;59(*Suppl* 2):S46–51.
362. McCarthy PM, James KB, Savage RM, *et al.* Implantable left ventricular assist device. Approaching an alternative for end-stage heart failure. Implantable LVAD Study Group. *Circulation* 1994;90(5 *Pt* 2):II83–6.
363. Frazier OH, Macris MP, Myers TJ, *et al.* Improved survival after extended bridge to cardiac transplantation. *Ann Thorac Surg.* 1994;57(6):1416–22.
364. McCarthy PM, Portner PM, Tobler HG, *et al.* Clinical experience with the Novacor ventricular assist system. *J Thorac Cardiovasc Surg.* 1991;102:578–87.
365. Vetter HO, Kaulbach HG, Schmitz C, *et al.* Experience with the Novacor left ventricular assist system as a bridge

to cardiac transplantation, including the new wearable system. *J Thorac Cardiovasc Surg*. 1995;109:74–80.
366. Evans RW, Orians C, Ascher NL. The potential supply of organ donors: an assessment of organ procurement effects in the United States. *JAMA* 1992;267:239–46.
367. Walker AM, editor. *Transplant Protocols*. Chestnut Hill, MA: Epidemiology Resources; 1990.
368. Bolman RM, Elick B, Olivari MT, *et al*. Improved immunosuppression for heart transplantation. *J Heart Transplant*. 1985;4:315–8.
369. Bolman RM, Olivari MT, Saffitz J, *et al*. Current results with triple therapy for heart transplantation. *Transplant Proc*. 1987;19:249–51.
370. Olivari MT, Kubo SH, Braunlin EA, *et al*. Five-year experience with triple-drug immunosuppression therapy in cardiac transplantation. *Circulation* 1990;82(*Suppl* 4):264–8.
371. Wan S, DeSmet JM, Antoine M, *et al*. Steroid administration in heart and heart-lung transplantation: is the timing adequate? *Ann Thorac Surg*. 1996;61(2):674–8.
372. Bolman RM, Cance CG. Intravenous cyclosporine for heart transplantation. *Transplant Proc*. 1989;21(1):2488.
373. Macris MP, Frazier OH, VanBuren CT, *et al*. Improved immunosuppression for heart transplant patients using intravenous doses of cyclosporine. *Transplantation* 1989;47: 311–4.
374. Schroeder TJ, Myre SA, Melvin DB, *et al*. Efficacy and safety of constant-rate intravenous cyclosporine infusion immediately after heart transplantation. *J Heart Transplant*. 1989;8:5–10.
375. Bolling SF, Deeb GM, Miska PT. Comparison of polyclonal antibody sera for early prophylaxis following cardiac transplantation. *J Surg Res*. 1989;47:292–6.
376. Carey JA, Frist WH. Use of polyclonal antilymphocytic preparations for prophylaxis in heart transplantation. *J Heart Transplant*. 1990;9:297–300.
377. Copeland JG, Icenogle TB, Williams RJ, *et al*. Rabbit antithymocyte globulin: a 10-year experience in cardiac transplantation. *J Thorac Cardiovasc Surg*. 1990;99:852–60.
378. Costanzo-Nordin MR, O'Sullivan EJ, Hubbell EA, *et al*. Longterm follow-up of heart transplant recipients treated with murine antihuman mature T-cell monoclonal antibody (OKT3): the Loyola experience. *J Heart Transplant*. 1989;8:288–95.
379. Costanzo-Nordin MR, O'Sullivan EJ, Johnson MR, *et al*. Prospective randomized trial of OKT3- versus horse antithymocyte globulin-based immunosuppressive prophylaxis in heart transplantation. *J Heart Transplant*. 1990;9:306–15.
380. Emery RW, Joyce LD, Pritzker MR. Induction immunosuppression for patients bridged to transplantation. *J Heart Transplant*. 1990;9:316–20.
381. Gay, WA, O'Connell JG, Burton NA, *et al*. OKT3 monoclonal antibody in cardiac transplantation: experience with 102 patients. *Ann Surg*. 1988;208:287–90.
382. Macris MP, Frazier OH, Lammermeier D, *et al*. Clinical experience with muromonab-CD3 monoclonal antibody (OKT3) in heart transplantation. *J Heart Transplant*. 1989; 8:281–7.
383. Prieto M, Lake KD, Pritzker MR, *et al*. OKT3 induction and steroid free maintenance immunosuppression for treatment of high risk heart transplant recipients. *J Heart Lung Transplant*. 1991;10:901–11.
384. Barr ML, Sanchez JA, Seche LA, *et al*. Anti-CD3 monoclonal antibody induction therapy immunological equivalency with triple-drug therapy in heart transplantation. *Circulation* 1990;82(*Suppl* 4):291–4.
385. Kirklin JK, Bourge RC, White-Williams C, *et al*. Prophylactic therapy for rejection after cardiac transplantation: a comparison of rabbit antithymocyte globulin and OKT3. *J Thorac Cardiovasc Surg*. 1990;99(4):716–24.
386. Kormos RL, Herlan DB, Armitage JM, *et al*. Monoclonal versus polyclonal therapy for prophylaxis against rejection after heart transplantation. *J Heart Transplant*. 1990;9:1–10.
387. Moore CK, Renlund DG, Rasmussen LG, *et al*. Long-term morbidity of cyclosporine with corticosteroid-free maintenance immunosuppression in cardiac transplantation. *Transplant Proc*. 1990;22:25–9.
388. O'Connell JB, Bristow MR, Rasmussen LG, *et al*. Cardiac allograft function with corticosteroid-free maintenance immunosuppression. *Circulation* 1990;82(*Suppl* 4):318–21.
389. Renlund DG, O'Connell JB, Gilbert EM, *et al*. A prospective comparison of murine monoclonal CD3 (OKT3) antibody-based and equine antithymocyte globulin-based rejection prophylaxis in cardiac transplantation. *Transplantation* 1989;47:599–605.
390. Renlund DG, O'Connell JB, Bristow MR. Early rejection prophylaxis in heart transplantation: is cytolytic therapy necessary? *J Heart Transplant*. 1989;8(3):191–2.
391. Swinnen LJ, Costanzo-Nordin MR, Fisher SG, *et al*. Increased incidence of lymphoproliferative disorder after immunosuppression with the monoclonal antibody of OKT3 in cardiac transplant recipients. *N Engl J Med*. 1990; 323:1723–8.
392. Oh CS, Stratta RJ, Fox BC, *et al*. Increased infections associated with the use of OKT3 for treatment of steroid-resistant rejection in renal transplantation. *Transplantation* 1988;45:68–73.
393. Miller LW, Schlant RC, Kobashigawa J, *et al*. Task Force 5: complications. *J Am Coll Cardiol*. 1993;22(1):41–53.
394. Billingham ME, Cary NRB, Hammond ME, *et al*. A working formulation for the standardization of nomenclature in the diagnosis of heart and lung rejection. *J Heart Transplant*. 1990;9(6):587–93.
395. Hosenpud JD, Norman DJ, Pantley GA. Low-dose oral prednisone in the treatment of acute cardiac allograft rejection not associated with hemodynamic compromise. *J Heart Transplant*. 1990;9:292–6.
396. Miller LW. Treatment of cardiac allograft rejection with intravenous steroids. II. *J Heart Transplant*. 1990;9(3):283–7.
397. Costanzo-Nordin MR, Silver MA, O'Connell JB, *et al*. Successful reversal of acute cardiac allograft rejection with OKT3 monoclonal antibody. *Circulation* 1987;76(*Suppl* 5):71–80.
398. Gilbert EM, Eiswirth CC, Renlund DG, *et al*. Use of Orthoclone OKT3 monoclonal antibody in cardiac transplantation: early experience with rejection prophylaxis and treatment of refractory rejection. *Transplant Proc*. 1987;21 (*Suppl* 1):45–53.
399. Sweeney MS, Sinnott JT, Cullison JP, *et al*. The use of

OKT3 for stubborn heart allograft rejection: an advance in clinical immunotherapy? *J Heart Transplant*. 1987;6:324–8.

400. Kirklin JK, Bourge RC, Naftel DC, *et al*. Treatment of recurrent heart rejection with mycophenolate mofetil (RS-61443): initial clinical experience. *J Heart Lung Transplant*. 1994;13(3):444–50.
401. Andreone PA, Olivari MT, Elick B, *et al*. Reduction of infectious complications following heart transplantation with triple-drug immunotherapy. *J Heart Transplant*. 1986; 5:13–9.
402. Mason JW, Stinson EB, Hunt SA, *et al*. Infections after cardiac transplantation: relation to rejection therapy. *Ann Intern Med*. 1976;85:69–72.
403. Grattan MT, Moreno-Cabral CE, Starnes VA, *et al*. Cytomegalovirus infection is associated with cardiac allograft rejection and atherosclerosis. *JAMA* 1989;261:3561–6.
404. McDonald K, Rector TJ, Braunlin EA, *et al*. Association of coronary artery disease in cardiac transplant recipients with cytomegalovirus infection. *Am J Cardiol*. 1989;64: 359–62.
405. Kriett JM, Kaye MP. The registry of the international society for heart transplantation: seventh official report—1990. *J Heart Transplant*. 1990;9:323–30.
406. Shennib H, Massard G. Airway complications in lung transplantation [review]. *Ann Thorac Surg*. 1994;57(2): 506–11.
407. Trulock EP. Management of lung transplant rejection [review]. *Chest* 1993;103(5):1566–76.
408. Reitz BA, Wallwork JL, Hunt SA, *et al*. Heart-lung transplantation: successful therapy for patients with pulmonary vascular disease. *N Engl J Med*. 1982;306:557–64.
409. Toronto Lung Transplant Group. Unilateral lung transplant for pulmonary fibrosis. *N Engl J Med*. 1986;314:1140–5.
410. Judson MA. Clinical aspects of lung transplantation [review]. *Clin Chest Med*. 1993;14(2):335–57.
411. Davis RD Jr., Pasque MK. Pulmonary transplantation. *Ann Surg*. 1995;221(1):14–28.
412. Jenkinson SG, Levine SM. Lung transplantation [review]. *Disease-A-Month* 1994;40(1):1–38.
413. Griffith BP, Bando K, Hardesty RL, *et al*. A prospective randomized trial of FK506 versus cyclosporine after human pulmonary transplantation. *Transplantation* 1994; 57(6):848–51.
414. Keenan RJ, Konishi H, Kawai A, *et al*. Clinical trial of tacrolimus versus cyclosporine in lung transplantation. *Ann Thorac Surg*. 1995;60(3):580–4.
415. Ramirez JC, Patterson GA, Winton TL, *et al*. Bilateral lung transplantation for cystic fibrosis. The Toronto Lung Transplant Group. *J Thorac Cardiovasc Surg*. 1992;103(2): 287–94.
416. Bryan CL, *et al*. Corticosteroid therapy does not potentiate bronchial anastomatic complications in a single lung transplantation. *Am Rev Respir Dis*. 1991;143(*Suppl* 1):A460.
417. Cooper JD, *et al*. Results of single and bilateral lung transplantation in 131 consecutive recipients. *J Thorac Cardiovasc Surg*. 1994;107:460–71.
418. Keenan RJ, Konishi H, Kawai A, *et al*. Clinical trial of tacrolimus versus cyclosporine in lung transplantation. *Ann Thorac Surg*. 1995;60(3):580–5.
419. Maurer JR. Therapeutic challenges following lung transplantation. *Clin Chest Med*. 1990;11(2):279–90.
420. Paradis IL, Williams P. Infection after lung transplantation [review]. *Semin Respir Infect*. 1993;8(3):207–15.
421. Snydman DR, Werner BG, Heinze-Lacey B. Use of cytomegalovirus immune globulin to prevent cytomegalovirus disease in renal transplant recipients. *N Engl J Med*. 1987;317:1049–54.
422. Duncan SR, Paradis IL, Williams P, *et al*. Prevention of cytomegalovirus infections in lung transplant recipients. *Am Rev Respir Dis*. 1992;145:A705 [abstract presented at International Conference of American Lung Association and American Thoracic Society, 1992; Miami Beach].
423. Kramer MR, Stoehr C, Lewiston NJ, *et al*. Trimethoprim-sulfamethoxazole prophylaxis for pneumocystis carinii infections in heart-lung and lung transplantation—how effective and for how long? *Transplantation* 1992;53:586–9.
424. Theodore J, Starnes VA, Lewiston NJ. Obliterative bronchiolitis. *Clin Chest Surg*. 1990;2(2):309–21.
425. Paradis I, Yousem S, Griffith B. Airway obstruction and bronchiolitis obliterans after lung transplantation [review]. *Clin Chest Med*. 1993;14(4):751–63.
426. Tzakis AG, Todo S, Reyes J, *et al*. Clinical intestinal transplantation: focus on complications. *Transplant Proc*. 1992;24(3):1238–40.
427. Todo S, Tzakis A, Reyes J, *et al*. Small intestinal transplantation in human with or without the colon. *Transplantation* 1994;57(6):840–8.
428. Watson AJM, Lear PA. Current status of intestinal transplantation. *Gut* 1989;30:1771–82.
429. Hasuike Y, Shaked A, Monden M, *et al*. Selective mesenteric lymphoid irradiation eliminates the effector cells of lethal graft-versus-host disease while protecting radiosensitive intestinal tissue. *Transplant Proc*. 1993;25(1):1196–7.
430. Hurlbut D, Zhong R, Wang P, *et al*. Intestinal permeability and bacterial translocation following orthotopic intestinal transplantation in the rat. *Transplant Proc*. 1990;22 (6):2451.
431. Fabrega AJ, Lopez-Boado M, Gonzalez S. Problems in the longterm renal allograft recipient. *Crit Care Clin*. 1990;6 (4):979–1005.
432. Kiok MC. Neurologic complications of pancreas transplants. *Neurol Clin*. 1988;6(2):367–76.
433. Van Thiel DH, Dindzans VJ, Gavaler JS, *et al*. The postoperative problems and management of the liver transplant recipient. *Prog Liver Dis*. 1990;9:657–85.
434. Slavis SA, Novick AC, Steinmuller DR, *et al*. Outcome of renal transplantation in patients with a functioning graft for 20 years or more. *J Urol*. 1990;144(1):20–2.
435. Braun WE. Long-term complications of renal transplantation. *Kidney Int*. 1990;37(5):1363–78.
436. Rubin RH, Tolkoff-Rubin NE. The impact of infection on the outcome of transplantation. *Transplant Proc*. 1991; 23(4):2068–74.
437. McCarthy JM, Karim MA, Kruger H, *et al*. The cost impact of cytomegalovirus disease in renal transplant recipients. *Transplantation* 1993;55:1277–82.
438. Pouteil-Noble C, Ecchard R, Landrivon G, *et al*. Cytomegalovirus infection—an etiologic factor for rejection. *Trans-*

plantation 1993;55:851–7.
439. Ho M. Epidemiology of cytomegalovirus infections. *Rev Infect Dis*. 1990;12(*Suppl* 7):S701–10.
440. Rubin RH. Impact of cytomegalovirus infection on organ transplant recipients. *Rev Infect Dis*. 1990;12 (*Suppl* 7): S754–66.
441. Boland GJ, Hene RJ, Ververs C, *et al*. Factors influencing the occurrence of active CMV infections after organ transplantation. *Clin Exp Immunol*. 1993;94:306–12.
442. Balfour HH, Chace BA, Stapleton JR, *et al*. A randomized, placebo-controlled trial of oral acyclovir for the prevention of cytomegalovirus disease in recipients of renal allografts. *N Engl J Med*. 1989;21:1381–7.
443. Elkins CC, Frist WH, Dummer S, *et al*. Cytomegalovirus disease after heart transplantation: is acyclovir prophylaxis indicated? *Ann Thorac Surg*. 1993;56:1267–73.
444. Legendre C, Ducloux D, Ferroni A, *et al*. Acyclovir in preventing cytomegalovirus infection in kidney transplant recipients: a case-controlled study. *J Med Virol*. 1993;(*Suppl* 1):118–22.
445. Merigan TC, Renlund DG, Keay S, *et al*. A controlled trial of ganciclovir to prevent cytomegalovirus disease after heart transplantation. *N Engl J Med*. 1992;326(18): 1182–6.
446. Hibberd PL, Tolkof-Rubin NE, Cosimi AB, *et al*. Symptomatic cytomegalovirus disease in cytomegalovirus antibody positive renal transplant recipients treated with OKT3. *Transplantation* 1992;53:68–72.
447. Lumbreras C, Otero JR, Herrero JA, *et al*. Ganciclovir prophylaxis decreases frequency and severity of cytomegalovirus disease in seropositive liver transplant recipients treated with OKT3 monoclonal antibodies. *Antimicrob Agents Chemother*. 1993;37:2490–2.
448. Martin M. Antiviral prophylaxis of CMV infection in liver transplantation. *Transplant Proc*. 1993;25:10–4.
449. Nicol DL, MacDonald AS, Belitsky P, *et al*. Reduction by combination prophylactic therapy with CMV hyperimmune globulin and acyclovir of the risk of primary CMV disease in renal transplant recipients. *Transplantation* 1993;55(4):841–6.
450. Martin M. Prophylactic cytomegalovirus management strategies. *Transplant Proc*. 1995;27(5 *Suppl* 1):23–8.
451. Morales JM. Reversible acute renal failure caused by the combined use of foscarnet and cyclosporine in organ transplanted patients. *Nephrol Dial Transplant*. 1995;10(6):883–8.
452. Snydman DR, Werner BG, Dougherty NN, *et al*. Cytomegalovirus immune globulin prophylaxis in liver transplantation. *Ann Intern Med*. 1993;119:984–91.
453. Snydman DR, Werner BG, Heinze-Lacey B, *et al*. Use of cytomegalovirus immune globulin to prevent cytomegalovirus disease in renal transplant recipients. *N Engl J Med*. 1987;317(17):1049–54.
454. Nalesnik MA, Locker J, Jaffe R, *et al*. Clonal characteristics of posttransplant lymphoproliferative disorders. *Transplant Proc*. 1988;20(*Suppl* 1):280–3.
455. Hanto DW, Frizzera G, Gajl-Peczalska KJ, *et al*. Epstein-Barr virus-induced B-cell lymphoma after renal transplantation: acyclovir therapy and transition from polyclonal to monoclonal B-cell proliferation. *N Engl J Med*. 1982; 306:913–8.
456. Penn I. Cancers complicating organ transplantation. *N Engl J Med*. 1990;323(25):1767–9.
457. Penn I. The changing patterns of posttransplant malignancies. *Transplant Proc*. 1991;23(1):1101–3.
458. Hibberd PL, Rubin RH. Antiviral therapy—an anti-malignancy strategy for transplant recipients? *Clin Transpl* 1992;6(*Special Iss*.):240–5.
459. Brumbaugh J, Baldwin JC, Stinson EB, *et al*. Quantitative analysis of immunosuppression in cyclosporine-treated heart transplant patients with lymphoma. *J Heart Transplant*. 1985;4:307–11.
460. Penn I. Cancers after cyclosporine therapy. *Transplant Proc*. 1988;20(*Suppl* 1):276–9.
461. Emery RW, Lake KD. Post-transplantation lymphoproliferative disorder and OKT3 [letter]. *N Engl J Med*. 1991;324 (20):1437.
462. Cosimi AB, Rubin RH. Post-transplantation lymphoproliferative disorder and OKT3 [letter]. *N Engl J Med*. 1991;324 (20):1438.
463. Abramowicz D, Goldman M, De Pauw L, *et al*. Posttransplantation lymphoproliferative disorder and OKT3 [letter]. *N Engl J Med*. 1991;324(20):1439.
464. Benkerrou M, Durandy A, Brousse N, Fischer A. Therapy for transplant-related lymphoproliferative diseases. *Rev Fr Hematol*. 1993;35:55–9.
465. Davis CL, Harrison KL, McVicar JP, *et al*. Antiviral prophylaxis and the Epstein Barr virus-related post-transplant lymphoproliferative disorder. *Clin Transpl*. 1995;9:53–9.
466. Petterson E, Hovi T, Ahonen T, *et al*. Prophylactic oral acyclovir after renal transplantation. *Transplantation* 1985;39:279–81.
467. Lynfield R, Herrin JT, Rubin RH. Varicella in pediatric renal transplant recipients. *Pediatrics* 1992;90:216–20.
468. Pereira BJG, Milford EL, Kirkman RL, *et al*. Transmission of hepatitis C virus by organ transplantation. *N Engl J Med*. 1991;325(7):454–60.
469. Chan TM, Lok AS, Cheng IL, *et al*. A prospective study of hepatitis C virus infection among renal transplant recipients. *Gastroenterol*. 1993;104(3):862–8.
470. Kiberd BA. Should hepatitis C-infected kidneys be transplanted in the United States? *Transplantation* 1994;57 (7):1068–72.
471. Hibberd PL, Rubin RH. Clinical aspects of fungal infection in organ transplant recipients. *Clin Infect Dis*. 1994;19 (*Suppl* 1):S33–40.
472. Collins LA, Samore MH, Roberts MS, *et al*. Risk factors for invasive fungal infections complicating orthotopic liver transplantation. *J Infect Dis*. 1994;170(3):544–52.
473. Tollemar J, Andersson S, Ringden O, *et al*. A retrospective clinical comparison between antifungal treatment with liposomal amphotericin B (AmBisome) and conventional amphotericin B in transplant patients. *Mycoses* 1992;35(9–10):215–20.
474. Masur H. Prevention and treatment of pneumocystis pneumonia. *N Engl J Med*. 1992;37(26):1853–60.
475. Olsen SL, Renlund DG, O'Connell, *et al*. Prevention of pneumocystis carinii pneumonia in cardiac transplant recipients by trimethoprim sulfamethoxazole. *Transplantation* 1993;56(2):359–62.
476. Porter GA, Bennett WM, Sheps SG, *et al*. Cyclosporine associated hypertension. *Arch Intern Med*. 1990;150:280–3.

477. Scherrer U. Cyclosporine induced activation in hypertension after heart transplantation. *N Engl J Med.* 1990;323: 693–9.
478. Olivari MT, Antolick A, Ring WS. Arterial hypertension in heart transplant recipients treated with three-drug immunosuppressive therapy. *J Heart Transplant.* 1989;8:34–9.
479. Starling RC, Cody RJ. Cardiac transplant hypertension. *Am J Cardiol.* 1990;65:106–11.
480. Bennett WM, Porter GA. Cyclosporine-associated hypertension. *Am J Med.* 1988;85:131–3.
481. Jarowenko MV, Flechner SM, VanBuren CT, *et al.* Influence of cyclosporine on posttransplant blood pressure response. *Am J Kidney Dis.* 1987;10:98–103.
482. Sturrock ND, Struthers AD. Hormonal and other mechanisms involved in the pathogenesis of cyclosporin-induced nephrotoxicity and hypertension in man [editorial]. *Clin Sci.* 1994;86(1):1–9.
483. Murray, BM, Paller MS. Beneficial effects of renal denervation and prazosin on GFR and renal blood flow after cyclosporine in rats. *Clin Nephrol.* 1986;25(*Suppl* 1):S37–9.
484. Coffman TM, Carr DR, Yarger WE, *et al.* Evidence that renal prostaglandin and thromboxane production is stimulated in chronic cyclosporine nephrotoxicity. *Transplantation* 1986;43:282–5.
485. Kon V, Sugiura M, Inagami T, *et al.* Role of endothelin in cyclosporine-induced glomerular dysfunction. *Kidney Int.* 1990;37:1487–91.
486. Kurtz A, Bruna R, Kuhn K. Cyclosporine A enhances renin secretion and production in isolated juxtaglomerular cells. *Kidney Int.* 1988;33:947–53.
487. Ciresi DL, Lloyd MA, Sandberg SM, *et al.* The sodium retaining effects of cyclosporine. *Kidney Int.* 1992;41:1599–605.
488. Textor SC, Canzanello VJ, Taler SJ, *et al.* Cyclosporine-induced hypertension after transplantation [review]. *Mayo Clin Proc.* 1994;69(12):1182–93.
489. Curtis JJ. Management of hypertension after transplantation [review]. *Kidney Int.* 1993;43(*Suppl*):S45–9.
490. First MR, Neylan JF, Rocher LL, *et al.* Hypertension after renal transplantation [review]. *J Am Soc Nephrol.* 1994;4(8 *Suppl*):S30–6.
491. Miller LW, Pennington DG, McBride LR. Long-term effects of cyclosporine in cardiac transplantation. *Transplant Proc.* 1990;22(*Suppl* 1):15–20.
492. Curtis JJ. Hypertension following kidney transplantation [review]. *Am J Kidney Dis.* 1994;23(3):471–5.
493. Lake, KD. Management of post-transplant obesity and hyperlipidemia. In: Emery RW, Miller L, editors. *Handbook of Cardiothoracic Transplantation*. Philadelphia, PA: Hanley & Belfus; 1995. p. 147–64.
494. Pirsch JD, D'Alessandro AM, Sollinger HW, *et al.* Hyperlipidemia and transplantation: etiologic factors and therapy. *J Am Soc Nephrol.* 1992;2(12 *Suppl*):S238–42.
495. Pirsch JD, Friedman R. Primary care of the renal transplant patient. *J Gen Intern Med.* 1994;9(1):29–37.
496. Johnson CP, Gallagher-Lepak S, Zhu YR, *et al.* Factors influencing weight gain after renal transplantation. *Transplantation* 1993;56(4):822–7.
497. Palmer M, Schaffner F, Thung SN. Excessive weight gain after liver transplantation. *Transplantation* 1991;51(4):797–800.
498. Rubin S, Dale J, Santamaria C, *et al.* Weight change in cardiac transplant patients. *Can J Cardiovasc Nurs.* 1991;2(2):9–13.
499. Hricik DE, Mayes JT, Schulak JA. Independent effects of cyclosporine and prednisone on posttransplant hypercholesterolemia. *Am J Kidney Dis.* 1991;18:353–8.
500. Blum RL. Computer-assisted design of studies using routine clinical data: analyzing the association of prednisone and cholesterol. *Ann Intern Med.* 1986;104:858–68.
501. Becker DM, Chamberlain B, Swank R, *et al.* Relationship between corticosteroid exposure and plasma lipid levels in heart transplant recipients. *Am J Med.* 1988;85:632–8.
502. Zimmerman J, Fainaru M, Eisenberg S. The effects of prednisone therapy on plasma lipoproteins and apolipoproteins: a prospective study. *Metabolism* 1984;33:521–6.
503. Renlund DG, Bristow MR, Crandall BG, *et al.* Hypercholesterolemia after transplantation: amelioration by corticosteroid-free maintenance immunosuppression. *J Heart Transplant.* 1989;8:214–20.
504. Taylor DO, Thompson JA, Hastillo A, *et al.* Hyperlipidemia after clinical heart transplantation. *J Heart Transplant.* 1989;8(3):209–13.
505. Miller LW, McBride LR, Pennington DG. Safe withdrawal of steroids without use of induction therapy in cardiac transplantation [abstract]. *J Am Coll Cardiol.* 1990;15(2): 69.
506. Ballantyne CM, Podet EJ, Patsch WP, *et al.* Effects of cyclosporine therapy on plasma lipoprotein levels. *JAMA* 1989;262(1):53–6.
507. Stamler JS, Vaughan DE, Rudd MA, *et al.* Frequency of hypercholesterolemia after cardiac transplantation. *Am J Cardiol.* 1988;62(17):1268–72.
508. Superko HR, Haskell WL, DiRicco CD. Lipoprotein and hepatic lipase activity and high-density lipoprotein subclasses after cardiac transplantation. *Am J Cardiol.* 1990;66:1131–4.
509. Harris KPG, Russell GI, Parvin SD, *et al.* Alterations in lipid and carbohydrate metabolism attributable to cyclosporin A in renal transplant recipients. *Br Med J.* 1986;292:16.
510. Expert Panel on Detection, Evaluation, and Treatment of High Blood Cholesterol in Adults. Summary of the Second Report of the Nation Cholesterol Education Program (NCEP) Expert Panel on Detection, Evaluation, and Treatment of High Blood Cholesterol in Adults (Adult Treatment Panel II). *JAMA* 1993;269(23):3015–23.
511. Kobashigawa JA, Murphy FL, Stevenson LW, *et al.* Low-dose lovastatin safely lowers cholesterol after cardiac transplantation. *Circulation* 1990;82(*Suppl* 4):281–3.
512. Kuo PC, Kirshenbaum JM, Gordon J, *et al.* Lovastatin therapy for hypercholesterolemia in cardiac transplant recipients. *Am J Cardiol.* 1989;64(10):631–5.
513. Keogh A, Day R, Critchley L, *et al.* The effect of food and cholestyramine on the absorption of cyclosporine in cardiac transplant recipients. *Transplant Proc.* 1988;20:27–30.
514. Corpier CL, Jones PH, Suki WN, *et al.* Rhabdomyolysis and renal injury with lovastatin use. Report of two cases in cardiac transplant recipients. *JAMA* 1988;260(2):239–41.

515. East C, Alivizatos PA, Grundy SM, *et al*. Rhabdomyolysis in patients receiving lovastatin after cardiac transplantation. *N Engl J Med*. 1988;318(1):47–8.
516. Kobashigawa JA, Katznelson S, Laks H, *et al*. Effect of pravastatin on outcomes after cardiac transplantation. *N Engl J Med*. 1995;10621–7.
517. Jindal RM. Posttransplant diabetes mellitus—a review. *Transplantation* 1994;58(12):1289–98.
518. First MR. Transplantation for the nephrologist—long-term complications after transplantation. *Am J Kidney Dis*. 1993; 22(3):477–86.
519. Keown PA, Shackleton CR, Ferguson BM. Long-term mortality, morbidity, and rehabilitation in organ transplant recipients. In: Paul LC, Solez K, editors. *Organ Transplantation: Long-Term Results*. New York: Marcel Dekker; 1992. p. 57–84.
520. Ost L. Effects of cyclosporine on prednisolone metabolism. *Lancet* 1984;1:451.
521. Tyden G, Brattstrom C, Gunnarsson R, *et al*. Metabolic control at 2 months to 4.5 years after pancreatic transplantation, with special reference to the role of cyclosporine. *Transplant Proc*. 1987;19:2294.
522. Ried M, Gibbons S, Kwok D, *et al*. Cyclosporine levels in human tissues of patients treated for one week to one year. *Transplant Proc*. 1983;15:2434.
523. Jindal RM, Popsecu I, Schwartz ME, *et al*. Diabetogenicity of FK506 versus cyclosporine in liver transplant recipients. *Transplantation* 1994;58:370.
524. Muchmore JS, Cooper DKC, Ye Y, *et al*. Loss of vertebral bone density in heart transplant patients. *Transplant Proc*. 1991;23:1184–5.
525. Katz IA, Epstein S. Posttransplantation bone disease [review]. *J Bone Miner Res*. 1992;7(2):123–6.
526. Lukert BP, Raisz LG. Glucocorticoid-induced osteoporosis. *Ann Intern Med*. 1990;112:352–64.
527. Aschendorff C, Offner G, Winkler L, *et al*. Adult height achieved in children after kidney transplantation. *Am J Dis Child*. 1990;144:1138–41.
528. Landmann J, Renner N, Gachter A, *et al*. Cyclosporin A and osteonecrosis of the femoral head. *J Bone Joint Surg*. 1987;69:1226–8.
529. Russel JA, Blahey WB, Stuart TA, *et al*. Avascular necrosis of bone marrow transplant patients. *Med Pediatr Oncol*. 1989;17:140–3.
530. Mazanec DJ, Grisanti JM. Drug-induced osteoporosis. *Cleve Clin J Med*. 1989;56:297–303.
531. Penn I. Incidence and treatment of neoplasia after transplantation. *J Heart Lung Transplant*. 1993;12(6 Pt 2):S328–36.
532. Penn I. Malignancy [review]. *Surg Clin North Am*. 1994; 74(5):1247–57.
533. Hemmens VJ, Moore D. Photochemical sensitization by azathioprine and its metabolites. II. Azathioprine and nitroimidazole metabolites. *Photochem Photobiol*. 1986;43: 257–62.
534. Edwards DI. Mechanisms of cytotoxicity of nitroimidazole drugs. *Prog Med Chem*. 1981;18:87–116.

SELF-ASSESSMENT QUESTIONS—PART I

1. Mycophenolate mofetil inhibits lymphocyte proliferation by blocking which pathway of DNA synthesis?

   a. purine salvage
   b. de novo purine synthesis
   c. pyrimidine synthesis
   d. all of the above

2. Which of the following are common adverse effects of mycophenolate mofetil?
   1. seizures
   2. leukopenia
   3. gastrointestinal distress
   4. nephrotoxicity

   a. 1 only
   b. 1 and 2
   c. 2 and 3
   d. all of the above

3. The adverse effects of OKT3 during the first several doses (including fever, hypotension, nausea and/or vomiting, and headaches) are related to:

   a. an allergic reaction to the murine component of OKT3.
   b. cytokine release secondary to T-cell activation.
   c. sepsis.
   d. serum sickness.

4. Methods of immunologic monitoring of OKT3 include which of the following?
   1. $CD3^+$ T lymphocyte subsets
   2. skin testing
   3. OKT3 serum levels
   4. antimurine antibody formation

   a. 1 and 2
   b. 1 and 3
   c. 1, 3, and 4
   d. all of the above

5. A patient with an anti-OKT3 titer of less than 1:100 can receive another course of OKT3.

   a. true
   b. false

6. Azathioprine (AZA) is effective therapy for treating acute rejection following transplantation procedures.

   a. true
   b. false

7. All heart transplant patients receive 500 mg of what immunosuppressive agent during the operative procedure?

    a. methylprednisolone
    b. cyclosporine
    c. dexamethasone
    d. azathioprine (AZA)

8. The protein binding pattern of cyclosporine (CsA) in serum can best be described by which of the following?

    a. CsA is highly bound to albumin only.
    b. CsA is highly bound to lipoproteins only.
    c. CsA is highly bound to albumin and lipoproteins.
    d. CsA is not bound to serum proteins and occurs as free drug in serum.

9. Which statement best characterizes the pharmacokinetics of cyclosporine (CsA) and tacrolimus?

    a. *Both* CsA and tacrolimus are completely absorbed after oral administration.
    b. CsA is completely absorbed after oral administration, but tacrolimus has a mean bioavailability of 30%.
    c. The absorption of CsA after oral administration is highly dependent on bile flow into the duodenum, whereas the absorption of tacrolimus occurs independently of bile flow.
    d. Tacrolimus is eliminated by the kidney primarily as unchanged drug, whereas CsA undergoes extensive hepatic metabolism.

10. The usefulness of corticosteroids in organ transplantation results from which of the following actions?

    a. direct inhibitory effect on circulating lymphocytes
    b. modulation of specific cellular immune functions
    c. specific anti-inflammatory action in the transplanted organ
    d. a and b only

11. Which of the following statements about the use of corticosteroids after organ transplantation is NOT true?

    a. Corticosteroids are always discontinued three months after transplantation.
    b. Corticosteroids are administered for both prevention and treatment of rejection.
    c. Up to 80% of patients can discontinue corticosteroids after 3–12 months following transplantation.
    d. Deflazacort has been shown to be an effective immunosuppressive agent with fewer side effects than prednisone.

12. Relative to cyclosporine, tacrolimus has been associated with a lower incidence of each of the following adverse effects, *except*:

    a. hypertension.
    b. hyperkalemia.
    c. hirsutism.
    d. gingival hyperplasia.

13. Whole blood tacrolimus levels are measured by ELISA or by IMX assay and are usually kept in which target range?

    a. 200–300 ng/ml
    b. 350–400 ng/ml
    c. 0.5–2.0 ng/ml
    d. 5–20 ng/ml

SELF-ASSESSMENT QUESTIONS—PART II

1. HLA matching between donor and recipient is a component of donor organ allocation for which of the following organ transplant populations?

    a. heart
    b. liver
    c. kidney
    d. all of the above

2. Which cell-to-cell interaction is responsible for initiating the "nonself" recognition associated with acute cellular rejection?

    a. helper ($CD4^+$) T cell–allogenic cell interaction
    b. cytotoxic ($CD8^+$) T cell–allogenic cell interaction
    c. macrophage–allogenic cell interaction
    d. natural killer cell–allogenic cell interaction

3. Hyperacute rejection occurs in response to T lymphocyte–mediated immune responses.

    a. true
    b. false

4. Which of the following cytokines is largely responsible for T-cell activation during an episode of acute cellular rejection?

    a. IL-1
    b. IL-2
    c. INF-γ
    d. TNF-α

5. Which of the following is considered the *standard* method for diagnosing rejection of the pancreas in a simultaneous kidney-pancreas transplant?

a. pancreas biopsy
b. kidney biopsy
c. alterations in serum/urinary amylase
d. alterations in blood glucose

6. Which of the following agents has demonstrated efficacy as monotherapy for both the prevention *and* treatment of CMV disease after solid organ transplantation?

a. acyclovir
b. ganciclovir
c. immunoglobulin
d. b and c

7. The most common viral infection after transplantation is:

a. hepatitis C virus.
b. herpes simplex virus.
c. cytomegalovirus.
d. Epstein-Barr virus.

8. Which immunosuppressive agent(s) have the greatest risk of post-transplant lymphoproliferative disease associated with its/their use?

a. cyclosporine
b. tacrolimus
c. OKT3 and/or Atgam
d. mycophenolate mofetil

9. Liver transplantation is most controversial in treating which of the following diseases?

a. acute liver failure
b. hepatitis B virus
c. liver carcinoma
d. cystic fibrosis

10. There are no upper or lower age limits for heart transplant candidates.

a. true
b. false

11. Acute heart or renal transplant rejection is initially treated with which therapy?

a. ATG/OKT3 and/or prednisone
b. Steroid pulse and/or prednisone
c. CsA
d. Quadruple therapy

12. Acute liver rejection is not effectively treated by intensifying immunosuppressive therapy.

a. true
b. false

13. Eighty percent of all infections in heart transplant patients occur within ________________ (period of time) after receiving high-dose immunosuppressive therapy.

14. What is the most common postoperative complication for kidney transplant patients?

a. hypertension
b. hyperlipidemia
c. allograft rejection
d. viral infections

15. Graft-versus-host disease is a frequent complication for which of the following transplanted organs?

a. kidney
b. pancreas
c. small bowel
d. kidney, pancreas, and small bowel

16. The most common fungal pathogen among recipients of organ transplants is which of the following?

a. *Candida albicans*
b. *Aspergillus* sp.
c. *Pneumocystis carinii*
d. *Candida krusii*

17. The combination of sulfadiazine and pyrimethamine provides effective prophylaxis for *all* the following opportunistic pathogens *except*:

a. *Pneumocystis carinii*.
b. *Candida albicans*.
c. *Toxoplasma gondii*.
d. *Escherichia coli*.

18. Which of the following drugs is an appropriate treatment for primary nonfunction of the hepatic allograft?

a. cyclosporine
b. tacrolimus
c. University of Wisconsin solution
d. alprostadil

19. The use of an extracorporeal liver assist device (ELAD) may be appropriate for *all* of the following clinical situations *except*:

a. acute cellular rejection.
b. primary nonfunction of the hepatic allograft.
c. acute fulminant liver failure as a bridge to transplantation.
d. acute liver failure after a toxic drug overdose.

CHAPTER 9

Bone Marrow Transplantation

Timothy R. McGuire
Associate Professor, Pharmacy Practice
College of Pharmacy
University of Nebraska Medical Center
Omaha, NE

Types of BMT 214
Peripheral Stem Cell Transplantation 214
Tissue Typing 214
  HLA System 215
  Donor/Recipient Matching 215
Preparative Regimens 216
  Radiation and Chemotherapy 216
  Pretransplant Immunosuppressive Agents 217
  Donor Lymphocyte Depletion 217
Complications of BMT 217
  Acute GVHD and GVL Effect 217
    Pathophysiology of Acute GVHD 217
    Afferent and Efferent Phases of Acute GVHD 217
    Staging and Grading 218
    Mechanisms of GVL Effect 218
    Post-transplant Immunosuppressive Agents 219
      ATG and OKT3 219
      Corticosteroids 220
      Cyclosporine and Tacrolimus 220
      Anticytokine Antibodies 221
  Chronic GVHD 221
  Management of Infectious Complications 221
    Bacterial and Fungal Infections 222
    Viral Infections 222
    Long-Term Risk of Infection 224
Summary 224
References 224
Self-Assessment Questions 226

Allogenic bone marrow transplantation (BMT) is used to treat several malignant and nonmalignant diseases. BMT is the first-line therapy in chronic myelogenous leukemia (CML), and it is used to treat acute myelogenous leukemia (AML) in many patients in first remission. Allogenic BMT is the treatment of choice for AML patients who relapse and have an acceptable donor. Allogenic BMT is also used in the treatment of acute lymphocytic leukemia (ALL) in patients out of first remission and in aplastic anemia. Autologous BMT is used to rescue patients from marrow aplasia after they receive high-dose chemotherapy. Because there are few immunologically based pathologies associated with autologous transplantation, the primary focus of this chapter will be the immunologic complications associated with allogenic BMT. Potential complications of BMT related to the alteration of the immune system will be described, with special emphasis on acute and chronic graft-versus-host disease (GVHD), graft-versus-leukemia (GVL) effect, and infection.

Several good review articles exist, and the reader is referred to those for information on the history and noninfectious and nonimmunologic complications of BMT.[1–3]

After completing this chapter, the reader should be able to:

1. Define the three major types of bone marrow transplantation.
2. Discuss the use of peripheral stem cell transplantation versus bone marrow transplantation.
3. Discuss how bone marrow donors and recipients are matched.
4. Describe the common preparative regimens for bone marrow donors and recipients.
5. Discuss the pathophysiology, prevention, and management of acute graft-versus-host disease.
6. Discuss the potential infectious complications of bone marrow transplantation and their management.

TYPES OF BMT

BMT is the process by which bone marrow is taken from a donor and infused intravenously into an appropriately prepared recipient. There are three major types of BMT—autologous, syngenic, and allogenic. When the bone marrow donor and recipient are the same person, this process is called autologous BMT. Syngenic BMT is a rare procedure in which the donor and recipient are identical twins.

In autologous and syngenic BMT, the donor and recipient are immunologically identical, so the bone marrow transplant procedure rarely involves immunologic complications. In allogenic BMT, the donor and recipient are genetically, and therefore immunologically, distinct. Allogenic BMT can be further characterized by the degree of tissue matching and whether a familial relationship exists between the donor and recipient. The three types of donors most frequently used in allogenic BMT are human leukocyte antigen (HLA)-matched siblings, single-antigen-mismatched siblings, and HLA-matched unrelated donors.

PERIPHERAL STEM CELL TRANSPLANTATION

Peripheral stem cell transplantation (PSCT) is the transplantation of peripheral blood progenitor cells (PBPCs) rather than bone marrow. PBPCs normally circulate in the peripheral blood in very low numbers. However, after treating donors with hematopoietic growth factors (such as granulocyte colony-stimulating factor [G-CSF],) with or without chemotherapy, there is an increase by a factor of 10 in the number of circulating stem cells.[4,5] The administration of myelosuppressive doses of cyclophosphamide to donors before collection also mobilizes bone marrow, leading to a higher number of progenitor cells in the blood.[6] PBPCs are harvested from the donor by leukapheresis and given to the recipient, resulting in a more rapid engraftment.

PSCT has several potential advantages over BMT, including elimination of the need for general anesthesia during donor bone marrow harvest, reduced contamination of stem cells with malignant cells in patients with disease in the bone marrow, and more rapid engraftment. In addition, patients who receive pelvic radiation are often not suitable donors, because the radiation can cause fibrotic changes that make marrow recovery from the iliac crest difficult. Because of these advantages, several investigators have recommended that PSCT become the standard of care in autologous transplant procedures.[4,7]

In the allogenic setting the use of PBPCs is becoming more common. How the benefits to the recipient of an allogenic PSCT compare with those of BMT are not known. However, the benefits to the donor are relatively clear: reduced potential complications from general anesthesia and bone marrow harvest.[8] There is currently little data comparing BMT and PSCT and their relative risk of acute GVHD. There has been concern because there is a higher lymphocyte content in the PBPC product than in bone marrow and thus a potential for higher rates of acute GVHD. A small retrospective study comparing BMT with PSCT in HLA-matched siblings found more rapid engraftment and an equivalent incidence of acute GVHD with the use of PBPCs.[9] This study used historic bone marrow controls; a randomized study is required to definitively answer this question.

TISSUE TYPING

Matching recipient and donor tissue type is a critical step

in reducing immunologic complications after allogenic BMT. Matching the donor to the recipient is required to reduce the occurrence of rejection of the donor bone marrow (graft rejection) and an attack by donor T lymphocytes on the tissues of the recipient (GVHD). Immunologic matching reviews the group of genes on chromosome 6 of the major histocompatibility complex (MHC), which includes the HLA system (see chapter 3).

HLA System

There are three classes of MHC gene products (classes I, II, and III). The HLA system includes four gene loci (three class I and one class II loci), which produce glycoproteins critical to differentiating between self and nonself. The HLA class I antigens (HLA-A, HLA-B, and HLA-C) and the class II antigen (HLA-D) are cell surface glycoproteins that are highly variable. Their major function is to present foreign antigen to T lymphocytes. A mismatch of donor and recipient bone marrow at HLA-A, HLA-B, and/or HLA-D initiate the immune reaction associated with graft rejection and GVHD. A mismatch at the HLA-C loci has not been as predictive for acute GVHD and is not routinely typed before BMT.[10]

The presentation of foreign antigen is integral to the self versus nonself function of the HLA system. β_2-Microglobulin and class I antigens are presented along with foreign antigens to CD8$^+$ T lymphocytes. HLA class II proteins are presented by antigen-presenting cells to CD4$^+$ (helper) T cells. This specificity between HLA class and the cells they stimulate results from a stabilizing interaction between the CD8 and CD4 proteins and specific domains on the class I and class II molecules (Figure 9-1). When there is a mismatch between donor and recipient at HLA class I or HLA class II antigens, the HLA proteins of the recipient appear as foreign antigen to the donor T lymphocytes, causing GVHD.[11]

To reduce morbidity and mortality from acute GVHD after allogenic BMT, HLA-matching across class I and class II barriers is a critical step. To identify an HLA-matched donor, class I and class II antigens are identified by serologic or molecular testing before transplantation. [12,13]

The identity of minor histocompatibility antigens are largely unknown, so they are not matched before transplant by the serologic or molecular techniques used to identify the MHC antigens.[14] T-lymphocyte response against minor histocompatibility antigens is similar to the immune response generated against virally infected cells and thus is mediated by a MHC class I process. Minor histocompatibility antigens are processed in the cytoplasm with MHC class I and β_2-microglobulin molecules, and the complex is transported to the cell membrane, where it interacts with the T-cell receptor (TCR) on CD8$^+$ T lymphocytes. This binding of minor histocompatibility antigens and MHC class I complex with the TCR on CD8$^+$ T lymphocytes results in apoptosis (programmed cell death) and death of the target cell. The minor antigen designation does not indicate relative importance; minor antigen mismatches can lead to potentially lethal acute GVHD.[15]

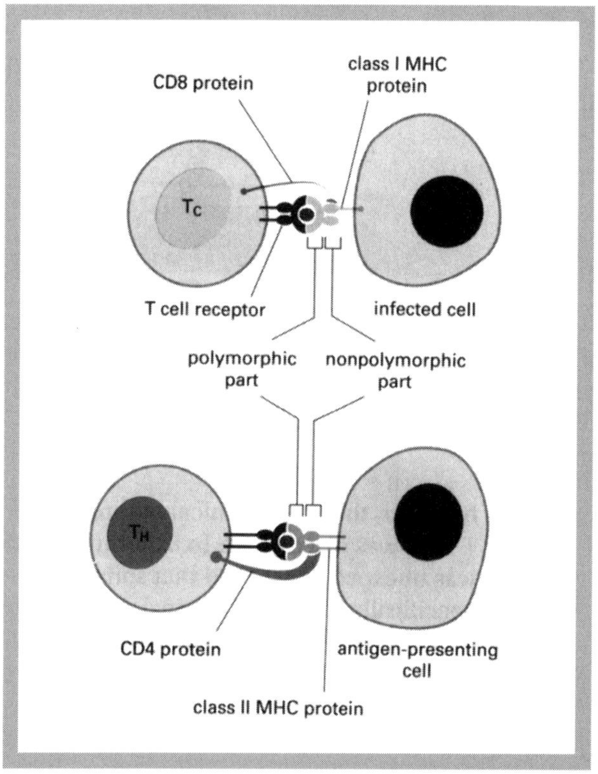

Figure 9-1. CD4 and CD8 interaction with MHC class I and class II molecules. MHC, major histocompatibility complex.

SOURCE: *Reprinted with permission from reference 11.*

Donor/Recipient Matching

Because a child obtains a set of HLA genes from both parents, the likelihood of siblings being HLA-matched is one in four. Finding unrelated individuals who are matched at the HLA loci is often difficult; under even the best circumstances, it may require screening tens of thousands of potential donors to find a suitable match.[10] The likelihood of a match between a given BMT candidate and an unrelated donor depends on the frequency of the patient's HLA type in the general population. BMT registries, which have logged millions of HLA types, have low numbers of nonwhite donors, making it difficult for African-American, Hispanic, and Asian patients to find an unrelated HLA-matched donor.

In addition to HLA-matched related and unrelated transplants, siblings mismatched at one HLA locus are used as donors and have survival rates similar to those in fully matched siblings.[11] The higher rates of acute GVHD in one-antigen-mismatched transplants are offset by a reduction in leukemic relapse as a result of a GVL effect (also described as an antitumor effect). Two and three antigen mismatches result in high rates of graft rejection and severe acute GVHD that is not sufficiently offset by GVL. GVHD and GVL are discussed in detail later in this chapter.

PREPARATIVE REGIMENS

BMT involves intense preparation of the recipient to prevent graft rejection. Preparation involves the administration of high-dose chemotherapy with or without radiation. Immunosuppressive agents such as ATG can be added to the preparative regimen to reduce the risk of graft rejection in high-risk allogenic transplantation. Although graft rejection is a potential source of mortality in BMT patients, the most common immunologic complication is acute GVHD. One of the manipulations that can be performed prior to transplant to reduce the risk of acute GVHD is T-cell depletion of the donor graft. This is performed by the in vitro treatment of the donor graft with antilymphocyte therapy. A form of in vivo purging can also be performed by administering lymphocidal therapy to the patient around the time the graft is infused.

Radiation and Chemotherapy

Patients undergoing an allogenic BMT receive bone marrow–ablative doses of chemotherapy and radiation the week preceding infusion of donor bone marrow. This serves several purposes: destruction of cancer cells, immunosuppression, and the creation of space in the marrow so that the new graft can take up residence.[16] Not only must the preparative regimen have activity against the cancer being treated, but it must also have significant immunosuppressive activity so that the donor marrow, which is immunologically distinct from the recipient, is not rejected when infused.

Several agents that are used in allogenic BMT preparative regimens have immunosuppressive activity. Total body irradiation (TBI) and cyclophosphamide are good immunosuppressives; busulfan, etoposide, cytarabine, carmustine, and cisplatin have lower immunosuppressive activity.[17] Preparative regimens used in allogenic BMT attempt to combine agents with complementary nonmarrow toxicities and include agents that provide sufficient immunosuppression. Table 9-1 lists examples of several preparative regimens used in allogenic BMT.[18–22]

Chemotherapy-only preparative regimens may be used in allogenic BMT, particularly in patients who have a higher risk of pneumonitis because of prior mediastinal radiation. The most common chemotherapy-only regimen consists of busulfan plus cyclophosphamide.[23,24] Radiation has several advantages when added to chemotherapy, including destruction of chemotherapy-resistant cancer cells, treatment of sanctuary sites, and immunosuppression. Concerns when administering preparative regimens that don't contain TBI include increased risk of relapse due to inadequate antitumor activity of the preparative regimen and increased risk of graft rejection as a result of the regimen's low immunosuppressive activity. Despite these concerns, equivalent results have been obtained with cyclophosphamide and busulfan combinations compared with TBI-containing regimens in chronic myelogenous leukemia.

Table 9-1. Allogenic BMT Preparative Regimens

AGENTS	DOSING REGIMENS (ROUTE)	DISEASE
Cyclophosphamide TBI	60 mg/kg per day for 2 days (IV) 1200–1575 rads over 6–7 days	Leukemias
Cyclophosphamide Busulfan	50 mg/kg per day for 4 days (IV) 4 mg/kg per day for 4 days (PO)	Leukemias
Cytarabine TBI	3 g/m^2 BID for 6 days (IV) 850–1200 rads over 6 days	ALL
Etoposide Cyclophosphamide TBI	1500 mg/m^2 for 1 day over 4 hr (IV) 60 mg/kg per day for 2 days (IV) 1200 rads over 6 days	MUD
Cyclophosphamide ATG	50 mg/kg per day for 4 days (IV) 30 mg/kg per day for 4 days (IV)	AA, second transplants

BMT, bone marrow transplant; IV, intravenous; TBI, total body irradiation; BID, twice per day; PO, orally; ALL, acute lymphocytic leukemia; MUD, matched unrelated donor transplant; AA, aplastic anemia; ATG, antithymocyte globulin.

Pretransplant Immunosuppressive Agents

There is a higher rate of graft rejection in patients undergoing HLA-matched unrelated transplants than those receiving HLA-matched related transplants. To increase the immunosuppressive activity of the preparative regimen and reduce graft rejection associated with matched unrelated BMT, traditional immunosuppressive agents, such as antithymocyte globulin (ATG), may be used as part of the BMT preparative regimen. The administration of ATG suppresses the residual immune function of the recipient, decreasing the risk of graft rejection.[22] ATG is further discussed later in this chapter.

Donor Lymphocyte Depletion

Purging donor bone marrow of T lymphocytes can effectively minimize the risk of acute GVHD. In patients undergoing HLA-matched related BMT receiving no post-transplant immunosuppression, the incidence of acute GVHD is about 80%. This incidence can be reduced to about 20% when 95% of donor T lymphocytes are removed from the graft. However, because T lymphocytes facilitate engraftment and can mount a GVL effect, the mortality associated with graft failure and leukemic relapse in many cases exceeds that caused by acute GVHD. In CML patients receiving T lymphocyte–depleted bone marrow, there is a fivefold increase in the risk of relapse compared with patients not receiving purged bone marrow. This reduction in antileukemic effect likely occurs from a reduction in acute GVHD and thus a reduction in GVL effect.[25]

COMPLICATIONS OF BMT

Acute GVHD and GVL Effect

Acute GVHD occurs when donor and recipient histocompatibility differences stimulate donor T lymphocytes. This stimulation results in the production of activated T lymphocytes and other activated white blood cells. These white blood cells cause direct and indirect tissue damage. The direct damage results from cell-to-cell interaction, whereas indirect damage occurs from the inflammatory cytokines released during white blood cell activation. There is also evidence for the early involvement of inflammatory cytokines released as a result of the preparative regimen–induced tissue damage. These cytokines can stimulate T lymphocytes in the donor graft, potentiating acute GVHD.[13,26] Several inflammatory cytokines increase the expression of MHC antigens and adhesion molecules, having the net effect of increasing histocompatibility differences between donor and recipient.[27]

Pathophysiology of Acute GVHD

Acute GVHD occurs when alloreactive cells in the donor graft attack the recipient's tissues, leading to damage of the skin, liver, and gut. The incidence and severity of acute GVHD are directly related to the number of donor T lymphocytes infused into the recipient, but there is a growing appreciation for the role of cytokines in the initiation and progression of acute GVHD.[26]

Cytokines are low-molecular-weight proteins that have profound immunologic effects at picomolar concentrations. They usually act locally and are able to regulate the intensity and duration of the immune response. The cytokine network is a redundant system, with many of the cytokine receptors sharing common signaling pathways.[28] For example, the binding of two inflammatory cytokines, tumor necrosis factor alpha (TNF-α) and interleukin 1-beta (IL-1β), to their receptors leads to similar biological effects because they activate the same signal-transducing pathways. The biological activity of these two cytokines include endogenous pyrogen activity, activation of coagulation pathways, increased MHC expression, and increased synthesis of other inflammatory cytokines.[11,28]

The ability of different cytokines to produce overlapping inflammatory effects leads to an amplification of tissue damage associated with their unregulated release. The massive and unregulated release of inflammatory cytokines in acute GVHD has been characterized as a cytokine storm.[13,26] The cytokine storm, which occurs during acute GVHD, may result from tissue damage from the preparative regimen and alloreactive stimulation of white blood cells in the donor marrow.[13]

Afferent and Efferent Phases of Acute GVHD

Acute GVHD can be described as having an afferent and an efferent phase. In the afferent phase, there is an initial stimulation and expansion of donor T lymphocytes sensitized to recipient tissue. Tissue destruction during this phase is mediated by helper T cells, which increase the activity of antigen-presenting cells, resulting in more efficient antigen presentation. Stimulation of antigen presentation leads to the release of inflammatory cytokines that increase immune-mediated tissue damage. During the afferent phase, there is a clonal expansion of allosensitized cytotoxic T lymphocytes as a result of helper T cell–derived IL-2.[13]

The afferent phase of acute GVHD begins shortly after the infusion of donor bone marrow. As previously discussed, there is a direct correlation between the number of mature donor T lymphocytes infused and the incidence and severity of acute GVHD. Because post-transplant immunosuppressive drugs affect donor T lymphocyte number and function in the recipient, the incidence, severity, and time to onset of acute GVHD is altered compared with patients not receiving post-transplant immunosuppression. Sullivan *et al.* demonstrated that severe acute GVHD occurs in all patients not receiving post-transplant immunosuppression in as little as a few days after donor bone marrow infusion. In contrast, patients who receive appropriate post-transplant immunosuppression have a 25–40% incidence of grade II–IV acute GVHD, usually occurring two to five weeks after transplant.[3,29]

The efferent phase of acute GVHD is characterized by the supraphysiologic production and release of inflammatory cytokines. The net effect of this cascade of cytokines is the activation of additional alloreactive cells (T and B lymphocytes and monocytes) and further destruction of recipient tissue. During this second stage of acute GVHD, cell death from the direct effects of immune cells on target tissue and damage from inflammatory cytokines produces the clinical effects associated with acute GVHD. This may explain why combination immunosuppressive therapy, which inhibits cell-mediated and cytokine-mediated cytotoxicity, is most effective in treating acute GVHD.[30]

Staging and Grading

Acute GVHD is a major source of morbidity and mortality after allogenic BMT. Patients who develop severe acute GVHD that is unresponsive to immunosuppression usually die from infection or from primary organ dysfunction. The high infection rate associated with acute GVHD results from a combination of immune dysregulation and the destruction of protective barriers, such as skin and mucosa. Organ dysfunction (skin, gut, and liver) occurs because of the direct cytotoxic effects on target tissue by activated T lymphocytes.[26,30] The severity of acute GVHD is assessed by determining the number of organs involved and the extent of involvement of each organ. Organ involvement includes skin (rash to desquamation), gut (mild to severe diarrhea), and liver (impaired liver function). Acute GVHD is graded from I to IV, with grades II–IV being considered most clinically important. Staging and grading of acute GVHD is presented in Table 9-2. The detailed staging and grading system illustrated in Table 9-2 is superior to a simplified system that designates acute GVHD as being absent, moderate, or severe. The detailed system allows for a more accurate assessment of patient outcome.[31] A more extensive discussion of the staging and grading of acute GVHD is beyond the scope of this chapter; the reader is referred to reference 13.

Mechanisms of GVL Effect

The GVL effect can benefit the bone marrow recipient by decreasing leukemic relapse. The GVL effect produces an antitumor (antileukemic) effect and is thought to occur by the generation of natural killer (CD56⁺) cells and

Table 9-2. Staging and Grading System for Acute GVHD[13]

ORGAN INVOLVED	DEGREE OF INVOLVEMENT	STAGE	OVERALL GRADE
Skin	Rash Coverage (% BSA)		Grade I: only **skin 1–2+**
	<25%	1+	
	25–50%	2+	
	>50%	3+	
	Desquamation	4+	
Liver	Bilirubin Elevation (mg/dl)		Grade II: skin 1–3, **liver 1+**, and intestine 1+
	2–3	1+	
	3–6	2+	
	6–15	3+	Grade III: skin 2–3+, **liver 2–3+**, and intestine 2–3+
	>15	4+	
			Grade IV: skin 2–4+, **liver 2–4+**, and intestine 2–4+
Intestine	Diarrhea (ml/day)		Grade II: skin 2–3+, liver 1+, and **intestine 1+**
	>500	1+	
	>1000	2+	
	>1500	3+	Grade III: skin 2–3+, liver 2–3+, and **intestine 2–3+**
	Pain/Ileus	4+	
			Grade IV: skin 2–4+, liver 2–4+, and **intestine 2–4+**

GVHD, graft-versus-host disease; BSA, body surface area. ***Bold*** *indicates overall clinical grade.*

cytotoxic T ($CD8^+$) lymphocytes produced during GVHD. It is difficult to inhibit GVHD without eliminating the beneficial effects of the GVL reaction. Because relapse remains the major source of post-transplant mortality in leukemia patients, it is important to maintain the GVL effect to increase the cure rate. A graft-versus-tumor effect has not been demonstrated in patients being treated for breast cancer or other solid tumors but is currently under investigation.

Attempts have been made to separate graft-versus-host and GVL effects. It has been proposed that GVHD and GVL are produced by different T-lymphocyte subsets, so it might be possible, by selective T-lymphocyte purging of donor marrow, to maintain the GVL effect while reducing the incidence of acute GVHD. The GVL effect results from the activation of $CD8^+$ and $CD4^+$ cells, which increases IL-2 production, leading to the expansion of cytotoxic T lymphocytes and natural killer cells. The cytotoxic T lymphocytes and natural killer cells reduce the rate of relapse after transplantation by destroying residual tumor cells.

As described previously, acute GVHD involves both $CD4^+$ and $CD8^+$ cells, so it is unlikely that acute GVHD and GVL can be easily separated based on selective T-cell depletion. Unique cells involved in GVHD and not GVL have yet to be conclusively identified. There is interest in a $CD4^-$, $CD8^-$, and $CD3^+$ natural suppressor cell, which in cell culture and under IL-2 stimulation inhibits acute GVHD while maintaining the GVL effect.[32] Work is also being performed on inhibiting $CD25^+$ (IL-2–receptor) cells with IL-2–receptor antibodies; this may allow the prevention of acute GVHD without losing the GVL effect.[33] It may also be possible to add back T lymphocytes eliminated during purging procedures. Preliminary data suggests that adding back lymphocytes after the period of greatest acute GVHD risk may stimulate the GVL effect without a high incidence of severe acute GVHD.[34]

Post-transplant Immunosuppressive Agents

Immunosuppressive therapy must be given to avoid acute GVHD. Drug therapy employs a handful of immunosuppressive drugs, usually in combination. Examples of immunosuppressive regimens are listed in Table 9-3. Drugs used to induce nonspecific immunosuppression include ATG, OKT3, and corticosteroids. Although these therapies are effective in the treatment and prevention of acute GVHD, their use results in a higher risk of serious infection. In addition to these relatively nonspecific therapies, there are a group of drugs with specific activity, including cyclosporine (CsA), tacrolimus (FK506), and several biotechnologically derived anticytokine agents that may improve response and reduce toxicity associated with post-transplant immunosuppression.

ATG and OKT3

ATG is produced by injecting human thymus tissue subcutaneously into an equine host. When the equine host is sensitized, the globulin fraction of blood is collected and purified. ATG is a nonspecific preparation that causes antibody-mediated clearance of circulating lymphocytes, neutrophils, and platelets. The destruction and retrafficking of T lymphocytes leads to the immunosuppression associated with the preparation.

Table 9-3. Immunosuppressive Regimens for Acute GVHD Prophylaxis

DRUG REGIMEN	DOSE (ROUTE)	FREQUENCY	COMMENTS
CsA	3–5 mg/kg per day (IV)	day 1–day 180	Tapered if no GVHD
Methotrexate	15 mg/m² per day (IV)	day 1	May hold for mucositis
	10 mg/m² per day (IV)	days 3, 6, and 11	
CsA	3–5 mg/kg per day (IV)	day -2–day 180	Tapered if no GVHD
Prednisone	0.5–1 mg/kg per day (PO)	day 7–day 57	Slow taper to day 180
Methotrexate	10 mg/m² per day (IV)	days 1, 3, and 6	
CsA	3–5 mg/kg per day (IV)	day 1–day 180	
Methylprednisolone	0.5–1.0 mg/kg per day (IV)	day 5–day 16	
ATG	10 mg/kg per day (IV)	day 5–day 16	
Tacrolimus	0.04 mg/kg per day (IV) CI; then 0.2 mg/kg per day (PO) divided in two daily doses q 12 h	when oral dose tolerated	DLT; renal dysfunction

CsA, cyclosporine; CI, continuous infusion; DLT, dose-limiting toxicity.

OKT3, a monoclonal antibody of mouse origin, binds to the CD3 antigen on T lymphocytes and causes a rapid but transient lymphopenia. Anti-CD3 antibodies react with 100% of peripheral blood T lymphocytes but only 10% of thymocytes. The administration of OKT3 results in the redistribution of $CD3^+$ cells from the peripheral blood into a nonvascular compartment. This redistribution is facilitated by increased adherence to vascular endothelium.[35] In addition, opsonization of $CD3^+$ cells leads to clearance by the reticuloendothelial system. It has also been demonstrated that OKT3 binding to the CD3 receptor induces apoptosis in activated T lymphocytes.[36] Although there is a rapid decline in lymphocyte numbers after administration of OKT3, the counts return within hours. The lymphocytes that return to the circulation do not have the CD3 receptor. Because of the close association and interaction between the CD3 receptor and the TCR, these CD3-negative lymphocytes have impaired alloreactivity.

Both ATG and OKT3 are potent and effective agents in the prevention and treatment of acute GVHD. These antibody products are performing a type of in vivo purging when used prophylactically just before and after transplant. The reduction in the severity and incidence of acute GVHD by administering these agents is further evidence of the pivotal role T lymphocytes play in acute GVHD. However, because CD3 is a pan-TCR, OKT3 has a global inhibitory effect on lymphocyte function and is associated with a significant risk of infection. In addition, both OKT3 and ATG can initially stimulate immune cells to release many of the proinflammatory cytokines involved in acute GVHD, including IL-1, IL-6, and TNF-α.[37] The importance of these inflammatory cytokines to the side effect profile of ATG and OKT3 is clear (i.e., they mediate fever and chills), but their importance in antagonizing the immunosuppressive activity of these antibodies is not known. Because of concerns about the mitogenic activity of OKT3, nonmitogenic anti-CD3 monoclonal antibody is under investigation that utilizes a subclass of IgG that is not associated with the constitutional symptoms caused by ATG and OKT3 administration.[38]

The toxicities of ATG and OKT3 are somewhat different but reflect either the administration of a foreign protein (ATG-equine, OKT3-murine) or a direct extension of binding to target antigens. For example, the fever, chills, rigors, and serum sickness associated with ATG and OKT3 administration result from a combination of foreign protein administration and release of cytokines after antibody binds to cytokine-secreting cells (mast cells, monocytes, and T lymphocytes). Thrombocytopenia associated with ATG occurs from reticuloendothelial cell clearance after antibody binding to platelets.

Corticosteroids

Corticosteroids are potent regulators of gene expression. They inhibit the transcription and translation of a number of inflammatory cytokine genes, such as IL-1 and TNF-α, important in the development of acute GVHD. Corticosteroids also inhibit granulocyte chemotaxis and degranulation, thus inhibiting granulocyte movement into organs undergoing alloreactive changes and decreasing the production of tissue-destructive free radicals. In addition, corticosteroids inhibit the presentation of MHC class II molecules by macrophages, leading to reduced alloreactivity. At the high doses used to treat acute GVHD, corticosteroids are effective lymphocidal drugs, reducing the number of cells that mediate acute GVHD.[39] Because of these varied and potent immunosuppressive effects in both the early and later stages of acute GVHD, high-dose corticosteroids are the treatment of choice for patients who develop grade II–IV acute GVHD.

Cyclosporine and Tacrolimus

CsA and tacrolimus block the transcription of IL-2, IL-4, and interferon alpha, thus blocking the early events in T-lymphocyte activation.[40] Both CsA and tacrolimus perform this function by reversibly binding to cytosolic proteins generally known as immunophilins (cyclophilin and FK binding protein). These are ubiquitous proteins whose full function is not well understood, but when bound to CsA and tacrolimus, they inhibit calcineuron activity. Calcineuron is a protein phosphatase involved in the signaling pathway associated with IL-2 gene expression (Figure 9-2).[41] The cleaving of a phosphate group from a nuclear regulatory protein increases IL-2 gene transcription. The inhibition of calcineuron by CsA inhibits the cleaving of this phosphate group and reduces IL-2 mRNA transcription. The binding of CsA and tacrolimus to their target immunophilins results in a specific and reversible immunosuppression.

The interaction between CsA and tacrolimus and their respective immunophilins is reversible, with alloreactivity returning within a few days of stopping the drug. Because these agents inhibit the IL-2–dependent proliferation of T lymphocytes, CsA and tacrolimus may have their major effects in preventing acute GVHD by inhibiting the early IL-2–dependent processes that initiate acute GVHD. Presumably, CsA and tacrolimus are less effective in treating acute GVHD when high numbers of activated T lymphocytes already exist and lymphocidal therapy is required. However, there have been impressive responses with tacrolimus in patients with severe acute GVHD that is resistant to steroid-CsA combinations. The 100-fold higher affinity tacrolimus has for its immunophilin compared with CsA may explain these responses.[42]

Prophylactic use of tacrolimus plus methotrexate for the prevention of acute GVHD has been reported in matched unrelated transplants; this study cited a 42% incidence of grade II–IV acute GVHD. Similar patients treated with CsA and methotrexate reported rates approaching 80%.[43,44]

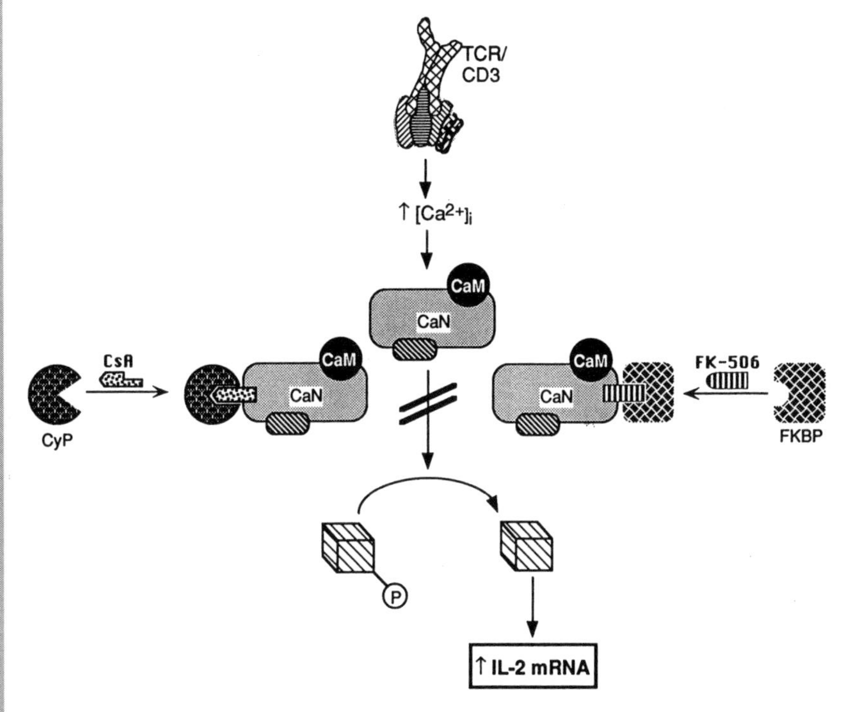

Figure 9-2. Mechanism of action of cyclosporine (CsA) and tacrolimus (FK506). CaN, calcineurin; CaM, calmodulin; FKBP, FK506 binding protein; CyP, cyclophilin; TCR, T-cell receptor; IL-2, interleukin 2.

SOURCE: *Reprinted with permission from: Sigal NH, Dumont FJ. Immunosuppression. In: Paul WE, editor.* Fundamental Immunology. *3rd ed. New York: Raven; 1993. p. 903–15.*

Anticytokine Antibodies

Monoclonal antibodies directed against inflammatory cytokines are currently being investigated. They include IL-2–receptor, IL-1–receptor, and TNF-α antagonists. Humanized anti-TAC is an IgG1 monoclonal antibody specific to the α subunit of the IL-2 receptor. Unlike CsA, which inhibits IL-2 gene transcription, this antibody blocks the effects of preformed IL-2, and this antibody may be an effective agent in treating acute GVHD. Anasetti *et al.* demonstrated an improvement in 40% of patients with steroid-resistant acute GVHD after treatment with IL-2 receptor monoclonal antibody.[45] The IL-1 receptor antagonist, a naturally occurring competitive inhibitor of IL-1, has been used in 17 patients with steroid-resistant acute GVHD. In over 60% of these patients, the severity of acute GVHD improved by at least one grade.[46] Recombinant soluble TNF-α receptor has been investigated in a mouse model for acute GVHD and demonstrated a 50% reduction in mortality when mice were treated soon after transplantation.[47]

Currently, these and several other biotechnologically derived cytokine antagonists are being evaluated for the prevention and treatment of acute GVHD. The preliminary results described above would suggest that these agents will have the same disappointing results seen with other agents when used in steroid-resistant acute GVHD but may be an effective class of agents for the prevention and early treatment of acute GVHD.

Chronic GVHD

Chronic GVHD has been defined as GVHD occurring after day 100 following BMT. Chronic GVHD is actually a different disease entity from acute GVHD. Unlike acute GVHD, chronic GVHD can affect nearly any organ and has many of the characteristics of an autoimmune disease.[48] Chronic GVHD usually occurs in patients who have had prior acute GVHD; less commonly it can occur in patients without a history of acute GVHD (de novo GVHD). The treatment that has most consistently reduced the severity of chronic GVHD is the combination of corticosteroids and CsA. Other agents used to treat chronic GVHD include thalidomide, azathioprine, and cyclophosphamide.[49,50]

The major cause of mortality in patients with chronic GVHD is infection.[48] Patients with chronic GVHD have a severe combined immune deficiency characterized by defective T-cell number and function, defective B-cell function with abnormal antibody production, abnormal neutrophil chemotaxis, and increased suppressor cell activity.[50,51] In addition to the severe immune dysfunction, chronic GVHD produces disease syndromes affecting the skin, liver, gastrointestinal tract, eyes, mouth, sinuses, respiratory tract, vagina, muscle, nervous system, urological system, and hematopoietic system.[50]

Management of Infectious Complications

Patients undergoing allogenic BMT are at high risk for infection as a result of the myelosuppressive activity of the preparative regimen and the immunosuppression associated with the procedure. Infections occur at various times after transplantation and depend on the presence of risk factors. The various methods of immunosuppression can result in neutropenia, which predisposes patients

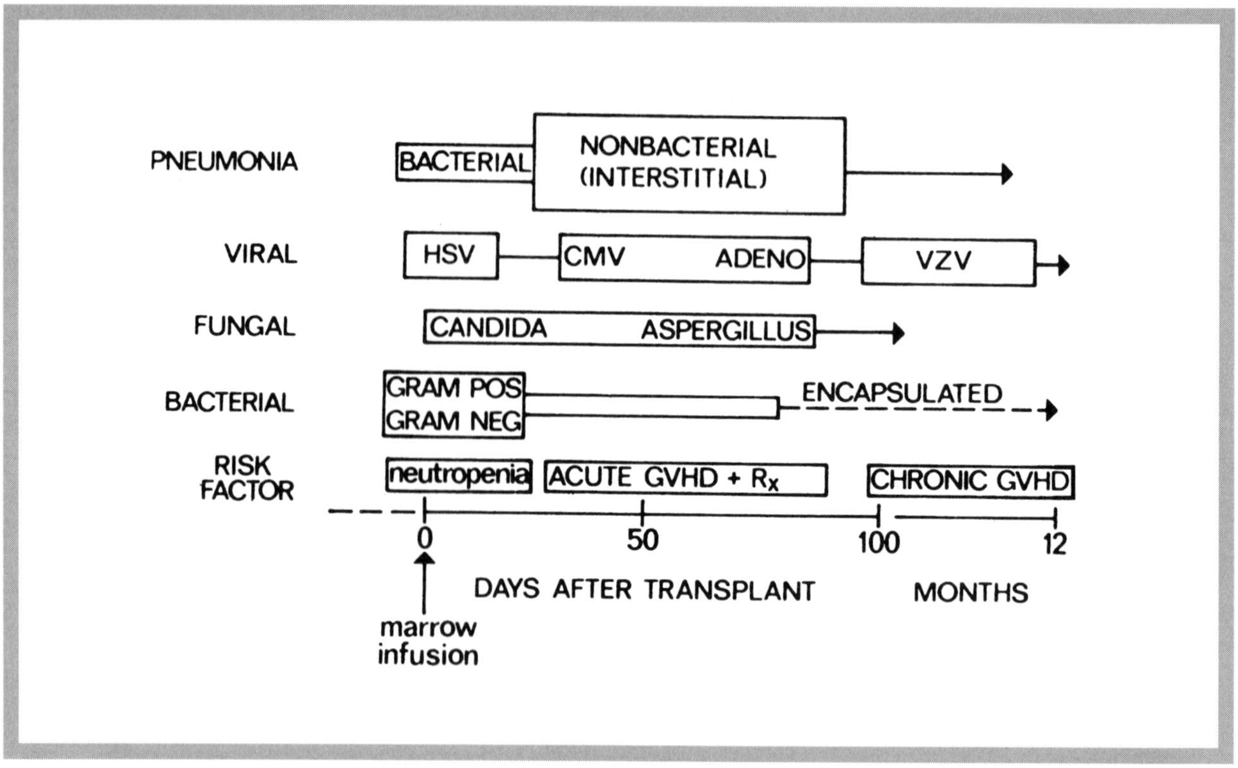

Figure 9-3. Infections after allogenic bone marrow transplantation. HSV, herpes simplex virus; CMV, cytomegalovirus; Adeno, adenovirus; VZV, varicella-zoster virus; GVHD, graft-versus-host disease; R_x, immunosuppressive therapy.

SOURCE: *Reprinted with permission from: Meyers JD. Infections in marrow recipients. In: Mandell GL, et al., editors.* Principles and Practice of Infectious Diseases. *3rd ed. New York: Churchill Livingstone; 1990. p. 2291–4.*

to bacterial and fungal infections. Figure 9-3 shows the infection time line after allogenic BMT.

Bacterial and Fungal Infections

The initial fever associated with neutropenia is assumed to be due to bacterial infection and requires the use of appropriate antibacterials with activity against gram-negative bacteria, particularly *Pseudomonas aeruginosa.* Antibacterials are usually used empirically after the patient develops neutropenic fever. In addition, an agent with gram-positive activity is often added. If fever persists despite empiric antibacterials, amphotericin B is added to treat presumed fungal infections. Fluconazole, although it has good activity against *Candida albicans*, lacks activity against nonalbican yeast and all molds (including *Aspergillus* sp.), making it less than optimal as an empiric agent in patients at high risk for systemic fungal infections.

Because of the high morbidity and mortality associated with fungal infections, prophylactic antifungals have been advocated.[52,53] However, because of the relatively low incidence of fungal infections in many institutions and the established use of empiric antifungals, prophylactic therapy is not routinely used. There are populations for which preventive antifungals are indicated, including patients colonized with *Aspergillus* sp. In addition, sporadic outbreaks of *Aspergillus* sp. can be devastating in BMT units, and when this occurs, prophylactic antifungal therapy is a reasonable intervention.

Viral Infections

In addition to bacterial and fungal infections, patients are at risk for Herpes simplex virus (HSV) reactivation. The HSV infections that occur after allogenic BMT are often severe, causing significant morbidity and adding many days to hospitalization. Acyclovir is used to prevent reactivation of latent virus. The effectiveness of intravenous acyclovir at doses of 250 mg/m^2 every 12 hours for prevention of HSV infections is nearly complete.[54] In addition, oral acyclovir at doses of 200 mg five times daily protects against HSV reactivation in patients able to take oral medications.[55]

After an initial period of risk associated with neutropenia and mucositis (the first two to three weeks following BMT), allogenic BMT patients are at continuing risk of viral and bacterial infection because of a chronic immune deficiency.[56,57] The source of chronic immunosuppression includes GVHD prevention and treatment regimens and chronic GVHD itself, which increases infectious risk due to barrier dysfunction and abnormal T-lymphocyte function.[58] Chronic GVHD also requires the prolonged use of relatively high doses of corticosteroids, which further impairs T-lymphocyte function.

Allogenic BMT patients are at high risk for cytomegalovirus (CMV) infections. CMV is a herpesvirus that is relatively difficult to treat with currently available antivirals. The median time to onset of CMV disease is about 60 days after transplant. About 60% of patients who present for transplantation are CMV seropositive. As with many other viruses, CMV remains latent in the body and can reactivate when a patient becomes immunosuppressed. CMV is often associated with gastrointestinal disease or pneumonia, but other organ systems can be involved, including bone marrow, liver and—more uncommonly—eyes (retinitis) and bladder (hemorrhagic cystitis). The complication most feared is CMV pneumonia, with historic case fatality rates of 85–90%.[59] Recent treatments have reduced mortality from CMV pneumonia, but it remains high, at about 50%.[60]

Because treatment of CMV pneumonia remains less than optimal, methods of preventing CMV disease have been aggressively instituted in the allogenic BMT setting. Patients who are CMV seronegative at the time of transplantation and who receive bone marrow from a seronegative donor can have their risk of CMV pneumonia nearly eliminated by using CMV-negative blood products.[59] Recent data on the use of filtered blood products suggests that rates of CMV pneumonia are similar to those seen after screening blood products.[61] This may be a method to reduce the incidence of CMV pneumonia in seronegative patients receiving seronegative bone marrow without depleting increasingly precious CMV-negative blood products. In seronegative patients who receive a graft from a seropositive donor, the screening of blood products is unlikely to be helpful because of the large amount of CMV that is transferred to the recipient from the donor bone marrow. While these patients are not usually given CMV-screened blood products, they do receive high-dose prophylactic acyclovir (500 mg/m^2 every eight hours) to reduce CMV disease rates. The ability of acyclovir to prevent CMV is controversial, given its low activity against CMV in vitro and its lack of effectiveness in treating CMV disease. The use of high-dose acyclovir in preventing CMV in allogenic BMT patients is based on a single nonrandomized study and remains a point of controversy. However, because this study reported a reduction in 100-day mortality in patients given prophylactic acyclovir, seropositive patients are usually given high-dose therapy.[62]

Although the use of high-dose prophylactic acyclovir during the first month following transplant has been reported to reduce rates of CMV pneumonia, the low activity of acyclovir against CMV has led many clinicians to use newer protocols that include ganciclovir. Waiting to use ganciclovir until engraftment occurs minimizes its marrow-suppressive effect on the new graft. Ganciclovir has significantly greater activity than acyclovir against CMV and may be superior in protecting against CMV pneumonia. Schmidt *et al.* studied the use of ganciclovir therapy in patients with CMV-positive broncheoaveolar lavage after bone marrow engraftment.[63] Patients who had a positive lavage and didn't receive ganciclovir were at a significantly higher risk for CMV disease. In a recent study by Einselle *et al.*, the method of detecting CMV was clinically important. The more sensitive polymerase chain reaction, which can measure minute quantities of CMV mRNA, allowed earlier initiation of gancyclovir and reduced CMV disease and decreased mortality.[64] Table 9-4 lists several of the antiretroviral regimens used to prevent and treat CMV disease.[65]

Table 9-4. CMV Prophylactic and Treatment Regimens

DRUG AND DOSE (ROUTE)	FREQUENCY AND DURATION	EFFICACY
Prophylaxis		
Acyclovir 500 mg/m^2 per dose (IV)	q 8 h, day –5 to day 30	40–50% reduction in CMV pneumonia
Gancyclovir 5 mg/kg per dose (IV)	q 12 h for 14 days, then daily until engraftment to day 100 ± IVIG	
IVIG	once per week to day 100	Unproven efficacy in CMV-positive patients
CMV-screened blood products		Protective in CMV-negative patients with negative graft
Treatment		
Ganciclovir 5 mg/kg per dose (IV)	q 12 h for 14–21 days	Reduces mortality by 40%
Foscarnet 60 mg/kg per dose (IV)	q 8 h for 14–21 days	Poor response in patients with CMV pneumonia

CMV, cytomegalovirus; IVIG, intravenous immune globulin.

When CMV disease occurs despite preventive therapy, ganciclovir combined with intravenous immunoglobulin is the treatment of choice. The usefulness of ganciclovir in the treatment of CMV pneumonia is conceptually straightforward because it has good activity against the virus and substantial ability to clear the virus. However, the activity of nonspecific intravenous immunoglobulin with relatively low amount of anti-CMV immunoglobulin is more difficult to understand. The activity of the nonspecific immunoglobulin preparations has been explained by some investigators as a modulation of the autoimmune aspects of CMV disease. The pathophysiology of CMV pneumonia may involve the cytopathic consequences of CMV to the lungs and a continuing autoimmune process that destroys lung tissue.

The new oral antivirals valacyclovir and famciclovir exhibit better absorption than acyclovir. In cancer patients receiving traditional chemotherapy regimens, they have been as effective as acyclovir. Because of improved bioavailability, the oral agents may be used to prevent and treat viral infections after BMT, including HSV and varicella-zoster virus (VZV).[66] It is doubtful that these agents will have a role in the treatment of CMV disease, given the low activity of acyclovir against the virus. However, valacyclovir and famciclovir may be useful in outpatient prophylaxis of CMV.

BMT patients are at high risk for VZV infection, with median time to onset of about six months after transplantation. VZV is treated as soon as it is diagnosed, regardless of severity, because of the risk of systemic disease. When the initial presentation is severe or there is evidence of progression, including coalescence of vesicular lesions, patients are given intravenous acyclovir at a dose of 500 mg/m^2 every eight hours for 10–14 days. Acyclovir inhibits systemic spread of the disease and speeds crusting by several days compared with untreated patients. Patients less severely affected can be given oral acyclovir at a dose of 800 mg four times daily. With the advent of valacyclovir and famciclovir, oral therapy may become a more popular method of treating allogenic BMT patients with VZV, avoiding the inconvenience of intravenous therapy.[65]

Long-Term Risk of Infection

Patients have a continuing risk of bacterial sepsis during the first two years after transplantation. This risk results from the immune dysfunction that occurs as a result of chronic GVHD and abnormal lymphocyte function associated with the allogenic BMT process. Although gram-negative bacterial infections are a continuing problem, encapsulated organisms are particularly important pathogens. *Pneumococcus* sp. are important pathogens in ambulatory allogenic BMT patients, probably as a result of chronically low complement levels. *Pneumocystis carinii* continues to be a pathogen in ambulatory BMT patients. To protect against infection by *Pneumococcus* and *Pneumocystis* sp., patients are often given oral antibiotics for up to a year after transplantation. Both trimethoprim–sulfamethoxazole and oral penicillin VK have been used. The role of other oral antibiotics with a greater antibacterial spectrum, such as the fluoroquinolones, has not been precisely defined, and concerns exist given the potential risk of superinfection.

SUMMARY

The optimal management of patients undergoing allogenic bone marrow transplantation (BMT) requires the careful balancing of immunosuppression to avoid graft rejection and severe acute graft-versus-host disease (GVHD) while maintaining sufficient immune function to limit infection and maintain a graft-versus-leukemia (GVL) effect. Sources of immunosuppression include the preparative regimen, post-transplant immunosuppressive therapy, and acute and chronic GVHD. It may be possible to separate the acute graft-versus-host and GVL reactions, leading to a reduction in the mortality from severe acute GVHD and tumor relapse. These areas of research may allow more frequent application of allogenic BMT in older patients and those without a matched sibling donor. Morbidity and mortality from infectious causes in allogenic BMT patients are highest during the first two months following transplant but can occur for up to two years because of abnormalities in T-lymphocyte subsets and a decline in complement levels.

REFERENCES

1. Thomas ED, Storb R, Clift RA, *et al.* Bone marrow transplantation. *N Engl J Med.* 1975;292:832–43, 895–902.
2. Thomas ED. Frontiers in bone marrow transplantation. *Blood Cells* 1991;17:259–67.
3. Yee GC. Bone marrow transplantation. In: DiPiro J, *et al.*, editors. *Pharmacotherapy*. 3rd ed. Norwalk, CT: Appleton and Lange; 1996. p. 2651–75.
4. Kessinger A, Armitage JO, Smith DM, *et al.* High dose therapy and autologous peripheral stem cell transplant for patients with lymphoma. *Blood* 1989;74:1260–5.
5. Gianni AM, Siena S, Bregni M, *et al.* Granulocyte macrophage colony stimulating factor to harvest circulating hematopoietic stem cells for autotransplantation. *Lancet* 1989;2:580–4.
6. Elias AD, Ayash L, Anderson KC, *et al.* Mobilization of peripheral blood progenitor cells by chemotherapy and GMCSF for hematologic support and high-dose intensification of breast cancer. *Blood* 1992;79:3036–44.
7. Juttner CA, To LB, Ho J, *et al.* Early hemopoietic recovery after autografting using peripheral blood stem cells in ANL. *Transplant Proc*. 1988;20:40–3.
8. Botrin MM, Buckner CD. Major complications of marrow harvesting for transplantation. *Exp Hematol.* 1983;11:916–21.
9. Bensinger WI, Clift R, Martin P, *et al.* Allogeneic periph-

eral stem cell transplantation in patients with advanced hematologic malignancies: a retrospective comparison with marrow transplantation. *Blood* 1996;88:2794–800.
10. Beatty PG, Dahlberg S, Mickelson EM, *et al.* Probability of finding HLA-matched unrelated marrow donors. *Transplantation* 1988;45:714–8.
11. Alberts B, Bray B, Lewis J, *et al.* The immune system. In: Alberts B, editor. *Molecular Biology of the Cell.* 3rd ed. New York: Garland; 1994. p. 1195–254.
12. Beatty PG, Clift RA, Mickelson EM, *et al.* Marrow transplantation from related donors other than HLA-identical siblings. *N Engl J Med.* 1985;313:765–71.
13. Ferrara JL, Deeg HT. Graft-versus-host disease. *N Engl J Med.* 1991;324:667–74.
14. Vogelsang GB, Hess AD. Graft-versus-host disease: new directions for a persistent problem. *Blood* 1994;84:2061–7.
15. Fowlis GA, Fairchild S, Tomonari K, *et al.* Toward identification of minor histocompatibility antigens in mouse and man. *Trans Proc.* 1992;24:1689–91.
16. Van Bekkum DW. Conditioning regimens for marrow grafting. *Semin Hematol.* 1984;21:81–90.
17. Gassman W, Uharek U, Wottge HU, *et al.* Comparison of cyclophosphamide, cytarabine, and etoposide as immunosuppressive agents before allogeneic bone marrow transplantation. *Blood* 1988;72:1574–9.
18. Clift RA, Buckner CD, Appelbaum FA, *et al.* Allogeneic marrow transplantation in patients with chronic myeloid leukemia in chronic phase. A randomized trial of two irradiation regimens. *Blood* 1991;77:1660–5.
19. Santos GW, Tutschka PJ, Brookmeyer CD, *et al.* Marrow transplantation for acute nonlymphocytic leukemia after treatment with busulfan cyclophosphamide. *N Engl J Med.* 1983;309:1347–53.
20. Coccia PF, Strandjord SE, Warkentin PI, *et al.* High dose cytosine arabinoside and fractionated total body irradiation: an improved preparative regimen for bone marrow transplantation of children with acute lymphocytic leukemia in second remission. *Blood* 1988;71:888–93.
21. Bacigalupo A, Lint MV, Valbonesi M, *et al.* Thiotepa and cyclophosphamide followed by granulocyte colony stimulating factor mobilized allogeneic peripheral blood cells in adults with advanced leukemia. *Blood* 1996;88:353–7.
22. Strob R, Longton G, Anasetti C, *et al.* Changing trends in marrow transplantation for aplastic anemia. *Bone Marrow Transplant.* 1992;10(*Suppl* 1):45–52.
23. Tutschka PJ, Copeland EA, Klein JP. Bone marrow transplantation for leukemia following a new busulfan and cyclophosphamide regimen. *Blood* 1987;70:1382–8.
24. Ghalie R, Reynolds J, Valentino LA, *et al.* Busulfan containing pre-transplant regimens for the treatment of solid tumors. *Bone Marrow Transplant.* 1994;14:437–42.
25. Martin PJ, Horowitz MM. T-cell depletion of donor marrow. In: Atkinson K, editor. *Clinical Bone Marrow Transplantation.* 1st ed. New York: Cambridge; 1994. p. 52–61.
26. Antin JH, Ferrara JL. Cytokine dysregulation and acute graft-versus-host disease. *Blood* 1992;80:2964–8.
27. Rosenberg AS, Singer A. Cellular basis of skin allograft rejection: an in vivo model of immune mediated tissue destruction. *Ann Rev Immunol.* 1992;10:333–58.
28. Durum SK, Oppenheim JJ. Proinflammatory cytokines and immunity. In: Paul WE, editor. *Fundamental Immunology.* 3rd ed. New York: Raven; 1993. p. 801–36.
29. Sullivan KM, Deeg HJ, Sanders J, *et al.* Hyperacute graft-versus-host disease in patients not given immunosuppression after allogeneic marrow transplantation. *Blood* 1986;67:1172–4.
30. Deeg HJ, Storb R. Graft-versus-host disease: pathophysiology and clinical aspects. *Ann Rev Med.* 1984;35:11–24.
31. Ferrara JL. Pathogenesis of graft-versus-host disease and graft-host tolerance. In: Atkinson K, editor. *Clinical Bone Marrow Transplantation.* 1st ed. New York: Cambridge; 1994. p. 52–61.
32. Holda JH, Maier T, Claman HN. Natural suppressor activity in graft vs host spleen and normal bone marrow is augmented by IL-2 and interferon-gamma. *J Immunol.* 1986;137:3538–43.
33. Datta AR, Barrett AJ, Jiang YZ, *et al.* Distinct T-cell populations distinguish chronic myelogenous leukemia cells from lymphocytes in the same individual: a model for separating graft-versus-host disease from graft-versus-leukemia reactions. *Bone Marrow Transplant.* 1994;14:517–24.
34. Naparstek E, Or R, Nagler A, *et al.* T-cell depleted allogeneic bone marrow transplantation for acute leukemia using campath-1 antibodies and posttransplant administration of donor's peripheral blood lymphocytes for preventing relapse. *Br J Hematol.* 1995;89:506–15.
35. Buysmann S, Bemelman FJ, Schellekens PT, *et al.* Activation and increased expression of adhesion molecules on peripheral blood lymphocytes is a mechanism for the immediate lymphocytopenia after administration of OKT3. *Blood* 1996;87:404–11.
36. Janssen O, Wesselborg S, Kabelitz D. Immunosuppression by OKT3 induction of programmed cell death (apoptosis) as a possible mechanism of action. *Transplantation* 1992; 53:233–4.
37. Rameshwar P, Gascon P. Release of interleukin-l and interleukin-6 from human monocytes by antithymocyte globulin: requirement for de novo synthesis. *Blood* 1992; 80:2531–8.
38. Anasetti C, Martin PJ, Storb R, *et al.* Treatment of acute graft versus host disease with anti-mitogenic anti-CD3 monoclonal antibody. *Transplantation* 1992;54:844–51.
39. Sackstein R, Borenstein M. The effects of corticosteroids on lymphocyte recirculation in humans. *J Invest Med.* 1995; 43:68–77.
40. Emmel EA, Verweij CL, Durand DB. Cyclosporin A specifically inhibits function of nuclear proteins involved in T-cell activation. *Science* 1989;246:1617–20.
41. Zav´yalov VP, Demesyuk AI, Lundell J, *et al.* Some new aspects of molecular mechanisms of cyclosporine effect on immune response. *APMIS* 1995;103:401–15.
42. Masaoka T, Shibata H, Kakishita E, *et al.* Phase II study of FK506 for allogeneic bone marrow transplantation. *Transplant Proc.* 1991;23:3228–31.
43. Nash RA, Pineiro LA, Storb R, *et al.* FK506 in combination with methotrexate for prevention of graft-versus-host disease after marrow transplantation from matched unrelated donors. *Blood* 1996;88:3634–41.
44. Hansen JA, Gooley T, Clift R, *et al.* Unrelated donor marrow transplantation for patients with chronic myelogenous leukemia [abstract]. *Blood* 1995;86:123a.

45. Anasetti C, Hansen JA, Waldmann TA, *et al.* Treatment of acute GVHD with humanized anti-TAC: an antibody that binds to the IL-2 receptor. *Blood* 1994;84:1320–7.
46. Antin JH, Weinstein HJ, Guinan EC, *et al.* Recombinant human IL-1 receptor antagonist in the treatment of steroid resistant graft versus host disease. *Blood* 1994;84:1342–8.
47. Xun CQ, Thompson JS, Jennings CD, *et al.* Effect of total body irradiation, busulfan cyclophosphamide, or cyclophosphamide conditioning on inflammatory cytokine release and development of acute and chronic graft versus host disease in H2-incompatible transplanted SCID mice. *Blood* 1994;83:2360–7.
48. Siadak M, Sullivan KM. The management of chronic graft versus host disease. *Blood Rev.* 1994;8:154–60.
49. Vogelsang GB, Farmer ER, Hess AD, *et al.* Thalidomide for the treatment of chronic graft versus host disease. *N Engl J Med.* 1992;326:1055–8.
50. Atkinson K. Chronic graft versus host disease. *Bone Marrow Transplant.* 1990;5:69–82.
51. Shulman HM, Sullivan KM, Weiden PL, *et al.* Chronic graft versus host disease syndrome in man. A long-term clinicopathological study of 20 Seattle patients. *Am J Med.* 1980;69:204–17.
52. Uzun O, Anaissie EJ. Antifungal prophylaxis in patients with hematologic malignancies: a reappraisal. *Blood* 1995;86:2063–72.
53. Crawford SW. Bone marrow transplantation and related infections. *Semin Respir Infect.* 1993;8:183–90.
54. Saral R, Burns WH, Laskin OL, *et al.* Acyclovir prophylaxis of herpes simplex infections. A randomized double blind, controlled trial in bone marrow transplant patients. *N Engl J Med.* 1981;305:63–7.
55. Wade JC, Newton B, Flournoy MC. Oral acyclovir for prevention of herpes simplex reactivation after marrow transplantation. *Ann Intern Med.* 1984;100:823–88.
56. Witherspoon RP, Storb R. Immunologic aspects of marrow transplantation. *Immunol Allergy Clin North Am.* 1989;9:187–208.
57. Lum LG, Munn NA, Schanfield MS, *et al.* The detection of specific antibody formation to recall antigens after human bone marrow transplantation. *Blood* 1986;67:582–7.
58. Azogui O, Gluckman E, Fradelizi D. Inhibition of IL-2 production after human allogeneic bone marrow transplantation. *J Immunol.* 1983;131:1205–8.
59. Meyers JD. Infection in bone marrow transplant patients. *Am J Med.* 1986;81:27–38.
60. Ljungman P, DeBock R, Cordonnier A, *et al.* Practices of cytomegalovirus diagnosis, prevention, and treatment in allogeneic bone marrow transplant recipients: a report from the working party for infectious disease of the EBMT. *Bone Marrow Transplant.* 1993;12:399–403.
61. Bowden RA, Slichter SJ, Sayers M, *et al.* A comparison of filtered leukocyte reduced and cytomegalovirus seronegative blood products for the prevention of transfusion associated cytomegalovirus infection after marrow transplantation. *Blood* 1995;86:3598–603.
62. Meyers JD, Reed EC, Shepp DM, *et al.* Acyclovir for prevention of cytomegalovirus infection and disease after allogeneic marrow transplantation. *N Engl J Med.* 1988; 318:70–5.
63. Schmidt GM, Horak DA, Niland JC, *et al.* A randomized, controlled trial of prophylactic ganciclovir for cytomegalovirus pulmonary infection in recipients of allogeneic bone marrow transplantation. *N Engl J Med.* 1991;324:1005–11.
64. Einsele H, Ehninger G, Hebart H, *et al.* Polymerase chain reaction monitoring reduces the incidence of cytomegalovirus disease and the duration and side effects of antiviral therapy after bone marrow transplantation. *Blood* 1995;86:2815–20.
65. Wingard JR. Viral infections in leukemia and bone marrow transplant patients. *Leuk Lymphoma* 1993;11:115–25.
66. Easterbrook P, Wood MJ. Successors to acyclovir. *J Antimicrob Chemother.* 1994;34:307–11.

SELF-ASSESSMENT QUESTIONS

1. Which of the following are the major cellular elements involved in acute graft-versus-host disease (GVHD)?

   a. granulocytes
   b. $CD4^+$ and $CD8^+$ T lymphocytes
   c. $CD34^+$ cells
   d. mast cells
   e. b and c

2. Which of the following cytokines have not been considered important in acute GVHD pathogenesis?

   a. prostaglandin E_2
   b. interleukin 2
   c. tumor necrosis factor alpha
   d. interleukin 1
   e. a and d

3. Which of the following organs is not affected by acute GVHD?

   a. gastrointestinal tract
   b. kidney
   c. liver
   d. brain
   e. b and d

4. Which of the following best describes graft-versus-leukemia (GVL) effect?

   a. a reduction in leukemia due to $CD34^+$ cells in the donor graft
   b. leukemia that develops as a result of post-transplant immunosuppression
   c. a reduction in leukemia relapse as a result of acute GVHD
   d. none of the above

5. Which of the following immunosuppressive agents is lymphocidal?

a. cyclosporine
b. rapamycin
c. tacrolimus
d. corticosteroids
e. a and c

6. The therapeutic difference between tacrolimus and cyclosporine can be explained by increased tissue penetration of tacrolimus.

a. true
b. false

7. Which of the following is the initial therapy for chronic GVHD?

a. cyclosporine
b. OKT3
c. tacrolimus
d. prednisone
e. a and d

8. Which of the following increases the risk of bacterial and fungal infections?

a. neutropenia
b. mucositis
c. severe diarrhea
d. corticosteroids
e. all of the above

9. Which of the following methods of prophylaxis for cytomegalovirus (CMV) is used in CMV-negative patients with a CMV-positive donor?

a. use of only CMV-negative blood products
b. ganciclovir starting day of transplant until engraftment
c. use of intravenous immunoglobulin daily until day 60
d. acyclovir starting just before transplant and continuing until discharge
e. none of the above

10. Which of the following is a risk factor for developing herpes zoster?

a. chronic GVHD
b. cyclosporine and corticosteroids
c. drug rash
d. use of bactrim for pneumocystis prophylaxis
e. a and b

CHAPTER 10

Immunotherapy of Cancer

Jill K. Bruton, Pharm.D.
Clinical Practice Specialist
Bone Marrow Transplantation
University of Texas M.D. Anderson Cancer Center
Houston, TX

Tumor Immunology 230
- Tumor-Associated Surface Antigens 231
  - Viral Tumor-Associated Antigens 231
  - Prostate-Specific Antigen and Cancer Antigen 125 231
- Antitumor Immune Mechanisms 232
  - Antitumor Antibodies and Complement 232
  - Cytotoxic T Lymphocytes 232
  - Natural Killer Cells 232
  - Killer Cells 232
  - Macrophages 232
  - Lymphokine-Activated Killer Cells 233
  - Antibody-Dependent Cellular Cytotoxicity 233
- Tumor Escape Mechanisms 233

Cancer Immunotherapy 233
- Mechanisms for Manipulating the Immune System 233
  - Tumor Vaccines 234
  - Immunostimulants 234
    - Bacillus Calmette-Guérin 234
    - Levamisole 235
- Biological Response Modifiers 236
  - Interferons 236
    - Interferon Alpha 237
      - Hairy Cell Leukemia 237
      - Chronic Myelogenous Leukemia 238
      - Kaposi's Sarcoma 239
      - Hepatitis 239
      - Renal Cell Carcinoma 240
      - Melanoma 240
      - Multiple Myeloma 241
      - Colorectal Cancer 242
    - Interferon Gamma and Interferon Beta 242
    - Toxicities 242

**The contributions made by Suzanne Fields to this chapter are gratefully acknowledged.*

Interleukins . . . 243
Interleukin 2 (T-Cell Growth Factor) . . . 244
Toxicities . . . 246
Biological Response Modifier Combinations . . . 247
Colony-Stimulating Factors . . . 249
Erythropoietin . . . 249
Granulocyte-Macrophage Colony-Stimulating Factor and Granulocyte Colony-Stimulating Factor . . . 250
Bone Marrow Transplant . . . 250
Neutropenia . . . 252
Myelodysplastic Syndrome . . . 254
Interleukin 1 . . . 255
Interleukin 3 . . . 255
Macrophage Colony-Stimulating Factor . . . 255
PIXY-321 . . . 255
Interleukin 6 . . . 255
Interleukin 11 . . . 256
Tumor Necrosis Factor . . . 256
Adoptive Cellular Immunotherapy . . . 256
Summary . . . 258
References . . . 258
Self-Assessment Questions . . . 267

The many unanswered questions about the role of the immune system in combating cancer have led to extensive research into ways to manipulate the immune system for therapeutic effect. It is known that immunodeficient patients are predisposed to developing some types of malignancies. Perhaps vaccines will be able to prevent proliferation of cells inclined to become cancerous. The expanding knowledge of tumor cell immunology and cancer development has led to varied attempts to utilize the immune system for treating or preventing cancer cell growth.

The pharmacist's role in cancer immunotherapy can be significant. The areas of immunology and biotechnology are developing and changing rapidly. In addition, many emerging products are prepared by recombinant DNA technology and will be very expensive. An appropriate balance between therapeutic effectiveness and cost containment will be an important consideration for cancer immunotherapy. Biological agents can also be helpful in managing adverse effects. A working knowledge of the therapeutic effects and side effects of these agents will be critical for pharmacists involved in the care of the patient with cancer.

After reading this chapter, the reader should be able to:

1. Discuss the antitumor effects of interferon alpha.
2. Discuss the side effects of interferon alpha.
3. Discuss the antitumor effects of interleukin 2.
4. Discuss the side effects of interleukin 2.
5. Discuss the therapeutic effects of recombinant colony-stimulating factors.
6. Discuss the side effects of recombinant colony-stimulating factors.

This chapter describes tumor immunology and the role of the immune system in cancer development and treatment, including the function of tumor-associated antigens and antitumor immune mechanisms (e.g., natural killer cells). Tumor vaccines and immunostimulants (Bacillus Calmette-Guérin and levamisole) used to manipulate the human immune system for the treatment of cancer are discussed briefly. Interferons, interleukins, colony-stimulating factors, and tumor necrosis factor are described in detail, with information about their antitumor mechanisms, method of administration, dosing, tumors against which each agent is used, and toxicities. The chapter concludes with a brief discussion of adoptive cellular immunotherapy.

TUMOR IMMUNOLOGY

Tumor cells are normal host cells that undergo malignant transformation and begin to divide uncontrollably, resulting in invasion of surrounding tissues or distant spread of disease. In the normal cell, growth and differentiation are regulated by genes known as proto-oncogenes. Genetic changes induced by viruses, chemical carcinogens, radiation, or other cellular mechanisms cause proto-oncogenes to be transformed into oncogenes, which stimulate neoplastic cell growth. If these newly transformed cells were recognized by the body as foreign, the body's natural immune system could play a role in the limitation of tumor development. Some malignant cells possess cell surface markers (tumor-associated antigens [TAAs]) that may help the immune system distinguish foreign cells from host cells. During the past decade, cancer immunology research has been greatly intensified in an attempt to treat malignancies by boosting the human immune system.

The role of the immune system in cancer treatment was first investigated in the early 1900s, when it was discovered that laboratory rats developed a strong immune response against transplanted tumors. Following this discovery, numerous attempts at host immunomodulation were made, but the results were quite disappointing. The observed immune response was attributed to the presence of normal histocompatibility antigens on cell surfaces rather than to the presence of specific TAAs. Cancer immunotherapy was virtually abandoned because researchers were unable to demonstrate TAAs on tumor cell surfaces and because the areas of cancer surgery and radiation therapy were developing rapidly. However, with the demonstration of TAAs on methylcholanthrene-induced sarcomas in laboratory mice by Foley and by Prehn and Main in the 1950s, the study of cancer immunotherapy was revived.[1,2]

Tumor-Associated Surface Antigens

To produce an antitumor immune response, the body must be able to distinguish host cells (self) from abnormal malignant cells (foreign). The presence of TAAs enhances the detection of malignant cells. Cytotoxic T lymphocytes (CTLs) recognize TAAs as foreign and initiate T-cell–mediated killing of tumor cells. Human genes *MAGE-1* and *MAGE-3* encode for tumor-specific antigens on melanoma cells, which are recognized by CTLs. Genes of the *MAGE* family are expressed in a significant number of tumors of various histological types. However, MAGE genes are silent in normal tissues, except for the testis and placenta. *MAGE-1* or *MAGE-3* genes are expressed in 40% of primary melanomas and 79% of metastatic melanomas. Four antigens have been identified that are encoded by *MAGE-1* or *MAGE-3* and presented by major histocompatibility complex (MHC) class I molecules human leukocyte antigen (HLA)-A1, A2, or Cw1601. These antigens may be used as targets for specific antitumor immunization of patients with cutaneous melanoma.[3]

Many TAAs are present on the surface of normal cells as well as tumor cells. For example, oncofetal antigens, such as carcinoembryonic antigen (CEA) and alpha-fetoprotein (AFP), are normally present in fetal and embryonic tissue during fetal development or during periods of cell differentiation in adults. Although these antigens are not immunogenic, they have been detected in the serum of patients with malignancies and other medical conditions. AFP levels are frequently elevated in patients with hepatomas, testicular carcinomas, and acute hepatitis, and in pregnant women. CEA levels may be elevated in patients with adenocarcinoma of the gastrointestinal tract, pancreas, breast, and lung as well as in several nonmalignant conditions, such as ulcerative colitis, alcoholic cirrhosis, pancreatitis, and emphysema. Heavy smokers have also been reported to have elevated CEA levels. Therefore, using the oncofetal antigens as a screening tool for malignancy is not very practical. Measuring CEA levels may be useful, however, for monitoring the clinical course in some patients with documented malignancies. Patients frequently exhibit a rise in serum CEA level with disease recurrence before the recurrence is actually clinically detectable (e.g., colon cancer).[4]

Viral Tumor-Associated Antigens

Viral antigens, induced by both RNA and DNA viruses located on the surface of tumor cells, are another type of TAA. Viral antigens have been associated with malignancies such as Burkitt's lymphoma and nasopharyngeal carcinoma (Epstein-Barr virus), cervical carcinoma (human papilloma virus), hepatocellular carcinoma (hepatitis B virus), and T-cell leukemia and lymphoma (human T-cell lymphotropic virus type I). Viral TAAs are shared by all tumors that are induced by a single type of virus (immunologic cross-reactivity) and are able to induce both humoral and cell-mediated immune responses in humans. In contrast, cell surface antigens on chemically induced tumors are unique to each tumor, making it difficult to use immunotherapy in the diagnosis and treatment of these tumors.[5]

Prostate-Specific Antigen and Cancer Antigen 125

Tumor cells may also express tissue-specific antigens or differentiation antigens on the cell surface that are similar to the surface antigens expressed by normal cells during tissue differentiation.[5] Because these antigens also occur on normal cells, the body does not mount an immune response against them. These antigens may, however, be used as targets for tumor-directed immunotherapy or as diagnostic markers. Prostate-specific antigen (PSA) and cancer antigen (CA) 125 are two tumor-derived markers that have been evaluated as methods for detecting and monitoring response in patients with prostate cancer and cancers originating in gynecologic tissues, respectively.

Routine screening for prostate cancer with the PSA test is controversial. The accuracy of PSA testing is in question. False-positive results may be seen in patients with benign prostatic hypertrophy or prostatitis. An elevated PSA test subjects the patient to further testing with ultrasonography and needle biopsy. There are potential complications associated with needle biopsy (e.g., bleeding and infection), and many patients experience anxiety and discomfort. The biggest concern surrounding PSA screening is the lack of evidence that early detection of prostate cancer results in improved patient outcomes. Randomized, controlled trials are currently being conducted. Furthermore, the potential complications of treatment (e.g., impotence, incontinence, and death) may outweigh the potential benefits of screening. Many prostate cancers are indolent in nature and are not considered clinically significant.[6] The American Cancer Society and the American Urological Association both support PSA screening; however, several groups oppose PSA screening, and the American College of Physicians is reviewing their recommendations.[6] The decision to obtain a PSA test should be made jointly by the physician and the informed patient. The PSA test should also accompany, not replace, the digital rectal examination.

CA125 in combination with pelvic examination and ultrasonography have been extensively studied as screening methods for ovarian cancer. CA125 has not proved to be suitable as a screening method for the early detection of ovarian cancer due to the high number of false positives. It is also not recommended for use in distinguishing benign from malignant pelvic masses. The United States Food and Drug Administration (FDA) has approved CA125 for use in assisting the detection of residual epithelial ovarian cancer in patients who have undergone primary therapy and who would be considered for a second-look operation. Tumor markers such as CA125 should only serve as a supplement to other diagnostic methods.[7]

Antitumor Immune Mechanisms

Both humoral and cellular immune mechanisms are involved in the body's antitumor response. These mechanisms are discussed in detail in chapters 1 and 2. Spontaneous tumor regression, increased frequency of tumor development in immunosuppressed hosts, and tumor infiltration with histiocytes, plasmacytes, lymphocytes, and eosinophils are all evidence for the involvement of the immune system in tumor cell death.[8] The host effector mechanisms involved in tumor immunity include antitumor antibodies, complement, CTLs, natural killer (NK) cells, killer (K) cells, macrophages, lymphokine-activated killer (LAK) cells, and antibody-dependent cell-mediated cytotoxicity (ADCC).

Antitumor Antibodies and Complement

Although the humoral immune response against tumor cells is minimal, it may play a role in the host immune response. Tumor antigens stimulate the release of immunoglobulins G and M (IgG and IgM), which bind to the surface of tumor cells. In the presence of complement, these antibodies destroy tumor cells via direct cell lysis or tumor opsonization and phagocytosis.[9] Antibody-coated target cells may also be eliminated from the body by ADCC mechanisms, which are discussed in a later section.

Cytotoxic T Lymphocytes

CTLs contain antigen-specific receptors that recognize TAAs on the surface of tumor cells. However, for the CTLs to recognize foreign antigens, the TAA must be coupled with a class I MHC antigen. The CTL receptor then binds to the MHC–foreign antigen complex, initiating a T cell–mediated immune response. The dependence of the immune response on the presence of both a self component (MHC) and a foreign antigen is termed MHC restriction. T cell–mediated killing can be intensified by the release of cytokines (e.g., interleukin [IL]-1, IL-2, IL-4, and interferon gamma [IFN-γ]) from activated CTLs that stimulate the activity of other effector cells of the immune system or have direct effects (e.g., IFN-γ).[10] For a detailed discussion of the MHC, see chapter 3.

Natural Killer Cells

NK cells, also known as large granular lymphocytes, are lymphocytes found in the spleen, lymph nodes, bone marrow, and peripheral blood that can lyse various tumor cells. The exact mechanism by which NK cells kill tumor cells is still unknown. However, it may involve the release of cytotoxins from granules within the NK cells. NK cells are stimulated by various agents, including interferon alpha (IFN-α), IL-2, Bacillus Calmette-Guérin (BCG), tumor necrosis factor (TNF), and some chemotherapy agents. Prostaglandins, on the other hand, inhibit the activity of NK cells. NK cells also destroy tumor cells via ADCC because of the presence of crystallizable fragment (Fc) receptors on the cell membrane. There is also evidence that NK cells may help minimize the metastatic spread of tumor cells.[5,8–10]

Killer Cells

Both K cells and NK cells have been referred to as null cells because they lack either T- or B-cell surface markers. K cells differ from NK cells in that they require the presence of cell surface antibodies to destroy tumor cells. K cells express on their cell surfaces Fc and antibody receptors that bind to IgG antibodies, resulting in target cell lysis via ADCC mechanisms.[11]

Macrophages

Macrophages are cytotoxic effector cells that may be activated by various agents, including endotoxin, immune complexes, and lymphokines (IL-1 and macrophage-activating factors [MAFs], one of which is IFN-γ). MAF is produced by antigen-stimulated T lymphocytes and attracts macrophages to the area of the tumor. These T lymphocytes also release migration inhibitory factor, which prevents the migration of macrophages away from the tumor-infiltrated area. Once macrophages are activated, they selectively kill tumor cells via cell lysis and phagocytosis. The secretion of TNF by activated macrophages may also contribute to their cytotoxicity. Macrophages also express Fc receptors on their surfaces, enabling them to attack antibody-coated target cells.[5,9,12]

Lymphokine-Activated Killer Cells

LAK cells are a heterogeneous population of cells, primarily NK cells and T cells, that become cytotoxic in the presence of IL-2. These cells are found in peripheral blood, bone marrow, lymph nodes, and various other sites. LAK cells appear to be more selective for tumor cells than for normal cells. Furthermore, cells that are resistant to NK cells have demonstrated sensitivity to cytotoxic LAK cells.[8,12–15] In clinical trials, LAK cells stimulated in vitro by IL-2 have demonstrated activity in patients with metastatic disease.

Antibody-Dependent Cellular Cytotoxicity

Some cytotoxic effector cells express Fc receptors on their surface (e.g., NK cells, K cells, granulocytes, and macrophages). These receptors are attracted to and bind to tumor antigens that have been coated with IgG. Once the K cell is attached to the target cell via the Fc receptors, the tumor cell is then lysed by mechanisms that are poorly understood (Figure 10-1). ADCC may be initiated or stimulated by various cytokines, including IL-2, IL-1, TNF, granulocyte-macrophage colony-stimulating factor (GM-CSF), and macrophage colony-stimulating factor (M-CSF).[8]

Tumor Escape Mechanisms

Immune responses against tumor cells have been clearly demonstrated both in vitro and in vivo. However, these host defense mechanisms appear to be ineffective in preventing initiation and proliferation of many tumors. Several possible explanations for tumor cell evasion of the immune system have been proposed, one of which involves the kinetics of tumor cell growth. Low quantities of tumor cells may not be sufficient to stimulate a host immune response. As a result, resistant tumor cells may have time to develop before the tumor is large enough to be recognized by the immune system. Another explanation of tumor cell evasion is that a tolerance to tumor antigens develops from prior exposure; a complementary explanation holds that tumor surface cell antigens are lost through the process of antigenic modulation (see chapter 11). A fourth explanation is that tumor cell surface antigens are masked by certain molecules that appear on the surface of tumor cells, such as sialic acid–containing mucopolysaccharides. A fifth possibility is that tumor cells may secrete tumor antigens that form complexes with circulating antibodies. These complexes may then block Fc receptors on the surface of host effector cells or induce suppressor cells, resulting in suppression of CTLs.[5] A final explanation for tumor cell evasion is that tumor cells may produce products that suppress the immune system. Prostaglandins and transforming growth factor beta (TGF-β) are two tumor products that inhibit the activity of immune effector cells.[5,12]

In summary, tumor cells are normal cells that undergo malignant transformation and may be recognized by the host immune system as foreign because TAAs are present. Both humoral and cellular immune mechanisms are involved in the body's response to the tumor. However, there are also various mechanisms by which tumor cells evade destruction by immune effector cells. Increased understanding of the host immune response and of tumor cell evasion mechanisms may, in the future, allow malignancies to be treated by manipulating the host immune system.

CANCER IMMUNOTHERAPY

Mechanisms for Manipulating the Immune System

The ability to differentiate normal cells from tumor cells on the basis of antigenic differences described thus far should permit tumor-directed immunotherapy. Unfortu-

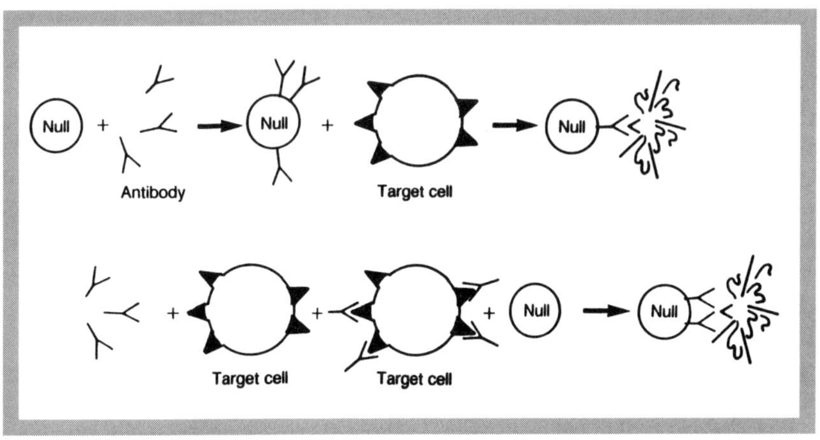

Figure 10-1. Antibody-dependent cell-mediated cytotoxicity is initiated by the attachment of effector cells to aggregated antibody on target cells.

SOURCE: *Reprinted with permission from Sell S. Cell-mediated immunity in vitro. In:* Immunology, Immunopathology and Immunity. *4th ed. New York: Elsevier; 1987. p. 162.*

nately, in the studies conducted to date, immunotherapy has demonstrated minimal activity in patients with advanced disease. As a result, the role of immunotherapy in the treatment of malignancy may be in the adjuvant setting (microscopic disease only) or in combination with other treatment modalities (chemotherapy, radiation, or surgery).

The human immune system can be manipulated to treat cancer through the following mechanisms: (1) vaccination of cancer patients with tumor cell preparations, (2) direct administration of biological response modifiers (BRMs) or immunostimulants in an attempt to modulate the patient's immune system, and (3) ex vivo manipulation of a patient's immune effector cells with BRMs to increase their cytotoxicity (adoptive cellular immunotherapy).

Tumor Vaccines

The rationale behind immunization and the use of various types of vaccines is discussed extensively in chapter 6. Because TAAs are present on tumor cells, the use of vaccines in the treatment or prevention of cancer has been explored. Active immunization with viral antigens has been successful in preventing the development of virally induced tumors in animals (e.g., feline leukemia virus in cats and Marek's disease in chickens).[5] Administering the hepatitis B vaccine to humans may produce similar results because of the association between hepatitis B virus infections of the liver and hepatocellular carcinoma.

Tumor vaccines may be produced from autologous tumor cells or allogenic tumor cell lines in an attempt to attain active specific stimulation of the immune system. To increase the immunogenicity of the vaccine, the tumor cells may be altered with enzymatic, chemical, or radiation procedures. Concomitant administration of nonspecific immunostimulants (e.g., BCG) may also be used in an attempt to increase the immune response. The use of tumor vaccines has been investigated as adjuvant therapy in patients with melanoma. A number of vaccines have been developed, which are all intended to induce or augment immunity against melanoma-associated antigens. Phase II trials of patients with American Joint Committee on Cancer (AJCC) stage IV disease treated with melanoma vaccines had a reported response rate of 13–23%.[16–18] Patients with AJCC stage III and stage IV disease treated with melanoma vaccine demonstrated enhanced survival compared with historical controls.[16,19,20] Several phase III trials are investigating adjuvant immunotherapy with melanoma vaccine in patients with AJCC stage IIB and stage III melanoma.[21] The results of two double-blind randomized trials have been reported. The first trial involved 122 patients with resected AJCC stage III melanoma who were pretreated with low-dose cyclophosphamide followed by BCG with or without the melanoma vaccine ganglioside GM_2. Although no significant difference was found in overall survival, there was a significant increase in disease-free survival in the vaccine group.[22] In the second trial, 250 patients with resected AJCC stage III melanoma received either vaccine (vaccinia melanoma oncolysate) or virus alone for one year. Results failed to demonstrate a statistically significant difference in either disease-free or overall survival between the two groups. However, there was a trend toward enhanced survival in patients treated with vaccine.[23]

More research is required before conclusions concerning the efficacy of tumor vaccines can be reached. Inherent problems in vaccine development include the need for an intact host immune system, the inability to affect large tumor cell masses, the inter- and intrapatient variation of TAAs, and the presence of similar surface antigens on both normal and tumor cells.[24]

Passive stimulation of the immune system via the administration of tumor-directed monoclonal antibodies (MoAbs) is also being investigated (see chapter 11).

Immunostimulants

Nonspecific stimulation of the immune system with bacterial and viral agents, as well as other antigenic agents, has been investigated in the treatment of various malignancies. The antitumor activity of host immunomodulation was serendipitously discovered by Coley around the turn of the century when he observed regression of sarcoma in a patient following erysipelas (an acute superficial form of cellulitis usually caused by infection with group A streptococci).[8] After this observation he began to treat patients with "Coley's toxins," which were combinations of bacterial toxins, and some tumor regressions were reported. Numerous immunostimulants are currently under investigation for the treatment of cancer.

Bacillus Calmette-Guérin

BCG is a live attenuated strain of *Mycobacterium bovis* that nonspecifically stimulates the host immune system. Clinical trials have been conducted with BCG in patients with acute leukemia, melanoma, and colon, breast, renal cell, and bladder cancers. However, the only significant responses have been seen with direct intravesical BCG administration in the treatment of superficial bladder cancer. Cell-mediated inflammatory responses, alone or in combination with ADCC mechanisms, have been proposed as possible antitumor mechanisms of intravesical BCG. However, recent data suggest that T cell–mediated immunologic mechanisms are primarily responsible for BCG's antitumor activity. Increased levels of various cytokines, including IL-l, IL-2, TNF, and IFN-γ, have been detected in patients' urine following intravesical BCG administration.[25,26] Criteria required for a tumor response include small tumor size, immunocompetence of the host, drug administration in close proximity to the tumor, and administration of adequate numbers of *M. bovis*.[27]

In a large trial conducted by the Southwest Oncology Group, intravesical BCG was shown to be more effective than intravesical doxorubicin in the treatment of superficial bladder carcinoma. Complete responses were achieved in 71% of patients treated with BCG and in 47% of those treated with intravesical doxorubicin.[28] Tumor recurrence occurred in 37% of the patients receiving doxorubicin and in 15% of those receiving BCG, and the mean time to recurrence was twice as long in the BCG group (22 months versus 10 months). In addition, patients with stage Ta and Tl tumors (high-risk patients) receiving BCG had less tumor recurrence than those receiving doxorubicin (57% versus 79%). Intravesical BCG administration was also superior to intravesical thiotepa and intravesical doxorubicin for the prophylaxis of disease progression and recurrence in superficial bladder carcinoma; the percent recurrence was 13% with BCG, 36% with thiotepa, and 43% with doxorubicin.[29]

Currently, two BCG products are commercially available for the intravesical treatment of bladder carcinoma in situ: TheraCys® (Connaught) and Tice® BCG (Organon). The regimen recommended by both manufacturers consists of induction therapy administered once a week for six weeks followed by maintenance therapy. Patients who do not respond to an initial six-week course of treatment should receive a second six-week course, because several studies have demonstrated responses in patients who receive a second course of therapy.[30–32] The maintenance regimen recommended by Connaught consists of one intravesical instillation 3, 6, 12, 18, and 24 months after the induction regimen. The Tice® BCG product should be administered monthly for 6–12 months.

The most common side effects associated with BCG therapy (Table 10-1) usually occur after the third or fourth BCG dose and increase in severity with subsequent doses. Systemic symptoms usually begin 2–4 hours after BCG instillation and subside within 24–72 hours. Concurrent administration of diphenhydramine and antipyretics may palliate some of the systemic side effects.[33,34] Systemic BCG infections manifested by pneumonitis or granulomatous hepatitis have been reported in less than 1% of patients receiving intravesical BCG. Fatal disseminated mycobacterial infection and sepsis following BCG therapy have been reported in six patients to date.[35,36] As a result, it is recommended that BCG never be given at the time of surgical manipulation of the genitourinary tract, to patients who are immunosuppressed, or after a traumatic bladder catheterization. Antituberculous antibiotics should be administered at the first signs of systemic BCG infection.

Table 10-1. Side Effects Associated with Bacillus Calmette-Guérin Therapy

Irritable bladder symptoms
- Dysuria
- Frequency
- Urgency
- Gross hematuria
- Cystitis

Flu-like syndrome
- Fever
- Malaise
- Chills
- Myalgias
- Nausea and vomiting
- Anorexia

BCG contains viable attenuated mycobacteria. Therefore, all of the materials used for drug preparation and administration should be immediately disposed of as biohazardous waste. The preparation of BCG and other sterile products under the same biological safety cabinet could potentially result in the contamination of the sterile product and transmission of the organism to the patient. This was the suspected cause of two cases of BCG-associated meningitis in two children receiving intrathecal chemotherapy for leukemia.[37] The biological safety cabinet should be carefully cleaned after preparation of BCG and before any sterile products are prepared. Patients should be counseled to mix their urine with an equal volume of household bleach and allow it to sit for 15 minutes before flushing during the first six hours after drug administration. They should also be instructed to sit while voiding after BCG therapy.

Levamisole

Levamisole is an anthelmintic agent that was originally developed for veterinary and human use in the treatment of parasitic worms. However, in the past two decades the immunologic effects of levamisole have been described and clinical trials have been conducted in several malignant diseases. In the studies to date, levamisole has demonstrated the most clinical activity in the adjuvant treatment of colorectal cancer. The exact mechanism by which levamisole stimulates the immune system is unknown and is probably quite complex. Levamisole appears to primarily affect the cells involved in cell-mediated immunity, because B lymphocytes and antibody production do not change after drug administration. Direct antitumor activity has also not been reported with levamisole.[38]

Clinical trials conducted in the adjuvant treatment of colon cancer have demonstrated limited activity for single-agent levamisole.[39,40] However, the combination of levamisole and 5-fluorouracil (5-FU) has demonstrated significant clinical activity (Table 10-2). In a small European study, patients with colorectal cancer were randomized into three treatment groups: (1) supportive care only, (2) 5-FU only, and (3) levamisole plus 5-FU. After a minimum of five years of follow-up, the patients receiving

Table 10-2. Clinical Trials of Levamisole Plus 5-Fluorouracil (5-FU) as Adjuvant Therapy for Colon Carcinoma

REFERENCE	NO. OF PATIENTS	TREATMENT	DISEASE RECURRENCE (%)
41[a]	45	Control	44
	42	5-FU	52
	44	5-FU/Levamisole	32
42[b], 43	315	Observation	56
	310	Levamisole	55
	304	5-FU/Levamisole	39

[a]*Included patients with stage A, B, or C disease.*
[b]*Included only patients with stage C disease.*

levamisole plus 5-FU had a significant survival advantage over the patients in the 5-FU group and the control group (32% disease recurrence versus 52% and 44%, respectively).[41]

These results have since been confirmed in a large multicenter study in the United States.[42,43] In this study, patients with surgically resected Dukes stage C colon cancer were randomized to observation alone, levamisole alone, or combination levamisole and 5-FU. At follow-up after five years, 39% of the patients in the levamisole and 5-FU group had relapsed, compared with 55% in the levamisole-only group and 56% in the control group. The combination of 5-FU and levamisole also provided a significant survival advantage compared to observation only, with a 33% reduction in mortality rate for the combination. As a result, the combination of 5-FU and levamisole is now recommended as standard therapy for patients with resected Dukes stage C colon cancer.

Levamisole is administered orally in a dose of 50 mg every eight hours for three days every two weeks in combination with 5-FU. Therapy should start three to five weeks after surgery and continue for one year.[38,42] Side effects reported with levamisole therapy include nausea, vomiting, metallic or altered taste, fever, malaise, dermatitis, mood elevation, insomnia, headache, and occasionally blood dyscrasias (granulocytopenia, leukopenia, and thrombocytopenia).[38,42]

Numerous other agents, including *Corynebacterium parvum*, bestatin, tuftsin, endotoxin, OK432 viruses, and various chemicals, are also being investigated as nonspecific stimulants of the host immune system.

Biological Response Modifiers

BRMs are natural or synthetic agents that modify a patient's biological response to tumor cells based on differences in their biological effects. These agents can be divided into three major categories: (1) agents that modulate a patient's immunologic mechanisms and lead to suppression of tumor cell growth, (2) agents that have direct antitumor effects, and (3) agents that modify the interaction between host and tumor via mechanisms other than immunologic or direct antitumor effects.[44] Many of the BRMs have more than one mechanism of antitumor activity, and these mechanisms may vary, depending on dose and schedule of administration. As a result, the exact mechanism responsible for BRM antitumor activity may be difficult to elucidate. However, the evolution of genetic engineering techniques now allows large-scale production of BRMs, and our understanding of the mechanisms of action and clinical utility of these agents is increasing rapidly.

Interferons

The IFNs are a group of glycoproteins produced in response to viral infections or other IFN inducers. There are three types of IFN: alpha (α), beta (β), and gamma (γ). IFN-α and IFN-β are produced by a variety of cell types and cause similar biological effects because of competitive binding at a common cell surface receptor. IFN-γ, on the other hand, binds to a distinct cell surface receptor and is produced by T lymphocytes. The IFNs create their biological effects through a variety of different mechanisms, including antiviral, antiproliferative, cytostatic, immunomodulatory, and differentiating effects.

The antitumor mechanisms of the IFNs may occur via direct or indirect effects on tumor cells. IFNs have demonstrated direct antiproliferative effects both in vivo and in vitro.[45, 46] These effects are due to lengthening of all phases of the cell cycle and suppression of the *c-myc* oncogene, which prevents cells from entering the division process. The IFNs also induce 2′-5′- oligoadenylate synthetase, protein kinase, and phosphodiesterase—three enzymes that inhibit RNA, DNA, and protein synthesis, resulting in increased inhibition. Enzyme inhibition contributes to both the antiviral and the antitumor effects of the IFNs. The IFNs also exert various immunomodulatory effects that enhance their antitumor activity. After administration of IFN, patients have demonstrated enhanced NK, K, and LAK cell activity, increased T-cell cytotoxicity, and augmented macrophage activity via enhanced MHC class I expression. All the IFNs enhance MHC class I expression, but IFN-γ also enhances MHC class II antigen expression. As a result, IFN-γ demonstrates greater immunomodulatory activity than either IFN-α or IFN-β.[45,47] All the antitumor effects of the IFNs depend on the timing, dose, route of administration, and duration of exposure to the biological agent.

IFN may be administered intramuscularly, intravenously, or subcutaneously in a variety of doses and sched-

Table 10-3. Therapeutic Uses of Interferon Alpha

Hairy cell leukemia*
Kaposi's sarcoma*
Condylomata acuminata*
Chronic hepatitis C*
Chronic myelogenous leukemia*
Chronic hepatitis B*
Melanoma
Renal cell carcinoma
Multiple myeloma
Non-Hodgkin's lymphoma
Malignant glioma
Ovarian cancer
Carcinoid tumors
Cutaneous T-cell lymphomas

**Uses approved by the Food and Drug Administration.*

ules. The antitumor effects appear to be dose responsive, as hematologic malignancies respond to lower IFN doses (5 million units (MU)/m^2 three times weekly or 3 MU daily), and solid tumors respond to higher doses (6–35 MU). Continuous dosing daily or three times per week appears to be more effective than administering doses on intermittent schedules.[48] Patients with minimal disease demonstrate greatest responsiveness to IFN therapy. Presently, IFN-α is approved by the FDA for the treatment of hairy cell leukemia, chronic myelogenous leukemia, Kaposi's sarcoma (KS), condylomata acuminata (genital warts), and chronic hepatitis C and hepatitis B. IFN-γ is approved only for treating chronic granulomatous disease. However, the IFNs are also being used in clinical trials to treat numerous other malignancies (Table 10-3).

Interferon Alpha

Hairy Cell Leukemia—IFN-α was originally approved by the FDA in 1986 for treating hairy cell leukemia (HCL). Recombinant IFN-α was found to eradicate hairy cells from the bone marrow and improve peripheral hematologic parameters. This was a significant advantage over previously used treatment modalities, such as splenectomy and low-dose chlorambucil. The effective dose of IFN-α was found to be 2 MU subcutaneously three times a week for 12 months. Trials that used this dose had objective (complete plus partial) response rates of approximately 70–80%, with complete response rates (normalization of blood counts [i.e., hemoglobin, neutrophil count, and platelet count] and less than 5% hairy cells in the bone marrow) of approximately 5–10% and partial response rates (normalization of blood counts only) of approximately 70%.[49–51] A lower dose of IFN-α was evaluated in an attempt to minimize toxicity. Twenty-two patients with hairy cell leukemia were treated with IFN-α2b 0.2 MU/m^2 for 6–12 months. The overall response rate was only 54% and responses were generally poor.[52] Low-dose IFN-α has also been shown to be ineffective for the treatment of relapse after previous IFN-α therapy.[53]

After two studies failed to show a benefit from extended treatment over one year, the investigators determined that 12 months of IFN-α treatment was optimal and reduced toxicity. In the first trial, 90 patients were randomized after 12 months of IFN-α to either observation or 6 additional months of treatment. No statistically significant difference in relapse rate was observed (26% in the observation group versus 18% in the treatment group.)[54] Relapses for both groups appeared at 1–19 months after IFN-α was discontinued. Extended therapy appeared to prolong the response while on IFN-α therapy but not for any added duration after discontinuation.[54] Following 24 months of IFN-α therapy in 35 patients with HCL, disease progression occurred in approximately 50% of patients at a median of 10 months after the drug was discontinued.[55] This same study was updated in 1990 with 195 patients accrued.[56] The relapse rate was comparable to those reported for 12-month treatment duration, showing no advantage for prolonged therapy.[51]

Treatment with IFN-α produces a rapid improvement in peripheral blood and bone marrow counts within the first 3–6 months after initiation of treatment. Improvements may continue for as long as one year.[50, 57] The improvement of peripheral blood counts combined with a decrease in bone marrow infiltration of hairy cells results in an improvement of performance status for the majority of patients. In one study, 95% of patients had a normal performance status after 12 months of IFN-α therapy.[58]

IFN-α has proved beneficial in the treatment of HCL. However, the majority of responses are partial responses, and most patients will eventually experience disease progression after completion of treatment.[58] Long-term follow-up of five years was reported on an initial cohort of 69 patients treated with IFN-α2b (Intron® A, Schering, Kenilworth NJ) 2 MU three times per week for 12 months.[59] The initial overall response rate was 91%, with a complete response rate of 13%. Forty-seven of 61 evaluable patients relapsed at a median time of 31 months after completion of treatment. At the time of relapse, patients were re-treated with IFN-α2b or treated with pentostatin or 2-chlorodeoxyadenosine (2-CdA). Ten patients never required retreatment. The five-year survival for the original group of 69 patients is 85%. This trial demonstrated that repeated courses of IFN can re-induce objective responses and that treatment with 2′-deoxycoformycin (pentostatin) and 2-CdA after IFN-α2b treatment can be successful. A distressing finding at this five-year follow-up was the incidence of secondary malignancies. Thirteen of the original 69 patients have developed a second malignancy.[59] It will be important to continue long-term follow-up on additional groups of IFN-treated patients.

In an attempt to increase the complete response rate and extend the duration of response, IFN-α maintenance treatment was tested as well as new agents used alone or in conjunction with IFN-α. Investigators evaluated whether a low-dose IFN-α maintenance regimen would extend duration of response.[60] Ninety-three patients with HCL were initially treated with 3 MU IFN-α three times per week for 12 months. Responding patients either continued with IFN-α maintenance treatment 1 MU three times per week or observation. The median duration of treatment was 30 months, and no relapses were seen in this group. This is compared to a relapse rate of 66% among patients in the observation group. The maintenance regimen was considered to be reasonably well tolerated, with only three patients discontinuing the drug because of side effects. Another study confirmed the results of this study using a low-dose regimen of 0.5 MU three times per week.[61] Further investigation of low-dose maintenance regimens and comparison of risk, benefit, and cost are warranted.

The Italian Cooperative Group evaluated the use of splenectomy as consolidation treatment.[58] Investigators found a benefit in progression-free survival, though not statistically significant, in patients who initially achieved a partial response to IFN-α treatment and then underwent splenectomy compared with patients who were randomized to observation (53% versus 22% at four years). Splenectomy provided no advantage for patients who achieved an initial complete response with IFN-α.

The nucleosides pentostatin and 2-CdA have been evaluated in the treatment of HCL. Pentostatin has proved to be an active agent, with overall response rates of 80–100% and complete response rates of 60–90%, which are often durable.[51] The recommended dosing regimen is 4 mg/m^2 intravenously every other week for three to six months until maximum response is attained. Pentostatin has been associated with significant toxicity, including renal dysfunction and serious infections. The incidence of infections has been reduced with the use of the recommended lower dose. A randomized trial comparing pentostatin and IFN-α has been conducted in patients with previously untreated HCL.[62] Results showed pentostatin to have a significantly higher complete response rate (76% versus 11%) and a significantly longer relapse-free survival. Patients who did not respond to IFN-α after six months were crossed over to the pentostatin arm and demonstrated an impressive complete response rate of 66%. Both treatment arms were well tolerated. However, another randomized trial of pentostatin versus IFN-α in previously splenectomized patients failed to show a statistically significant difference in response rate. Pentostatin-induced remissions were significantly longer.[63] Pentostatin has also been evaluated in sequential[64] and alternating cycles[65] with IFN-α. Alternating cycles did not prove to be of any benefit, as no patients achieved a complete response. The sequential cycle, on the other hand, was successful, with a durable complete response rate of 90% and a low incidence of infection. Pentostatin has also demonstrated the ability to re-induce durable complete responses in patients who have progressed after IFN-α therapy.[66] Although results of these trials are promising, additional studies with extended follow-up will be necessary to assess potential long-term adverse consequences, such as late infections and secondary malignancies, and to determine pentostatin's ability to cure HCL.

Another nucleoside, 2-CdA, has demonstrated impressive response rates in HCL after only one course of treatment. A durable complete response rate of approximately 80% has been observed after a single seven-day infusion of 0.1 mg/kg per day. Only minimal toxicity has been reported with this regimen.[51] Both pentostatin and 2-CdA have been approved by the FDA for treatment of HCL.

Further studies are needed to determine the individual role each of these three agents (IFN-α, pentostatin, and 2-CdA) will play in the front-line treatment plan for patients with HCL.

Chronic Myelogenous Leukemia—Chronic myelogenous leukemia (CML) begins as a benign chronic phase and progresses into an accelerated or blastic phase. To date, the only curable treatment has been allogenic bone marrow transplantation (BMT). Conventional chemotherapy has not demonstrated the ability to prevent progression to blast crisis. IFN-α has been investigated in the treatment of CML and has demonstrated long-term cytogenetic remissions (complete disappearance of the Philadelphia chromosome). The Philadelphia chromosome is a hallmark finding in CML. It is a cytogenetic abnormality representing reciprocal translocation of genetic material between chromosome 22 and chromosome 9. Complete disappearance of the Philadelphia chromosome represents elimination of the leukemic clone.

The initial single-agent, single-arm studies of IFN-α in CML revealed a dose-response relationship. Studies showed that larger doses (greater than 4 MU/m^2 per day) were associated with a higher response rate than smaller doses.[67] In patients given 5 MU/m^2 per day, 74% demonstrated a hematologic response and 33% had a cytogenetic response, with 26% of those experiencing a complete cytogenetic response. Durable cytogenetic remissions lasting two to eight years were observed in 90% of patients with complete cytogenetic response.[68,69]

Randomized trials compared the efficacy of IFN-α and conventional chemotherapy (busulfan or hydroxyurea). Results showed both treatment groups to be equally effective at producing hematologic remissions. One trial by the Italian Cooperative Study Group[70] demonstrated durable cytogenetic remissions and improved survival in patients treated with IFN-α compared with those treated with chemotherapy (72 months versus 52 months, respectively).

Studies evaluated the use of IFN-α as a means of maintaining remissions induced by chemotherapy. IFN-α was administered as maintenance treatment following induction chemotherapy. Results of these studies showed no benefit of chemotherapy followed by IFN-α compared to IFN-α alone.[67]

Combination regimens of IFN-α and chemotherapy have been compared to IFN-α alone. The combination regimen of cytarabine plus IFN-α was found to induce a greater number of hematologic responses (55% versus 28%, respectively), and there was a trend toward more cytogenetic responses (15% versus 5%). The combination regimen also demonstrated an improved three-year survival rate compared with IFN-α alone (75% versus 48%).[71]

IFN-α has also been investigated in the BMT setting. Researchers evaluated the use of IFN-α after BMT to induce cytogenetic remissions in relapsed patients or to prevent relapse after BMT in high-risk patients. Results of a small treatment after relapse trial indicate that patients with a cytogenetic relapse only do better than patients with both a cytogenetic and a hematologic relapse (71% versus 40% survival).[72] However, more studies are needed with larger patient populations to determine the efficacy of IFN-α in this setting and its effect on survival.

IFN-α has recently received FDA approval for the treatment of CML. Newly diagnosed patients with low-risk prognostic features (lack of peripheral blood and marrow basophilia, no other cytogenetic abnormalities, white race, and less than 60 years of age) are thought to have the best response. Time to cytogenetic response is approximately 3–12 months after initiation of treatment; however, complete cytogenetic response may require 6 months to four years of IFN-α therapy.

Kaposi's Sarcoma—Approximately 35–50% of patients with acquired immunodeficiency syndrome (AIDS)-related KS also experience an objective response to IFN-α therapy with fewer opportunistic infections and prolonged survival.[73–75] The recommended doses of IFN-α monotherapy for KS are 18–36 MU (or 30 MU/m^2) three times weekly. Tumor response to IFN-α in KS appears to be dose related. A review of trials using IFN-α as single-agent therapy showed a mean objective response rate of 30%, with the largest number of responses seen with doses greater than or equal to 20 MU/m^2 per day.[76] Many patients are unable to tolerate the side effects associated with high-dose therapy, however, and require dosage reduction. Response to IFN-α is also correlated with the patient's degree of immunosuppression. Patients most likely to respond are those with CD4$^+$ T-lymphocyte counts above 200, no opportunistic infections, less extensive disease, and no constitutional symptoms (e.g., fever, night sweats, or weight loss).[77] IFN-α suppresses the human immunodeficiency virus (HIV) in vitro and in vivo.[74,75] Several studies have been conducted with the combination of zidovudine and IFN-α in an attempt to potentiate antiviral activity and minimize toxicities.[78,80] Antitumor responses of 45–50% have been obtained with the combination regimen, accompanied by decreased serum HIV p24 antigen levels and increased CD4$^+$ T-lymphocyte counts. The combination regimen appears to be more efficacious than IFN-α monotherapy, with longer remission durations and improved survival.[77] A review of trials with zidovudine and IFN-α revealed the maximally tolerated dose of IFN-α was 5–18 MU/day.[76] The recommended combination regimen is zidovudine 600 mg/day plus IFN-α 9–18 MU/day. The dose-limiting toxicities in these studies included neutropenia, anemia, thrombocytopenia, and hepatotoxicity. The addition of GM-CSF and granulocyte colony-stimulating factor (G-CSF) reduced neutropenia, allowed larger doses of zidovudine to be given, and did not adversely affect antitumor activity.[77]

IFN-β and IFN-γ have also been reported to produce some antitumor and antiviral effects in patients with AIDS-related KS.[81,82] However, the antitumor responses have not been clinically meaningful.

Although the combination of zidovudine and IFN-α does appear to prolong survival in patients with KS, it is not curative therapy. Therefore, new therapeutic approaches to AIDS-related KS must continue to be explored.

Hepatitis—Patients with chronic hepatitis B or hepatitis C (non-A, non-B hepatitis) are at increased risk for hepatocellular carcinoma. Because of their antiviral activity, IFNs have demonstrated clinical activity in the treatment of hepatitis B and hepatitis C. IFN-α has been approved by the FDA for the treatment of both hepatitis B and hepatitis C.

Marcellin and colleagues [83] reviewed several controlled trials comparing treatment with IFN-α to no treatment in patients with chronic hepatitis C. Results of these trials revealed treatment to be better than no treatment and that a 3-MU dose was more effective than a 1-MU dose. Approximately 50% of treated patients had normalization of alanine aminotransferase (ALT) levels with loss of hepatitis C virus RNA in the serum and improvement in liver histology, with regression of lobular and periportal inflammation. Unfortunately, it has been demonstrated that approximately 50% of responding patients will relapse, showing increasing ALT levels within two to six months after IFN-α has been discontinued.[83,84] At most, 20% will have a sustained response six months after discontinuation of therapy.[83]

The current recommended IFN-α dosing regimen is 3 MU subcutaneously three times per week for 24 weeks. More intensive regimens using higher doses and longer durations have demonstrated a slight improvement in sustained response rate, but these regimens are of questionable benefit.[83] Factors that seem to predict a positive response to IFN-α treatment include younger age, low serum hepatitis C virus RNA level, a short duration of infection, and absence of cirrhosis.[83,84]

The use of IFN-α in combination with other agents is currently being evaluated. Additional trials with long-term follow-up to assess the impact of IFN-α on the incidence of cirrhosis and hepatocellular carcinoma are warranted. Given that approximately 50% of patients who develop acute hepatitis C will advance to the chronic stage, the use of IFN-α in acute hepatitis C should be evaluated in large trials to determine if it can prevent progression to the chronic stage.

Treatment of chronic hepatitis B infection with IFN-α results in interruption of hepatitis B virus (HBV) replication and thus loss of markers for HBV replication (HBV DNA and hepatitis B e antigen [HBeAg]), and normalization of serum aminotransferase levels. Response, defined as loss of HBeAg and HBV DNA, is seen in approximately 30–35% of patients.[85] This response is usually associated with an initial rise in serum aminotransferase levels and then a normalization of liver enzymes. Loss of hepatitis B surface antigen (HBsAg) is seen in approximately 6% of treated patients immediately after therapy.[85] Loss of HBsAg may occur early or may take several years after loss of HBeAg. Loss of HBsAg may indicate complete recovery from hepatitis B infection.[83]

The relapse rate is relatively low (approximately 3–14%) within the first year after IFN-α therapy.[86] In general, most patients who relapse will respond to a second course of treatment. The duration of chronic hepatitis B remissions obtained in patients treated on four different IFN-α protocols (various doses) was evaluated.[87] Overall, 23 patients (36%) responded initially to IFN-α therapy with loss of HBeAg and improved serum aminotransferases. Furthermore, 65% of the responding patients also became negative for HBsAg after losing the HBeAg. At a median follow-up of 4.3 years, only 3 of the 23 initial responders had relapsed.

The optimal dose and duration of treatment has been controversial. Varying doses and schedules have been used; however, a dose of 5 MU daily or 10 MU three times per week for 4–6 months should provide response with tolerable toxicity. Approximately 20% of patients require a dose reduction, and 5% require early discontinuation of treatment because of side effects.[85]

In an attempt to improve response rate, IFNs have been evaluated in combination with steroid therapy. Several studies have been conducted, and the combination has failed to show a benefit over IFN-α alone.[88] Further studies with long-term follow-up are needed to determine the impact IFNs will have on the incidence and mortality of cirrhosis and hepatocellular carcinoma.

Renal Cell Carcinoma—The role of IFNs in the therapy of advanced renal cell carcinoma has been reviewed by Quesada.[89] The overall response obtained with various treatment regimens was 16%. It also appears that frequent administration of IFNs (e.g., daily or three times weekly) are more effective than cyclic schedules (e.g., 3–4 week rest intervals between doses). Prolonged drug administration over several months may be necessary to obtain a tumor response. Clinical characteristics of patients most likely to respond to IFN-α therapy include a performance status of better than 90%, prior nephrectomy, no prior therapy, and metastases confined to the lung and mediastinal lymph nodes. Further studies need to be conducted to determine the optimal dose, the efficacy of IFNs in combination with other biological or chemotherapeutic agents, and the impact IFNs have on survival in patients with metastatic renal cell carcinoma.

Melanoma—IFN-α has been used to treat malignant melanoma. Phase II trials of IFN-α in patients with melanoma demonstrated an objective response rate of 11–27%, which is comparable to single-agent chemotherapy.[76] The majority of responses are partial, with a remission duration of approximately four months. However, there is a small percentage of patients who develop complete durable responses. Robinson and colleagues[90] administered IFN-α2b at a dose of 10 MU/m^2 subcutaneously three times per week for 12 weeks. Four of 59 patients attained a complete response, and six patients had a partial response.

Variable doses and schedules of IFN-α have been used. There does not appear to be a definite dose-response relationship. Doses ranging from 10 to 100 MU/m^2 have similar response rates.[76,91] However, it has been shown that uninterrupted therapy given either daily or on alternate days should be used over intermittent schedules, and treatment should be continued for at least three months.

IFN-α has been combined with other chemotherapeutic agents, such as cyclophosphamide and dacarbazine, in an attempt to enhance its cytotoxic effects. Combinations of IFN-α and cyclophosphamide have not proved to be of major benefit. Trials evaluating the combination of dacarbazine and IFN-α have demonstrated contradictory results.[92,93] Randomized controlled trials comparing the combination of dacarbazine and IFN-α versus IFN-α alone are currently being conducted and should establish whether or not there is a true synergism between these two agents.

The combination of IFN-α and recombinant IL-2 (rIL-2) did not prove to be of significant benefit over rIL-2 alone in a randomized trial conducted in melanoma patients.[94] Another trial evaluated the combination of IFN-α and rIL-2 in escalating doses.[95] Although an improved response rate was seen in the higher-dose groups, the higher dose did not increase the survival rate or duration of response and was associated with increased toxicity. Additional trials that evaluated the combination of rIL-2 and IFN-α in melanoma patients used different dosing regimens and showed variable response rates (0–56%).[95] The use of both rIL-2 and IFN-α in combination with chemotherapy regimens is now under investigation. A combination of rIL-2, carmustine (BCNU), dacarbazine, cisplatin, tamoxifen, and IFN-α resulted in an overall response rate of 57% (24 of 34) in patients with melanoma. There were 10 complete responses and 14 partial responses, with a median duration of more than nine and more than seven months, respectively.[96]

Intralesional IFN-α has been used with some success. An overall response rate of 18% with a complete response rate of 6% has been demonstrated.[97]

IFN-α has proved to be more effective in patients with minimal tumor burden. This is the basis for evaluating the role of IFN-α therapy in the adjuvant setting after surgery in patients at high risk for relapse. Several different groups are currently investigating IFN-α administered at different dosing regimens (low, moderate, and intensive dose) for periods ranging from three months to two years.[91] Results of one such trial have recently been reported. The Eastern Cooperative Oncology Group investigated the use of IFN-α2b (Intron®A) administered at maximum tolerated doses for one year to prevent relapse and death of patients at high risk after curative surgery for melanoma.[98] Eligible patients had surgically resected primary cutaneous melanoma without prior systemic adjuvant therapy and without evidence of distant metastatic disease. Patients were randomly assigned to receive either IFN-α at 20 MU/m² per day intravenously five days per week for 4 weeks, followed by three times weekly at 10 MU/m² per day subcutaneously for 48 weeks, or close observation. Results demonstrated that adjuvant therapy with IFN-α significantly reduced the incidence of melanoma recurrence and prolonged overall survival by approximately one year. The estimated five-year relapse-free survival rate was 46% for patients treated with IFN-α and 37% for patients on the observation arm. The impact of IFN-α on overall survival has been sustained over a median follow-up of seven years. Toxicity of IFN-α therapy was considered significant but tolerable in the majority of patients. Severe (grade 3) toxicity was evident in 67% of all patients at some point during the year of treatment. Life-threatening toxicity occurred in 9% of patients, and two had lethal hepatic toxicity. Dose delays and/or reductions due to toxicity were required in 37% of patients during induction phase and in 36% during the maintenance phase. The encouraging results from this trial provide a strong rationale for continued investigation with different regimens of IFN-α therapy.

Multiple Myeloma—Single-agent IFN-α therapy produces overall response rates of approximately 15–20% in patients with multiple myeloma that is refractory to standard therapy.[99–101] Response rates may be somewhat higher in patients who are treatment naive, but they are still lower than the response rates obtained with standard chemotherapy regimens. In an attempt to increase response rates, the combination of IFN therapy and chemotherapeutic agents is being investigated in clinical trials. An objective response rate of 71% was obtained in 30 patients with previously untreated multiple myeloma when IFN-α was added to standard melphalan-prednisone therapy.[102]

In a phase III trial, patients receiving combined IFN-α, melphalan, and prednisone experienced greater tumor response than patients receiving only combined melphalan and prednisone (95% versus 68%, respectively).[103] Furthermore, the response duration and median survival were longer in the patients receiving IFN-α, melphalan, and prednisone combined.

However, another randomized trial by the Cancer and Leukemia Group B[104] failed to show any advantage with the addition of IFN-α2b to standard melphalan and prednisone in newly diagnosed patients with multiple myeloma. Response rate, duration of response, and median survival were similar in both groups. Toxicity was greater in the group receiving melphalan, prednisone, and IFN-α but was usually mild to moderate in nature. Similar results were also seen by Corrado and colleagues[105] with the combination of melphalan, prednisone, and IFN-α2b. IFN has also been added to combination chemotherapy regimens. One randomized trial compared IFN-α2b plus VMCP (vincristine, melphalan, cyclophosphamide, and prednisolone) chemotherapy to VMCP alone.[106] Response rates and overall survival were comparable between the two groups. The only statistically significant difference was in the proportion of patients with progressive disease, which was significantly lower in group receiving the IFN-α2b and VMCP (10.6%) than in the group that received VMCP alone (22.9%). Toxicity was also found to be significantly higher in the first group. These same investigators conducted a metanalysis on all trials that combined IFN-α and induction chemotherapy. A small but significant advantage was seen in the combination group for response rates and progression-free and overall survivals. However, this small benefit in response must be weighed against the increased toxicity seen with combination regimens.

Maintenance therapy with IFN-α after induction therapy with standard chemotherapy regimens has also been investigated. In this study, patients were randomized to maintenance treatment with IFN-α (3×10^6 IU/m² three times weekly) or no treatment following disease stabilization with various standard induction regimens.[107] The patients receiving IFN-α maintenance therapy experienced longer response (26 months versus 14 months) and longer survival (52 months versus 39 months) than the control patients. These results have been confirmed by additional trials. Two trials found improvements in progression-free and overall survivals with IFN-α maintenance,[106,108] whereas another trial found benefit in progression-free survival but not in overall survival.[109] Ludwig and colleagues[106] evaluated the effect of the induction regimen on response to maintenance treatment with IFN-α. They found that patients who received both IFN-α in the induction regimen and as maintenance had the longest duration of response and had prolonged survival compared with patients who had chemotherapy alone as induction. However, there are other trials that have failed to demonstrate any benefit of IFN-α maintenance in terms of response duration or overall survival.[110,111] A metanalysis was also conducted with data from IFN-α maintenance trials involving more than 900 patients.[106] A significant benefit was observed in progression-free and overall survival of patients receiving IFN-α maintenance compared with patients randomized to observation.

Continued studies are needed to define the role of IFN-α in maintenance therapy for multiple myeloma. Because some of the previous studies demonstrated an improvement in remission duration but not in overall survival, it is important to include quality-of-life assessments and cost analyses in future studies. This will help to determine whether the increased toxicity and expense to the patient is worth the potential gain in progression-free survival with the possibility of not affecting overall survival.

Colorectal Cancer—IFN-α in combination with 5-FU has demonstrated significant activity in the treatment of advanced colorectal cancer. In the pilot study, 32 previously untreated patients were treated with 5-FU (5-day continuous infusion followed by weekly bolus therapy) in combination with IFN-α 9 MU administered subcutaneously three times per week.[112] Sixty-three percent of patients achieved a partial response, but three toxic deaths were associated with the treatment regimen. Unfortunately, the response rates were not reproducible in subsequent trials, which demonstrated response rates of 26–42%, very few complete responses, and significant toxicity. These trials failed to demonstrate an advantage of the combination of 5-FU and IFN-α compared with other 5-FU regimens.[113–116] A phase III randomized trial comparing the combination of 5-FU and leucovorin versus the combination of 5-FU and IFN-α demonstrated equivalent efficacy but increased toxicity with the 5-FU and IFN-α regimen.[117]

In an attempt to improve response rate, the triple-drug regimen of 5-FU, folinic acid, and IFN-α was evaluated. A randomized multicenter trial compared the combinations of 5-FU and folinic acid, 5-FU and IFN-α, and 5-FU plus IFN-α and folinic acid in patients with advanced colorectal cancer.[118] An interim analysis revealed that the triple-drug regimen of 5-FU, IFN-α, and folinic acid provided no significant advantage over 5-FU and folinic acid alone. The toxicity of the triple-drug regimen was found to be unacceptably high, with a 10% treatment-related mortality. This arm of the study was closed, and the study continues with 5-FU and IFN-α versus 5-FU and folinic acid. Other smaller trials also found that the triple-drug regimen provided no advantage over single-agent 5-FU or 5-FU plus folinic acid and was associated with greater toxicity.[119–121]

In contrast, two trials evaluating the triple-drug regimen had response rates of 54 and 51%, with some complete responses in both trials.[122,123] All the studies looking at combinations of IFN-α, 5-FU, and folinic acid have used varying doses and schedules, making direct comparison difficult outside comparative trials.

Therapy with IFN-α has also produced partial responses in patients with non-Hodgkin's lymphoma, cutaneous T-cell lymphoma, malignant glioma, ovarian cancer, carcinoid tumors, and bladder cancer. Further trials need to be conducted to evaluate the utility of IFN-α therapy in these types of malignancies.

Interferon Gamma and Interferon Beta

IFN-γ is approved for use in the treatment of chronic granulomatous disease. Fewer patients with chronic granulomatous disease developed serious infections while receiving IFN-γ (50 mg/m^2 three times weekly) than did patients receiving placebo (22% versus 46%, respectively).[124] Furthermore, there was a reduction in the total number of serious infections in the IFN-γ group (20 infections) than in the placebo group (56 infections). The use of concomitant prophylactic antibiotics in some patients did not negate the beneficial effects of IFN-γ. As a result, it is now strongly recommended that patients with chronic granulomatous disease receive prophylactic IFN-γ to reduce the development of serious infections.

IFN-γ may also be useful in the treatment of infections caused by such intracellular pathogens as *Mycobacterium*, *Leishmania*, *Toxoplasma*, *Rickettsia*, and *Chlamydia* species. IFN-γ activates endothelial cells, fibroblasts, epithelial cells, hepatocytes, and macrophages to kill intracellular pathogens. Clinical studies have evaluated IFN-γ for treatment of *Mycobacterium avium* complex, leprosy caused by *Mycobacterium leprae*, and protozoal infections, such as leishmaniasis and toxoplasmosis. The use of IFN-γ in combination with other antimicrobial agents had some encouraging responses in patients with these infections. The role of IFN-γ in the treatment of multiresistant tuberculosis and fungal infections is also being explored.[125]

IFN-γ has demonstrated antitumor activity in various malignancies, including ovarian carcinoma, renal cell carcinoma, melanoma, CML, and mycosis fungoides. Additional studies with IFN-γ alone and in combination with other BRMs or chemotherapeutic agents need to be conducted to determine its precise role in the treatment of cancer. Phase I studies with IFN-β are in progress, but it is too early to determine whether this agent has significant antitumor activity.

Toxicities

The toxicities experienced with IFNs vary, based on the type of IFN (α, β, or γ), dose, route of administration, and patient characteristics (such as age and performance status).[45,126] The most common acute toxicity associated with IFN therapy is an acute flu-like syndrome consisting of fever, chills, headaches, myalgias, malaise, nasal congestion, dizziness, and tachycardia. The fevers associated with IFN-α usually occur within six hours of drug administration and may persist for four to eight hours. They occur most commonly with doses of 18 MU or more and may be ameliorated by administering acetaminophen. Instructing patients to administer their IFNs at bedtime may also palliate some of the acute flu-like side effects. Antihistamines may help minimize the nasal congestion problems associated with IFNs. Because patients develop tachyphylaxis to most of the acute symptoms of IFNs with continued dosing, palliative agents should be necessary only for the first 7–10 days of therapy. However, patients receiving IFNs on an intermittent schedule may not develop tolerance to the acute flu-like symptoms. Gradually escalating the dose at first over a 7- to 10-day period may help minimize the acute toxicities of therapy. In contrast to the fevers associated with IFN-α, the fever that follows IFN-γ peaks at 6–12 hours after drug administration and lasts longer. Furthermore, continuous daily administration of IFN-γ does not result in disappearance of the acute febrile response.

Patients receiving daily doses of 20 MU of IFNs or more may also experience extreme fatigue that manifests as weakness, tiredness, or lack of desire and motivation. These symptoms may be worse in older patients or patients with a poor performance status. If the symptoms are severe enough, they may warrant dosage reductions or drug discontinuation. However, administering the dose on an intermittent schedule (e.g., two to three times weekly) may help to minimize the fatigue. Daily doses greater than 10 MU may also produce anorexia and weight loss in up to 50% of patients. Gastrointestinal toxicities, such as nausea, vomiting, diarrhea, and aberrant taste (metallic or salty), may further contribute to the anorexia and weight loss associated with therapy. Antiemetics and antidiarrheals may help minimize some of these side effects.[45,126]

IFN therapy may also be accompanied by various major organ toxicities. For example, extremely high doses of IFNs (100 MU or more) may result in central nervous system toxicities, including somnolence, lethargy, confusion, and mental slowing. Psychotic reactions and visual or auditory hallucinations have also been reported with doses of 20 MU/m^2 or more. These symptoms resolve when therapy is discontinued. Hematologic toxicities, such as leukopenia, thrombocytopenia, and normocytic, normochromic anemia, are also associated with IFN therapy but are rarely the dose-limiting toxicities. Elevations in serum glutamic-oxaloacetic transaminase (SGOT) and serum glutamic-pyruvic transaminase (SGPT) occur in approximately one-third of patients receiving IFN-α. With IFN-γ, alkaline phosphatase and lactic dehydrogenase levels may be elevated as well as SGOT and SGPT levels. Serum triglycerides may also be increased with IFN-γ. Finally, dermatologic toxicities are reported with IFNs, including mild thinning or loss of hair, transient skin rashes, and excessive growth of eyelashes.[45,126]

The development of serum-neutralizing and -nonneutralizing antibodies after the administration of IFNs has been reported. The formation and measurement of neutralizing IFN antibodies vary from patient to patient and may be influenced by several factors, including route of drug administration, duration of treatment, cumulative dose, tumor type, and antibody assay methodology.[127,128] There is some evidence that the IFN-α2a preparation may be more immunogenic than IFN-α2b. In 559 patients receiving IFN-α2a, 27.4% developed neutralizing antibodies, whereas only 2.4% of 423 patients receiving IFN-α2b developed antibodies.[129,130] Variability in IFN doses and assay methodology as well as patient heterogeneity may have influenced these results. However, a more recent study conducted among patients receiving IFNs for hepatitis used a single-assay method to compare antibody development with IFN-α2a and IFN-α2b. In this study, 20.2% of the patients treated with IFN-α2a developed neutralizing antibodies; only 6.9% of the patients receiving IFN-α2b did.[131] The clinical effect of neutralizing IFN antibody development remains controversial. However, some evidence suggests that antibody development is associated with decreased antitumor response.[45,55,127,132,133] The possibility of antibody development with prolonged drug administration in diseases such as hairy cell leukemia, CML, KS, and chronic hepatitis was thought to be a problem at first. However, a small study conducted recently demonstrated that the presence of IFN antibodies during long-term therapy is transient and that long-term effectiveness of IFNs will probably not be affected by neutralizing antibody development in most patients.[134] Additional studies of antibody development and drug effectiveness need to be conducted to determine their true significance in IFN therapy.

Interleukins

The ILs are a group of glycoproteins, secreted primarily by activated lymphocytes and macrophages, that are involved in the body's immune response. These agents exert their antitumor effects indirectly via complex interactions with host immune effector cells. Currently, 12 ILs have been described, and some of the IL receptors have been defined. Both the primary cellular sources and the principal effects of these soluble cytokines are discussed in greater detail in chapter 2. Recombinant DNA technology has allowed large-scale production of several IL products. Recombinant forms of IL-1, IL-2, IL-3, IL-4, IL-6, and IL-11 are currently being used in clinical trials. IL-2 is discussed in detail in this section, and IL-1, IL-3, IL-6, and IL-11 are discussed in the section on colony-stimulating factors.

Interleukin 2 (T-Cell Growth Factor)

IL-2, also known as T-cell growth factor, is produced by T lymphocytes and stimulates lymphocytic proliferation (increases in B, T, NK, and LAK cells).[135] IL-2 also increases the production of various other lymphokines, including TNF, IFN-γ, and GM-CSF, which further contributes to its tumoricidal activity. Figure 10-2 depicts the cell regulatory activities of IL-2. Numerous clinical trials have been conducted using various dosing schedules and routes of administration of rIL-2. The patients included in the clinical trials had advanced-stage cancer and failed to respond to standard therapy or were untreatable with standard therapy. The two rIL-2 products used in the clinical trials were aldesleukin (Proleukin®, Chiron Corp, Emeryville, CA) and teceleukin (Tecin®, Hoffman-LaRoche). Originally, the activity of the two different products was measured in Cetus and Nutley (Roche) units, respectively. However, in 1988 a standard international unit (IU; 1 Cetus unit = 6 IU, 1 Roche unit = 3 IU) was authorized by the World Health Organization.[136]

Table 10-4 summarizes the studies conducted with rIL-2 therapy alone in patients with advanced malignancies.[137–150] The primary tumor types that have responded to therapy with recombinant rIL-2 include renal cell carcinoma and melanoma. Objective responses of 20–30% have been reported, and a small subset of patients (less than 5%) has obtained a complete remission with rIL-2 therapy.

Encouraging results of phase II trials with rIL-2 led to the eventual FDA approval of rIL-2 (aldesleukin) for treatment of metastatic renal cell carcinoma. Approval in the United States was based on results of 255 patients entered on seven phase II clinical trials in 21 different institutions. Patients in this trial were treated according to the National Cancer Institute (NCI) regimen developed by Rosenberg and colleagues.[137,151] This is also the regimen approved by the FDA. Patients were treated with aldesleukin 600,000 or 720,000 IU/kg administered by intravenous bolus every eight hours over five days for up to 14 doses. A period of five to nine days of rest was given, followed by another identical cycle. Courses were repeated every 6–12 weeks. Results of the 255 patients treated with this regimen are reviewed by Fyfe and colleagues.[152] The overall objective response rate was 14%, with 12 (5%) complete responses and 24 (9%) partial responses. Responses were observed in patients with intact primary tumors or visceral and bone metastases, and even in patients with large tumor burden or bulky disease. The most

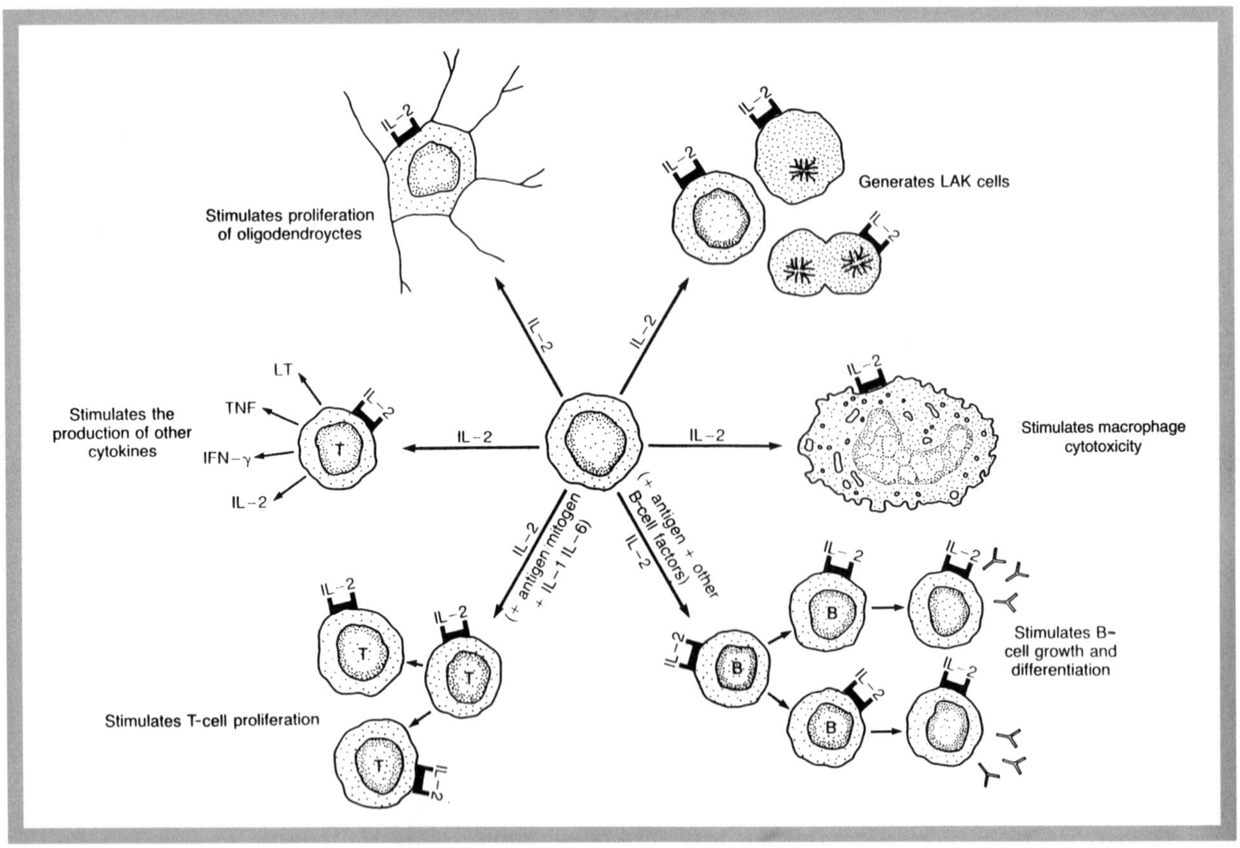

Figure 10-2. Biological and regulatory activities of interleukin 2. LAK, lymphokine-activated killer; LT, leukotrienes; TNF, tumor necrosis factor; IFN, interferon.

SOURCE: Reprinted with permission from Bakwill FR. Cytokines in Cancer Therapy. *Oxford: Oxford University Press; 1989. p. 93.*

Table 10-4. Selected Clinical Trials Using IL-2 Alone in Patients with Cancer

TREATMENT REGIMEN	NO. OF EVALUABLE PATIENTS	CR (%)	PR (%)	COMMENT	REFERENCE
0.01–0.1 MU/kg[a] IVB q 8 hr or 1–6 MU/m[2b] IVB q 8 hr	130	3	14	Responses in renal cell and melanoma only	137
1–3 MU/m² per day[b] CI or IVB 4 days/week for 4 weeks	23	0	13	Responses in renal cell only	138
10 MU/m[2a] IVB three times weekly	41	2	10	All patients had renal cell carcinoma	139
3–10 MU/m[2a] CI for 24 hr weekly for 6 weeks	16	0	6	Responses in renal cell only	140
0.01–1 MU/m[2a] IVB weekly	17	0	0	Treatment duration ranged from 3 to 33 weeks	141
1.5–3 MU/m[2a] IVB 5 days/ week for 4 weeks	26	0	12	Responses reported in lymphoma, CLL, and melanoma only	142
0.001–30 MU/m[2b] CI for 24 hr weekly for 4 weeks, then twice weekly for 4 weeks	33	0	6	Responses in melanoma only	143
0.1 MU/kg[a] IVB q 8 hr for 14 doses	46	4	17	All patients had melanoma	144
1–16.4 MU/m[2a] for five doses in a 6-day period	31	0	13	All patients had melanoma. First dose intrasplenic, remaining four doses given IV at different intervals	145
0.3–30 MU[b] IVB, CI, or SC weekly for 4 weeks	17	0	0	Pharmacokinetic study	146
3 MU/m² per day[a]	42	6	13	All patients had renal cell carcinoma	147
0.5 MU twice daily IV followed by 1 MU SC 6 days/week[c]	11	18	9	All patients had renal cell carcinoma. Prolonged IL-2 administration (21–240 days)	148
0.5–5 MU/m² per day[a] SC 5 days/week	15	0	0	All patients had renal cell carcinoma. One patient had a minor response	149
0.001–10 MU/m[2b] IM, IV, SC weekly	14	0	7	Response in patient with non-Hodgkin's lymphona	150

IL-2, interleukin 2; IVB, intravenous bolus; CI, continuous infusion; SC, subcutaneous; IM, intramuscular; CR, complete response; CLL, chronic lymphocytic leukemia; IV, intravenously.
[a]Cetus Corporation IL-2.
[b]Hoffman-LaRoche IL-2.
[c]Biogen IL-2.

encouraging result was the durability of the responses. The median duration of response for patients achieving a partial remission was 25 months, and for those achieving complete remission it was estimated to be approximately 40 months. The median survival time for all 255 patients was 15.8 months.[153]

The only prognostic factor shown to be predictive for response was an Eastern Cooperative Oncology Group (ECOG) performance status of zero. High-dose rIL-2 treatment was associated with severe acute toxicities, most of which were related to capillary leak syndrome. Hypotension was the most common toxicity. The majority of acute toxicities were rapidly reversible; however, there was a 4% treatment-related mortality.

Because of the high incidence of severe toxicities observed with the high-dose intravenous bolus regimen, investigators looked at continuous infusion administration of rIL-2 in an attempt to decrease toxicity while maintaining efficacy. The most common regimen was a dose of 18 MIU/m^2 per day as a continuous infusion for 120 hours for the first induction cycle and 108 hours for the second cycle. This was followed by maintenance cycles every three weeks. In general, the response rates and toxicities reported in the continuous-infusion trials were similar to those of the high-dose intravenous bolus regimens.

A randomized phase II trial was conducted by Weiss and colleagues.[154] Forty-six patients were randomized to receive intravenous bolus rIL-2, and 48 patients were randomized to receive continuous infusion rIL-2. Response rates were similar between the two groups, with an objective response rate of 20% in the intravenous bolus arm and 15% in the continuous infusion arm. No significant difference in durability of response or toxicities could be identified between the two groups. It would appear that continuous infusion rIL-2 is as effective as intermittent bolus administration and may have similar toxicity, but more direct comparative trials are needed.[136]

The administration of rIL-2 by subcutaneous injection was also evaluated, with the intent of moving treatment to the outpatient setting and further reducing toxicity. This method of administration had a comparable response rate of 23% with two (8%) complete remissions.[155] Toxicity was generally mild and no significant hypotension or capillary leak was observed. This regimen may prove to be useful in the outpatient setting; however, randomized trials are needed.

To evaluate the issue of dose and schedule of administration, the NCI Surgery Branch is conducting a large prospective randomized trial in patients with metastatic renal cell carcinoma. Patients are randomized to receive the high-dose rIL-2 regimen of 720,000 IU/kg administered by intravenous bolus every eight hours, a second intravenous bolus regimen but with a lower dose of 72,000 IU/kg of rIL-2, or an outpatient subcutaneous regimen. Results of this trial will be important in determining whether lower doses of rIL-2 are as effective as higher doses but with less toxicity and whether the impact on survival will be the same.

Toxicities

High-dose rIL-2 therapy has been associated with a variety of toxic effects that are frequently quite serious and require intensive patient care management. These toxicities appear to be related to dose and dosing schedule, because the greatest toxicities are seen with high-dose continuous infusion therapy. Combination regimens using rIL-2 therapy have also been associated with serious toxicities, but most of those toxicities might be attributed to rIL-2.[156, 157] The side effects of rIL-2 therapy usually resolve spontaneously after therapy is discontinued.

Toxicities associated with high-dose rIL-2 therapy are listed in Table 10-5. One of the most common side effects that occurs with rIL-2 therapy is a capillary or vascular leak syndrome.[157] Because of an increase in vascular permeability, patients may experience an accumulation of fluid in any organ system. Interstitial edema, fluid retention, and pulmonary lymphoid infiltrates frequently cause patients to require supplemental oxygen; 5–10% of patients may require ventilatory support.[157] The capillary leak syndrome may also cause a decrease in intravascular volume in many patients, leading to severe hypotension, which may be further compounded by the decrease in myocardial contractility that is associated with rIL-2. As a result, most patients require blood pressure support with fluid supplementation and pharmacologic agents. However, one must be extremely careful with fluid supplementation in patients receiving rIL-2, because impaired renal perfusion may cause increased capillary permeability with fluid accumulation and renal abnormalities (e.g., decreased urine output). Overly aggressive fluid supplementation can lead to pulmonary edema and respiratory distress, weight gain, and cerebral edema, which can contribute to lethargy and confusion.[135,136]

Several theories have been proposed as possible mechanisms for the capillary leak syndrome.[157] The first theory is that rIL-2 has a direct effect on blood vessel integrity and results in increased vascular permeability. Another is that rIL-2 causes the production or release of substances that have direct effects on vascular permeability. A third theory suggests that LAK cells, either stimulated in vivo or administered concomitantly, may be directly or indirectly responsible for the capillary leak syndrome. It may eventually be determined that a combination of these mechanisms contributes to the development of the capillary leak syndrome.

Systemic symptoms, such as fever, rigors, chills, and malaise, usually occur two to four hours after rIL-2 administration and are probably secondary to the release of various other cytokines, including IL-1, IL-6, TNF, and IFN-γ.[157, 158] These side effects may be minimized with the concomitant administration of acetaminophen, nonster-

Table 10-5. Toxicities Associated with rIL-2 Therapy

Capillary leak syndrome Interstitial edema Fluid retention Lymphoid infiltrates	**Neuroendocrine toxicities** Elevated corticotropin, cortisol, prolactin, and growth hormone Hypothyroidism
Systemic symptoms Fever Chills Rigors Malaise	**Hematologic toxicities** Lymphopenia and lymphocytosis Anemia Thrombocytopenia Eosinophilia
Dermatologic toxicities Diffuse macular erythema Desquamating rash Burning, pruritis	**Bacterial sepsis** **Hepatotoxicity** Intrahepatic cholestasis Elevated liver function enzymes Prolonged prothrombin time
Gastrointestinal toxicities Nausea and vomiting Diarrhea Anorexia Stomatitis	**Cardiotoxicity** Atrial and ventricular arrhythmias Myocardial infarction Decreased myocardial contractility
Neurologic toxicities Hallucinations Disorientation Personality and behavior changes	**Nephrotoxicity** Prerenal azotemia Oliguria

oidal anti-inflammatory agents, and meperidine for symptomatic relief. Nonsteroidal anti-inflammatory agents must be administered cautiously in patients receiving rIL-2, however, because they may increase the risk of renal function abnormalities.[157] Diffuse macular erythema, which may progress to a desquamating rash, has also been reported with rIL-2 therapy.[159] Antipruritics, such as diphenhydramine, may help alleviate the burning and pruritus associated with rIL-2 dermatologic toxicities. Gastrointestinal toxicities, including nausea, vomiting, diarrhea, anorexia, and stomatitis, commonly occur with rIL-2 administration and may be managed with antiemetics, antidiarrheals, and topical oral anesthetics.

Neurological toxicities manifested as hallucinations, disorientation, personality changes, and behavioral changes occur relatively frequently with rIL-2 and warrant immediate discontinuation of the drug. These symptoms generally resolve after therapy is discontinued, but they may actually progress at first.[157,158] rIL-2 also affects the neuroendocrine system, resulting in elevated levels of adrenocorticotropic hormone, cortisol, prolactin, and growth hormone.[160] Hypothyroidism has been reported in several patients when rIL-2 was administered in combination with LAK cells.[157] Hematologic toxicities, including anemia, thrombocytopenia, eosinophilia, and initial lymphopenia followed by lymphocytosis, have all been associated with rIL-2 therapy.[157,158] There is also some evidence that rIL-2 may adversely affect neutrophil activity, resulting in increased patient susceptibility to infection.[161] As many as 10–30% of patients receiving rIL-2 develop bacterial infections. The organisms cultured most frequently are *Staphylococcus aureus* and *Staphylococcus epidermidis*.[157] Most of these infections are related to indwelling central venous catheters. In an attempt to decrease the morbidity and mortality associated with rIL-2 therapy, prophylactic antistaphylococcal antibiotics are now administered routinely during rIL-2 treatment courses.

Biological Response Modifier Combinations

The combination of IFN-α and rIL-2 demonstrated synergistic activity in experimental animal models. This led to the investigation of the combination in patients with cancer. Trials have used both high-dose and low-dose rIL-2 in combination with IFN-α by different doses and routes of administration. Response rates have been variable, ranging between 0 and 56% for melanoma and between 9 and 42% for renal cell carcinoma.[162]

In an early phase I trial, Rosenberg and colleagues[163] evaluated the combination of rIL-2 at doses of 2.6–11.7 MIU/m^2 given by intravenous bolus and IFN-α at 3–6 MU/m^2. In patients with melanoma, 13 of 39 (33%) patients responded (3 complete and 10 partial responses). The response rate appeared to increase with increasing dose, with no responses observed with the low-dose rIL-2/IFN-α combination. In patients with renal cell carcinoma, 11 of 35 (31%) patients responded (4 complete and 7 partial responses). A long-term follow-up evaluation of these patients with the addition of another 95 patients was conducted as part of a phase I/II study evaluating the combination regimen.[162] IFN-α 3–6 MU/m^2 was administered intravenously in combination with rIL-2 in escalating doses of 2.6–15.6 MIU/m^2 by intravenous bolus administration. Among 189 patients, the total response rate was 23%, with 18 complete responses and 25 partial responses. The highest response rate was noted in the group with the highest IFN-α dose in combination with intermediate-dose rIL-2. The median duration of follow-up evaluation was 65.8 months. After more than 60 months, one melanoma patient and nine renal cell carcinoma patients still showed ongoing response. The five-year survival rate was 25% for patients with renal cell carcinoma, 6% for melanoma patients, and zero for all other patients. In general, toxicity observed in this trial was similar to that observed for either agent alone; however, there was an increase in toxicity at the higher dose levels. Overall, the response rate and five-year survival rate were not significantly better than those observed with high-dose rIL-2 alone, and the combination was associated with more toxicity, especially at higher doses. Two prospective randomized trials comparing high-dose intravenous bolus rIL-2 alone versus rIL-2 plus IFN-α could not detect a significant difference in response rate, toxicity, or median survival between the two groups.[164,165]

Trials evaluating IFN-α in combination with rIL-2 given as a continuous infusion have demonstrated comparable results to the intravenous bolus rIL-2 combination regimens. Response rates have varied from zero to 35% with a median duration of 12 months. Toxicities were similar to those seen with intravenous bolus rIL-2.[136]

Low-dose rIL-2 administered subcutaneously in combination with IFN-α has been investigated as an outpatient regimen. One group demonstrated a comparable response rate of 25% with 9 (6%) complete remissions and 29 (19%) partial remissions. Treatment-related toxicity was considered low to moderate and appeared to be less than that seen with either intravenous bolus or continuous infusion rIL-2.[166] Large randomized phase III trials are needed to compare these combination regimens with single-agent rIL-2 to evaluate efficacy, toxicity, and quality of life.

Combinations of rIL-2 and chemotherapy agents, such as cyclophosphamide and dacarbazine, have been conducted primarily in melanoma patients. Response rates range from 15 to 24%; however, no trial has proven the combination regimen to be more effective than high-dose rIL-2 alone.[136] There has recently been increased interest in a triple-drug regimen of rIL-2, IFN, and 5-FU. Initial phase I and phase II trials demonstrated overall response rates of 47–48%, with some complete responses and only mild to moderate systemic toxicity.[167,168] Additional trials are needed to confirm these results.

rIL-2 has also been evaluated in the treatment of other malignancies and by different methods of administration. Patients with metastatic small-cell lung cancer were treated with rIL-2 after receiving four cycles of chemotherapy. Additional tumor regression was observed in 5 of 24 patients (21%).[169] Intraventricular administration of rIL-2 (6 MIU) has resulted in clearance of tumor cells from the cerebrospinal fluid in 9 patients with leptomeningeal carcinoma originating from metastatic melanoma and lung cancer.[170]

Responses have been observed in patients with malignant glioma administered intracavitary rIL-2 and LAK cells via Ommaya reservoir.[171]

Intraperitoneal administration of rIL-2 with or without LAK cells is being investigated in patients with ovarian cancer, but the results are still quite preliminary.[172,173] Low-dose rIL-2 (200 U) injected perilymphatically produced complete or partial disappearance of tumor in six of eight patients with recurrent squamous cell carcinoma of the head and neck.[174] Responses have also been noted in patients with intermediate or low-grade lymphoma, non-small-cell lung cancer, colon cancer, breast cancer, and bladder cancer by intravesical administration.[175]

The use of rIL-2 in the BMT setting has been investigated. Preclinical studies demonstrated that incubation of murine bone marrow with rIL-2 in vitro leads to the generation of K cells that are cytotoxic to cancer cells. Systemic administration of rIL-2 after syngenic BMT with activated bone marrow cells produced graft-versus-leukemia (GVL) effects in mice.[176] These findings led to the investigation of rIL-2 in human clinical trials. Because allogenic BMT in patients with acute myeloid leukemia (AML) produces a significantly lower relapse rate than autologous BMT, it was concluded that immune mechanisms such as GVL must contribute to disease control after allogenic BMT.[177] rIL-2 was therefore evaluated in patients undergoing autologous BMT for AML in an attempt to induce a GVL effect.

In a trial by Benyunes and colleagues,[178] patients with AML were treated with rIL-2 with or without LAK cells after autologous BMT in an attempt to eradicate residual disease and reduce relapses. rIL-2 was administered by continuous infusion at a dose of 3 MU/m^2 per day for 5 days and was started at a median of 51 days after autologous BMT. rIL-2 had no serious toxic effect on the graft, which is similar to what has been previously reported.[179] At a median of more than 34 months after BMT, 3 patients relapsed and 10 patients remained in complete remission. The actuarial disease-free survival for all patients is 64% at four years.[177] The authors of the study could not recommend LAK cell therapy in this setting because it caused the development of unacceptable thrombocytopenia.

Soiffer and colleagues demonstrated that a low dose of rIL-2 (6×10^5 IU/m^2 per day) could be administered to outpatients for a prolonged period of time (90 days) after both autologous and allogenic T cell–depleted BMT. Patients receiving rIL-2 after allogenic BMT did not have an increased incidence of graft-versus-host disease (GVHD) and did demonstrate a lower risk of relapse compared with historical controls.[180,181]

In a phase I trial, autologous bone marrow cells were cultured in vitro with rIL-2 and then reinfused back to AML patients who had received conditioning chemotherapy. rIL-2 was administered subcutaneously at escalating doses of 2–6 $\times 10^5$ U/m^2 per day from days 0 to 7 following transplant. Side effects from this regimen were generally mild, with fever being the most common side effect observed. The neutrophil and platelet count recovery was delayed when compared with those of patients receiving unmanipulated syngenic or allogenic BMT. Two patients died from infection, three patients relapsed, and five patients continued to be in remission 18–32 months after transplant.[182] Comparative trials of rIL-2 versus no rIL-2 after autologous BMT are needed to determine the true impact on relapse rate and disease-free survival.

Colony-Stimulating Factors

The hematopoietic CSFs are a group of growth factors that are essential for the proliferation, differentiation, maturation, and functional activity of various hematopoietic stem cells. The complex interactions of these agents and their precise role in the human immune system are discussed in chapter 2. The CSFs currently manufactured by recombinant DNA technology are erythropoietin (EPO), GM-CSF, G-CSF, M-CSF, multipotential CSF (multi-CSF or IL-3), IL-1, IL-4, IL-5, IL-6, and IL-11.[183] Of these, only EPO, GM-CSF, and G-CSF are commercially available. The CSFs have been used clinically as a supportive measure to reduce the duration of neutropenia and the incidence of neutropenic complications related to chemotherapy. Trials with CSFs have also demonstrated clinical benefit following autologous, allogenic, and peripheral blood progenitor cell (PBPC) transplantation. In addition, CSFs have been used to mobilize autologous and donor PBPCs for transplantation and in patients with engraftment failure following transplantation.

Erythropoietin

EPO is a glycoprotein hormone that regulates the proliferation and maturation of red blood cells. A recombinant EPO product (rEPO) was the first CSF to be approved by the FDA. rEPO was approved for the treatment of anemia of chronic renal failure at a dose of 50–100 U per kilogram of body weight intravenously three times per week. Studies found that rEPO caused a rise in the hematocrit, decreased or eliminated transfusion requirements, and resulted in an improved quality of life for patients with end-stage renal disease.[184]

Similar to the anemia of chronic renal failure, the anemia associated with cancer and chemotherapy has been linked to inappropriately low serum EPO concentrations in relation to hemoglobin concentration. The inverse linear relationship between hemoglobin and serum EPO concentrations observed in iron-deficiency anemia is not demonstrated in patients with cancer.[185] Baseline endogenous EPO levels are thought to correspond to response to rEPO. Patients with plasma EPO levels between 100 and 500 U/L are more likely to respond to moderate doses of rEPO than patients with EPO levels of more than 500 U/L.[184] rEPO has recently been approved for the treatment of chemotherapy-induced anemia. In a randomized, placebo-controlled trial, three groups of patients with cancer and anemia were evaluated (patients not receiving chemotherapy and patients receiving chemotherapy with or without cisplatin). Patients were administered rEPO 100–150 U/kg subcutaneously three times per week. In all three groups, patients who received rEPO had a significant increase in hematocrit, and significantly more rEPO-treated patients had correction of their anemia than did patients receiving placebo. A significant difference in the number of red blood cell transfusions could not be detected in the first month of treatment. In months two and three, there were fewer transfusions for all patients receiving rEPO, but this difference was only statistically significant for patients also in the cisplatin chemotherapy group. Quality of life was also assessed in this trial and was found to be significantly improved in all three patient groups receiving rEPO compared with that of placebo-treated patients.[185] Another trial evaluated rEPO for treatment of anemia in patients receiving only cisplatin-based chemotherapy. Results showed a significant increase in hemoglobin over baseline in rEPO-treated patients compared with that of placebo-treated patients. Furthermore, patients in the rEPO group required significantly fewer blood transfusions than patients in the placebo group (20% versus 56%, respectively).[186]

rEPO has also been studied for use after BMT to improve erythroid recovery and decrease transfusion requirements. Two randomized trials in allogenic transplant patients used rEPO doses of 100–200 U/kg starting from the day of the transplant. Results of these studies demonstrated a significant decrease in red blood cell transfusion requirements compared with placebo-treated patients.[187,188] Results of studies in autologous BMT patients have not demonstrated any significant benefit with the use of rEPO.[189]

The use of rEPO is being investigated in numerous other treatment settings, including aplastic anemia, the anemia of chronic diseases, myelodysplastic syndrome, and the anemia associated with malignancy.[190,191]

Granulocyte-Macrophage Colony-Stimulating Factor and Granulocyte Colony-Stimulating Factor

GM-CSF stimulates the production and activity of neutrophils, basophils, eosinophils, monocytes, and early erythroid and megakaryocytic progenitor cells.[192] Recombinant GM-CSF (rGM-CSF) has been derived from three different sources: bacteria (*Escherichia coli*), yeast (*Saccharomyces cerevisiae*), and mammalian cells (Chinese hamster ovary [CHO] cells). The product manufactured by *E. coli* is nonglycosylated, the yeast product is partially glycosylated, and the CHO cell–derived product is fully glycosylated. Clinically significant differences in the therapeutic effectiveness and toxicity of these rGM-CSF products have yet to be established.[193] However, some preliminary evidence suggests that patients may develop antibodies to the yeast-derived rGM-CSF product because the yeast sugars serve as haptens and the antibodies react with the unprotected glycosylation sites.[194] GM-CSF antibody development may cause decreased GM-CSF serum concentrations, possibly by increasing plasma clearance. A first-dose effect syndrome characterized by symptomatic hypoxia and hypotension has also been described following *E. coli*–derived rGM-CSF in a small subset of patients.[195] The true incidence and mechanism of the first-dose effect of rGM-CSF need to be determined.

rGM-CSF has FDA approval for use in the acceleration of myeloid engraftment in patients undergoing autologous BMT for the treatment of non-Hodgkin's lymphoma, acute lymphoblastic leukemia, and Hodgkin's disease. It is also indicated for acceleration of myeloid recovery after allogenic BMT from HLA-matched related donors. Additional indications for treatment with rGM-CSF include mobilization of hematopoietic progenitor cells, acceleration of myeloid engraftment following peripheral blood progenitor cell transplantation, engraftment failure or delay following allogenic or autologous BMT, and in patients 55 years of age or older following induction chemotherapy for AML to decrease the duration of neutropenia and incidence of severe infections. The recommended dose is 250 μg/m^2 per day.[196]

G-CSF differs from GM-CSF in that it is more lineage specific and selectively stimulates neutrophil production and activity. Table 10-6 further describes the differences between the biological effects of GM- and G-CSF.[197] The currently available recombinant G-CSF (rG-CSF) product is derived from *E. coli* and is nonglycosylated. Both rGM- and rG-CSF have been used in a variety of malignant and nonmalignant treatment settings, including leukopenia associated with AIDS or AIDS-related therapy, bone marrow failure secondary to myelodysplasia or aplastic anemia, idiopathic and congenital neutropenias, and leukopenia associated with cancer chemotherapy and BMT.[198] rG-CSF initially received FDA approval for the treatment of neutropenia associated with myelosuppressive anticancer drugs at a recommended dose of 5 μg/kg per day. rG-CSF is also indicated for chronic administration in patients with congenital neutropenia, cyclic neutropenia, or idiopathic neutropenia. It has also been approved for use in patients with nonmyeloid malignancies undergoing myeloabalative chemotherapy followed by marrow transplantation to reduce the duration of neutropenia and neutropenia-related clinical sequelae (e.g., febrile neutropenia). The recommended dosage for this patient population is 10 μg/kg per day. Recently, rG-CSF has received approval for the mobilization of hematopoietic progenitor cells into the peripheral blood for collection by leukapheresis. The recommended dosage is 10 μg/kg per day continued for at least four days prior to the first leukapheresis procedure and continued until the last leukapheresis. [199]

Bone Marrow Transplant—Both rGM- and rG-CSF have been investigated for use in patients undergoing either autologous or allogenic BMT. Several review articles concerning the use of hematopoietic growth factors in BMT have been published.[200–204] Table 10-7 describes clinical trials conducted with rGM-CSF after BMT.[205–216] The initial trials were relatively small, nonrandomized studies that compared results to historical controls. Overall, both rGM- and rG-CSF were found to have a significant impact on neutrophil recovery after autologous BMT.[203] A

Table 10-6. Comparison of Biological Effects of G-CSF and GM-CSF

PROLIFERATION/ DIFFERENTIATION	G-CSF	GM-CSF
Granulocytes		
Neutrophil	Effect	Effect
Eosinophil	No effect	Effect
Monocyte-macrophage	No effect	Effect
Neutrophil migration	Enhanced	Inhibited
True lymphokine (product of T cells)	No	Yes
Chromosomal localization	17q	5q
Detectable in serum	Yes	No

SOURCE: *Reprinted with permission from Gabrilove JL. Introduction and overview of hematopoietic growth factors.* Semin Hematol. *1989;26(Suppl 2):3. G-CSF, granulocyte colony-stimulating factor; GM-CSF, granulocyte-macrophage colony-stimulating factor.*

Table 10-7. Selected Clinical Trials of GM-CSF Following Bone Marrow Transplantation

NUMBER OF PATIENTS		DAYS TO NEUTROPHILS ≥0.5 × 10⁹/L		DAYS TO NEUTROPHILS ≥1.0 × 10⁹/L		DAYS FEBRILE		INFECTION (%)		GM-CSF DOSE/DAY	REFERENCE
Tx	CONTROLS	Tx	CONTROLS	Tx	CONTROLS	Tx	CONTROLS	Tx	CONTROLS		
20	20	13	16	NR	NR	NR	NR	NR	NR	8 μg/kg	205
12	19	17	24.9	NR	NR	5	4.7	58	68	100–400 μg/m²	206
19	23	15.8	19.2	NR	NR	NR	NR	16	35	2–32 μg/kg	207
41	47	14	21	NR	NR	NR	NR	39	47	250 μg/m²	208
65	63	19	26	26	33	8	8	17	30	NR	209
39	40	15	28	18	33	NR	NR	46.2	70	250 μg/m²	210
36	33	12	16	15	24	NR	NR	2.7	18	10 μg/kg	211
30	31	14	20	NR	NR	8	6	33.3[a]	32.2	250 μg/m²	212
12	12	NR	NR	16	27	NR	NR	17	8	10 μg/kg	213
41	43	14	17.3	NR	NR	NR	NR	NR	NR	250 μg/m²	214
29	28	15.8	19.9	NR	NR	11	13	45	53.5	5.5 μg/kg	215
28	25	17	21	NR	NR	NR[b]	NR	NR[b]	NR	10 μg/kg	216

NR, not reported; Tx, treatment.
[a]Percentage of patients with infections other than bacteremia; there was no significant difference in number of positive blood cultures.
[b]No significant difference in duration of fever or frequency of infection between GM-CSF and placebo.

marked reduction in the median duration of neutropenia (days of absolute neutrophil count [ANC] below 500/mm³) was observed, and rG-CSF was found to also reduce the period of severe neutropenia (defined as days of ANC below 200/mm³).[217] However, no effect was observed on the nadir (ANC below 100/mm³) or the initial period of agranulocytosis. This indicated that early marrow progenitor cells are not affected by recombinant rGM- or rG-CSF.[203,218] Initial trials also demonstrated a reduction in the number of documented infections, febrile days, and days in the hospital.[200,203,219]

Randomized phase III trials of rGM-CSF after autologous BMT confirmed the acceleration of neutrophil recovery seen with the phase I/II trials. Other clinical endpoints, such as number of documented infections, febrile days, and days in the hospital, were reduced in some trials but not in others.[209–212] Only Linke *et al.*[210] and Advani *et al.* [211] were able to demonstrate a significant decrease in the number of documented infections in patients treated with rGM-CSF. In addition to accelerated recovery, another trial also demonstrated a reduction in cost to patients treated with rGM-CSF compared with those who were not.[213]

Stahel and colleagues conducted a randomized study of rG-CSF 10 or 20 μg/kg per day versus placebo after autologous BMT.[220] In patients treated with rG-CSF, they found significant reductions in time to neutrophil recovery and median number of days with fever. They also noted a decrease in the number of days in the hospital and days on intravenous antibiotics, but these decreases were not statistically significant. There were no differences in either clinical results or neutrophil recovery between the two doses of rG-CSF. Another randomized trial using rG-CSF after autologous BMT found a similar acceleration in time to neutrophil recovery; however, no significant difference was detected for days with fever, use of intravenous antibiotics, and days of hospitalization.[221] There have been no statistically significant differences noted in treatment-related mortality or overall survival in patients treated with either rGM- or rG-CSF compared with placebo.[203]

After rGM- and rG-CSF demonstrated favorable results following autologous BMT, both agents were investigated in patients undergoing allogenic BMT. rGM-CSF has been more extensively studied than rG-CSF. Initial phase I and II trials found rGM-CSF to be well tolerated at doses up to 250 μg/m² per day. Compared with historical controls, patients treated with rGM-CSF recovered their neutrophil counts an average of five days earlier, had fewer days with fever, and were discharged from the hospital sooner. rGM-CSF demonstrated no effect on the incidence or severity of GVHD, the rate of graft failure, or the incidence of relapse.[204] Randomized phase III trials with rGM-CSF were initiated based on these encouraging results from the phase I/II trials. The time to achieve an absolute neutrophil count of more than 500 neutrophils/mm^3 was shortened in the patients treated with rGM-CSF in all trials.[205,214–216] However, clinical effectiveness was demonstrated in only some of the trials. Reduction in the incidence of infection was noted in three of the four trials,[214–216] and decrease in hospital stay was noted in only one trial.[216] There were no differences observed in the incidence of GVHD, relapse, or survival between rGM-CSF and placebo in all four trials.[205, 214–216] Only limited data is available at this time from phase III randomized trials of rG-CSF, but it suggests that rG- and rGM-CSF have similar efficacy after allogenic BMT.[204]

Autologous transplantation of peripheral blood stem cells (PBSCs) rather than bone marrow has increased markedly over the past few years. Pretreatment with rGM- or rG-CSF has been shown to increase the number of hematopoietic stem cells circulating in the peripheral blood, which would reduce the number of leukapheresis treatments needed.[203,204] The use of rGM- or rG-CSF–mobilized PBSCs reduced the time to neutrophil count recovery compared with bone marrow infusion. More impressively, the time to recover platelets to 20,000 platelets/mm^3 was almost two weeks shorter than with bone marrow.[204] A randomized trial evaluated rG-CSF after autologous PBSC transplant to determine whether rG-CSF could further accelerate engraftment. Patients who received rG-CSF were found to have a reduction in the median time to a neutrophil count greater than 500 neutrophils/mm^3 compared with the control group. The rG-CSF treatment group also demonstrated significant reductions in the median duration of post-transplant hospitalization and the median number of days on nonprophylatic antibiotics. No statistically significant differences were found in time to platelet engraftment, number of febrile days, progression-free survival, or overall survival.[222] It was therefore determined that rG-CSF could enhance the neutrophil recovery associated with PBSC transplant.

The use of PBSCs in allogenic transplantation is currently under investigation. Initially, there was concern that PBSCs, which contain approximately a factor of ten more T cells than bone marrow, would increase the incidence of GVHD.[204] A pilot study evaluated the use of rG-CSF–mobilized PBSCs for allogenic transplantation.[223] Eight patients with hematologic malignancies received unmodified PBSCs from HLA-identical siblings. The donors received rG-CSF 16 μg/kg per day subcutaneously for the five days preceding PBSC collection. It was well tolerated by all donors, with only mild bone pain and flu-like symptoms. All patients engrafted, and a rapid neutrophil recovery (500 neutrophils/mm^3) before day 16 and a platelet recovery to 20,000 platelets/mm^3 by day 12 post-transplant were seen in seven of the eight patients. The incidence and severity of acute GVHD was not more than what would be expected with allogenic BMT. Two patients experienced grade 2 acute GVHD, and another patient progressed to grade 3. Based on these results and other similar reports, phase III studies comparing PBSCs with marrow for allogenic transplantation have been initiated.

Further randomized trials with rGM- and rG-CSF in transplantation are needed to address issues such as dose and schedule of administration; potential differences in efficacy and/or tolerability between rGM- and rG-CSF; and cost versus benefit, especially in the allogenic setting, where clinical endpoints such as incidence of infection, hospitalization, and number of days on intravenous antibiotics are not routinely affected and improvement in neutrophil recovery is not as dramatic as in autologous transplantation. Finally, it will also be important to determine whether rGM- and rG-CSF will have any impact on survival. To date, no trials have demonstrated any significant difference in overall survival.

rGM-CSF has also been used to stimulate hematopoiesis in patients with marrow graft failure after BMT. Marrow graft failure is defined as either a failure to reach 100 neutrophils/mm^3 by day 28 after transplant or as a drop in neutrophils to less than 500 neutrophils/mm^3 for longer than seven days after initial engraftment.[204] One trial treated patients with marrow failure after autologous, allogenic, or syngenic BMT with rGM-CSF doses of 60–1000 μg/m^2 per day.[224] Fifty-seven percent (21 of 37) of patients obtained an absolute neutrophil count of 500 neutrophils/mm^3 or more within two weeks of starting treatment. Survival at 100 days was 59% in patients treated with rGM-CSF, compared with 32% in historic controls, and survival at one year was 50 and 23%, respectively. None of the patients who received chemically purged bone marrow responded to the rGM-CSF, whereas all the patients who received nonpurged bone marrow or bone marrow purged with monoclonal antibodies responded to treatment with rGM-CSF. Another trial treated 140 patients with graft failure with rGM-CSF 250 μg/m^2 per day for 14 days. Survival at 100 days for allogenic BMT patients was 50% in the rGM-CSF group and 28% in the historical control group. In autologous BMT patients, survival to day 100 was 72% in the rGM-CSF group, compared with 59% for historical controls.[225]

Neutropenia—Both rGM- and rG-CSF have been shown to reduce the duration of neutropenia and the intensity of the nadir associated with standard chemotherapy regimens.[226] Table 10-8 summarizes clinical trials conducted with rGM- and rG-CSF in chemotherapy-induced neutropenia.[227–239] rG-CSF reduced the incidence of febrile neutropenia by approximately 50% in three prospective, randomized, placebo-controlled trials [234–236] In two of the trials, which involved patients with small-cell lung cancer, rG-CSF administration also resulted in significant reductions in antibiotic use and hospitalization.

Results of randomized trials using rGM-CSF have been less consistent. In one randomized, placebo-controlled trial, patients with non-Hodgkin's lymphoma who received rGM-CSF after chemotherapy demonstrated

Table 10-8. Selected Clinical Trials of G-CSF and GM-CSF in Chemotherapy-Induced Neutropenia

TYPE OF MALIGNANCY	G-CSF OR GM-CSF DOSE/DAY	NUMBER OF PATIENTS		DURATION OF NEUTROPENIA (DAYS)		REFERENCE
		Tx	CONTROL	Tx	CONTROL	
Various	20–60 μg/kg G-CSF	18	11	6	12	227
Acute leukemia	200 μg/m² G-CSF	48	50	20	28	228
Various	0.3–10 μg/kg G-CSF	31	ND	[a]	ND	229
Urogenital cancer	2 μg/kg G-CSF	32	38	1	6.7	230
Sarcoma	4–64 μg/kg GM-CSF	12	12	3.5	7.4	231
Ovarian	1.5–6 μg/kg GM-CSF	9	6	[b]	[b]	232
Acute myeloid leukemia	250 μg/kg GM-CSF	18	39	22.5	25.2	233
SCLC	230 μg/m² G-CSF	101	110	1[c]	6	234
SCLC	230 μg/m² G-CSF	65	64	6[d]	15	235
NHL	230 μg/m² G-CSF	41	39	NR[e]	NR	236
NHL	400 μg GM-CSF	87	85	NR[f]	NR	237
SCLC	5–20 μg/kg GM-CSF	NR	NR	NR[g]	NR	238
Germ cell	10 μg/kg GM-CSF	32	29	NR	NR	239

ND, not done; NR, not reported; Tx, treatment; SCLC, small cell lung cancer; NHL, non-Hodgkin's lymphoma.
[a]*Only 9 of 31 patients developed neutropenia (absolute neutrophil count [ANC] <1000). Median duration, 3.7 days.*
[b]*Neutropenia decreased significantly in the GM-CSF group.*
[c]*Median duration of neutropenia (ANC <1000).*
[d]*Median duration of neutropenia over six cycles of chemotherapy (ANC <1000).*
[e]*Incidence of neutropenia significantly reduced with G-CSF.*
[f]*Statistically significant decrease in incidence of neutropenia with GM-CSF with courses 3–6.*
[g]*Recovery from neutropenia was significantly faster with GM-CSF dosages, compared with observation ($P < 0.01$).*

faster neutrophil recovery, decreased incidence of febrile neutropenia, and reduced hospitalization. However, only 72% of patients were able to tolerate the rGM-CSF.[237] In another trial involving patients with small-cell lung cancer, rGM-CSF treatment resulted in faster neutrophil recovery but had no significant effect on incidence of febrile neutropenia, days in hospital, or days on intravenous antibiotics.[238] An additional trial failed to demonstrate a significant difference between rGM-CSF and placebo in terms of neutrophil recovery, incidence of febrile neutropenia, and days in hospital.[239] None of the randomized trials with rGM- or rG-CSF have detected a difference in infectious mortality, response rates, or survival.[240]

The American Society of Clinical Oncology (ASCO) has published clinical practice guidelines for the use of CSFs based on review of the medical literature.[240] ASCO guidelines concerning the use of CSFs after chemotherapy to reduce the incidence of febrile neutropenia therefore recommend that CSFs be reserved for use in patients with a 40% or greater likelihood of experiencing febrile neutropenia. Cost analyses were conducted, and results suggested that CSF administration would rarely be cost effective if baseline risk of febrile neutropenia is less than 20%. However, chemotherapy regimens with an expected risk of febrile neutropenia of greater than 40% without CSF support may benefit economically from use of CSF.[241]

The ASCO guidelines' recommended dosing for rG-CSF is 5 μg/kg per day and for rGM-CSF is 250 μg/m² per day for patients receiving chemotherapy. The preferred route of administration is subcutaneous because it is more convenient and potentially more active. It is also recommended that the dose be rounded off to the nearest vial size to increase convenience to the patient, reduce cost, and prevent waste.[240]

The use of rGM- and rG-CSF to maintain or increase dose intensity of standard chemotherapy regimens, in an attempt to increase response rates, has been investigated. CSFs may be used to maintain treatment intensity by preventing the need for dose reductions secondary to myelosuppression and preventing delays between chemotherapy cycles. One representative trial involved breast cancer patients being treated with doxorubicin therapy and supported by rG-CSF. The addition of rG-CSF resulted in such a decrease in time to neutrophil recovery that repeat courses of doxorubicin could be administered every two weeks rather than every three weeks. Treatment with rG-CSF also allowed for dose escalation of doxorubicin.[242] Another trial evaluated small cell lung cancer patients receiving chemotherapy with or without rG-CSF and found that patients treated with rG-CSF had fewer dose reductions and dose delays than patients in the control group. As a result, patients in the rG-CSF group received 9% more chemotherapy than those in the control group. Unfortunately, this did not lead to an improvement in response rate or survival.[235] Further investigation is needed to determine whether maintaining treatment intensity with CSFs, by decreasing dose reductions and treatment delays, will result in improved response rates and survival.

Dose intensification of chemotherapy with the use of CSFs has been shown to increase response rates in some malignancies, such as breast cancer. Whether or not this results in improved survival rates remains to be determined.[226]

Myelodysplastic Syndrome—rGM-CSF has been evaluated in patients with myelodysplastic syndrome (MDS) and was found to increase the numbers of circulating neutrophils, eosinophils, monocytes, and lymphocytes. It has only minimal activity in increasing platelet counts and does not appear to reduce platelet or red blood cell transfusion requirements.[243] Preliminary results from one randomized trial of rGM-CSF versus placebo in patients with AML showed an increase in neutrophil, eosinophil, and lymphocyte counts in the GM-CSF–treated group. Hemoglobin and platelet levels were not affected by the rGM-CSF. There were fewer infections in the patients given rGM-CSF, but this did not result in an improvement in survival. Four patients in each group transformed to acute leukemia.[244]

rG-CSF has been evaluated in MDS. Treatment with rG-CSF demonstrated the ability to increase the absolute neutrophil count in a large majority of patients and increase the reticulocyte count in a smaller number of patients.[243] Results of a long-term study of 3–16 months of rG-CSF for treatment of MDS showed that 10 of 11 patients had increases in leukocyte and absolute neutrophil counts. Patients who maintained an absolute neutrophil count above 1500 neutrophils/mm^3 had a significantly decreased incidence of bacterial infections. Three patients progressed to acute leukemia while on maintenance rG-CSF; however, it is difficult to determine if this was related to rG-CSF or simply the natural history of the disease.[245]

Due to a lack of evidence for clinical benefit, ASCO guidelines do not recommend the chronic administration of a CSF to patients with MDS. However, it may be appropriate to initiate intermittent treatment with a CSF in neutropenic patients with infections.[240]

A number of studies have investigated the use of CSFs in treating aplastic anemia. CSFs have been used in an attempt to increase production of mature cells from the remaining deficient pool of precursor cells.[246] Results of these studies suggest that rGM- and rG-CSF can elevate neutrophil levels in some patients with moderate aplastic anemia. Patients who had more pluripotent stem cells than baseline levels in their bone marrow had a higher likelihood of responding or had a greater response to CSFs. The neutrophil response may be dose dependent and requires continuous administration of CSFs. There has been no consistent effect on platelet or hemoglobin levels and no effect on transfusion requirements. Infections appear to occur less often in patients treated with rGM- or rG-CSF, but it is not known whether this will improve overall survival.[243,246] More studies are needed to address issues such as when to initiate treatment with CSF, length of therapy (i.e., continuous versus only during infections), and the effects on survival.

A final setting in which clinical trials have been conducted with rG-CSF is the treatment of congenital or cyclic neutropenia.[198,247] In the studies to date, patients have experienced a significant and sustained increase in their neutrophil count and a decrease in subsequent infections.

Both rGM- and rG-CSF are relatively well tolerated by patients at the usual recommended doses. The primary side effects associated with rG-CSF include bone pain, myalgias, and skin rash. In the phase II and III trials, approximately one-fourth of patients experienced bone pain.[248] This bone pain was reported more frequently with higher doses (20 µg/kg per day and more) and could usually be controlled with non-narcotic analgesics. Transient hypotension after rG-CSF administration was reported in approximately 4% of the patients in the phase III trials.

rGM-CSF has been associated with more serious toxicities, especially at higher doses. At lower doses (10 µg/kg or less), mild side effects, such as low-grade fever, myalgias, phlebitis or pain at the injection site, bone pain, headache, and nausea, have been reported.[193,249] Most of these symptoms may be palliated with acetaminophen and supportive care measures. At higher doses (15 µg/kg or more), more serious toxicities have occurred. Pleural or pericardial effusions and ascites secondary to a capillary leak syndrome were reported in the early dose-ranging trials with rGM-CSF.[207,231,250,251] Therefore, in patients with pre-existing congestive heart failure, pleural effusions, or pericardial effusions, rGM-CSF should be administered cautiously, because these conditions may be aggravated during therapy. Other side effects that occur with higher-dose therapy include severe myalgias and arthralgias, eosinophilia, and elevated liver function tests. Toxicities also appear to be greater with intravenous administration than with subcutaneous administration, especially if the rate of administration is rapid.

Interleukin 1

IL-1 is a broad-acting cytokine that plays an important role as a regulator of hematopoiesis. It induces and synergizes with a variety of other cytokines to amplify the hematopoietic response.[252–254] IL-1 has the ability to accelerate hematopoiesis in normal cells after exposure to radiation or chemotherapy. Phase I and II trials of IL-1 after autologous BMT have demonstrated an improvement in the number of days to neutrophil engraftment compared with historic controls.[255–257] The shortened time to engraftment seemed to correlate with a decreased incidence of infection in one of the trials.[257] Platelet recovery was also evaluated in one trial, and no difference was found in time to platelet count of 50,000 platelets/µl between IL-1–treated patients and historic controls.[255] Side effects associated with IL-1 administration include fever, headache, myalgias, arthralgias, and tachycardia. The dose-limiting toxicity in the phase I/II trials was hypotension.

Interleukin 3

IL-3, also known as multi-CSF, is a multilineage hematopoietic growth factor that stimulates the proliferation and differentiation of early progenitor cells, resulting in an increase in red blood cells, platelets, monocytes, basophils, eosinophils, and mast cells. Clinical trials with IL-3 have focused on its use following bone marrow transplantation, as a PBPC-mobilizing agent, and as a sequential agent with rGM- or rG-CSF.[252] Trials of IL-3 alone after combination chemotherapy have had mixed results in ameliorating chemotherapy-induced cytopenias. One trial demonstrated a significant reduction in mean number of days of neutropenia with IL-3 treatment, but the treatment had no effect on platelet count nadir.[258] Biemsa *et al.*[259] evaluated ovarian cancer patients treated with combination chemotherapy followed by IL-3. Results showed a significant decrease in platelet transfusion requirements and less treatment delays between cycles secondary to neutropenia for patients treated with IL-3.

The use of IL-3 alone after high-dose chemotherapy and autologous BMT was evaluated in a phase I trial. Treatment with IL-3 did not demonstrate a significant difference in time to platelet or neutrophil engraftment compared with historic controls who received rGM-CSF.[260] However, the sequential administration of IL-3 and rGM-CSF following autologous BMT was reported to reduce platelet transfusion requirements compared with historical controls who received rGM-, rG-CSF, or IL-3 alone.[261] Sequential administration of IL-3 followed by rGM-CSF has also been evaluated for mobilization of PBPCs and demonstrated an increase in the peak number of $CD34^+$ cells collected.[262]

Macrophage Colony-Stimulating Factor

M-CSF stimulates the production and activity of monocytes and macrophages and the release of numerous cytokines (G-CSF, GM-CSF, IFNs, IL-1, and TNF-α).[193] In animal models, M-CSF has demonstrated tumoricidal activity against melanoma and antimicrobial activity against bacteria and fungi. M-CSF also causes terminal differentiation of AML cells in vitro.[263] On the basis of this activity, phase I trials are being conducted with M-CSF. In a phase I trial of M-CSF in patients with metastatic melanoma, one patient experienced an antitumor response. At all dosage levels, patients experienced an increase in circulating monocytes and a transient decrease in platelet counts after M-CSF.[264] M-CSF has also shortened the duration of absolute neutropenia after BMT compared with historical controls.[265,266] Significant antifungal activity has been reported with M-CSF in the BMT setting.[267] However, another trial reported by Nemunaitis *et al.*[268] evaluated the use of M-CSF in 46 patients with invasive fungal infections. They found no effect on neutrophil, monocyte, or lymphocyte counts during the study. At follow-up evaluation, 12 patients were alive and free of fungal disease; 34 patients did not survive. There was a significant difference in survival of patients who received M-CSF compared with historical controls, who only received antifungal antibiotics. However, the differences in survival were due to an increased survival rate for patients with a Karnofsky score above 20%. Toxicity associated with M-CSF was primarily thrombocytopenia, which occurred in 11 of 46 patients. Additional studies with M-CSF are warranted.

PIXY-321

Based on the different but complementary hematopoietic effects of GM-CSF and IL-3, a fusion product named PIXY-321 was developed. This is a genetically engineered molecule that combines yeast-derived GM-CSF with IL-3 by the use of an amino-acid linker protein.[252] In phase I/II clinical trials of PIXY-321 after combination chemotherapy, PIXY-321 demonstrated the ability to reduce the duration of neutropenia and to reduce or eliminate the cumulative thrombocytopenia often seen with repeated cycles of chemotherapy.[252,269] The use of PIXY-321 following high-dose chemotherapy and autologous BMT demonstrated a decrease in time to platelet engraftment for PIXY-321–treated patients, compared with historic control patients treated with rGM-CSF (17 days versus 26 days, respectively). Time to neutrophil engraftment was similar between the two groups.[270] Phase III trials of PIXY-321 have been initiated in the areas of chemotherapy-induced cytopenias and BMT.

Interleukin 6

IL-6 is a cytokine with effects on T cells, myeloid cell differentiation, regulation of acute-phase reactants, and the development and maturation of megakaryocytes.[252] In a clinical phase I/II trial, IL-6 was evaluated in patients receiving chemotherapy for advanced sarcoma. Patients who received postchemotherapy IL-6 had higher median platelet nadirs than patients who did not receive IL-6.[271] Phase I/II trials of IL-6 in combination with either rGM- or rG-CSF following high-dose chemotherapy and autologous BMT have also been conducted. Fay *et al.*[272] evaluated the concomitant administration of IL-6 at doses of 0.5 or 1 µg/kg per day and rGM-CSF at 3 or 5 µg/kg per day following autologous BMT. The median time to reach an absolute neutrophil count of 500 neutrophils/mm^3 was 11 days, with a median of 12 days to platelet engraftment. The combination of IL-6 and rG-CSF following autologous BMT was evaluated in patients with breast cancer.[273] There was no significant difference in median time to an absolute neutrophil count of 500 neutrophils/mm^3 or median time to platelet engraftment between patients who received both IL-6 and rG-CSF and those who received rG-CSF alone. The use of IL-6 in combination with rGM- or rG-CSF following dose-intensive therapy is still under investigation.

Interleukin 11

IL-11 enhances the growth of IL-3–dependent megakaryocytic colony formation, promotes maturation of late human megakaryocytic progenitors, and induces production of acute-phase proteins.[252] A phase I trial evaluated IL-11 at doses ranging from 10 to 100 µg/kg per day in breast cancer patients receiving cyclophosphamide and doxorubicin.[274] Results demonstrated prevention of severe cumulative thrombocytopenia, which was optimal at doses of 25 and 50 µg/kg per day. Bone marrow samples obtained after 14 days of IL-11 administration showed a significant increase in megakaryocyte numbers in patients receiving 50 µg/kg per day or more. A recent randomized trial administered IL-11 (25–50 µg/kg) or placebo subcutaneously every day for 14–21 days starting from the day after chemotherapy ended. All patients except three also received rG-CSF. The mean number of platelet transfusions and the median duration of grade 3 thrombocytopenia was lower in the IL-11–treated patients. The number of patients who did not require any platelet transfusions was significantly higher in the group that received IL-11 50 µg/kg, compared with placebo groups. Adverse effects included edema, dizziness, tachycardia, atrial arrhythmias, syncope, palpitations, hypotension, dyspnea, fever, chills, headache, rash, and conjunctival injection.[275] More randomized trials are needed to determine whether the postchemotherapy addition of IL-11 to rG-CSF significantly improves hematopoietic recovery and reduces platelet transfusions.

Tumor Necrosis Factor

TNF is a cytokine that is produced and released by host effector cells during an immune response. Two different genes for TNF have been sequenced and produced via recombinant DNA technology: TNF-α (cachectin) and TNF-β (lymphotoxin).[276] Various biological effects, including inflammatory reactions, anorexia, and septic shock syndrome, are elucidated by TNF because of immune cell activation and the release of other cytokines, such as IL-1 and G-CSF.[277,278] TNF also produces antitumor effects via mechanisms that are not fully understood, but direct tumor cell cytotoxicity due to free-radical induction, DNA fragmentation, and nuclear membrane breakdown have all been proposed.[278] Several phase I and II clinical trials using various doses, schedules, and routes of administration of both recombinant TNF products have been conducted. Unfortunately, significant antitumor activity of TNF has not been reported in most of these studies.[279–284] Combination trials of TNF with other cytokines has not demonstrated a significant increase in response rate.[285] Intravenous administration of TNF is associated with a number of potentially severe toxicities, including fever, chills and rigors, myalgias, nausea, vomiting, and fatigue. Hypotension following intravenous bolus administration was the dose-limiting side effect in most phase I trials. Infusion of TNF may also cause hepatotoxicity with elevation of serum transaminases, nephrotoxicity with increase in blood urea nitrogen and serum creatinine, and pulmonary toxicity consisting of decreased lung diffusion capacity. Other side effects include thrombocytopenia, leukopenia, headache, and altered lipid metabolism.[285] Because of the high incidence of systemic side effects and the lack of clinical response, research with TNF has begun to focus more on local treatment. Alternative methods of administration include intraperitoneal therapy for gynecological malignancies, which proved beneficial for reducing malignant ascites, and isolated limb perfusion for melanoma. In a multicenter pilot study, the combination of TNF-α, IFN-γ, and melphalan for isolated limb perfusion produced a complete response rate of 90% and a partial response rate of 10% in patients with melanoma. The median survival is 28 or more months. Systemic toxicities included fever, chills, moderate hypotension, severe pulmonary toxicity in 10 of 58 patients, mild to severe liver toxicity (grade 3 or 4 in 10 of 58 patients), and transient neutropenia.[286] Because of the high response rates seen in this study, isolated limb perfusion with TNF and melphalan may be the treatment of choice for in-transit melanoma metastases of the limbs. The Surgery Branch of the NCI is currently conducting a prospective randomized trial comparing isolated limb perfusion with melphalan alone versus the triple-drug combination of TNF, IFN-α, and melphalan. Results of this trial will verify whether the addition of TNF significantly improves response rates and whether this justifies the increased risk of severe toxicity.

Adoptive Cellular Immunotherapy

Adoptive cellular immunotherapy (ACI) may be defined as the transfer of cells that have been boosted with BRMs in vitro to patients with cancer in an attempt to elicit an antitumor response.[5,24] Two primary techniques are currently being used in clinical trials with ACI. In the first method, peripheral blood leukocytes are removed from patients by apheresis and cultured in vitro with rIL-2. The result is the generation of LAK cells. The LAK cells are then administered to the patient either intravenously or intraperitoneally, usually along with the concomitant administration of rIL-2 to maintain cytotoxicity. The second method, which produces tumor-infiltrating lymphocytes (TILs), is similar, but the lymphocytes cultured in vitro with IL-2 are obtained from tumor specimens rather than from peripheral blood. This type of immunotherapy is extremely labor-intensive for both hospital and laboratory personnel and is also quite expensive. Clinical trials using ACI with a combination of IL-2 and LAK cells have demonstrated objective response rates of 20–25%. Most responses have occurred in renal cell carcinoma, melanoma, and colon cancer.[287–295] Both continuous infusion and intermittent bolus schedules have been used for IL-2 administration.

The efficacy of high-dose IL-2 alone was compared to the combination of IL-2 plus LAK cells in patients with renal cell carcinoma and melanoma.[296] It was concluded that the addition of LAK cells did not result in any significant improvement in response rate and the toxicity profile was similar for the two regimens. A number of other trials confirmed this result.

Data from trials comparing continuous infusion of IL-2 alone or in combination with LAK cells in 327 patients with advanced renal cell carcinoma were analyzed.[297] No statistically significant differences were observed in response rates between IL-2 alone and IL-2 with LAK cells (15 and 18%, respectively). In addition, no significant differences were noted for the number of complete responders, duration of response, progression-free survival, and overall survival between the two groups.

At this time, the data do not support an added benefit of LAK cells to the efficacy of high-dose bolus or continuous infusion of IL-2 and do not justify the additional expense associated with this therapy.

The combination of IL-2 and TILs has also been used to treat advanced malignancies.[298,299] In a promising study conducted at the NCI, an overall response rate of 55% was obtained in patients with metastatic melanoma, and one patient experienced a complete remission. Patients who failed with other IL-2 regimens responded to the combination IL-2 and TIL therapy.[294]

Initial trials of IL-2 and TIL combination therapy appeared to be more effective than IL-2 plus LAK; however, this has not been confirmed by later trials. Results of TILs in patients with renal cell carcinoma were not as promising, with only four objective responses observed in 31 patients.[299,300] Results to date do not demonstrate a significant improvement of IL-2 plus TILs over IL-2 alone; however, alternative treatment regimens designed to enhance the response to TIL therapy are currently under investigation.

TILs modified by retroviral gene transduction have been used in five patients with metastatic melanoma in an attempt to optimize therapy and define the in vivo distribution and survival of TIL cells.[301] Three of the five patients experienced tumor regression after gene-modified TIL therapy, and the side effects were similar to those reported with combined TIL and IL-2 therapy. Furthermore, it appears that TIL cells survive in the circulation for almost 200 days and in tumor cells for as long as two months after administration. As a result, it may be possible to use TILs as vehicles for tumor-directed therapy or for introducing other genes to correct inherited genetic defects. Clinical experiments using TIL cells carrying retrovirally transduced TNF genes are now under way at the NCI.

Another type of ACI is being performed in patients with CML who have relapsed following allogenic transplantation. Researchers have administered infusions of lymphocytes from the original marrow donor to relapsed patients in an attempt to induce a GVL reaction. There has been indirect clinical evidence that GVL is important in the treatment of leukemia. Patients who develop GVHD have a decreased risk of relapse, relapse rates are higher after identical twin transplants, and the risk of relapse increases after infusion of allogenic bone marrow that has been depleted of T cells.[302,303]

Cytogenetic remissions have been induced following donor lymphocyte infusions in patients with relapsed CML. Porter and colleagues[303] treated 11 patients with relapsed CML after allogenic BMT with IFN-α and infusions of donor lymphocytes. IFN-α was given at a dose of 5 MU/m^2 per day subcutaneously for 6–12 weeks prior to the first cell infusion and continued for 4 weeks after the last infusion. Six of eight patients with stable CML after relapse had a complete cytogenetic remission, with disappearance of the Philadelphia chromosome. Remissions were sustained at a median follow-up of 461 days. Three patients with accelerated CML after relapse did not enter a remission. Six patients developed grade 1 acute GVHD and three other patients progressed to grade 3. All patients with a cytogenetic remission developed GVHD. Five of the eight patients who were followed for more than 100 days developed limited chronic GVHD, which was controlled by immunosuppressive therapy. Another complication of donor lymphocyte infusion is bone marrow suppression. In this trial, five patients had transient absolute granulocyte counts below 500 granulocytes/mm^3 and one patient died of aspergillus infection after developing grade 3 acute GVHD and pancytopenia. In a larger trial, Kolb *et al.*[304] treated 84 relapsed CML patients with donor lymphocyte infusions. Fifty-four (72%) of 75 evaluable patients achieved a complete cytogenetic response. The three-year survival rate after lymphocyte infusion was 67%.

Donor lymphocyte infusion has shown to be an effective therapy in patients with CML who have relapsed after allogenic BMT. Further studies are needed to determine the effect of this treatment on survival and length of remissions.

SUMMARY

The immunotherapy of cancer encompasses a broad range of agents used to treat and prevent cancers as well as to treat side effects associated with anticancer therapy. Many of these agents are still under clinical study to determine optimum dose and regimen or to discover new therapeutic uses.

Tumor-associated antigens heighten the potential for selectively identifying cancer cells for destruction through the cellular and humoral immune systems. Vaccines, immunostimulants, and biological response modifiers have been and are currently under investigation for their antitumor effects.

Biological response modifiers include the interferons, interleukins, and colony-stimulating factors. Each agent may be used alone in therapy or in combination with other biological or antineoplastic agents.

REFERENCES

1. Foley EJ. Antigenic properties of methylcholanthrene-induced tumors in mice of the strain of origin. *Cancer Res.* 1953;13:835–7.
2. Prehn RT, Main JM. Immunity to methylcholanthrene-induced sarcomas. *J Natl Cancer Inst.* 1957;18:769–78.
3. Brasseur F, Rimoldi D, Lie'nard D, *et al.* Expression of MAGE genes in primary and metastatic cutaneous melanoma. *Int J Cancer* 1995;63:375–80.
4. Martin EW, Minton JP, Carey LC. CEA-directed second-look surgery in the asymptomatic patient after primary resection of colorectal carcinoma. *Ann Surg.* 1985;202:310–7.
5. Abbas AK, Lichtman AH, Pober JS. Immunity to tumors. In: Wonsiewicz MJ, editor. *Cellular and Molecular Immunology*. Philadelphia, PA: WB Saunders; 1991. p. 336–52.
6. Woolf SH. Screening for prostate cancer with prostate-specific antigen. An examination of the evidence. *N Engl J Med.* 1995;331(21):1401–5.
7. Tuxen MK, Soletormos G, Dombernowsky P. Tumour review: tumour markers in the management of patients with ovarian cancer. *Cancer Treat Rev.* 1995;21(3):215–45.
8. Morton DL, Economou J. Cancer immunology and immunotherapy. In: Haskell CM, editor. *Cancer Treatment*. 3rd ed. Philadelphia, PA: WB Saunders; 1990. p. 102–19.
9. Benjamin E, Sunshine G, Leskowitz S. Tumor immunology. In: *Immunology: A Short Course*. 3rd ed. New York: Wiley-Liss; 1996. p. 399–417.
10. Stevenson HC. Adoptive cellular immunotherapy of cancer: an overview. In: Stevenson HC, editor. *Adoptive Cellular Immunotherapy of Cancer*. New York: Marcel Dekker; 1989. p. 1–18.
11. Sell S. The immune system II: organs. In: Dolan J, Langan C, editors. *Immunology, Immunopathology and Immunity*. 5th ed. Stamford, CT: Appleton and Lange; 1996. p. 48–92.
12. Dawson M, Moore M. Tumor immunology. In: Roitt I, Brostoff J, Male D, editors. *Immunology*. 2nd ed. London: Gower Medical; 1989. p. 18.1–18.18.
13. Borden EC, Sondel PM. Lymphokines and cytokines as cancer treatment. *Cancer* 1990;65:800–14.
14. Parkinson DR. Interleukin-2 in cancer therapy. *Semin in Oncol.* 1988;15(*Suppl* 6):10–26.
15. Vose BM. Immunomodulating agents. In: Byers VS, Baldwin RW, editors. *Immunology of Malignant Disease*. Lancaster, PA: MTP Press; 1987. p. 70–82.
16. Morton DL, Foshag LF, Hoon DS, *et al.* Prolongation of survival in metastatic melanoma after active specific immunotherapy with a new polyvalent melanoma vaccine. *Ann Surg.* 1992;216:463–82.
17. Berd D, Maquire HC Jr, McCue P, *et al.* Treatment of metastatic melanoma with an autologous tumor-cell vaccine: clinical and immunological results in 64 patients. *J Clin Oncol.* 1990;8:1858–67.
18. Mitchell MS, Harel W, Kan-Mitchell J, *et al.* Active specific immunotherapy of melanoma with allogeneic cell lysates: rationale, results, and possible mechanisms of action. *Ann NY Acad Sci.* 1993;690:153–66.
19. Hersey P, Edwards A, Coates A, *et al.* Evidence that treatment with vaccinia melanoma lysates (VMCL) may improve survival of patients with stage II melanoma: treatment of stage II melanoma with viral lysates. *Cancer Immunol Immunother.* 1987;25:257–65.
20. Barth A, Hoon DSB, Foshag LJ, *et al.* Polyvalent melanoma cell vaccine induces delayed-type hypersensitivity and in vitro cellular immune response. *Cancer Res.* 1994; 54:3342–5.
21. Barth A, Morton DL. The role of adjuvant therapy in melanoma management. *Cancer* 1995;75:726–34.
22. Livingston PO, Wong GYC, Adluri S, *et al.* Improved survival in stage III melanoma patients with GM_2 antibodies: a randomized trial of adjuvant vaccination with GM_2 ganglioside. *J Clin Oncol.* 1994;12:1036–44.
23. Wallack MK, Sivanandham M, Balch CM, *et al.* A phase III, randomized, double-blind, multi-institutional trial of vaccinia melanoma oncolysate (VMO) active specific immunotherapy for patients with stage II (VICC) melanoma. *Cancer* 1995;75:34–42.
24. Stevenson HC, Tsang KY. Tumor immunology. In: Virella G, Goust JM, Fudenberg HH, editors. *Introduction to Medical Immunology*. 2nd ed. New York: Marcel Dekker; 1990. p. 513–33.
25. Bohle A, Nowc CH, Ulmer AJ, *et al.* Elevations of cytokines interleukin-1, interleukin-2, and tumor necrosis factor in the urine of patients after intravesical bacillus Calmette-Guerin immunotherapy. *J Urol.* 1990;144:59–64.
26. Prescott S, James K, Hargreave TB, *et al.* Radio-immunoassay detection of interferon-gamma in urine after intravesical Evans BCG therapy. *J Urol.* 1990;114:1248–51.
27. Droller MJ. Biologic response modifiers in genitourinary neoplasia. *Cancer* 1987;60:635–44.
28. Lamm DL, Crissmann J, Blumenstein B, *et al.* Adriamycin versus BCG in superficial bladder cancer: a Southwest

Oncology Group study. *EORTC GU Group Monograph* 1989;6:263–70.
29. Martinez-Pineiro JA, Leon JJ, Martinez-Pineiro L Jr, *et al.* Bacillus Calmette-Guerin versus doxorubicin versus thiotepa: a randomized prospective study in 202 patients with superficial bladder cancer. *J Urol.* 1990;143:502–6.
30. Khanna OP, Son DL, Mazer H, *et al.* Multicenter study of superficial bladder cancer treated with intravesical bacillus Calmette-Guerin or adriamycin. *Urology* 1990;35:101–8.
31. Coplen DE, Marcus MD, Myers JA, *et al.* Long-term follow-up of patients treated with 1 or 2, 6-week courses of intravesical bacillus Calmette-Guerin: analysis of possible predictors of response free of tumor. *J Urol.* 1990;144:652–7.
32. Sarosdy MF, Lamm DL. Long-term results of intravesical bacillus Calmette-Guerin therapy for superficial bladder cancer. *J Urol.* 1989;142:719–22.
33. Orihuela E, Herr HW, Pinsky CM, *et al.* Toxicity of intravesical BCG and its management in patients with superficial bladder tumors. *Cancer* 1987;60:326–33.
34. Lamm DL, Steg A, Boccon-Gibod L, *et al.* Complications of bacillus Calmette-Guerin immunotherapy: review of 2602 patients and comparison of chemotherapy complications. *EORTC GU Group Monograph* 1989;6:335–55.
35. Rawls WH, Lamm DL, Lowe BA, *et al.* Fatal sepsis following intravesical bacillus Calmette-Guerin administration for bladder cancer. *J Urol.* 1990;144:1328–30.
36. Deresiewicz RL, Stone RM, Aster JC. Fatal disseminated mycobacterial infection following intravesical bacillus Calmette-Guerin. *J Urol.* 1990;144:1331–4.
37. Stone MM, Vannier AM, Storch SK, *et al.* Brief report: meningitis due to iatrogenic BCG infection in two immunocompromised children. *N Engl J Med.* 1995;333: 561–3.
38. Mutch RS, Hutson PR. Levamisole in the adjuvant treatment of colon cancer. *Clin Pharm.* 1991;10:95–109.
39. Chlebowski RT, Nystrom S, Reynolds R, *et al.* Long-term survival following levamisole or placebo adjuvant treatment of colorectal cancer: a Western Cancer Study Group trial. *Oncology* 1988;45:141–3.
40. Arnaud JP, Buyse M, Nordlinger B, *et al.* Adjuvant therapy of poor prognosis colon cancer with levamisole: results of an EORTC double-blind randomized clinical trial. *Br J Surg.* 1989;76:284–9.
41. Windle R, Bell PRF, Shaw D. Five-year results of a randomized trial of adjuvant 5-fluorouracil and levamisole in colorectal cancer. *Br J Surg.* 1987;74:569–72.
42. Moertel CG, Fleming TR, MacDonald JS, *et al.* Levamisole and fluorouracil for adjuvant therapy of resected colon carcinoma. *N Engl J Med.* 1990;322:352–8.
43. Moertel CG, Fleming TR, Macdonald JS, *et al.* Fluorouracil plus levamisole as effective adjuvant therapy after resection of stage III colon carcinoma: a final report. *Ann Intern Med.* 1995;122(5):321–6.
44. Clark JW, Longo DL. Biologic response modifiers in cancer therapy. In: Magrath I, editor. *New Directions in Cancer Treatment.* Berlin: Springer-Verlag; 1989. p. 297–316.
45. Clark JW, Longo DL. Interferons in cancer therapy. *Princ Pract Oncol Update* 1987;4:1–16.
46. Nelson BE, Borden EC. Interferons: biological and clinical effects. *Semin Surg Oncol.* 1989;5:391–401.
47. Peters M. Mechanisms of action of interferons. *Semin Liver Dis.* 1989;9:235–9.
48. Spiegel RJ. Alpha interferons: a clinical overview. *Urology* 1989;34(*Suppl* 4):75–9.
49. Thompson JA, Fefer A. Interferon in the treatment of hairy cell leukemia. *Cancer* 1987;59:605–9.
50. Cheson BD, Martin A. Clinical trials in hairy cell leukemia: current status and future directions. *Ann Intern Med.* 1987;106:871–8.
51. Savon A, Piro LD. Treatment of hairy cell leukemia. *Blood* 1992;79(5):1111–20.
52. Moormeier JA, Ratain MJ, Westbrook CA, *et al.* Low-dose interferon alpha-2b in the treatment of hairy cell. *J Natl Cancer Inst.* 1989;81:1172–4.
53. Thompson JA, Kidd P, Rubin E, *et al.* Very low dose a-2b interferon for the treatment of hairy cell leukemia. *Blood* 1989;73:1440–3.
54. Golomb HM, Ratain MJ, Fefer A, *et al.* Randomized study of the duration of treatment with interferon alfa-2b in patients with hairy cell leukemia. *J Natl Cancer Inst.* 1988;80:369–73.
55. Berman E, Heller G, Kempin S, *et al.* Incidence of response and long-term follow-up in patients with hairy cell leukemia treated with recombinant interferon alfa-2a. *Blood* 1990;75:839–45.
56. Golomb HM, Fefer A, Golde DW, *et al.* Update of a multi-institutional study of 195 patients (Pts.) with hairy cell leukemia (HCL) treated with interferon alfa-2b (IFN). *Proc Am Soc Clin Oncol.* 1990;6:215.
57. Ratain MJ, Golomb HM, Bardawil RG, *et al.* Durability of responses to interferon alfa-2b in advanced hairy cell leukemia. *Blood* 1987;69:872–7.
58. Grever M, Kopecky K, Foucar MK, *et al.* Randomized comparison of pentostatin versus interferon alfa-2a in previously untreated patients with hairy cell leukemia. Final report from the Italian Cooperative Group for HCL. *Ann Oncol.* 1994;5(8):725–31.
59. Spielberger RT, Mick R, Ratain MJ, *et al.* Interferon treatment for hairy cell leukemia—an update on a cohort of 69 patients treated from 1983 to 1986. *Leuk Lymphoma* 1994;14(1):89–93.
60. Troussard X, Flandrin G. Hairy cell leukemia—an update on a cohort of 93 patients treated in a single institution. Effects of interferon in patients relapsing after splenectomy and in patients with or without maintenance treatment. *Leuk Lymphoma* 1994;14(1):99–105.
61. Nielsen B, Braide I. Three years' continuous low-dose interferon-treatment of hairy-cell leukemia evaluation of response and maintenance dose. *Eur J Haematol.* 1992;49: 174–9.
62. Grever M, Kopecky K, Foucar MK, *et al.* Randomized comparison of pentostatin versus interferon alfa-2a in previously untreated patients with hairy cell leukemia: an intergroup study. *J Clin Oncol.* 1995;13(4):974–82.
63. Rai KR, *et al.* Comparison of pentostatin and alpha interferon in splenectomized patients with active hairy cell leukemia: an intergroup study. *Leuk Lymphoma* 1994;14(1): 107–8.
64. Habermann TM, Andersen JW, Cassileth PA, *et al.* Sequential administration of recombinant interferon alfa and deoxycoformycin in the treatment of hairy cell leukemia.

Br J Haematol. 1992;80:466–71.
65. Martin A, Nerenstone S, Urba WJ, *et al.* Treatment of hairy cell leukemia with alternating cycles of pentostatin and recombinant leukocyte-A interferon: results of a phase II study. *J Clin Oncol.* 1990;8:721–30.
66. Annino L, Ferrari A, Giona F, *et al.* Deoxycoformycin induces long-lasting remissions in hairy cell leukemia: clinical and biological results of two different regimens. *Leuk Lymphoma* 1994;14(1):115–9.
67. Wetzler M, Kantarjian H, Kurzrock R, *et al.* Interferon-a therapy for chronic myelogenous leukemia. *Am J Med.* 1995;99:402–11.
68. Talpaz M, Kantarjian H, Kurzock R, *et al.* Interferon-alpha produces sustained cytogenetic responses in chronic myelogenous leukemia: Philadelphia chromosome-positive patients. *Ann Intern Med.* 1991;114:532–8.
69. Kantarjian H, Deisseroth A, Kurzock R, *et al.* Chronic myelogenous leukemia: a concise update. *Blood* 1993;82: 691–703.
70. The Italian Cooperative Study Group on Chronic Myeloid Leukemia. Interferon alfa-2a as compared with conventional chemotherapy for the treatment of chronic myeloid leukemia. *N Engl J Med.* 1994;330:820–5.
71. Kantarjian H, Keating MJ, Estey EH, *et al.* Treatment of advanced stages of Philadelphia chromosome-positive chronic myelogenous leukemia with interferon-alpha and low-dose cytarabine. *J Clin Oncol.* 1992;10:772–8.
72. Arcese W, Mauro FR, Serenci M, *et al.* Interferon therapy for Ph´ chronic myelogenous leukemia patients relapsing after T-cell depleted allogeneic bone marrow transplantation. *Eur J Cancer* 1991;27(*Suppl* 4):S28–30.
73. Volberding PA, Mitsuyasu RT, Golando JP, *et al.* Treatment of Kaposi's sarcoma with interferon alfa-2b (Intron® A). *Cancer* 1987;59:620–5.
74. DeWit R, Boucher CAB, Veenhof KHN, *et al.* Clinical and virological effects of high-dose recombinant interferon-a in disseminated AIDS-related Kaposi's sarcoma. *Lancet* 1988;2(8622):1214–7.
75. Lane HC, Feinberg J, Davey V, *et al.* Anti-retroviral effects of interferon-a in AIDS-associated Kaposi's sarcoma. *Lancet* 1988;2(8622):1218–22.
76. Dorr RT. Interferon in malignant and viral diseases. *Drugs* 1993;45(2):177–211.
77. Orfanos CE, Husak R, Wolfer U, *et al.* Kaposi's sarcoma: a re-evaluation. *Recent Results Cancer Res.* 1995;139:275–96.
78. Kovacs JA, Deyton L, Davey R, *et al.* Combined zidovudine and interferon-a therapy in patients with Kaposi sarcoma and the acquired immunodeficiency syndrome (AIDS). *Ann Intern Med.* 1989;111:280–7.
79. Krown SE, Gold JWM, Niedzwiecki D, *et al.* Interferon-a with zidovudine: safety, tolerance, and clinical and virologic effects in patients with Kaposi sarcoma associated with the acquired immunodeficiency syndrome (AIDS). *Ann Intern Med.* 1990;112:812–21.
80. Stadler R, Bratzke B, Schaart F, *et al.* Long-term combined rIFN-alpha-2a and zidovudine therapy for HIV-associated Kaposi's sarcoma: clinical consequences and side effects. *J Invest Dermatol.* 1990;95(*Suppl* 6):S170–5.
81. Miles SA, Wang H, Cortes E, *et al.* Beta-interferon therapy in patients with poor-prognosis Kaposi sarcoma related to the acquired immunodeficiency syndrome (AIDS): a phase II trial with preliminary evidence of antiviral activity and low incidence of opportunistic infections. *Ann Intern Med.* 1990;112:582–9.
82. Heagy W, Groopman J, Schindler J, *et al.* Use of IFN-g in patients with AIDS. *J Acquir Immune Defic Syndr.* 1990;3: 584–90.
83. Marcellin P, Benhamou JP. Treatment of chronic viral hepatitis. *Baillieres Clin Gastroenterol.* 1994;8(2):233–53.
84. Bhandari BN, Wright TL. Hepatitis C: an overview. *Ann Rev Med.* 1995;46:309–17.
85. Wong DKH, Cheung Am, O'Rourke K, *et al.* Effect of alpha-interferon treatment in patients with hepatitis B e antigen-positive chronic hepatitis B. *Ann Intern Med.* 1993; 119:312–23.
86. Wong JB, Koff RS, Tine F, *et al.* Cost-effectiveness of interferon-2b treatment for hepatitis B e antigen-positive chronic hepatitis B. *Ann Intern Med.* 1995;122:664–75.
87. Korenman J, Baker B, Waggoner J, *et al.* Long-term remission of chronic hepatitis B after alpha-interferon therapy. *Ann Intern Med.* 1991;114:629–34.
88. Krogsgaard K. Does corticosteroid pretreatment enhance the effect of alfa interferon treatment in chronic hepatitis B? *J Hepatol.* 1994;20:159–62.
89. Quesada JR. Role of interferons in the therapy of metastatic renal cell carcinoma. *Urology* 1989:34(*Suppl*):80–3.
90. Robinson WA, Mughal TI, Thomas MR, *et al.* Treatment of metastatic malignant melanoma with recombinant interferon alpha-2. *Immunobiology* 1986;172:275–82.
91. Kirkwood JM. Studies of interferons in the therapy of melanoma. *Semin Oncol.* 1991;18(5 *Suppl* 7):83–90.
92. Vorobiof DA, Falkson G, Voges CW. DTIC versus DTIC and recombinant interferon alfa 2b (rIFNa2b) in the treatment of patients with advanced malignant melanoma. *Proc Am Soc Clin Oncol.* 1989;8:284. Abstract 1105.
93. Bajetta E, Negretti E, Giannotti B, *et al.* Phase II study of interferon alpha-2a (rIFN alpha-2a) and dacarbazine (DTIC) in metastatic melanoma. *Proc Am Soc Clin Oncol.* 1989;8:286. Abstract 1113.
94. Sparano JA, Fisher RI, Sunderland M, *et al.* Randomized phase III trial of treatment with high-dose interleukin-2 either alone or in combination with interferon alfa-2a in patients with advanced melanoma. *J Clin Oncol.* 1993; 11:1969–77.
95. Marcincola FM, White DE, Wise AP, *et al.* Combination therapy with interferon alfa-2a and interleukin-2 for the treatment of metastatic cancer. *J Clin Oncol.* 1995;13(5): 110–22.
96. Richards JM, Mehta N, Ramming K, *et al.* Sequential chemo-immunotherapy in the treatment of metastatic melanoma. *J Clin Oncol.* 1992;10:138–43.
97. VonWussow P, Block B, Hartmann F, *et al.* Intralesional interferon-alpha therapy in advanced malignant melanoma. *Cancer* 1988:61:1071–4.
98. Kirkwood JM, Strawderman MH, Ernstoff MS, *et al.* Interferon alfa-2b adjuvant therapy of high-risk resected cutaneous melanoma: the Eastern Cooperative Oncology Group trial EST 1684. *J Clin Oncol.* 1996;14(1):7–17.
99. Costanzi JJ, Cooper MR, Scarffe JH, *et al.* Phase II study of recombinant alpha-2 interferon in resistant multiple myeloma. *J Clin Oncol.* 1985;3:654–9.

100. Wagstaff JK, Loynds P, Scarffe JH. A phase II study of rDNA human alpha-2 interferon in multiple myeloma. *Cancer Treat Rep*. 1985;69:495–8.
101. Quesada JR, Alexanian R, Hawkins M, *et al*. Treatment of multiple myeloma with recombinant alpha-interferon. *Blood* 1986;67:275–8.
102. Cooper MR, Fefer A, Thompson J, *et al*. Alpha-2 interferon/melphalan/prednisone in previously untreated patients with multiple myeloma: a phase I-II trial. *Cancer Treat Rep*. 1986;70:473–6.
103. Montuoro A, DeRosa L, DeBlasio A, *et al*. Alpha-2a-interferon/melphalan/prednisone versus melphalan/prednisone in previously untreated patients with multiple myeloma. *Br J Haematol*. 1990;76:365–8.
104. Cooper MR, Dear K, McIntyre OR, *et al*. A randomized clinical trial comparing melphalan/prednisone with or without interferon alfa-2b in newly diagnosed patients with multiple myeloma: a cancer and leukemia group B study. *J Clin Oncol*. 1993;11:155–60.
105. Corrado C, Pavlovsky S, Saslasky J, *et al*. Randomized trial comparing melphalan/prednisone with or without recombinant alpha-2 interferon (rIFN-2) in multiple myeloma [abstract]. *Proc Am Soc Clin Oncol*. 1989;8:1007.
106. Ludwig H, Cohen AM, Polliak A, *et al*. Interferon-alpha for induction and maintenance in multiple myeloma: results of two multicenter randomized trials and summary of other studies. *Ann Oncol*. 1995;6(5):467–76.
107. Mandelli F, Avvisati G, Amadori S, *et al*. Maintenance treatment with recombinant interferon alfa-2b in patients with multiple myeloma responding to conventional induction chemotherapy. *N Engl J Med*. 1990;322:1430–4.
108. Browman GP, Bergsagel D, Sicheri D, *et al*. Randomized trial of interferon maintenance in multiple myeloma: a study of the National Cancer Institute of Canada Clinical Trials Group. *J Clin Oncol*. 1995;13:2354–60.
109. Westin J, Rodjer S, Turesson I, *et al*. Interferon alfa-2b versus no maintenance therapy during the plateau phase in multiple myeloma: a randomized study. *Br J Haematol*. 1995;89:561–8.
110. Peest D, Deicher H, Coldeway R, *et al*. A comparison of polychemotherapy and melphalan/prednisone for primary remission induction, and interferon-alpha for maintenance treatment, in multiple myeloma. A prospective trial of the German Myeloma Treatment Group. *Eur J Cancer* 1995; 31A(2):146–51.
111. Salmon SE, Crowley JJ, Grogan TM, *et al*. Combination chemotherapy, glucocorticoids, and interferon alfa in the treatment of multiple myeloma: a Southwest Oncology Group Study. *J Clin Oncol*. 1994;12 (11):2405–14.
112. Wadler S, Wiernik PH. Clinical update on the role of fluorouracil and recombinant interferon alfa-2a in the treatment of colorectal cancer. *Semin Oncol*. 1990;17(*Suppl* 1):16–21.
113. Ferguson JE, Hulse P, Lorigan P, *et al*. Continuous infusion of 5-fluorouracil with alpha-2b interferon for advanced colorectal carcinoma. *Br J Cancer* 1995;72(1):193–7.
114. Kemeny N, Younes A. Alfa-2A interferon and 5-fluorouracil for advanced colorectal carcinoma: the Memorial Sloan-Kettering experience. *Semin Oncol*. 1992;19(2 *Suppl* 3):171–5.
115. Wadler S, Lembersky B, Atkins M, *et al*. Phase II trial of fluorouracil and recombinant interferon alfa-2a in patients with advanced colorectal carcinoma: an Eastern Cooperative Oncology Group study. *J Clin Oncol*. 1991;9(10):1806–10.
116. Pazdur R, Moore DF Jr, Bready B. Modulation of fluorouracil with recombinant alfa interferon: M.D. Anderson clinical trial. *Semin Oncol*. 1992;19(2 *Suppl* 3):176–9.
117. Corfu-A Study Group. Phase II randomized study of two fluorouracil combinations with either interferon alfa-2a or leucovorin for advanced colorectal cancer. *J Clin Oncol*. 1995;13(4):921–8.
118. Kohne CH, Wilke H, Hecker H, *et al*. Interferon-alpha does not improve the antineoplastic efficacy of high-dose infusional 5-fluorouracil plus folinic acid in advanced colorectal cancer. First results of a randomized multicenter study by the Association of Medical Oncology of the German Cancer Society (AIO). *Ann Oncol*. 1995;6(5):461–6.
119. Marshall ME, Tangen CM, Berenberg JL, *et al*. Treatment of advanced colorectal carcinoma with 5-fluorouracil, leucovorin and Roferon-A: a Southwest Oncology Study Group Study. *Cancer Biother*. 1994;9(4):301–6.
120. Brunetti I, Falcone A, Bertuccelli M, *et al*. Double 5-fluorouracil modulation with folinic acid and recombinant alpha-2B-interferon-A phase I-II study in metastatic colorectal cancer patients. *Am J Clin Oncol*. 1994;17(3): 210–4.
121. Sobrero A, Nobile MT, Guglielmi A, *et al*. Phase II study of 5-fluorouracil plus leucoyorin and interferon alpha 2b in advanced colorectal cancer. *Eur J Cancer* 1992;28A(4–5):850–2.
122. Grem JL, Jordan E, Robson ME, *et al*. Phase II study of fluorouracil, leucovorin, and interferon alfa-2a in metastatic colorectal carcinoma. *J Clin Oncol*. 1993;11(9):1737–45.
123. Cascinus S, Fedeli A, Fedeli SL, *et al*. Double biochemical modulation of 5-fluorouracil by leucovorin and cycle low dose interferon alpha-2b in advanced colorectal cancer patients. *Ann Oncol*. 1992;3(6):489–91.
124. International Chronic Granulomatous Disease Cooperative Study Group. A controlled trial of interferon gamma to prevent infection in chronic granulomatous disease. *N Engl J Med*. 1991;324:509–16.
125. Gallin JI, Farber JM, Holland SM, Nutman TB. Interferon-gamma in the management of infectious diseases. *Ann Intern Med*. 1995;123:216–24.
126. Quesada JR, Talpaz M, Rios A, *et al*. Clinical toxicity of interferons in cancer patients: a review. *J Clin Oncol*. 1986; 4:234–43.
127. Figlin RA. Biotherapy with interferon—1988. *Semin Oncol*. 1988;15:3–9.
128. Koeller JM. Biologic response modifiers: the interferon alfa experience. *Am J Hosp Pharm*. 1989;46(*Suppl* 2):S11–5.
129. Jones GJ, Itri LM. Safety and tolerance of recombinant alfa-2b (Roferon-A) in cancer patients. *Cancer* 1986;57 (*Suppl* 2):1709–15.
130. Spiegel RJ, Spicehandler JR, Jacobs SL, *et al*. Low incidence of serum neutralizing factors in patients receiving recombinant alfa-2b interferon (Intron-A). *Am J Med*. 1986;80:223–7.
131. Antonelli G, Currenti M, Turriziani O, *et al*. Neutralizing

antibodies to interferon-a: relative frequency in patients treated with different interferon preparations. *J Infect Dis*. 1991;163:882–5.

132. Freund M, VonWussow P, Diedrich H, *et al*. Recombinant human interferon (IFN) in chronic myelogenous leukemia: dose dependency of response and frequency of neutralizing anti-interferon antibodies. *Br J Haematol*. 1989; 72:350–6.
133. Steis RG, Smith II JW, Urba WJ, *et al*. Resistance to recombinant interferon alfa-2a in hairy-cell leukemia associated with neutralizing anti-interferon antibodies. *N Engl J Med*. 1988;318:1409–13.
134. Steis RG, Smith II JW, Urba WJ, *et al*. Loss of interferon antibodies during prolonged continuous interferon-a2a therapy in hairy cell leukemia. *Blood* 1991;77(Feb 15): 792–8.
135. Kintzel PE, Calis KA. Recombinant interleukin-2: a biological response modifier. *Clin Pharm*. 1991;10:110–28.
136. Bruton JK, Koeller JM. Recombinant interleukin-2. *Pharmacotherapy* 1994;14(6):635–56.
137. Rosenberg SA, Lotze MT, Yang JC, *et al*. Experience with the use of high-dose interleukin-2 in the treatment of 652 cancer patients. *Ann Surg*. 1989;210:474–84.
138. Sosman JA, Kohler PC, Hank J, *et al*. Repetitive weekly cycles of recombinant human interleukin-2: responses of renal cell carcinoma with acceptable toxicity. *J Natl Cancer Inst*. 1988;80:60–3.
139. Bukowski RM, Goodman P, Crawford D, *et al*. Phase II trial of high-dose intermittent interleukin-2 in metastatic renal cell carcinoma: a Southwest Oncology Group study. *J Natl Cancer Inst*. 1990;82:143–6.
140. Richards JM, Barker E, Latta J, *et al*. Phase I study of weekly 24-hour infusions of recombinant human interleukin-2. *J Natl Cancer Inst*. 1988;80:1325–8.
141. Atkins MB, Gould JA, Allegretta M, *et al*. Phase I evaluation of recombinant interleukin-2 in patients with advanced malignant disease. *J Clin Oncol*. 1986;4:1380–91.
142. Allison MAK, Jones SE, McGuffey P. Phase II trial of outpatient interleukin-2 in malignant lymphoma, chronic lymphocytic leukemia, and selected solid tumors. *J Clin Oncol*. 1989;7:75–80.
143. Creekmore SP, Harris JE, Ellis TM, *et al*. A phase I clinical trial of recombinant interleukin-2 by periodic 24-hour intravenous infusions. *J Clin Oncol*. 1989;7:276–84.
144. Parkinson DR, Abrams JS, Wiernik PH, *et al*. Interleukin-2 therapy in patients with metastatic malignant melanoma: a phase II study. *J Clin Oncol*. 1990;8:1650–6.
145. Thatcher N, Dazzi H, Johnson RJ, *et al*. Recombinant interleukin-2 (rIL-2) given intrasplenically and intravenously for advanced malignant melanoma: a phase I and II study. *Br J Cancer* 1989;60:770–4.
146. Thompson JA, Lee DJ, Cox WW, *et al*. Recombinant interleukin 2 toxicity, pharmacokinetics, and immunomodulatory effects in a phase I trial. *Cancer Res*. 1987;47: 4202–7.
147. Negrier S, Philip T, Stoter G, *et al*. Interleukin-2 with or without LAK cells in metastatic renal cell carcinoma: a report of a European multicenter study. *Eur J Cancer Clin Oncol*. 1989;25(*Suppl* 3):S21–S28.
148. Marumo K, Muraki J, Ueno M, *et al*. Immunologic study of human recombinant interleukin-2 (low-dose) in patients with advanced renal cell carcinoma. *Urology* 1989;33:219–25.
149. Whitehead RP, Ward D, Hemingway L, *et al*. Subcutaneous recombinant interleukin-2 in a dose escalating regimen in patients with metastatic renal cell adenocarcinoma. *Cancer Res*. 1990;50:6708–15.
150. Urba WJ, Steis RG, Longo DL, *et al*. Immunomodulatory properties and toxicity of interleukin 2 in patients with cancer. *Cancer Res*. 1990;50:185–92.
151. Rosenberg SA, Lotze MT, Muul LM, *et al*. A progress report on the treatment of 157 patients with advanced cancer using lymphoxine-activated killer cells and interleukin-2 or high dose interleukin-2 alone. *N Engl J Med*. 1987; 316:889–97.
152. Fyfe G, Fisher RI, Rosenberg SA, *et al*. Results of treatment of 255 patients with metastatic renal cell carcinoma who received high-dose recombinant interleukin-2 therapy. *J Clin Oncol*. 1995;13(3):688–96.
153. Fyfe GA, Fisher RI, Rosenberg SA, *et al*. Long-term response data for 255 patients with metastatic renal cell carcinoma treated with high-dose recombinant interleukin-2 therapy [letter]. *J Clin Oncol*. 1996;14(8):2410–1.
154. Weiss GR, Margolin KA, Aronson FR, *et al*. A randomized phase II trial of continuous infusion interleukin-2 or bolus injection interleukin-2 plus lymphokine-activated killer cells for advanced renal cell carcinoma. *J Clin Oncol*. 1992;10:275–81.
155. Sleijfer DT, Janssen RAJ, Buter J, *et al*. Phase II study of subcutaneous interleukin-2 in unselected patients with advanced renal cell cancer on an outpatient basis. *J Clin Oncol*. 1992;10:1119–23.
156. Chang AE, Rosenberg SA. Overview of interleukin-2 as an immunotherapeutic agent. *Semin Surg Oncol*. 1989;5: 385–90.
157. Siegel JP, Puri RK. Interleukin-2 toxicity. *J Clin Oncol*. 1991;9:694–704.
158. Crum E. Biological-response modifier-induced emergencies. *Semin Oncol*. 1989;16:579–87.
159. Gaspari AA, Lotze MT, Rosenberg SA, *et al*. Dermatologic changes associated with interleukin 2 administration. *JAMA* 1987;258:1624–9.
160. Denicoff KD, Durkin TM, Lotze MT, *et al*. The neuroendocrine effects of interleukin-2 treatment. *J Clin Endocrinol Metab*. 1989;69:402–10.
161. Klempner MS, Noring R, Mier JW, *et al*. An acquired chemotactic defect in neutrophils from patients receiving interleukin-2 immunotherapy. *N Engl J Med*. 1990;322: 959–65.
162. Marincola FM, White DE, Wise AP, *et al*. Combination therapy with interferon alfa-2a and interleukin-2 for the treatment of metastatic cancer. *J Clin Oncol*. 1995;13(5): 1110–22.
163. Rosenberg SA, Lotze MT, Yang JC, *et al*. Combination therapy with interleukin-2 and alpha-interferon for the treatment of patients with advanced cancer. *J Clin Oncol*. 1989;7(12):1863–74.
164. Atkins MB, Sparano J, Fisher RI, *et al*. Randomized phase II trial of high-dose interleukin-2 either alone or in combination with interferon alfa-2b in advanced renal cell carcinoma. *J Clin Oncol*. 1993;11(4):661–70.
165. Sparano JA, Fisher RI, Sunderland M, *et al*. Randomized

phase III trial of treatment with high-dose interleukin-2 either alone or in combination with interferon alfa-2a in patients with advanced melanoma. *J Clin Oncol*. 1993;11: 1969–77.
166. Atzpodien J, Hanninen EL, Kirchner H, *et al*. Multiinstitutional home-therapy trial of recombinant human interleukin-2 and interferon alfa-2 in progressive metastatic renal cell carcinoma. *J Clin Oncol*. 1995;13:497–501.
167. Atzpodien J, Kirchner H, Hannien EL, *et al*. Interleukin-2 in combination with interferon-alpha and 5-fluorouracil for metastatic renal cell cancer. *Eur J Cancer* 1993;29 A(5):56–8.
168. Sella A, Zukiwski A, Robinson E, *et al*. Interleukin-2 with interferon-alpha and 5-fluorouracil in patients with metastatic renal cell cancer [abstract]. *Proc Am Soc Clin Oncol*. 1994;13:237.
169. Clamon G, Herndon J, Perry MC, *et al*. Interleukin-2 activity in patients with extensive small-cell-lung cancer: a phase II trial of Cancer and Leukemia Group B. *J Natl Cancer Inst*. 1993;85:316–20.
170. Moser RP, Bruner JM, Grimm EA. Biologic therapy for brain tumors. *Cancer Bull*. 1991;43:117–26.
171. Hayes RL. The cellular immunotherapy of primary brain tumors. *Rev Neurol*. 1992;148:454–66.
172. Stewart JA, Belinson JL, Moore AL, *et al*. Phase I trial of intraperitoneal recombinant interleukin-2/lymphokine-activated killer cells in patients with ovarian cancer. *Cancer Res*. 1990;50:6302–10.
173. Chapman PB, Kolitz JE, Hakes TB, *et al*. A phase I trial of intraperitoneal recombinant interleukin-2 in patients with ovarian carcinoma. *Invest New Drugs* 1988;6:179–88.
174. Cortesina G, DeStefani A, Grovarelli M, *et al*. Treatment of recurrent squamous cell carcinoma of the head and neck with low doses of interleukin-2 injected perilymphatically. *Cancer* 1988;62:2482–5.
175. Sznol M, Hawkins MJ. Interleukin-2 in malignancies other than melanoma and renal cell carcinoma. In: Atkins MB, Mier JW, editors. *Therapeutic Applications of IL-2*. New York: Marcel Dekker; 1993. p. 177.
176. Charak BS, Choudhary GD, Tefft M, *et al*. Interleukin-2 in bone marrow transplantation: preclinical studies. *Bone Marrow Transplant*. 1992;10:103–11.
177. Klingemann HG, Phillips GL. Is there a place for immunotherapy with interleukin-2 to prevent relapse after autologous stem cell transplantation for acute leukemia? *Leuk Lymphoma* 1995;16:397–405.
178. Benyunes MC, Massumoto C, York A, *et al*. Interleukin-2 with or without lymphokine-activated killer cells as consolidative immunotherapy after autologous bone marrow transplantation for acute myelogenous leukemia. *Bone Marrow Transplant*. 1993;12:159–63.
179. Blaie BD, Olive D, Stoppa AM, *et al*. Hematologic and immunologic effects of the systemic administration of recombinant interleukin-2 after autologous bone marrow transplantation. *Blood* 1990;76(6):1092–7.
180. Soiffer RJ, Murray C, Cochran K, *et al*. Clinical and immunologic effects of prolonged infusion of low-dose recombinant interleukin-2 after autologous and T-cell-depleted allogeneic bone marrow transplantation. *Blood* 1992; 79(2):517–26.
181. Soiffer RJ, Murray C, Gonin R, *et al*. Effect of low-dose interleukin-2 on disease relapse after T-cell-depleted allogeneic bone marrow transplantation. *Blood* 1994;84(3): 964–71.
182. Klingemann HG, Eaves CJ, Barnett MJ, *et al*. Transplantation of patients with high risk acute myeloid leukemia in first remission with autologous marrow cultured in interleukin-2 followed by interleukin-2 administration. *Bone Marrow Transplant*. 1994;14:389–96.
183. Metcalf D. Haemopoietic growth factors, I. *Lancet* 1989;1 (8642):825–7.
184. Erslev AJ. Erythropoietin. *N Engl J Med*. 1991;324(19): 1339–44.
185. Abels RI. Use of recombinant human erythropoietin in the treatment of anemia in patients who have cancer. *Semin Oncol*. 1992;19(3 *Suppl* 8):29–35.
186. Cascinu S, Fedeli A, Del Ferro E, *et al*. Recombinant human erythropoietin treatment in cisplatin-associated anemia: a randomized, double-blind trial with placebo. *J Clin Oncol*. 1994;12(5):1058–62.
187. Steegman JL, Lopez J, Otero MJ, *et al*. Erythropoietin treatment in allogenic BMT accelerates erythroid reconstitution: results of a prospective controlled randomized trial. *Bone Marrow Transplant*. 1992;10:541–6.
188. Klaesson S, Ringden O, Ljungman P, *et al*. Reduced blood transfusions requirements after allogenic bone marrow transplantation: results of a randomized, double-blind study with high-dose erythropoietin. *Bone Marrow Transplant*. 1994;13:397–402.
189. Miller CB, Mills S. Erythropoietin after bone marrow transplantation. *Heme Onc Clin North Am*. 1994;8(5):975–92.
190. Groopman JE, Molina JM, Scadden DT. Hematopoietic growth factors: biology and clinical applications. *N Engl J Med*. 1989;321:1449–59.
191. Metcalf D. Haemopoietic growth factors. II. Clinical applications. *Lancet* 1989;1(8643):885–7.
192. Robinson BE, Quesenberry PJ. Hematopoietic growth factors: overview and clinical applications. Part 2. *Am J Med Sci*. 1990;300(4):237–44.
193. Wallerstein R Jr, Deisseroth A. Hematopoietic growth factors in cancer treatment. *Prin Pract Oncol Updates* 1990;4: 1–16.
194. Gribben JG, Devereux S, Thomas NSB, *et al*. Development of antibodies to unprotected glycosylation sites on recombinant human GM-CSF. *Lancet* 1990;335:434–7.
195. Lieschke GJ, Cebon J, Morstyn G. Characterization of the clinical effects after the first dose of bacterially synthesized recombinant human granulocyte-macrophage colony-stimulating factor. *Blood* 1989;74:2634–43.
196. Immunex Corp. Leukine Package Insert. Seattle, WA. October, 1996.
197. Gabrilove JL. Introduction and overview of hematopoietic growth factors. *Semin Hematol*. 1989;26(*Suppl* 2):1–4.
198. Golde DW. Overview of myeloid growth factors. *Semin Hematol*. 1990;27(*Suppl* 3):1–7.
199. Amgen, Inc. Neupogen Package Insert. Thousand Oaks, CA. December, 1994.
200. Aurer I, Ribas A, Gale RP. What is the role of recombinant colony stimulating factors in bone marrow transplantation? *Bone Marrow Transplant*. 1990;6:79–87.
201. Mertelsmann R, Herrmann F, Hecht T, *et al*. Hematopoietic growth factors in bone marrow transplantation. *Bone*

Marrow Transplant. 1990;6:73–7.

202. Goldstone AH, Khwaja A. The role of haemopoietic growth factors in bone marrow transplantation. *Leuk Res.* 1990;14:721–9.
203. Harmenberg J, Hoglund M, Hellstrom-Lindberg EG. G- and GM-CSF in oncology and oncological haematology. *Eur J Haematol.* 1994;52:1–28.
204. Appelbaum FK. Allogenic marrow transplantation and the use of hematopoietic growth factors. *Stem Cells* 1995;13: 344–50.
205. Powles R, Smith C, Milan S, *et al.* Human recombinant GM-CSF in allogeneic bone marrow transplantation for leukaemia: double-blind placebo-controlled trial. *Lancet* 1990;336:1417–20.
206. Devereaux S, Linch DC, Gribben JG, *et al.* GM-CSF accelerates neutrophil recovery after autologous bone marrow transplantation for Hodgkin's disease. *Bone Marrow Transplant.* 1989;4:49–54.
207. Brandt SJ, Peters WP, Atwater SK, *et al.* Effect of recombinant human granulocyte-macrophage colony-stimulating factor on hematopoietic reconstitution after high-dose chemotherapy and autologous bone marrow transplantation. *N Engl J Med.* 1988;318:869–76.
208. Gorin NC, Coiffier B, Hayat M, *et al.* RHU GM-CSF shortens aplasia duration after ABMT in non-Hodgkin's lymphoma: a randomized placebo-controlled double-blind study. *Bone Marrow Transplant.* 1991;7(*Suppl* 2):82.
209. Nemunaitis J, Rabinowe SN, Singer JW, *et al.* Recombinant granulocyte-macrophage colony-stimulating factor after autologous bone marrow transplantation for lymphoid cancer. *N Engl J Med.* 1991;324:1773–8.
210. Linke H, Boogaerts MA, Carella AM, *et al.* A controlled trial of recombinant human granulocyte-macrophage colony-stimulating factor after total body irradiation, high-dose chemotherapy, and autologous bone marrow transplantation for acute lymphoblastic leukemia or malignant lymphoma. *Blood* 1992;80(9):2188–95.
211. Advani R, Chao NJ, Horning SJ, *et al.* Granulocyte-macrophage colony-stimulating factor (GM-CSF) as an adjunct to autologous hemopoietic stem cell transplantation for lymphoma. *Ann Intern Med.* 1992;116:183–9.
212. Khwaja A, Linch DC, Goldstone AH, *et al.* Recombinant human granulocyte-macrophage-colony-stimulating factor after autologous bone marrow transplantation for malignant lymphoma: a British National Lymphoma Investigation double-blind, placebo-controlled trial. *Br J Haematol.* 1992;82:317–23.
213. Gulati SC, Bennett CL. Granulocyte-macrophage-colony-stimulating factor (GM-CSF) as adjunct therapy in relapsed Hodgkins disease. *Ann Intern Med.* 1992;116:177–82.
214. Nemunaitis J, Rosenfeld C, Ash R, *et al.* Phase III double-blind trial of rhGM-CSF (Sargramostin) following allogeneic bone marrow transplant (BMT). *Blood* 1993;82(10 *Suppl* 1):286a.
215. DeWitte T, Gratwohl A, Van Der Lely N, *et al.* Recombinant human granulocyte-macrophage colony-stimulating factor accelerates neutrophil and monocyte recovery after allogeneic T-cell-depleted bone marrow transplantation. *Blood* 1992;79:1359–65.
216. Hiraoka A, Masaoka T, Mizoguchi H, *et al.* Recombinant human non-glycosylated granulocyte-macrophage colony-stimulating factor in allogeneic bone marrow transplantation: double-blind placebo-controlled phase III clinical trial. *Jpn J Clin Oncol.* 1994;24:205–11.
217. Marrtelsmann R, Herrmann F, Hect T, *et al.* Hematopoietic growth factors in bone marrow transplantation. *Bone Marrow Transplant.* 1990;6:73–7.
218. Peters WP. The myeloid colony-stimulating factors: introduction and overview. *Semin Hematol.* 1991;28(*Suppl* 2): 1–5.
219. Taylor KM, Jagannath S, Spitzer G, *et al.* Recombinant human granulocyte colony-stimulating factor hastens granulocyte recovery after high-dose chemotherapy and autologous bone marrow transplantation in Hodgkin's disease. *J Clin Oncol.* 1989;7(12):1791–9.
220. Stahel RA, Jost LM, Cerny T, *et al.* Randomized study of recombinant human granulocyte colony-stimulating factor after high-dose chemotherapy and autologous bone marrow transplantation for high-risk lymphoid malignancies. *J Clin Oncol.* 1994;12(9):1931–8.
221. Schmitz N, Dreger P, Zander AR, *et al.* Results of a randomized, controlled, multicentre study of recombinant human granulocyte colony-stimulating factor (filgrastim) in patients with Hodgkin's disease and non-Hodgkin's lymphoma undergoing autologous bone marrow transplantation. *Bone Marrow Transplant.* 1995;15:261–6.
222. Klumpp TR, Mangan KF, Goldberg SL, *et al.* Granulocyte colony-stimulating factor accelerates neutrophil engraftment following peripheral-blood stem-cell transplantation: a prospective, randomized trial. *J Clin Oncol.* 1995;13(6): 1323–7.
223. Bensinger NI, Weaver CH, Appelbaum FR, *et al.* Transplantation of allogeneic peripheral blood stem cells mobilized by recombinant human granulocyte colony stimulating factor (rh-G-CSF). *Blood* 1995;85:1655–8.
224. Nemunaitis J, Singer JW, Buckner CD, *et al.* Use of recombinant human granulocyte-macrophage colony-stimulating factor in graft failure after bone marrow transplantation. *Blood* 1990;76:245–53.
225. Biermah P, Appelbaum F, Oeffe D, *et al.* Granulocyte-macrophage colony stimulating factor (GM-CSF) for engraftment failure (EF) following autologous (AUTO) or allogeneic (ALLO) bone marrow transplantation (BMT). *Blood* 1992;80(*Suppl* 1):269.
226. Neidhart JA. Hematopoietic colony-stimulating factors. Uses in combination with standard chemotherapeutic regimens and in support of dose intensification. *Cancer* 1992; 70:913–20.
227. Neidhart J, Mangalik A, Kohler W, *et al.* Granulocyte colony-stimulating factor stimulates recovery of granulocytes in patients receiving dose-intensive chemotherapy without bone marrow transplantation. *J Clin Oncol.* 1989;7: 1685–92.
228. Ohno R, Tomonaga M, Kobayashi T, *et al.* Effect of granulocyte colony-stimulating factor after intensive induction therapy in relapsed or refractory acute leukemia. *N Engl J Med.* 1990;323:871–7.
229. Morstyn G, Campbell L, Lieschke G, *et al.* Treatment of chemotherapy-induced neutropenia by subcutaneously administered granulocyte colony-stimulating factor with optimization of dose and duration of therapy. *J Clin Oncol.*

1989;7:1554–62.
230. Kotake T, Miki T, Akaza H, *et al.* Effect of recombinant granulocyte colony-stimulating factor (rG-CSF) on chemotherapy-induced neutropenia in patients with urogenital cancer. *Cancer Chemother Pharmacol.* 1991;27:253–7.
231. Antman KS, Griffin JD, Elias A, *et al.* Effect of recombinant human granulocyte-macrophage colony-stimulating factor on chemotherapy-induced myelosuppression. *N Engl J Med.* 1988;319:593–8.
232. deVries EGE, Biesma B, Willemse PHB, *et al.* A double-blind placebo-controlled study with granulocyte-macrophage colony-stimulating factor during chemotherapy for ovarian carcinoma. *Cancer Res.* 1991;51:116–22.
233. Bettelheim P, Valent P, Andreeff M, *et al.* Recombinant human granulocyte-macrophage colony-stimulating factor in combination with standard induction chemotherapy in de novo acute myeloid leukemia. *Blood* 1991;77:700–11.
234. Crawford J, Ozer H, Stroller R, *et al.* Reduction by granulocyte colony-stimulating factor of fever and neutropenia induced by chemotherapy in patients with small-cell lung cancer (r-met Hu G-CSF). *N Engl J Med.* 1991;325:164–70.
235. Trillet-Lenoir V, Green J, Manegold C, *et al.* Recombinant granulocyte colony-stimulating factor reduces the infections complications of cytotoxic chemotherapy. *Eur J Cancer* 1993;29A:319–24.
236. Pettengell R, Gurney H, Radford JA, *et al.* Granulocyte colony-stimulating factor to prevent dose-limiting neutropenia in non-Hodgkin's lymphoma: a randomized controlled trial. *Blood* 1992;80:1430–6.
237. Gerhartz HH, Engelhard M, Meusers P, *et al.* Randomized double-blind, placebo-controlled phase III study of recombinant human granulocyte-macrophage colony-stimulating factor as adjunct to induction treatment of high-grade malignant non-Hodgkin's lymphomas. *Blood* 1993;82: 2329–39.
238. Hamm JT, Schiller J, Oken MM, *et al.* Dose ranging study of recombinant human granulocyte-macrophage colony-stimulating factor in small cell lung cancer [abstract]. *Proc Am Soc Clin Oncol.* 1993;12:335.
239. Nichols C, Bajorin D, Schmoll HJ, *et al.* VIP chemotherapy with/without GM-CSF for poor risk, relapsed, or refractory germ cell tumors (GCT): preliminary analysis of a randomized controlled trial [abstract]. *Proc Am Soc Clin Oncol.* 1991;10:167.
240. American Society of Clinical Oncology recommendations for the use of hematopoietic colony-stimulating factors: evidence-based, clinical practice guidelines. *J Clin Oncol.* 1994;12:2471–508.
241. Lyman GH, Lyman CG, Sanderson RA, *et al.* Decision analysis of hematopoietic growth factor use in patients receiving cancer chemotherapy. *J Natl Cancer Inst.* 1993;85: 488–93.
242. Bronchud MH, Howell A, Crowther D, *et al.* The use of granulocyte colony-stimulating factor to increase the intensity of treatment with doxorubicin in patients with advanced breast and ovarian cancer. *Br J Cancer* 1989;60: 121–5.
243. Nimer SD. The use of colony-stimulating factors in primary hematologic disorders. *Cancer* 1992;70:921–7.
244. Schuster MW, Larson RA, Thompson JA, *et al.* Granulocyte-macrophage colony-stimulating factor (GM–CSF) for myelodysplastic syndrome (MDS): results of a multi-center randomized controlled trial [abstract]. *Blood* 1990; 76(*Suppl* 1):318.
245. Negrin R, Haeuber D, Nagler A, *et al.* Maintenance treatment of patients with myelodysplastic syndromes using recombinant human granulocyte colony-stimulating factor. *Blood* 1990;76:36–43.
246. Lieschke GJ, Burgess AW. Granulocyte colony-stimulating factor and granulocyte-macrophage colony-stimulating factor. *N Engl J Med.* 1992;372(2):99–106.
247. Groopman JE, Molina JM, Scadden DT. Hematopoietic growth factors: biology and clinical applications. *N Engl J Med.* 1989;321:1449–59.
248. Amgen, Inc. Neupogen package insert. Thousand Oaks, CA. February, 1991.
249. Immunex Corporation. Leukine package insert. Seattle, WA. March, 1991. Hoechst-Roussel Pharmaceuticals, Inc. Prokine package insert. Somerville, NJ. March, 1991.
250. Steward WP, Austin R, Scarffe JH, *et al.* Phase I study of recombinant DNA granulocyte-macrophage colony-stimulating factor (rGM-CSF). *Br J Cancer* 1988;57:258.
251. Lieschke GJ, Maher D, Cebon J, *et al.* Effects of subcutaneously administered bacterially synthesized recombinant human granulocyte-macrophage colony stimulating factor in patients with advanced malignancy. *Ann Intern Med.* 1989;110:357–64.
252. Vose JM, Armitage JO. Clinical applications of hematopoietic growth factors. *J Clin Oncol.* 1995;13(4):1023–35.
253. Starnes HF Jr. Biological effects and possible clinical applications of interleukin-1. *Semin Hematol.* 1991;28(*Suppl* 2):34–41.
254. Dinavello CA. Interleukin-1 and interleukin-1 antagonism. *Blood* 1991;77:1627–52.
255. Wilson WH, Bryant G, Fox M, *et al.* Interleukin-1 administration before high-dose ifosfamide (I), CBDCA (C), and etoposide (E) recovery: a phase I/II study [abstract]. *Proc Am Soc Clin Oncol.* 1993;12:937a.
256. Weisdorf D, Katsanis E, Verfailie C, *et al.* Interleukin-1 alpha administered after autologous transplantation: a phase I/II clinical trial. *Blood* 1994;84:2044–9.
257. Nemunaitis J, Appelbaum FR, Lilleby K, *et al.* Phase I study of recombinant interleukin-1 beta in patients undergoing autologous bone marrow transplant for acute myelogenous leukemia. *Blood* 1994;83:3474–9.
258. Postmus PE, Gietema JA, Damsma O, *et al.* Effects of recombinant human interleukin-3 in patients with relapsed small-cell lung cancer treated with chemotherapy: a dose-finding study. *J Clin Oncol.* 1992;10:1131–40.
259. Biemsa B, Willemse PHB, Mulder NH, *et al.* Effects of interleukin-3 after chemotherapy for advanced ovarian cancer. *Blood* 1992;80:1141–8.
260. Nemunaitis J, Appelbaum FR, Singer JW, *et al.* Phase I trial with recombinant human interleukin-3 in patients with lymphoma undergoing autologous bone marrow transplantation. *Blood* 1993;82:3272–8.
261. Fay JW, Lazarus HM, Herzig R, *et al.* Sequential administration of interleukin-3 (rhIL-3) and granulocyte-macrophage colony stimulating factor after autologous bone marrow transplantation for malignant lymphoma: a phase I/II

trial multicenter trial. *Blood* 1994;84:2151–7.
262. Haas R, Ehrhardt R, Witt B, *et al.* Autografting with peripheral blood stem cells mobilized by sequential interleukin-3/granulocyte-macrophage colony-stimulating factor following high-dose chemotherapy in non-Hodgkin's lymphoma. *Bone Marrow Transplant.* 1993;12:643–9.
263. Bajorin DF, Cheung NKV, Houghton AN. Macrophage colony-stimulating factor: biological effects and potential applications for cancer therapy. *Semin Hematol.* 1991;28 (*Suppl* 2):42–8.
264. Bajorin DF, Jakubowski A, Cody B, *et al.* Recombinant macrophage colony stimulating factor (rhM-CSF): a phase I trial in patients with metastatic melanoma [abstract]. *Proc Am Soc Clin Oncol.* 1990;9:183.
265. Peters WP, Kurtzberg J, Rao M, *et al.* Effects of recombinant human macrophage colony stimulating factor (rHuM-CSF) on hematopoiesis following high dose chemotherapy and autologous bone marrow support [abstract]. *Blood* 1989;74(*Suppl*):269a.
266. Masaoka T, Shibata H, Ohno R, *et al.* Double-blind test of human urinary macrophage colony-stimulating factor for allogeneic and syngeneic bone marrow transplantation: effectiveness of treatment and 2-year follow-up for relapse of leukaemia. *Br J Haematol.* 1990;76:501–5.
267. Meyers JD, Buckner CD, Bianco JC, *et al.* Phase I/II trial of recombinant human macrophage-colony stimulating factor (M-CSF) in patients with invasive fungal infection. *Blood* 1990;76:158a. Abstract 625.
268. Nemunaitis J, Shannon-Dorcy K, Appelbaum FR, *et al.* Long-term follow-up of patients with invasive fungal disease who received adjunctive therapy with recombinant human macrophage colony-stimulating factor. *Blood* 1993; 82:1422–7.
269. Furman WL, Marina N, Luo X, *et al.* A pediatric phase I/II trial of subcutaneous (SQ) PIXY 321 administered after ifosfamide/carboplatin/etoposide (ICE) chemotherapy [abstract]. *Proc Am Soc Clin Oncol.* 1994;13:1429a.
270. Vose JM, Anderson J, Blerman PJ, *et al.* Initial trial of PIXY321 (GM-CSF/IL-3 fusion protein) following high-dose chemotherapy and autologous bone marrow transplantation (ABMT) for lymphoid malignancy [abstract]. *Proc Am Soc Clin Oncol.* 1993;12:1237a.
271. Demetri TD, Bukowski RM, Samuels B, *et al.* Stimulation of thrombopoiesis by recombinant human interleukin-6 (IL-6) pre and post chemotherapy in previously untreated sarcoma patients with normal hematopoiesis [abstract]. *Blood* 1993;82(*Suppl* 1):1452a.
272. Fay JW, Collins R, Pineiro L, *et al.* Concomitant administration of interleukin-6 (rh IL-6) and leucomax (rh GM-CSF) following autologous bone marrow transplantation: a phase I trial [abstract]. *Blood* 1993;82(*Suppl* 1):1707a.
273. Devine SM, Winton EF, Holland HK, *et al.* Simultaneous administration of interleukin-6 (rh IL-6) and Neupogen (rh G-CSF) following autologous bone marrow transplantation (ABMT) for breast cancer [abstract]. *Blood* 1994; 84(*Suppl* 1):343a.
274. Gordon M, Hoffman R, Battiato L, *et al.* Recombinant human interleukin eleven (Neumega rhIL-11) prevents cycles of cyclophosphamide and doxorubicin chemotherapy [abstract]. *Proc Am Soc Clin Oncol.* 1994;13:326a.
275. Elias L, Tepler I, Smith JW, *et al.* Randomized trial of recombinant human interleukin eleven (neumega rhIL-11 growth factor) in patients with severe chemotherapy-induced thrombocytopenia. *Blood* 1995;86(10 *Suppl* 1):498a.
276. Cerami A. Cachectin/TNF and the immune response. *Adv Oncol.* 1990;6:5–9.
277. Beutler B, Cerami A. Cachectin: more than a tumor necrosis factor. *N Engl J Med.* 1987;316:379–85.
278. Grunfeld C, Palladino MA. Tumor necrosis factor: immunologic, antitumor, metabolic, and cardiovascular activities. *Adv Intern Med.* 1990;35:45–72.
279. Sherman ML, Spriggs DR, Arthur KA, *et al.* Recombinant human tumor necrosis factor administered as a five-day continuous infusion in cancer patients: phase I toxicity and effects on lipid metabolism. *J Clin Oncol.* 1988;6: 344–50.
280. Chapman PB, Lester TJ, Casper ES, *et al.* Clinical pharmacology of recombinant human tumor necrosis factor in patients with advanced cancer. *J Clin Oncol.* 1987;5:1942–51.
281. Spriggs DR, Sherman ML, Michie H, *et al.* Recombinant human tumor necrosis factor administered as a 24-hour intravenous infusion. A phase I and pharmacologic study. *J Natl Cancer Inst.* 1988;80:1039–44.
282. Creagan ET, Kovach JS, Moertel CG, *et al.* A phase I clinical trial of recombinant human tumor necrosis factor. *Cancer* 1988;62:2467–71.
283. Schiller JH, Storer BE, Witt PL, *et al.* Biological and clinical effects of intravenous tumor necrosis factor-a administered three times weekly. *Cancer Res.* 1991;51:1651–8.
284. Blick M, Sherwin SA, Rosenblum M, *et al.* Phase I study of recombinant tumor necrosis factor in cancer patients. *Cancer Res.* 1987;47:2986–9.
285. Hieber U, Heim ME. Tumor necrosis factor for the treatment of malignancies. *Oncology* 1994;51:142–53.
286. Lienard D, Eggermont AMM, Schraffordt Koops H, *et al.* Isolated perfusion of the limb with high-dose tumour necrosis factor-alpha (TNF-alpha), interferon-gamma (IFN-gamma) and melphalan for melanoma stage III. Results of a multi-centre pilot study. *Melanoma Res.* 1994;4(*Suppl* 1):21–6.
287. Gaynor ER, Weiss GR, Margolin KA, *et al.* Phase I study of high-dose continuous-infusion recombinant interleukin-2 and autologous lymphokine-activated killer cells in patients with metastatic or unresectable malignant melanoma and renal cell carcinoma. *J Natl Cancer Inst.* 1990;82: 1397–402.
288. Dutcher JP, Creekmore S, Weiss GR, *et al.* A phase II study of interleukin-2 and lymphokine-activated killer cells in patients with metastatic malignant melanoma. *J Clin Oncol.* 1989;7:477–85.
289. Dutcher JP, Gaynor ER, Boldt DH, *et al.* A phase II study of high-dose continuous infusion interleukin-2 with lymphokine-activated killer cells in patients with metastatic melanoma. *J Clin Oncol.* 1991;9:641–8.
290. Clark JW, Smith JW II, Steis RG, *et al.* Interleukin 2 and lymphokine-activated killer cell therapy: analysis of a bolus interleukin 2 and a continuous infusion interleukin 2 regimen. *Cancer Res.* 1990;50:7343–50.
291. Wang J, Walle A, Gordon B, *et al.* Adoptive immunotherapy for stage IV renal cell carcinoma: a novel protocol utilizing periodate and interleukin-2-activated autolo-

gous leukocytes and continuous infusions of low-dose interleukin-2. *Am J Med.* 1987;83:1016–23.

292. Eberlein TJ, Schoof DD, Jung SE, *et al.* A new regimen of interleukin 2 and lymphokine-activated killer cells. Efficacy without significant toxicity. *Arch Intern Med.* 1988; 148:2571–6.
293. West WH, Tauer KW, Yannelli JR, *et al.* Constant-infusion recombinant interleukin-2 in adoptive immunotherapy of advanced cancer. *N Engl J Med.* 1987;316:898–905.
294. Rosenberg SA. Adoptive cellular therapy in patients with advanced cancer. *Biol. Ther Cancer Updates* 1991;1:1–15.
295. Hawkins MJ. PPO Updates IL-2/LAK. *Prin Pract Oncol.* 1989;3:1–14.
296. McCabe MS, Stablein D, Hawkins MJ. The modified group C experience-phase III randomized trials of IL-2/LAK in advanced renal cell carcinoma and advanced melanoma [abstract]. *Proc Am Soc Clin Oncol.* 1991;10:213.
297. Palmer PA, Vinke J, Evers P, *et al.* Continuous infusion of recombinant interleukin-2 with or without autologous lymphokine-activated killer cells for the treatment of advanced renal cell carcinoma. *Eur J Cancer Clin Oncol.* 1992;28A: 1038–44.
298. Kradin RL, Lazarus DS, Dubinett SM, *et al.* Tumor-infiltrating lymphocytes and interleukin-2 in treatment of advanced cancer. *Lancet* 1989;1(8638):577–80.
299. Rosenberg SA, Packard BS, Aebersold PM, *et al.* Use of tumor-infiltrating lymphocytes and interleukin-2 in the immunotherapy of patients with metastatic melanoma: a preliminary report. *N Engl J Med.* 1988;319:1676–80.
300. Bukowski RM, Sharfman W, Murthy S, *et al.* Clinical results and characterization of tumor-infiltrating lymphocytes with or without recombinant interleukin-2 in human metastatic renal cell carcinoma. *Cancer Res.* 1991;51:4199–205.
301. Rosenberg SA, Aebersold P, Cornetta K, *et al.* Gene transfer into humans—immunotherapy of patients with advanced melanoma, using tumor-infiltrating lymphocytes modified by retroviral gene transduction. *N Engl J Med.* 1990;323:570–8.
302. Marmont AM. The graft-versus-leukemia (GVL) effect after allogeneic bone marrow transplantation for chronic myelogenous leukemia (CML). *Leuk Lymphoma* 1993;11 (*Suppl* 1):221–6.
303. Porter DL, Roth MS, McGarigle C, *et al.* Induction of graft-versus-host disease as immunotherapy for relapsed chronic myeloid leukemia. *N Engl J Med.* 1994;330:100–6.
304. Kolb HJ, Schattenberg A, Goldman J, *et al.* Graft-versus-leukemia effect of donor lymphocyte transfusions in marrow grafted patients. *Blood* 1995;86:2041–50.

SELF-ASSESSMENT QUESTIONS

1. The mechanism of action of interferons includes induction of the enzymes 2,5-A synthetase, protein kinase, and phosphodiesterase. This results in what type of antitumor effect?

2. Interferon alpha has FDA approval for which of the following indications?

   a. chronic myelogenous leukemia
   b. Kaposi's sarcoma
   c. hairy cell leukemia
   d. hepatitis B
   e. a and c only
   f. all of the above

3. Which of the following is true of interferon alpha therapy for chronic myelogenous leukemia?

   a. Durable cytogenetic remissions have been seen in 90% of patients who achieved a complete cytogenetic response.
   b. Single-agent, single-arm studies demonstrated no dose-response relationship.
   c. Newly diagnosed patients with low-risk prognostic features are thought to have the best response.
   d. Time to cytogenetic response is approximately three weeks.
   e. a and c only
   f. all of the above

4. Which of the following statements is true regarding interferon alpha treatment for hepatitis?

   a. Interferon alpha is FDA approved for treatment of both hepatitis B and hepatitis C.
   b. At most, only 20% of patients with hepatitis C will have a sustained response six months after discontinuation of therapy.
   c. Factors that predict a positive response to interferon treatment in hepatitis C include younger age, low serum hepatitis C virus RNA level, a short duration of infection, and absence of cirrhosis.
   d. Treatment of chronic hepatitis B infection with interferon alpha results in interruption of hepatitis B virus replication and loss of markers (hepatitis B e antigen and hepatitis B virus DNA).
   e. a and c only
   f. all of the above

5. What is the most common acute toxicity associated with interferon alpha therapy?

6. Which of the following are true regarding side effects of interferon alpha?

   a. Gradual escalation of the dose over a 7- to 10-day period may help minimize acute toxicities.
   b. Nausea, anorexia, and weight loss are not common side effects.
   c. Administration of the dose on an intermittent schedule may help minimize symptoms of fatigue.
   d. Administration of low doses of interferon may result in central nervous system toxicities.
   e. a and c only
   f. all of the above

7. Interferon gamma demonstrates greater immunomodulatory activity than either interferon alpha or interferon beta because it enhances both MHC class I and class II antigen expression.

   a. true
   b. false

8. Name the two primary tumor types that have responded to therapy with recombinant IL-2.

9. Interleukin 2 exerts its antitumor effects directly and indirectly by stimulating natural killer cell production and various other cytokines.

   a. true
   b. false

10. What are the two recombinant interleukin 2 products currently used in clinical trials?

11. Which of the following are true regarding side effects of interleukin 2 therapy?

    a. Capillary leak syndrome is a common side effect and is a result of increased vascular permeability, which leads to fluid accumulation.
    b. Nausea, vomiting, and diarrhea are rarely seen with interleukin 2 therapy.
    c. If a patient experiences neurological symptoms (hallucinations, disorientation, and personality or behavioral changes), the drug should be discontinued immediately.
    d. Hypertension is generally more common than hypotension during interleukin 2 therapy.
    e. a and c only
    f. all of the above

12. Toxicities associated with interleukin 2 therapy are dose and schedule dependent.

    a. true
    b. false

13. Both granulocyte colony-stimulating factor (G-CSF) and granulocyte macrophage colony-stimulating factor (GM-CSF) stimulate neutrophil production; however, GM-CSF is more selective and lineage-specific.

    a. true
    b. false

14. FDA-approved indications for GM-CSF include which of the following?

    a. acceleration of myeloid engraftment after autologous and allogenic bone marrow transplant
    b. mobilization of hematopoietic progenitor cells
    c. engraftment failure after either allogenic or autologous bone marrow transplant
    d. to decrease duration of neutropenia following induction chemotherapy in patients 55 years of age or older with acute myelogenous leukemia
    e. a and c only
    f. all of the above

15. List the primary side effects associated with G-CSF therapy.

16. Interleukin 1 can produce acute symptoms of fever, hypotension, headache, myalgia, arthralgias, and tachycardia.

    a. true
    b. false

17. PIXY-321 is a fusion product that combines which two colony-stimulating factors?

18. Which of the following colony-stimulating factors is responsible for the proliferation and maturation of red blood cells?

    a. macrophage colony-stimulating factor
    b. granulocyte-macrophage colony-stimulating factor
    c. interleukin 1
    d. erythropoietin

19. Which of the following are true regarding the colony-stimulating factors?

    a. Interleukin 3 is also known as multi-CSF, a multilineage hematopoietic growth factor.
    b. Macrophage colony-stimulating factor stimulates the production and activity of monocytes and macrophages.
    c. Side effects associated with interleukin 11 include tachycardia, syncope, atrial arrhythmias, palpitations, and hypotension.
    d. Interleukin 6 and interleukin 11 stimulate the development and maturation of megakaryocytes.
    e. a and c only
    f. all of the above

20. Which of the following have been observed in clinical trials of granulocyte colony-stimulating factor for chemotherapy-induced neutropenia?

    a. reduced incidence of febrile neutropenia
    b. reduced time to platelet engraftment
    c. reduction in antibiotic use and hospital stay
    d. decreased number of red blood cell transfusions
    e. a and c only
    f. all of the above

CHAPTER 11

Monoclonal Antibodies

Val R. Adams, Pharm.D.
Assistant Professor
College of Pharmacy
University of Kentucky
Lexington, KY

Janet L. Karlix, Pharm.D.
Associate Professor
Department of Pharmacy Practice, College of Pharmacy
University of Florida
Gainesville, FL

Production of MoAbs ... 270
General Procedures for Producing MoAbs ... 271
Forming the Hybridoma ... 272
Selecting the Hybridoma ... 272
Screening for the Desired Hybridoma ... 272
Cloning ... 272
Large-Scale Production of MoAbs ... 272
Storing Hybridomas ... 273
Purification Procedures ... 273
Modified Production Procedures ... 273
Human MoAbs ... 273
Interspecies Hybridomas ... 274
EBV Transformation ... 274
Lymphoblastoid Cell Lines ... 274
Chimeric Antibodies ... 274
Bivalent Antibodies ... 275
MoAb Fragments ... 275
MoAb Applications ... 276
Laboratory Applications ... 276
Diagnostic Uses ... 276
Infectious Disease Diagnosis ... 276
Pregnancy Tests ... 277
Ovulation Tests ... 277
Oncologic Diagnosis ... 278
Cell and Tissue Typing ... 278
MoAbs for Tissue Typing ... 278

**The contributions made by Karl Kwok to this chapter are gratefully acknowledged.*

Drug Assays 279
Protein Purification 279
In Vivo Applications of MoAbs 279
Imaging 280
Therapeutic Uses 283
Transplantation 283
Cardiac Disease 283
Oncology 284
Applications with Immunoconjugates 287
Problems and Possible Solutions for MoAbTherapy in Oncology 289
Autoimmune Diseases 290
Toxin Reversal 290
Vaccines 290
Summary 291
References 291
Self-Assessment Questions 298

Monoclonal antibodies (MoAbs) are antibodies that are identical in structure and immunologic function, including specificity and binding affinity. They are produced from identical genes that typically originate from a single cell that has been cloned. Polyclonal antibodies differ in composition, structure, and immunologic function. The ability to produce MoAbs has been a key component in expanding our knowledge of the role of cell surface antigens and soluble proteins in biological fluids. This knowledge has ultimately led to important advances in our understanding of diseases and the development of therapeutic agents.

This chapter includes a brief discussion of the historical background of MoAbs, a description of their production techniques and applications in the laboratory, and a look at their imaging and therapeutic uses. The advantages and drawbacks associated with these applications are included.

After completing this chapter, the reader should be able to:

1. Discuss production techniques for creating MoAbs.
2. Describe current applications of MoAb imaging and therapy.
3. Discuss advantages of MoAb therapy.
4. Discuss drawbacks of MoAb antibody therapy.

For additional information, the reader is referred to:

- Clark M. General introduction. In: Birch JR, Lennox ES, editors. *Monoclonal Antibodies: Principles and Applications*. New York: Wiley-Liss; 1995. p.1–43.
- Scheinberg DA, Chapman PB. Therapeutic applications of monoclonal antibodies for human disease. In: Birch JR, Lennox ES, editors. *Monoclonal Antibodies: Principles and Applications*. New York: Wiley-Liss; 1995. p.45–105.

PRODUCTION OF MOABS

Hybridoma technology, which was developed in the 1970s, has revolutionized immunochemistry.[1] The ability to produce large amounts of MoAbs that recognize and interact with specific antigens make them ideal agents for a variety of applications. MoAbs are used extensively in laboratories to identify and quantify a given compound or to identify and classify cells or subsets of cells. Figure 11-1 shows a T cell and some of its unique surface proteins, such as CD4 and CD8. MoAbs that bind CD4 or CD8 can be used to classify subsets of T cells using flow cytometry techniques.[2] MoAbs can be tagged with a radioactive isotope and used for in vivo imaging. A product that utilizes this concept is Oncoscint CR/OV®.[3] MoAbs can also provide therapeutic results by binding cells or proteins in biological fluids or tissues. A good example is abciximab, which binds to a platelet glycoprotein receptor, resulting in antithrombotic effects.[3] Chemical compounds can be conjugated to MoAbs, which can deliver high levels of the compound at the desired site when given to patients. The ability to produce MoAbs that bind to specific antigens has led the way for antibody-directed therapy.

The discovery that antibodies bind to specific protein sites led scientists to develop methods to obtain certain immunoglobulins. The ability to obtain antibodies of the researcher's choice holds the promise of a magic

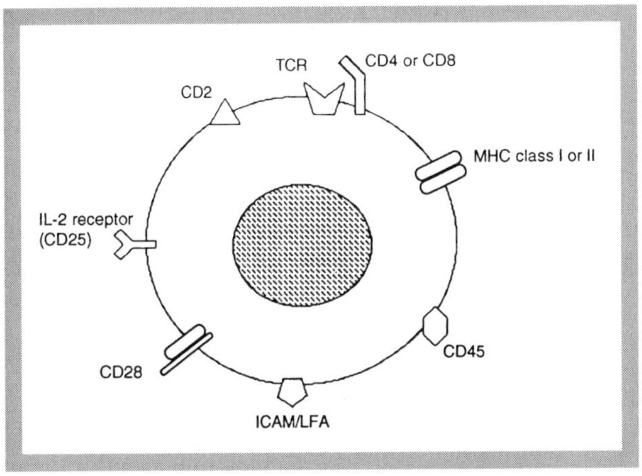

Figure 11-1. Antigens associated with human T cells. TCR, T-cell receptor; CD, cluster of differentiation; IL, interleukin; ICAM, intercellular adhesion molecule; LFA, lymphocyte function-associated antigen; MHC, major histocompatibility complex.

bullet. Theoretically, antibodies can be generated that bind to virtually any protein, whether it's part of a microbe or a tumor cell. In the first attempts, polyclonal antibodies were produced by injecting antigens into rabbits, goats, and horses. The host animal's immune system mounted a response to the antigen. After the animals were bled, the antibodies were extracted, isolated, and purified. This method provided antibodies that were useful for diagnostic and therapeutic uses, but it had several limitations. The antibody quality varied with each lot, and the quantity of any single antiserum was limited to only a few grams. Most of the antisera produced by this method also contained many other antibodies of unknown binding specificity.

In 1974, Georges Kohler and Cesar Milstein[1] of the Medical Research Council in Cambridge, England, developed a procedure to potentially obtain an unlimited quantity of a pure antibody with single specificity. Their research of somatic cells showed that malignant myeloma cells (a plasma cell tumor) were capable of immortal growth in vitro, whereas antibody-secreting B lymphocytes do not survive long in cultures. Through their studies they originated the hybrid myeloma (hybridoma) technique and produced MoAbs for the first time.

The first MoAbs were produced by obtaining antibody-secreting B lymphocytes from the spleen of a mouse immunized with sheep red blood cells (RBCs). These lymphocytes were then fused with genetically deficient mouse myeloma cells unable to grow under certain conditions. Equal numbers of spleen cells and myeloma cells were fused using inactivated Sendai virus, and samples were grown in selective medium. Only the cells that inherited the features of both parents by fusion survived in the medium. These so-called hybridomas produced monoclonal antisheep RBC antibodies while growing indefinitely in cell culture.[1] An improved version of Kohler and Milstein's procedure is used by many scientists today to obtain virtually unlimited quantities of a pure antibody with a single specificity.

General Procedures for Producing MoAbs

Procedures for producing murine (mouse origin) MoAbs have been described.[4–6] Minor modifications have been performed by different investigators to increase the yield and specificity of their MoAbs.[5–8] The overall scheme for the murine production of MoAbs is described in Figure 11-2.

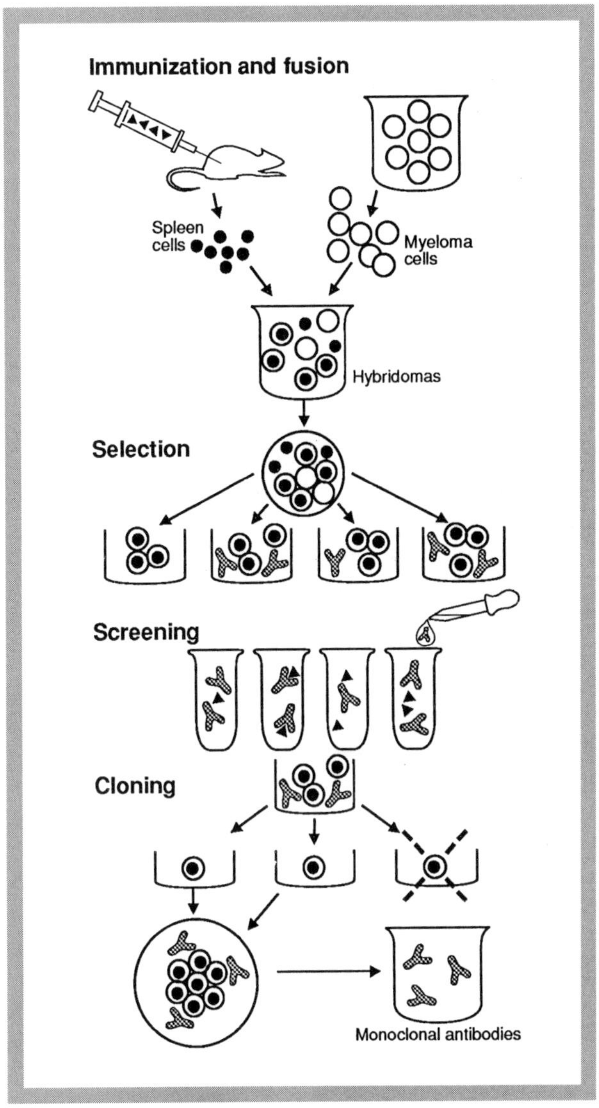

Figure 11-2. Production of murine monoclonal antibodies

SOURCE: *Reprinted with permission from Chisholm R. On the trail of the magic bullet.* High Technology Business *1983; 3[Jan]:61.*

Forming the Hybridoma

B lymphocytes secreting antibodies to a desired antigen must be obtained. To accomplish this, a mouse is vaccinated with the antigen (protein) that the desired MoAb will bind. The foreign protein stimulates the mouse's B lymphocytes to expand in number and produce antibodies against various epitopes. The mouse may be given additional antigen exposures to ensure a good yield of specific antibody-producing B lymphocytes.[6–8]

The mouse is sacrificed, and the spleen is removed so the lymphocytes from the spleen can be isolated. Only a few of the many B lymphocytes in the spleen are antigen specific and secrete the desired antibody. All the lymphocytes are mixed with myeloma cells in the presence of polyethylene glycol, which fuses the cellular membranes of the two cell types by making the membranes more adhesive.[6–8]

There are other techniques for fusion that use viruses and electrical fields.[9,10] The fusion results in a mixture of cells in which only a small percentage are the desired hybridomas (those containing the cell contents of both parental cells). Other components of the cell mixture include lymphocyte–lymphocyte fused cells, myeloma–myeloma fused cells, unfused myeloma cells, and unfused lymphocytes.

Selecting the Hybridoma

The large number of undesired cells in the mixture must be eliminated to select only the hybridomas. The mixture of spleen cells (lymphocytes), myeloma cells, and hybridoma cells are grown in a selective medium containing hypoxanthine, aminopterin, and thymidine (HAT). Aminopterin, a compound similar to methotrexate, blocks normal nucleic acid biosynthesis in cells. Hypoxanthine and thymidine can be used as substrates to produce nucleic acids via nucleotide salvage pathways in cells containing the enzymes hypoxanthine-guanine phosphoribosyltransferase (HGPRT) or thymidine kinase (TK). The myeloma cell line chosen for fusion is a mutant lacking HGPRT and TK enzymes. The unfused myeloma cells die because they are unable to use hypoxanthine or thymidine to bypass the nucleic acid synthesis block caused by aminopterin. The hybridoma cells grow as the chromosomes from the lymphocytes provide the information for producing the enzymes HGPRT or TK. The unfused lymphocytes are eliminated because of naturally poor growth in vitro. The surviving hybridomas are grown as small colonies in separate wells of a culture dish.[6–8]

Screening for the Desired Hybridoma

The cell cultures are allowed to grow for a few weeks (usually two to three weeks) and are then screened to select the hybridoma that is producing the desired antibody. There are many methods by which the specific hybridoma secreting the desired antibody can be identified. The most widely used methods are the radioimmunoassay (RIA) and enzyme-linked immunosorbent assay (ELISA) techniques, which are sensitive, quick, and easy to use. Other screening methods include flow cytometry and a cytotoxicity assay.[6–8]

In the RIA and ELISA techniques, the target antigen is chemically bound to the bottom of testing tray wells. The supernatant from each of the hybridoma cultures is added to corresponding antigen wells. Antibodies in the supernatant specific for the target antigen bind, and unbound antibodies are washed away. Radioactive or enzyme-labeled secondary antibodies specific for the primary antibodies are added to the wells, and the mixture is incubated and rewashed. The wells that show radioactivity or a color reaction contain the desired antibody. The corresponding wells of hybridoma cultures may be cloned to produce a clonal population of hybridoma cells that produced the desired MoAb.[6–8]

Cloning

The purpose of cloning is to ensure that all of the hybridoma cells are actually of one population. The various hybridomas in culture may secrete a mixture of antibodies that recognize different sites or epitopes on the target antigen. By diluting the hybridomas, only one cell is deposited into each well of a 96-well culture plate. The single cell grows into a colony of identical cells. The medium from each colony is screened for specific antibody production, and the desired hybridoma clone is selected according to its antibody specificity.[6–8]

Large-Scale Production of MoAbs

There are many methods for producing large quantities of desired MoAbs, and many more are being developed to provide for wide commercial applications of the antibodies.[8,10–12] The simplest production method is to grow the desired hybridoma in cell cultures and harvest the secreted antibodies from the supernatant. This method provides relatively low yield compared with other methods and is relatively expensive. However, it is useful for the production of small quantities of antibodies for research purposes.

Another method requires hybridoma cells to be injected into the peritoneal cavities of mice. These hybridoma cells, which grow quickly because of their neoplastic properties, secrete antibodies into the ascitic fluid in the peritoneal cavity. After 10–21 days, 2–5 ml of ascitic fluid is harvested from each mouse. High concentrations of antibody are achievable in the ascitic fluid, approximately 5–15 mg/ml. This method usually produces 10 to 100 times the concentration of MoAbs obtained from tissue culture. Hundreds to thousands of mice, however, are required to produce even 1 kg of MoAbs. Other disadvantages of this method include contamination of the peritoneal fluid with other proteins besides the desired antibodies and the cost of harvesting from large numbers of mice.[13]

In the early 1980s, the production requirements of MoAbs could generally be fulfilled by the methods available at that time. During this early period, only microgram to gram doses where required for a relatively small amount of testing. Today, hundreds of kilograms of MoAbs are required per year. This demand has spurred the development of new production techniques.

One recent technique uses cell growth chambers consisting of a mass of hollow fibers packed longitudinally into cylindrical cartridges called bioreactors. Each fiber is a hollow tube with a 200-μm inner diameter with a semipermeable membrane. The cells are grown in the space surrounding the fibers, and the fibers are used to deliver nutrients to the cells. Each of the bioreactors contains about 10 trillion cells. The hybridomas grow in high density and continuously produce MoAbs in concentrations of approximately 100–500 μg/ml in the media. MoAbs, in relatively pure form, can be produced at a rate of several milligrams per day from an average hybridoma cell line.[8,11] Several variations of this basic bioreactor have been designed. Recently, an efficient modification using small glass cylinders in a three-liter bioreactor was able to produce 6 g of purified MoAb in 36 days.[12]

Storing Hybridomas

Hybridoma cells may be frozen and stored for future use. Cells stored in liquid nitrogen have been shown to be viable after several years. Because a hybridoma occasionally stops secreting antibodies, it is important that a parental seed stock of hybridomas be kept frozen. The frozen seed stock can then be used to restart the cultures.[8]

Purification Procedures

MoAbs should be purified before in vivo use and commercial applications. MoAbs may be purified by precipitation with ammonium sulfate, gel filtration, electrophoresis, ion exchange, or affinity chromatography. Stability, affinity, activity, and formulation information should be obtained.[8]

Modified Production Procedures

MoAbs have been incorporated into several assays that are essential to both clinical and research laboratories. The application of MoAbs in vivo has been much slower because of side effects and lack of efficacy. In general, low efficacy can be contributed to one or more of the following causes. First, MoAb uptake by the reticuloendothelial system or poor tissue penetration may prevent specific binding by the MoAb. Second, when cytotoxicity is the goal, low efficacy can result if a MoAb subtype doesn't bind complement or binds to a cell surface protein that modulates (also known as antigenic modulation, defined as internalization or shedding of the protein-MoAb complex by the cell). Third, low efficacy can be due to an immune response against the MoAb. As with any antigen, the patient's immune system will eventually produce antibodies against the MoAb, inactivating it. This most commonly occurs with repeated doses of a MoAb. A patient's immune reaction to the MoAb is also a primary adverse event, which may be manifested as anaphylaxis.

Murine production is currently the predominant method of MoAb generation. A major concern with the use of murine MoAbs is the formation of human antimurine antibodies (HAMAs), which has been clinically observed and correlated with decreased efficacy and severe allergic reactions.[14] These limitations have stimulated scientists to create modified production procedures to improve efficacy and decrease adverse events. New procedures are primarily aimed at decreasing the HAMA response.

Human MoAbs

Combining human lymphocytes with human myeloma cells produces hybridoma cells that secrete human MoAbs. Reduced antigenicity and increased effector activity are the primary advantages human MoAbs have over murine antibodies. Patients receiving human MoAbs are less likely to form antibodies against them than those receiving murine MoAbs; however, cases of human-anti-human antibodies (HAHAs) have been reported.[15] The technology for producing human MoAbs still lags behind murine MoAb technology for several reasons. Ethical concerns prevent scientists from vaccinating humans with antigens for the sole purpose of increasing the number of antibody-producing B lymphocytes. Therefore, the standard method of using spleen cells is only feasible in the rare case in which a spleen is available from a hyperimmunized human.

The development of a permanent human myeloma cell line has been more difficult than originally imagined. A number of HAT-sensitive human myeloma fusion partners have been developed and used to form hybridomas. However, human myeloma cell lines are usually unsatisfactory because of their slow-growing nature and low yield of hybrids. Finally, human hybridomas are not easily grown in the ascites of tumor-bearing mice, so cell culture techniques to develop a clonable human hybridoma are needed.[8,16]

Four alternative approaches to the development of human MoAbs are being explored to decrease antigenicity: (1) interspecies fusion with mouse myeloma cells to create mouse-human hybridoma cells, (2) immortalization of B lymphocytes by Epstein-Barr virus (EBV) transformation, (3) use of lymphoblastoid derivatives and development of more stable myeloid fusion partners, and (4) application of chimeric antibodies and recombinant

DNA techniques. Most of these techniques have yielded usable MoAbs, but production limitations slow wide application of any one methodology.

Interspecies Hybridomas

Interspecies hybrids result when human lymphocytes are fused with mouse myeloma cells. These lymphocytes are derived from lymphatic tissue removed for therapeutic purposes from surgical patients who have been exposed to particular antigens. The technique results in relatively high fusion frequencies, and the resulting hybrids are capable of secreting high levels of human antibodies. Limitations encountered with the interspecies hybrids include rapid loss of human chromosomes or altered gene expression, which can result in unstable or decreased immunoglobulin production.[17]

EBV Transformation

This technique uses in vitro EBV infection of human B lymphocytes to induce polyclonal activation and immunoglobulin production. Antigen-specific cells can be preselected before transformation by EBV infection, or the EBV line may be cloned and then screened for antibody production. The production of human antibodies by this method has resulted in immunoglobulin M (IgM) antibodies, which have different properties than IgG antibodies. Other problems with this method include a low yield of antibodies and the risk that EBV might be released into the culture and then introduced into the patient.[18]

Lymphoblastoid Cell Lines

Lymphoblastoid cell lines are typically EBV-containing nonmalignant B cells, which may be better immortal fusion partners than human myeloma cell lines. However, hybridomas that use a lymphoblastoid cell line have lower fusion frequencies and produce lower levels of immunoglobulins than fusion partners from a murine myeloma cell line.[19–21] Other methods using EBV hybridomas and genetic engineering techniques may eventually circumvent some of the current problems.

Chimeric Antibodies

The desire to decrease antigenicity and improve efficacy of antibodies has led to the development of chimeric antibodies, immunoglobulin molecules created primarily by recombinant DNA techniques and gene transfection.[22–29] The process creates mouse-human antibodies consisting of mouse Fab (or hypervariable) regions and human Fc regions. The process for producing chimeric antibodies is summarized in Figure 11-3. DNA specific for the desired

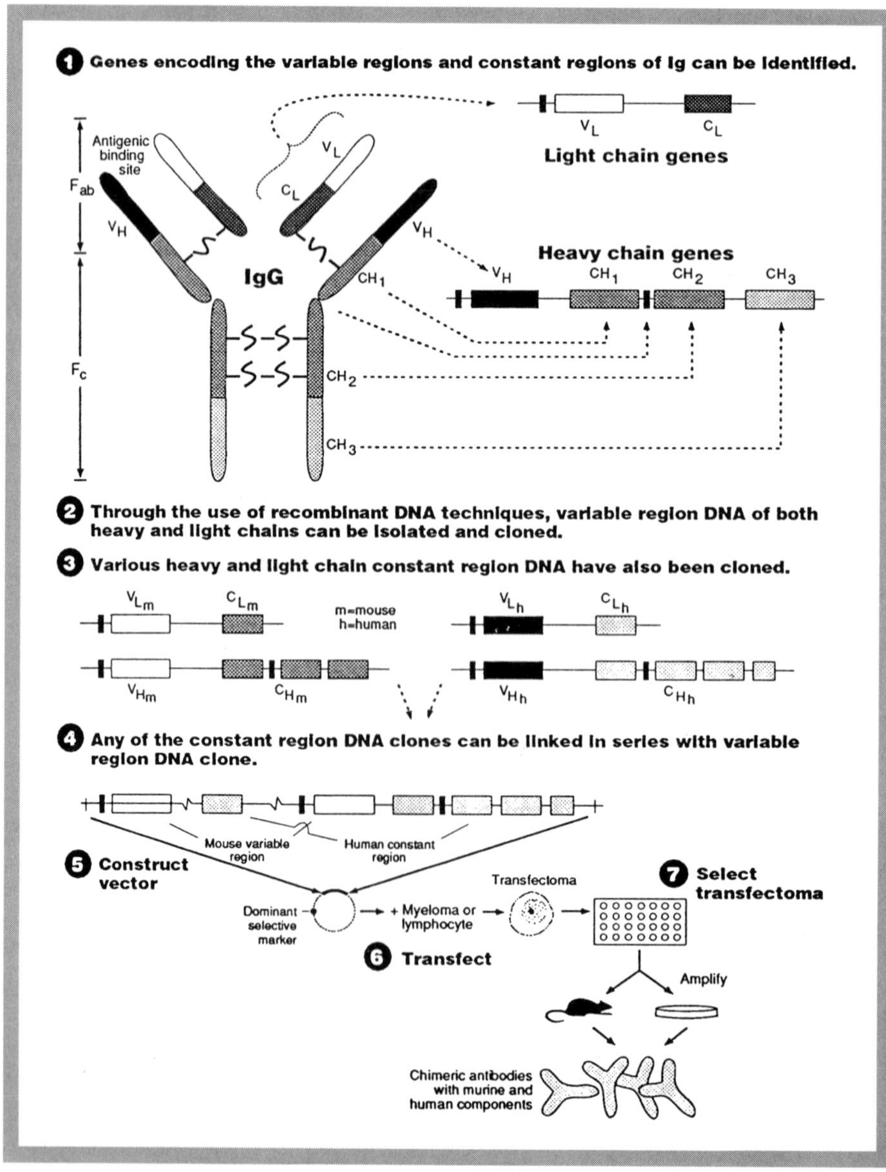

Figure 11-3. Production of chimeric antibodies

SOURCE: *Adapted with permission from Morrison SL. Transfectomas provide novel chimeric antibodies.* Science *1985;229:1203–4. Copyright 1985 by the AAAS.*

variable region is obtained from a murine B cell and then spliced to DNA that codes for the constant region of the human immunoglobulin. The chimeric gene containing the combined sequences is spliced into an expression vector containing a selectable marker. The vector is transfected into the appropriate recipient cell line. The stable transfectants that synthesize the genes of interest are identified, selected, and amplified by growth in culture or in the ascitic fluid of tumor-bearing mice.

Chimeric antibodies have recently been taken one step further. Small regions within the mouse Fab region have been isolated as the sections that actually bind antigen. These regions are known as hypervariable regions or complementarity-determining regions, because their amino acid sequence greatly differs from one antibody to another. Researchers have replicated the sequences for antigen-specific mouse hypervariable regions and placed these sequences into genes encoding for intact human immunoglobulin. The resulting chimeric antibody binds the antigen that the mouse antibody was directed against, but it is almost entirely human in composition.[30,31] Chimeric molecules are less antigenic than murine MoAbs, so their potential for adverse reactions is reduced and their potential for therapeutic effects is increased.[32]

Being able to choose the constant region is another advantage of chimeric antibodies. The constant region of a MoAb determines effector functions, such as binding of complement, uptake by cells of the reticuloendothelial system, and binding of other proteins. The constant region also partially determines the biodistribution and serum half-life of a MoAb.[33] Theoretically, it is possible to combine any murine variable region and human Fc portion to optimize the therapeutic potential.

The chimeric immunoglobulin can also be constructed so that the Fc portion is covalently bound to a nonimmunoglobulin protein.[27,28] The MoAb Fc portion may be bound to an enzyme so that antigen-antibody binding can be detected by adding an appropriate substrate, or it may be bound to a toxin and used as an immunotoxin.

Bivalent Antibodies

Bivalent antibodies are hybrids with two binding sites that can bind to different antigens. The bifunctional antibodies may be produced by chemical, biological, or genetic methods.[33–35] The chemical production of bivalent antibodies involves reducing two distinct MoAbs to monovalent fragments, mixing the fragments, and then oxidizing them to form whole antibodies with dual specificity. The resulting antibodies can bind two different antigens simultaneously. The biological production of bivalent antibodies requires making second-generation hybridomas. In this technique, two hybridomas are fused, resulting in cells that produce antibody molecules with both specificities. The genetic approach to making bivalent MoAbs involves inserting DNA for two different antibody genes into a cellular expression vector. The antibody genes are translated into MoAb chains, which then combine to form a whole MoAb. A linking molecule is often inserted to ensure binding of both chains. Bispecific antibodies represent an improvement in MoAb technology because they can bind two cell types together, such as cytotoxic T cells with tumor cells. The principal advantage of bispecific MoAbs is increased cytotoxicity.[35]

MoAb Fragments

In the past decade, the use of Fab and $F(ab')_2$ portions of MoAbs has included a broad range of immunological and biochemical investigations. MoAb fragments have been used to study antigen-antibody binding when the absence of Fc-associated effector functions was desirable.

The monovalent Fab is ideal for investigations in which Fc function or cross-linking of antigen are not desirable (Figure 11-4). The $F(ab')_2$ is bivalent and has substantially higher association constants to antigen than the Fab. $F(ab')_2$ can be compared with Fab and complete MoAb molecules to study the effects of receptor cross-linking on cellular activation. $F(ab')_2$ may be more desirable than Fab if a greater avidity to antigen is needed.[8]

MoAb fragments are produced by proteolytic cleavage in the hinge region, which splits the immunoglobulin into fragments. Cleavage by papain produces the monovalent Fab (45,000 molecular weight [MW]); cleavage by pepsin, in the absence of reducing agent, produces the $F(ab')_2$ (100,000 MW) (Figure 11-4). Monoclonal Fab fragments can also be produced by incorporating genes for the heavy and light chain variable regions into a recombinant expression system.[36,37]

The altered pharmacology and pharmacokinetics of Fab and $F(ab')_2$ fragments provide several advantages over whole MoAb antibodies. First, both fragments lack the Fc portion necessary for cytotoxic activity, which is advantageous when such activity is neither necessary nor desirable. A second advantage of Fab and $F(ab')_2$ is better tissue penetration and biodistribution characteristics, which is attributed to their lower molecular weight.[38–40] Third, MoAb fragments are cleared more quickly than the larger whole MoAb molecules. Fourth, patients who receive Fab or $F(ab')_2$ fragments are less likely to mount an immune response against these proteins than they are against whole MoAbs.

Recombinant techniques make it possible to link molecules to Fab, $F(ab')_2$, MoAb single chains,[41] or whole MoAbs. Various molecules, including toxins, chemotherapy, and radioactive compounds, have been connected to antibodies to enhance cytotoxicity. For example, a DNA sequence that codes for a MoAb Fab that binds an ovarian cancer antigen has been recombinantly linked to a pseudomonas exotoxin gene. The resulting single-chain immunotoxin can bind and kill cells expressing the ovarian antigen.[42] Recombinant technology may also provide

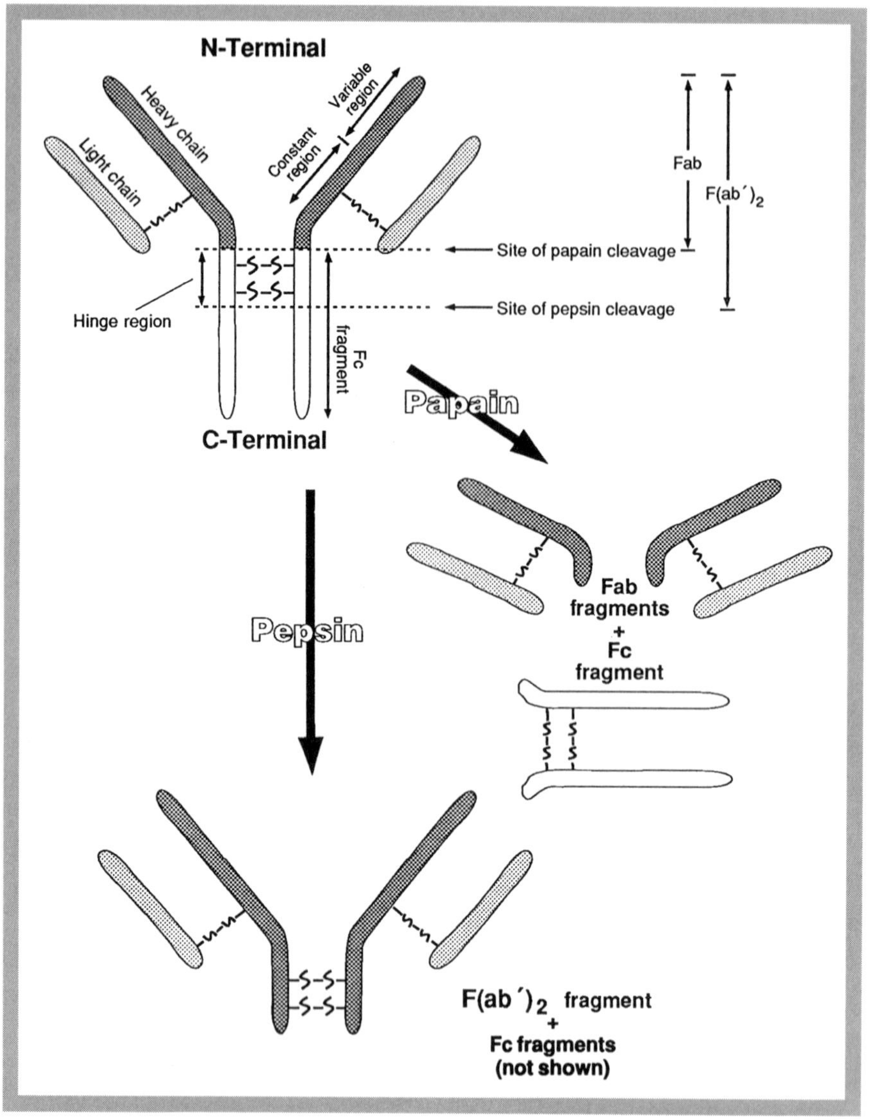

Figure 11-4. Schematic diagram of immunoglobulin molecule, with the cleavage sites for papain and pepsin for the production of Fab and F(ab´)$_2$ fragments

the means by which antibodies or antibody fragments can be generated from bacteria or plants (such as tobacco[43]) at a lower cost than that of hybridoma technology.

MOAB APPLICATIONS

Laboratory Applications

MoAbs are used in laboratories around the world on a daily basis. After technology increased their availability, they quickly became a frequently used tool for diagnosis, cell typing, drug assays, and protein purification.

Diagnostic Uses

MoAbs are employed today primarily as in vitro diagnostic reagents. Several hundred diagnostic tests have been developed and are being marketed, ranging from tests for detecting antibodies against human immunodeficiency virus type 1 (HIV-1) to over-the-counter home pregnancy tests.[44,45] Commercial MoAb diagnostic kits for use in laboratories are now available for tumor markers, pregnancy tests, and for such infectious diseases as chlamydia, herpes simplex, gonorrhea, hepatitis B, and bacterial infections.

The diagnostic use of MoAbs relies on their ability to detect the desired antigen. In general, most of the tests involve placing pure antibody in a test solution to which a sample of biologic fluid can be added. If the target antigen is present in the sample, an antibody-antigen reaction takes place. The techniques used to detect this reaction are RIA, ELISA, immunofluorescence (IF), and agglutination inhibition.

Infectious Disease Diagnosis

MoAb-based kits for detecting bacterial infections, viral infections, and fungal infections continue to be developed.[46] There are many MoAbs available against these microorganisms. Most of the currently available kits and laboratory studies use IF methods to detect antigen-antibody reactions. MoAbs directed against pathogens of sexually transmitted diseases are beginning to appear on the market for organism identification. Panels of MoAbs have been prepared that distinguish *Neisseria gonorrhea*, *Chlamydia trachomatis*, and herpes simplex viruses (HSVs) 1 and 2 from one another and from other common organisms.[46–49] Often a panel of several MoAbs directed at different antigenic components of the organism are needed in the test to capture the majority of different isolates of an organism. Each of the antibodies reacts with a single specificity to identify a particular antigenic determinant of one of the organisms. Alternatively, a single MoAb can be used, provided it binds to an antigenic site found in all of the serovars (immunotypes) of the organism.

Chlamydia trachomatis can be diagnosed by direct fluorescein-conjugated MoAbs.[50,51] The IF slide test can identify *Chlamydia trachomatis* bodies in scrapings of genital secretions and in tissue culture. The IF slide test's sensitivity and specificity of 92 and 97%, respectively, compare favorably with those of tissue cell culture techniques, which are assumed to be 100% accurate. The MoAb IF test is easier to perform, quicker, and less expensive than standard tissue culture techniques. IF slide test results are obtained in 30 minutes, whereas cell cultures take three to six days.

MoAbs are also available for detecting viral antigens.[52–56] A rapid laboratory diagnosis of cytomegalovirus (CMV) infections by a direct IF method is available.[53] The antibody produces dense IF with prominent lobular staining within the nucleus. A new diagnostic assay developed for CMV infections measures the presence of CMV-mediated early antigens in peripheral blood leukocytes during active CMV infection.[54] MoAbs and restriction endonuclease digestion have been used for distinguishing HSVs 1 and 2. Other MoAbs directed at viral antigens are being developed, including those that will be useful for screening blood to prevent hepatitis C.

A large area of diagnostic MoAb assay development has been the detection of antibodies in the serum of patients who have been exposed to HIV-1, which is responsible for the development of acquired immunodeficiency syndrome (AIDS). Most of these tests use ELISA methodology to detect the presence of anti-HIV antibodies rapidly.[56,57] The assays are being used to screen donated blood and to make initial diagnosis of HIV infections. A number of confirmation assays are being developed using MoAbs against viral elements, such as p24 core antigen. Measuring the p24 antigen also provides information about the activity of HIV.[58]

MoAbs developed for other infectious organisms raise the possibility of developing diagnostic assays for these organisms; a MoAb against *Rickettsia rickettsii* is one example.[47] MoAb immunoassays for *Plasmodium falciparum* are being examined for use to screen blood donors for malaria.[59] MoAbs are being used to detect *Pneumocystis carinii* in sputum, providing a rapid and less invasive technique for the diagnosis of *P. carinii* pneumonia. Pools of MoAbs with specificity for different viruses are used to diagnose respiratory infections, such as parainfluenza, influenza A and B, respiratory syncytial virus, and adenovirus.[60]

One of the early applications of MoAbs was in defining antigenic sites on viruses (e.g., those that cause influenza, measles, and rabies). MoAb reagents were capable of distinguishing among the strains of viruses isolated in different parts of the world. Determining the differences and similarities of viral epitopes will lead to better vaccines. These studies on viruses, as well as studies on bacteria and parasites, will have implications for the diagnostic use of MoAbs. Most importantly, information on common antigenic structures of microorganisms allows for improved sensitivity of diagnostic tests in this era of world travel.

The largest market for MoAb use is currently the self-care market. The number of MoAb home testing kits used as diagnostic aids has rapidly increased, largely because of advances in MoAb technology.

Pregnancy Tests

The first publicly available MoAbs were developed for pregnancy testing. Many companies are now manufacturing MoAb diagnostic assays for pregnancy and for ovulation.[45] Home pregnancy tests detect human chorionic gonadotrophin (HCG) in the patient's urine. Most older pregnancy tests used polyclonal antibodies of animal origin. These antibodies could interact with hormones and/or drugs and result in a false-positive reaction. Consequently, pregnancy kits using polyclonal antibodies were removed from the market in November 1992. The newer pregnancy kits use MoAbs that bind specifically with the β subunit of HCG. These kits use enzyme assays that result in a color change indicating a positive result, and they are unaffected by other hormones, drugs, vibration, or sunlight. The manufacturers of these kits report 99% accuracy with positive results, and some can be read within a minute after use.[61]

Ovulation Tests

Being able to predict ovulation allows a woman to identify the time during her menstrual cycle when she is fertile. This ability facilitates conception by enabling intercourse, intrauterine insemination, or in vitro fertilization to be optimally timed. MoAb-based tests are available to detect the surge in luteinizing hormone (LH) that precedes ovulation.[61] Because MoAbs used in these tests are specific for the β subunit of the LH molecule, cross-reactivity with other hormones is unlikely. A number of test kits are available that use ELISA.

The MoAb ovulation tests offer semiquantitative determinations of the LH level in the urine. Testing of the morning urine starts in advance of likely ovulation and is continued daily until ovulation occurs, as indicated by an increase in color intensity. Some kits include a dipstick coated with an antibody directed at the α subunit of LH and a test solution that contains a MoAb-enzyme complex specific for the β subunit of LH. If LH is present in the added urine, the α subunit of LH binds to the dipstick. The test solution, which recognizes the β subunit of the bound LH, is then added, forming a sandwich-like complex on the dipstick. After the dipstick has been rinsed, a color substrate in the test kit is added that reacts with the enzyme bound to the stick, imparting a blue color. The intensity of the blue color reflects the amount of LH in the urine sample. A kit contains either six or nine tests. The prediction rate of ovulation increases with the number of tests performed. The results of these tests can be affected by administration of exogenous hormones (estrogen-progestin combinations), which can alter LH contained in the menotropins, and by the administration of danazol, which suppresses LH production.[61]

Oncologic Diagnosis

Much of the work with MoAbs originated to diagnose, image, and treat cancers. In recent years, immunocytochemical techniques have been increasingly used to study the surface antigens of malignant cells. These studies have provided information on cell populations and their differentiation, and these techniques are extremely valuable in diagnosing and classifying hematologic malignancies.

MoAbs may be used as reagents for the immunochemical staining and diagnosis of neoplasms in pathologic specimens. Specific tumors shed characteristic antigens into the host circulation (see chapter 10). These tumor-associated antigens (TAAs) may allow for relatively noninvasive early detection of the cancer. Four recognized TAAs with widespread clinical applications are alpha-fetoprotein (AFP), HCG, carcinoembryonic antigen (CEA), and prostate-specific antigen (PSA). AFP and HCG are important markers for detecting and monitoring nonseminomatous germ cell tumors. Serum elevations of CEA are caused primarily by colon and gastrointestinal carcinomas. An elevated PSA level is a good marker of prostate cancer. Other anti-TAA MoAbs are being tested for potential applications.[62–64] A drawback to the clinical application of some of these MoAbs is their potential cross-reactivity with similar antigens found on normal cells. Continued research will lead to the development of MoAbs of greater specificity, resulting in improved tumor detection and fewer cross-reactions with normal tissues and, thus, an increased efficiency of these MoAbs for early detection of cancer.

Cell and Tissue Typing

There are more than 300 antigenic determinants on the surface of the human RBC membrane. These antigens, which are genetically linked, are grouped together to form the blood group systems. The term blood type refers to the antigenic phenotype, which is the serologic expression of the inherited blood group genes. Twenty-one blood groups are currently recognized. The antigens were first recognized by the analysis of the alloantibodies produced as a result of transfusions or pregnancy. Blood typing is important for avoiding the transfusion of antigen-incompatible blood and the early detection and prevention of hemolytic disease of the newborn.

MoAbs are used to study the function and structures of these antigens. MoAbs directed at blood groups A and B have been produced by hybridoma techniques.[65] Other blood group antigens have been isolated and studied; purified sources are relatively abundant. MoAb affinity chromatography can be used to purify the antigens, and the antigens can then be used to further immunize mice to produce reagents for blood typing. One role of MoAbs is to provide unlimited quantities of reagents for blood bank typing.

MoAbs have long been available for detecting the presence of Rh factors. One product detects the presence of anti-Rh factors. The antibody can be used to determine whether the pregnant woman has potentially dangerous Rh antibodies against an Rh^+ fetus. The antibody may also be administered prophylactically to an Rh^- woman who is carrying an Rh^+ fetus to avoid the risk of hemolytic anemia in the newborn.[2]

As a research tool, MoAbs have been invaluable in identifying human lymphocyte subpopulations.[66] MoAbs have enhanced our understanding of the structures and functions of the subclasses of both B and T lymphocytes. MoAbs are commonly used to identify subpopulations of T lymphocytes. Lymphocytes were found to possess numerous types of cell surface proteins, which were termed "clusters of differentiation" (CD). MoAbs specific to different types of cell surface proteins on lymphocytes have further elucidated the function of specific lymphocyte subsets. The OKT (Ortho) series of MoAbs was first developed by Reinherz, Kung, and Goldstein.[67] OKT antibodies recognize antigens on the surface of T lymphocytes. Mature T cells are detected by the MoAb OKT3, which recognizes the CD3 antigen. An anti-CD4 MoAb primarily binds helper/inducer T cells at the CD4 antigen, and an anti-CD8 MoAb binds cytotoxic/suppressor T cells at the CD8 antigen. Other MoAbs may bind tissues and cells other than T cells.

MoAbs can be used to determine the proportions and absolute numbers of T cells and T-cell subsets. The ratio of helper/inducer T cells to cytotoxic/suppressor T cells ($CD4^+/CD8^+$ ratio) in peripheral blood is significant in many disease states. For example, $CD4^+/CD8^+$ ratio is helpful in the diagnosis of immunodeficiency syndromes, such as AIDS. In patients with AIDS, the number of helper T cells in circulation is diminished. The diagnosis of AIDS can be made with a $CD4^+$ count of less than 200 cells/mm^3 or when the percentage of $CD4^+$ lymphocytes is less than 14% in patients known to be infected with HIV.[68] The absolute number of $CD4^+$ cells/mm^3 in AIDS patients can help clinicians predict what type of opportunistic infections are most likely and also provides information that can optimize the timing of prophylactic drug therapy. The ratios and/or absolute number of $CD4^+$ and $CD8^+$ cells are also altered in a number of other disease processes, such as infectious diseases, autoimmune diseases, allergies, aging, and transplantation.

MoAbs for Tissue Typing

The importance of identifying surface proteins on cells that play a major role in the acceptance or rejection of transplanted tissues has been known for some time. MoAbs can be used to define these molecules and their roles in graft tolerance. MoAbs, through their use in phenotyping of normal cells (such as lymphocytes) within the body, will help identify the roles that these cells play in homeostasis.

Human leukocyte antigens (HLAs) are important in the transplantation of organs, tissues, and bone marrow (see chapter 3).[69] The HLA complex is located on chromosome 6 of the human major histocompatibility complex (MHC) and is responsible for encoding self antigens. Tissue typing to determine HLAs can help to increase the chances of tissue engraftment and organ acceptance.

The HLAs were among the first human structures recognized by MoAbs. Many reagents have since been produced for recognizing HLAs. MoAbs to these antigens have given immunologists tools to analyze the structure, function, and role of the HLAs in diseases.[69] The role of MoAbs used for HLA typing is well established. Typically, anti-HLA antibodies that bind complement are used in these assays, and they identify the lysis of cells as their end point. However, newer technology (e.g., polymerase chain reaction [PCR]) is beginning to be used for HLA typing of transplant patients.

MoAbs are also useful for classifying leukemias and lymphomas based on their surface proteins. The antibody reagents can distinguish between T- and B-cell leukemia and can also provide information on T-cell malignancies. T-cell malignancies of early differentiation express CD10, CD9, or both, whereas more mature T-cell malignancies, such as cutaneous T-cell lymphomas, express CD4. The type of acute lymphocytic leukemia may also be determined by MoAbs. Analysis of different types of leukemias and lymphomas allow drug therapy to be optimized for individual patients.

Drug Assays

A number of standard laboratory methods have been developed for measuring drug concentrations: high-performance liquid chromatography, RIAs, and enzyme-multiplied immunoassay technique. MoAbs are valuable tools for drug assays. MoAb-based assays are very specific and highly sensitive. They are currently used to detect digoxin, phenobarbital, theophylline, and many other drugs. The use of MoAbs in drug assays has opened the door to home testing of serum and saliva drug levels. A number of kits are now available for office use by physicians to monitor drug therapy. These office kits are similar to the quantitative immunoassays used in many laboratories. MoAbs for different drugs are replacing many of the polyclonal reagents formerly used in larger drug-assaying systems.[70]

Protein Purification

Specific MoAbs make excellent reagents and biologic tools for assaying, purifying, and detecting proteins. As research tools, MoAbs can recognize specific amino acid sequences of polypeptides. MoAbs and DNA techniques have been used to define regions of immunogenic determinants on a protein and to elucidate the essential amino acid sequences that can serve as synthetic vaccines. MoAbs have been used to sort out cells with selected surface-binding proteins. Hematopoetic progenitor and stems cells used for bone marrow transplantation can be collected by passing blood through a column coated with antibodies to CD34. After treatment, the CD34^{+} cells are then injected back into the patient. They are also used to purify protein molecules. MoAbs can be placed on an affinity column; mixtures containing the target protein are then passed through the column. The desired protein molecule binds specifically to the MoAb while the impurities are washed through. The protein may then be isolated from the column. Many proteins, including AFP and interferons, can be purified by means of MoAbs.[71,72] This procedure is also used to purify factor VIII.

In Vivo Applications of MoAbs

Considerable MoAb antibody research has been directed at therapeutic uses in vivo for an expanding number of applications. For years investigators have attempted to use MoAbs as therapy for diverse human diseases, including cardiac, liver, and renal allograft failure; cancer diagnosis and therapy; graft-versus-host disease (GVHD); infections; coronary artery disease and infarction; and a number of autoimmune diseases. The therapeutic use of MoAbs in oncology has been studied extensively but has resulted in only limited success. In contrast, MoAb therapy to modulate the immune system in organ transplantation has resulted in considerable progress. The following discussion is not intended to summarize the hundreds of clinical studies reported; it reviews approaches taken with MoAbs to treat and diagnose diseases, the obstacles associated with their use, and areas where rapid progress is being made. Table 11-1 is a list of MoAbs that are on the market or have been named by the United States Adopted Names (USAN) Council.[3,73]

The USAN Council has developed guidelines for nonproprietary naming of MoAbs that provides information about them. First, MoAbs and fragments end in the suffix *-mab*. Second, there is a single letter to indicate the animal source, for safety reasons. They are as follows: *u*, human; *o*, mouse; *a*, rat; *e*, hamster; *i*, primate; and *xi* = chimera. The appropriate letter immediately precedes the suffix (i.e., *-umab* [human], *-omab* [mouse], *-ximab* [chimera]). Third, a single syllable describing the disease or subclass is incorporated into the name. The USAN Council has currently approved the following syllables: *-vir-*, viral; *-bac-*, bacterial; *-lim-*, immune (immunomodulator); *-cir-*, cardiovascular; and for tumors by subclass, *-col-*, colon; *-mel-*, melanoma; *-mar-*, mammary; *-pr(o)-*, prostate;

Table 11-1. MoAb Names Adopted by the USAN Council[3]

USAN (Trademarked name)	MANUFACTURER	THERAPEUTIC USE
Antiendotoxins		
Edobacomab (E5)	Xoma	Treatment of gram-negative sepsis/shock
Nebacumab (Centoxin)	Centocor	Treatment of gram-negative sepsis/shock
Antifibrin		
Technetium Tc 99m biciromab (Fibriscint)	Centocor	Diagnosis of deep vein thrombosis
Antimyosin		
Indium In 111 imciromab pentetate (Myoscint)	Centocor	Cardiac imaging agent
Antithrombotic		
Abciximab (ReoPro)	Eli Lilly	Decrease restenosis after angioplasty
Antiviral		
Sevirumab	Sandoz	Anti-CMV
Tuvirumab	Sandoz	Anti-HBV
Immunosuppressant		
Dacliximab (Zenapax)	Hoffmann-LaRoche	Anti-interleukin 2 antibody to reverse allograft rejection
Muromonab-CD3 (Orthoclone OKT3)	Ortho	Anti-CD3 antibody to prevent or reverse allograft rejection
Zolimomab aritox (Orthozyme CD5 Plus)	Xoma	Anti-CD5 antibody immunotoxin to reverse allograft rejection
Oncology		
Capromab pendetide	Cytogen	Anti-prostate carcinoma cell
Votumumab (OncoSPECT)	PerImmune	Anti-human carcinoma-associated antigen
Indium In 111 satumomab pendetide (OncoScint CR/OV)	Cytogen	Radiodiagnostic for ovarian and colorectal carcinoma
Indium In 111 altumomab pentetate (Hybri-CEAker)	Hybritech	Radiodiagnostic for tumors expressing carcinoembryonic antigen

MoAb, monoclonal antibody; USAN, United States Adopted Name; CMV, cytomegalovirus; HBV, hepatitis B virus.

-got-, testis; *-gov-*, ovarian; *-tum-*, miscellaneous. Fourth, a distinct syllable is selected as a prefix to create a unique name. The order is as follows: the unique prefix, target disease state, animal source, and the monoclonal root *-mab* (e.g., biciromab, satumomab, nebacumab, sevirumab). Separate words are added if the product is radiolabeled or conjugated to another chemical. Radiolabeled products name the isotope, the element symbol, and isotope number, followed by the name of the MoAb (e.g., technetium Tc 99m biciromab). MoAbs conjugated to toxins must contain *tox* as part of the name selected for the toxin (i.e., Zolimomab aritox). Finally, a separate name must be given to any linker or chelator used to connect a radioisotope or toxin to the MoAb (e.g., indium In 111 altumomab pentetate).[3,73]

Imaging

MoAbs have proven useful in vitro as diagnostic assays for drugs, infections, and diseases. The in vivo use of MoAbs for imaging is a powerful application as well. MoAbs may be covalently linked with radioisotopes or contrast agents for in vivo administration, for ex vivo detection by a gamma camera, or for a magnetic resonance imaging (MRI) scanner to localize damaged tissues or tumors.[74–76] Imaging with labeled MoAbs provides useful information regarding differential diagnosis, extent of disease or damage, and the progression or resolution of the disease. Initial applications of MoAb-targeted imaging have been mainly in oncology, cardiology, and infectious diseases.

The successful use of MoAb-targeted imaging must overcome several limitations.[77] Potential sources of problems include background interference or trapping of conjugated MoAbs, the type of ligands or coupling techniques needed to attach the dye or radioisotope to the MoAbs, the type of imaging material, and the pharmacokinetics of the MoAbs and imaging agents. The trapping or nonspecific binding of the conjugated MoAb is important for the resolution and specificity of the image. Trapping and nonspecific binding can occur during the initial infusion, as the body breaks down the bonds between the conjugated isotope and MoAbs, and as the MoAb is cleared. This trapping can increase the background interference or decrease the resolution of the image. Careful selection of the MoAb and type of ligand to strengthen the bonds between antibody and isotope can minimize this limitation.

The choice of isotope is important to optimize tumor visualization while exposing the patient's healthy tissues to the least amount of damaging radiation. Isotopes with a short half life (hours to days) are ideal for in vivo imaging to decrease the time of radiation exposure. However, fresh isotopes have to be coupled to the antibody before every treatment. Current methods employ conjugation of a chelating agent, such as diethylenetriamine penta-acetic acid, to the antibody.[78,79] The chelated antibody conjugate is stable and can be stored for long periods without loss of activity.[80] The radioisotope conjugate is formed by adding the radioisotope to the chelated antibody, resulting in a very tight covalent bond. Activation can be performed with a freshly generated isotope shortly before treatment.

For imaging purposes, ideal radioisotopes not only have short half-lives but also emit gamma rays that exit the body and can easily be detected ex vivo. The choice of conjugated isotope determines the type of equipment needed to visualize the image.[81,82] Previously, most MoAbs were linked to indium-111 (^{111}In), but there is increasing use of technetium-99m (^{99m}Tc) due to new chelation and linkage chemistries. ^{99m}Tc's main advantages are that most gamma cameras are calibrated in the photon range of ^{99m}Tc, and it is less expensive than other radioisotopes. However, the relatively short half-life of ^{99m}Tc (six hours) versus the longer half-life of ^{111}In (2.7 days) is a disadvantage because it does not permit imaging over a longer period. ^{99m}Tc-labeled MoAbs have been able to provide clear images without background interference in about three hours. Another quality desired in an isotope is ease of attachment to MoAbs. Iodine compounds (^{123}I, ^{131}I) have this characteristic. Although ^{131}I is an inexpensive radioisotope and is easy to complex with MoAbs, it has poor emission characteristics. In addition, isotopes that emit alpha and/or beta radiation, such as ^{131}I, are usually reserved for treatment rather than pure imaging because the massive particles emitted induce local radiation-mediated cellular toxicity. The emission characteristics and a list of advantages and disadvantages of ^{99m}Tc, ^{111}In, ^{123}I, and ^{131}I are provided in Table 11-2.[83]

Table 11-2. Radioisotopes Used for Imaging Studies

ISOTOPE	ENERGY (KeV)	HALF-LIFE	ADVANTAGES	DISADVANTAGES
^{99m}Tc	140	6 hr	Pure gamma radiation Inexpensive High photon flux	Complex chemistry Short half-life Relatively high counts in kidney and bladder Affinity for liver and RES
^{111}In	173[a] 247[a]	3 days	Pure gamma radiation Delayed imaging possible	Affinity for liver and RES
^{123}I	159	13 hr	Pure gamma radiation Ease of labeling	Dehalogenates Produced by cyclotron Expensive
^{131}I	364	8.05 days	Ease of labeling	Dehalogenates Low counts High radiation due to beta radiation and long half-life

RES, reticuloendothelial system.
[a]Particles given off at two levels of energy.

SOURCE: *Reprinted with permission from Serafini AN. From monoclonal antibodies to peptides and molecular recognition units: an overview.* J Nucl Med. *1993;34:533–6.*

The form of antibody may also be important.[84] Antibody fragments used in imaging have several potential advantages over intact antibodies. Indeed, fragments [such as Fab and $F(ab')_2$] are cleared from the blood substantially faster than the whole antibody.[40,85–87] Such rapid clearance eliminates the blood pool background for imaging and reduces the toxicity of therapy.[88] The lack of Fc receptor in fragments should eliminate nonspecific uptake by the reticuloendothelial system and entrapment in highly vascular organs. Their smaller size also facilitates more rapid diffusion out of the vascular space and might make them less immunogenic. Most studies with radioisotope conjugates have been done with intact MoAbs. The theoretical advantages of fragment conjugates are only beginning to be explored.

Cardiac imaging techniques with MoAbs have arisen from the development of antibodies to thrombus, fibrin, and myosin.[76] Cardiac myosin can be detected after cardiac injury and cellular death. The antimyosin MoAbs and MoAb fragments have been labeled with either ^{99m}Tc or ^{111}In to detect zones of acute myocardial necrosis and to determine the size of the infarction. Centocor's ^{111}In-labeled antimyosin product (Myoscint® [Imciromab]) currently has orphan drug approval.[89]

Clinical trials note that overall sensitivity for the diagnosis of acute infarction has been greater than 90% with little or no localization of the antibodies in regions of previous infarctions.[90,91] A diagnostic scan with ^{111}In-labeled antimyosin Fab antibodies can provide a diagnosis of subacute as well as acute myocardial necrosis.[92] The antimyosin MoAb-labeled imaging tool is useful in differentiating between severe ischemia and irreversible necrosis. Other trials are under way to yield a noninvasive approach to the diagnosis of myocarditis or cardiomyopathy.[93]

Antifibrin MoAbs[94,95] and antiplatelet MoAbs[96,97] are useful in delineating thrombi in both arteries and veins, and they are under investigation for detecting deep venous thrombosis[98] and thrombi in organs with high blood pool activity.[99] The choices of (1) antiplatelet or antifibrin MoAb, (2) types of antibody fragments, and (3) radionucleotide are still controversial. Antibodies have been suitable for imaging thrombus. Labeled Fab fragments are more advantageous than whole molecules because their lower molecular weight improves antibody penetration into the thrombus. Absence of the Fc portion decreases immune reaction and improves clearance of these antibodies. Future applications of these antibodies might include early detection of atherosclerotic plaque, monitoring of clot resolution after therapy with thrombolytics, and other noninvasive imaging techniques.

The use of antibodies in tumor imaging is not a new concept. Isotope-labeled polyclonal antibodies have been used in the past to visualize and localize tumors.[100] Progress in directing MoAbs to specific cell surface antigens on tumors should make it possible to use radiolabeled MoAbs to define tumor location, size, and extent.[100,101] Periodic injections of isotope-labeled MoAbs could provide information on the progression of the disease and the effectiveness of treatment. A number of MoAbs and MoAb fragments, primarily labeled with ^{111}In or ^{99m}Tc, are undergoing clinical trials in this country. The available MoAbs used for imaging are directed at melanomas and ovarian, breast, colon, and lung cancers.[40,102–107] The Food and Drug Administration (FDA) has approved indium In 111 satumomab pendetide (OncoScint CR/OV®, Cytogen) for imaging colorectal and ovarian cancers.[108] OncoScint CR/OV® targets TAG-72, an antigen expressed on the majority of adenocarcinomas. Other MoAbs that target malignancies, such as neuroblastoma, lymphoma, and ovarian, prostate, pancreatic, and gastrointestinal tumors, are being studied.[102,108–113]

In vivo imaging with MoAbs is the first step in developing antibodies for cancer therapy. The imaging tool allows investigators to determine the specificity of the MoAb for the intended tumor antigen and to overcome some of the limitations of in vivo use before using MoAbs that carry potentially harmful, highly active radioisotopes or cytotoxic ligands. Because the majority of these antibodies are murine-based products, a HAMA response can occur, which would contraindicate readministration.

The possible applications of MoAbs in the imaging of infectious diseases are numerous. Many MoAbs are already available that are directed toward different types of microorganisms. Current interest is in the imaging of deep-seated infections. Such imaging would allow the infection's location to be identified and might also allow the organism or organisms to be identified without invasive surgical procedures.[114]

Initial trials have determined the relative safety of these radiolabeled MoAbs; essentially no adverse reactions or toxicities have been observed. Further trials are under way to assess the efficacy of the labeled MoAbs in detection of tumors, and to determine the optimum dose, and generate data about biodistribution, clearance, and image enhancement.[101,115–117] Further trials are under way to compare results with MoAbs to those obtained by surgery or biopsy to identify persistent or metastatic disease.[118,119] Such imaging scans may eventually eliminate the need for exploratory surgery or help oncologists determine prognosis and plans for additional medical treatments. Concerns remain about the binding of the MoAbs to normal tissues and nonspecific organ distribution (primarily in the liver, spleen, kidneys, and the highly vascularized tissues) as well as lack of consistent binding to known tumor. This lack of consistent binding, which must be addressed before development and release of MoAbs for imaging purposes, occurs because the specific conjugation of MoAbs to isotopes can change the binding affinity of the antibody and/or the pharmacokinetics of either the MoAb or the isotope alone. Routine clinical use of MoAbs or MoAb fragments will improve with better conjugation methods and better choices of antibodies and isotopes for the desired application.

Therapeutic Uses

In vivo use of MoAbs for therapy currently involves a number of general strategies, including the application of MoAbs for (1) direct immunologic destruction of specified cells, (2) targeting molecules that are critical for growth or differentiation of specific cells, and (3) delivering therapeutic agents to specific tissues. The potential therapeutic applications in transplantation, cardiology, oncology, autoimmune disorders, toxin reversal, and infectious disease are discussed.

The choice of MoAb depends on a number of factors that may have an impact on their biodistribution, their ability to bind antigen, and their ability to elicit some therapeutic effect. One selection factor is the antibody class type (e.g., IgG versus IgM) and subclass (e.g., IgG2a versus IgG3). Because they cannot fix human complement, most murine MoAbs do not have the potential to kill tumor cells in the presence of either immune cells or complement. Certain subclasses of murine MoAbs, such as IgM and IgG3, can fix complement, however. The use of human or humanized MoAbs may overcome these limitations. Another selection factor is whether the MoAb should be used as a whole molecule or digested into fragments, such as Fab or $F(ab')_2$. Smaller proteins have better tissue penetration, but removal of the Fc portion eliminates the effector function of the MoAb. Finally, the antibody should be selected for its avidity to the target antigen, thus determining its degree of binding.[8]

Transplantation

Although the early focus of MoAb research was on cancer immunotherapy, the use of MoAbs in transplantation has been more successful. The clinical application guidelines of immunosuppressive therapy with OKT3[120] for the prophylaxis and treatment of transplant rejection is discussed in depth in chapter 8. In summary, the murine MoAb OKT3, which is reactive for the CD3 surface antigen of T lymphocytes, has proven effective in managing organ transplant rejection and preventing rejection in renal, renal-pancreatic, liver, and cardiac transplantation. Ortho's OKT3 (Muromonab-CD3®) is the only anti-CD3 MoAb that is commercially available; however, other anti-CD3 antibodies (e.g.,WT32 and 64.1) have been tested with positive results as well.[121]

Because T-cell stimulation and clonal proliferation require several surface protein receptor interactions, MoAbs have been developed against these receptors. Trials have been performed with antibodies against CD45, CD4, interleukin 2 (IL-2) receptor, CD11a, T-cell receptor (TCR), CD18, B7, and CD28. In addition, MoAbs designed to bind cytokines, such as IL-1 and TNF, have also undergone evaluation.[121] Because allograft rejection can be due to T or B cells, diagnostic procedures on biopsy specimens can indicate which cells should be targeted to reverse the rejection episode. MoAbs and immunotoxins directed at these pathogenic cells have proven very effective in reversing rejection episodes.

Initially, the goal of therapy was to remove all the T cells or make them nonfunctional; however, the realization that T-cell stimulation requires two signals redefines these goals. Blocking a signal can produce antigen-specific anergy and leave most T cells fully functional. The first T-cell signal occurs with the binding of the TCR to the MHC-antigen complex presented by an antigen-presenting cell (APC). The second signal occurs when CD28 is stimulated by its ligand, B7. MoAbs to CD28 or B7 can prevent the second signal. T cells that receive the first signal but not the second become nonfunctional and cannot be stimulated. In animal transplant models, antibodies that block the second signal given concurrently with donor-specific transfusions have been able to induce antigen-specific anergy that lasted over 100 days.[122] Antibodies that inhibit CD28 stimulation are beginning to be evaluated in humans.

Cardiac Disease

The therapeutic role of MoAbs in cardiovascular medicine is growing.[123] MoAbs may play a role in prophylactic prevention of thrombosis or as fibrinolytic or antithrombotic agents. Recently, abciximab (c7E3 Fab) was approved by the FDA to prevent ischemic complications after angioplasty.[124] Other applications of MoAbs being explored include detecting intravascular thrombi and targeting fibrinolysis by means of a fibrin-specific antibody-urokinase complex.[125]

Abciximab is a chimeric human-murine MoAb Fab that binds to the platelet glycoprotein IIb/IIIa receptor. Binding to this receptor provides it with greater antithrombotic effects than aspirin or heparin in animal models. It decreases ischemic complications during the first 30 postoperative days by 35% following coronary angioplasty or artherectomy in high-risk patients. It also reduces the incidence of restenosis during the first six months (27% in abciximab patients versus 35% in placebo patients).

Unbound abciximab is rapidly cleared from the circulation, but the platelet-bound portion can circulate for several days. As would be predicted, the humanized Fab fragment has low immunogenicity. Only 6% of patients form an antibody response to the drug. In general, abciximab is well tolerated; the only major side effect is bleeding complications (14% in abciximab patients versus 7% in placebo patients).

Fibrin-specific MoAbs are being developed to target thrombi (as discussed in the imaging section). A further application is to couple the MoAbs to streptokinase, urokinase, or tissue plasminogen activator.[126] Urokinase has been coupled to the fibrin-specific MoAb 64C5. In an in vitro fibrinolytic assay, the MoAb conjugate with urokinase increased the efficiency of plasmin lysis 100-fold. If these effects can be demonstrated in vivo, the dose of urokinase required for effective lysis of a thrombus will result in only minimal fibrinogenolysis, the major impediment to widespread application of this form of therapy.

One of the most widely used drugs in cardiac therapy is digoxin; however, digitalis intoxication is also one of the most frequently reported adverse drug reactions. Management of digitalis overdose has traditionally consisted of supportive measures. The use of digoxin-specific polyclonal antibodies in treating digoxin overdose is an established therapeutic alternative.[127] Digoxin-specific polyclonal antibodies have been prepared from sheep, and digoxin-immune Fab fragments are now available to treat digoxin or digitoxin intoxication. The digoxin-immune Fab fragment (Digibind® [Glaxo Wellcome]) is prepared from antibodies produced by sheep in response to immunization with a digoxin-albumin conjugate. The polyclonal antibodies are digested with papain and purified to produce the digoxin-specific Fab fragment. The Fab fragment is used because the goal of therapy is to bind the drug, inactivating it. The constant portion of the immunoglobulin, which contains the Fc receptor, is discarded. The Fab has a number of desirable properties over an intact molecule. Because of their smaller molecular size, Fab molecules may be distributed more quickly and in larger volumes and possess a shorter half-life; when administered intravenously, Fab particles are probably less antigenic than whole molecules.[128]

Oncology

Oncology is an area of vigorous MoAb research. In general, the research has been clinically disappointing. However, it has helped identify problems with MoAb therapy and challenged researchers to invent new methods to overcome obstacles. This section will discuss different approaches, drawbacks, and new methods of MoAb applications to oncology. A more comprehensive list of clinical studies and their results are reviewed elsewhere.[121]

Tumor cells express a number of surface antigens that are relatively specific for the neoplasm. MoAbs have been developed against a variety of these TAAs.[129–131] The MoAbs have been used as a single entity or labeled with radioactive isotopes, toxins, or chemotherapeutic agents. These trials are providing useful information on MoAbs, their relative specificity, pharmacokinetics, adverse reactions, efficacy, and possible limitations for wide clinical applications.[121,132]

Early trials using MoAbs to treat cancer involved the application of unconjugated whole antibodies. Studies in animal tumor models have demonstrated that passive administration of unmodified MoAbs can prevent tumor growth and lead to the regression of some established tumors.[133,134] The antitumor effects are believed to be mediated by host immune mechanisms involving the direct killing of tumor cells by complement activation or opsonization and elimination or MoAb-directed killing of target cells by immune effector cells (antibody-dependent cell-mediated cytotoxicity) (Figure 11-5). Immune effector cells include killer cells, natural killer cells, macrophages, and neutrophils. Another possible mechanism of the antitumor effects of MoAbs is the direct binding to or blockage of a vital growth receptor on tumor cells. Finally, the MoAbs may indirectly stimulate the production of host antibody against tumor antigens.

Many different growth factors (e.g., colony-stimulating factors and interleukins) are responsible for the growth and differentiation of cells (see chapter 2). Tumor cells seem to be immortal and may be stimulated by some autostimulatory growth factors. MoAbs directed at these factors or their receptors may interrupt the growth of the tumor.[135–137]

A number of factors must be considered when tumor antigens and appropriate MoAbs are selected. A prerequisite for tumor targeting is to select MoAbs that react

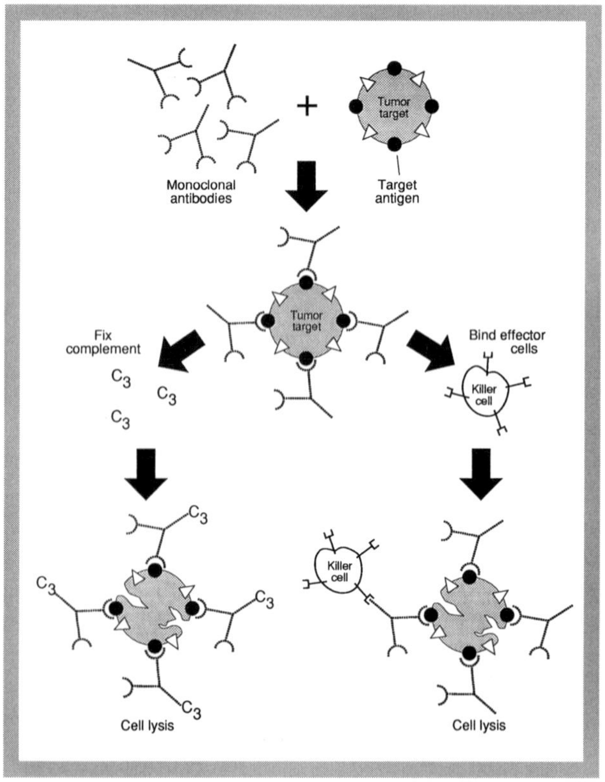

Figure 11-5. Antibody-dependent cellular cytotoxicity

SOURCE: *Adapted with permission from Lowder JN. The current status of monoclonal antibodies in the diagnosis and therapy of cancer.* Current Problems in Cancer *1986;10:503.*

specifically with antigens present in high levels on tumor cells but not expressed on most normal tissues. Specificity is a critical feature for potential applications of MoAbs. However, absolute specificity is neither necessary nor always desired. Specificity limited to one particular antigen may limit the application of the MoAb for treatment of other patients who have the same type of tumor but lack that specific antigen.

The ideal MoAb for in vivo treatment would target an antigen expressed exclusively on the surface of tumor cells, in high density, in both primary and metastatic lesions. The antigen would be neither secreted nor shed from the cell surface and would not modulate. In contrast, shedding and secretion of tumor antigen is desirable in diagnostic applications where it makes serum monitoring easier.

Some murine MoAbs have already undergone phase I or II trials to determine dosing, adverse effects, and host response. Some of the MoAbs used and responses to them are listed in Table 11-3. The early trials concentrated on treating leukemia, lymphoma, melanoma, and gastrointestinal carcinomas. Although some therapeutic responses with MoAbs used for immunocytotoxic effects in therapy have been reported, virtually all responses have been transient.[138] Several of the studies confirmed the binding of antibodies to malignant cells in the circulation, bone marrow, lymph nodes, and cutaneous skin nodules sites.[139]

Rather than target a general TAA, an alternative approach that creates a MoAb that recognizes the idiotypic region of a specific patient's B-cell lymphoma has been tried (Figure 11-6). This MoAb, or anti-idiotype antibody, is specific for the variable region of the surface immunoglobulin on the lymphoma cells of that patient. Anti-idiotype antibody therapy has been tried in a number of clinical trials for the treatment of B-cell lymphoma.[140] A recent trial used patient-specific anti-idiotype antibodies in combination with interferon alpha (IFN-α) in an attempt to improve the therapeutic outcome.[141] IFN-α can increase expression of some TAAs and has a different mechanism of action than the MoAbs that augment their activity. Other cytokines, such as interleukin 2 and granulocyte-macrophage colony-stimulating factor, have also been used with MoAbs to generate TAAs in an attempt to increase efficacy.[45,142–145] In general, response rates were low, and those who did respond quickly relapsed. The best response rate was reported with the use of patient-specific MoAbs and IFN-α, which resulted in a response in 8 of 11 patients and a long-lasting, complete response in 3 patients. Although this one small study reported a good response rate, the amount of work required to design patient-specific MoAbs limits the utility of this treatment.

A phase I study evaluating a murine MoAb to treat chronic lymphocytic leukemia (CLL) evaluated toxicity based on dose received and duration of infusion. In general, toxicity was minimal with lower doses and slower infusion rates but increased with higher doses and/or fast infusion rates. Patients receiving the murine MoAb at infusion rates above 5–10 mg experienced pulmonary toxicity manifested as dyspnea and wheezing. The cause of the dyspnea appears to be associated

Table 11-3. Results of Clinical Trials with MoAbs Against Human Tumors

TUMOR	MoAb/CLASS	EVALUABLE PATIENTS	RESPONSE
ALL	J5	4	0/4
T-ALL	Leu-1, others	6	1/6
AML	Several	3	0/3
CLL	T101/IgG2a	23	2/23
CTCL	T101/IgG2a, Leu-1	35	15/35
CTCL	^{131}I-T101	6	6/6
T cell	T101	5	1/5
B lymphoma	Anti-idiotype	10	5/10
	^{131}I-MB-1/IgG1	2	2/2
	AB89	1	0/1
Ovarian (IP)	^{131}I-HMFG1, -HMFG2, -AUAI, -H17E2	24	8/24
GI	17-1A/IgG2a	40	5/40
Melanoma	R24/IgG3	21	6/21
	96.5-RTA/IgG2a (ricin)	22	5/22
	96.5/IgG2a	5	0/5
	9.2.27/IgG2a	8	0/8
	48.7/IgG1	4	0/4

ALL, acute lymphocytic leukemia; T-ALL, T-cell lymphocytic leukemia; AML, acute myelogenous leukemia; CLL, chronic lymphocytic leukemia; CTCL, cutaneous T-cell lymphoma; IP, intraperitoneal; GI, gastrointestinal.

SOURCE: *Adapted with permission from Scheinberg DA, Houghton AN. Current status of antitumor therapy with monoclonal antibodies.* Oncology *1987;1:34.*

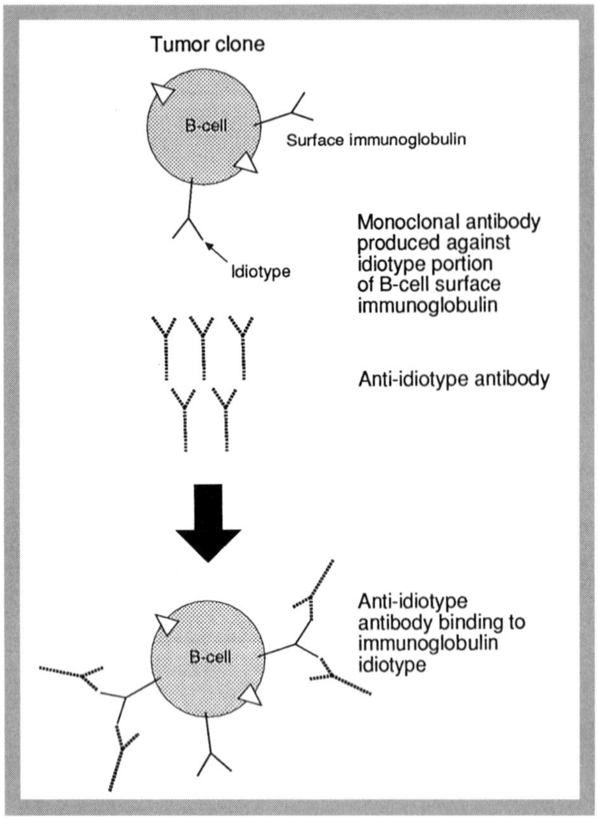

Figure 11-6. Antibodies directed against surface immunoglobulin of neoplastic B-cell lymphomas—"anti-idiotype antibodies"

with leukoagglutination and trapping in the lungs after antibody therapy.[146] Some of the more frequent toxicities observed with unmodified MoAbs were chills, fevers, flushing, urticaria, headaches, rigors, myalgias, pruritus, dyspnea, wheezing, nausea, vomiting, diarrhea, hypotension, and facial edema; rare toxicities included anaphylactic reactions, serum sickness, and facial palsy.[146,147] Tumor lysis, cytokine release, and/or a HAMA response may be responsible for many adverse effects. Pretreatment with different combinations of acetaminophen, diphenhydramine, meperidine, and prochlorperazine have been used to alleviate specific problems.[146–148] Immunosuppressive agents, such as cyclosporine, have also been employed to decrease these toxicities.

A number of phenomena identified in these trials may be responsible for decreasing MoAb activity. First, because these trials used murine MoAbs, the body could recognize these proteins as foreign and make its own antibodies against them after several injections. These HAMAs usually developed two to three weeks after initial murine MoAb exposure. With subsequent therapy, the HAMA could bind up the murine MoAbs before they reached their target cells, decreasing clinical effectiveness and possibly exposing the patient to an antibody-induced allergic or anaphylactic reaction.[14,149] Retreatment with a murine MoAb requires the clinician to measure antimurine antibodies. Experience with OKT-3 shows that antibody titers above 1:100–1:1000 may predispose the patient to greater adverse effects, including anaphylaxis and/or decreased efficacy with retreatment.

In another observed phenomenon, antigenic modulation, the surface antigen targeted by the MoAb disappears from the cell surface (Figure 11-7).[150] The modulation may result from the cell internalizing or shedding the antigen. This response may occur rapidly; surface antigens may disappear 2 hours after administration of the MoAb and reappear on the cell surface 24 hours later. If the tumor cell internalizes the antibody-antigen complex, the tumor can escape cytotoxicity associated with opsonization. However, this property may be exploited therapeutically with conjugated MoAbs, in which internalization of the toxic antibody-antigen complex leads to cell death.

Other problems recognized in the early trials include lymphoma cells that escape targeting via phenotypic alteration of the idiotype and the presence of blocking antigens in the peripheral circulation.[151,152] These blocking antigens are often seen in lymphomas in which neoplastic cells secrete their surface antigens.

Some major limitations, such as lack of uptake in solid tumors, HAMA responses, and nonspecific uptake by normal organs, are due to the antibody properties and are independent of the target. Other limitations, such as antigenic modulation and phenotype alteration, are target specific. Because of the limited efficacy of unconjugated murine MoAbs, other approaches were developed. MoAbs have been designed to carry and deliver radioisotopes, toxins, chemotherapy agents, or liposome-filled drugs to the tumor cells. In addition, many of the antibodies were

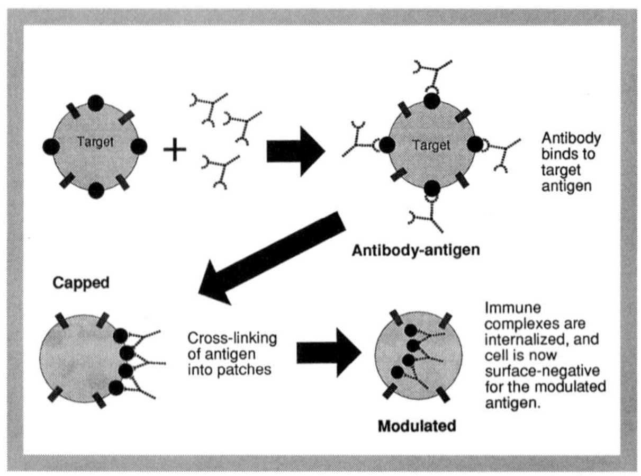

Figure 11-7. Antigenic modulation

SOURCE: *Adapted with permission from Lowder JN. The current status of monoclonal antibodies in the diagnosis and therapy of cancer.* Current Problems in Cancer *1986;10:505.*

humanized or had all or part of the Fc portion of the molecule removed.

Applications with Immunoconjugates—There are some general requirements for conjugating various toxic agents to antibodies. First, the conjugated form of the antibody should retain its antigen-binding capacity so it maintains its specificity for targeted tissue. The agents should also be covalently linked and stable to prevent random distribution of the cytotoxin. However, linkage to the antibody should not inhibit activity of the agent and should allow the agent to be liberated at its site of action. The conjugated MoAb or the cytotoxic agents should not accumulate in nontargeted tissues and should follow normal clearance from the body.

One of the earliest immunoconjugates used was a radioisotope conjugated to an antibody. Radioisotopes are a vital part of the development of MoAbs because of their use as research tools in clinical assays and for in vivo applications of imaging and cancer therapy.[101,153–155] Conjugation with radioisotopes is often done before other cytotoxic conjugation to demonstrate the specificity of the MoAb conjugate.

Radioisotopes have important advantages as conjugates for therapy. Radioisotopes provide cytotoxic activity without being internalized into the cells; they cause cytotoxicity to adjacent cells by ionizing radiation, thus affecting even tumor cells that don't express the target antigen. The range of the toxic effect depends on the isotope and its type of radiating energy. ^{131}I is the most commonly used radioisotope for therapy; however, other radioisotopes also hold therapeutic interest (beta particle emitters, such as yttrium-90,[156] rhenium-186,[157] and scandium-47, and alpha particle emitters, such as bismuth-212, lead-212).[158,159]

The primary disadvantage of radioisotopes is their toxic effects on nearby healthy tissue, especially at nonspecific sites where the MoAb conjugate might be retained (e.g., lung, spleen, or liver). Therefore, dosimetry studies are important for determining ratios between radiation doses received by targeted tissues and doses received by nonspecific organs.[160] The prior administration of unconjugated nonspecific MoAbs may reduce the indiscriminate collection of MoAb conjugates by vital organs.

Therapeutic trials in humans are being conducted with radioisotope conjugates.[161] Small phase I and II trials using radioisotopes have reported some success. However, only 0.001% of the dose per gram injected was taken up by solid tumors.[162,163] At this level of uptake, targeting radionuclides with MoAbs compares poorly with external beam radiation. To overcome this problem, investigators have used Fab- and $F(ab')_2$-labeled MoAbs. Better tissue penetration is achieved with these smaller proteins, but not enough to improve current therapy. Another approach that was successful in animals was to inject the MoAb directly into the artery that feeds the tumor, but this approach failed in human subjects.[162] The most reproducible positive therapeutic improvement over traditional therapy has been seen in patients with diffuse disease. This would be expected, because metastatic disease greatly diminishes the utility of external beam radiation.

^{131}I and other radioisotopes may be rapidly cleaved from amino acid residues on degraded MoAbs, leading to decreased tumor uptake and increased nonspecific tissue doses (i.e., thyroid uptake of ^{131}I). Nonspecific uptake of the radioactive iodine by the thyroid gland can be partially blocked by pretreating these patients with a saturated solution of potassium iodide. Blocking the reticuloendothelial system with unlabeled antibody may decrease nonspecific localization of radioisotope conjugates in the liver and spleen. The onset of hematologic toxicities is generally delayed, and patients may become profoundly neutropenic and thrombocytopenic.[164] An adjunctive measure to alleviate such marrow dysfunction is to rescue the patient with stored autologous bone marrow or colony-stimulating factors.

Toxin conjugates, or immunotoxins, are compounds formed by chemically linking antibodies to naturally occurring toxic polypeptides that inactivate protein synthesis.[165–169] The toxin may be a whole toxin of plant or bacterial origin, a subunit of a toxin, or a class of plant proteins know as hemitoxins. Table 11-4 lists examples of these types of toxins.

In its natural state, a toxin usually consists of A and

Table 11-4. Available Toxins to Conjugate with MoAbs

CATEGORY	EXAMPLES
Plant hemitoxins	Pokeweed antiviral protein Gelonin Saporin *Momordica charantia* inhibitor
Plant toxins	Ricin Abrin Modecin
Bacterial toxins	Diphtheria toxin Pseudomonas exotoxin A
Toxin subunits	Ricin A chain Abrin B chain
Toxin fragments	Diphtheria toxin fragment A

SOURCE: *Adapted with permission from Frankel AE, Houston LL, Issell BF. Prospects for immunotoxin therapy in cancer.* Annu Rev Med. *1986;37:129.*

B polypeptide chains. The B chain binds to the cell surface and may facilitate the translocation of the A chain through the cell membrane into the cytosol. The A chain then inactivates protein synthesis by one of two methods, depending on the origin of the toxin. Bacterial toxins (diphtheria and pseudomonas exotoxin A) disrupt protein synthesis by ribosylating elongation factor 2, whereas the plant toxins (ricin, abrin, and modecin) inactivate protein synthesis by inactivating the 60S subunit of ribosomes. Once in the cytoplasm, a single molecule of these extremely potent toxins can cause cell death.

Whole toxins are lethal to both tumor and normal cells. The A chain subunit, however, is essentially inactive unless attached to the cell surface and internalized. When the A chain of ricin is conjugated to a MoAb, toxicity should be limited to only those tumor cells specifically targeted by the MoAb. Because the conjugate lacks the ricin B chain, which allows intact ricin to bind to nearly all cells, any free A chains released from killed cells or detached from MoAbs should not be toxic to other cells. The proposed action of an immunotoxin is shown in Figure 11-8.

Other issues must be addressed before constructing immunotoxins. A MoAb that is very specific for the target cell must be selected. This MoAb should be internalized, delivering the toxin to its intracellular target. The nature of the antibody-toxin linkage is crucial because, when internalized, the toxin must be separated from the antibody to function properly. Innovative conjugation systems have been developed that incorporate an acid-labile ligand that cleaves inside the acidic environment of the lysosome after the conjugate has been phagocytized.

Clinically, immunotoxins may be used in (1) ex vivo therapy (e.g., against specific cancer cells to purge them from autologous bone marrow),[170] (2) intracavitary therapy (e.g., in ovarian carcinoma for intraperitoneal therapy of minimal residual disease),[171] and (3) in vivo systemic therapy to attack circulating tumor cells, metastatic tumors, and solid tumor disease[172] or cells involved in GVHD.

A number of investigators are studying ex vivo applications of ricin immunotoxin in bone marrow transplantation therapy.[173,174] The transplantation of the pluripotent stem cells in bone marrow is a proven method of restoring hematopoiesis after supralethal chemotherapy. The major impediments to the use of bone marrow transplants are (1) the presence of donor T cells that can cause GVHD in allogenic specimens and (2) the possible reinfusion of tumor cells in autologous marrow transplants. Anti-T-cell immunotoxins appear to offer an effective means of ex vivo T-cell depletion before allogenic bone marrow reinfusion. However, other problems, such as stem cell depletion, failure to engraft, rejection, and relapse, must be addressed in future clinical trials.[175]

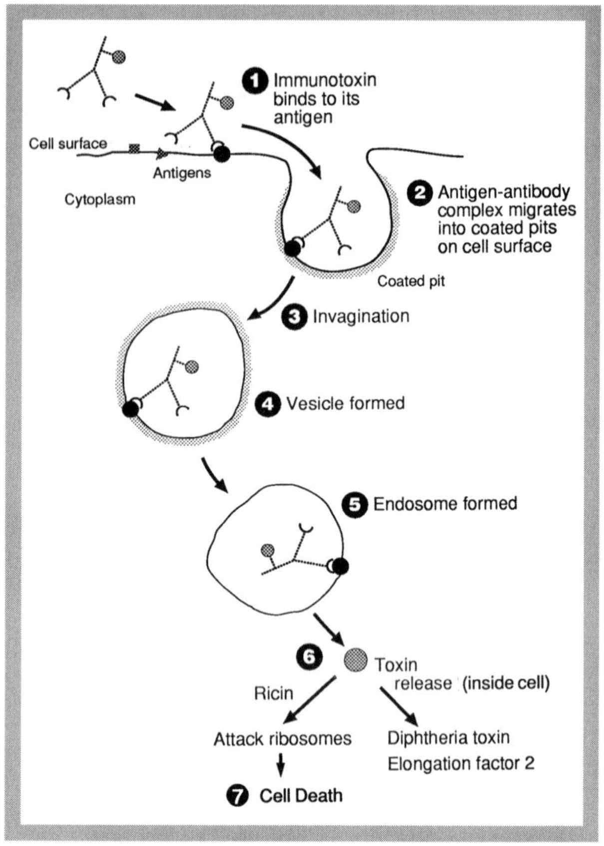

Figure 11-8. Proposed action of immunotoxin

SOURCE: *Adapted with permission from Frankel AE, Houston LL, Issell BF. Prospects for immunotoxin in therapy in cancer.* Ann Rev Med. *1986;37:132.*

The ex vivo use of immunotoxin to deplete residual cancer cells in autologous bone marrow is under investigation. Success thus far is limited; however, more trials are under way to evaluate the efficacy of this technique in patients undergoing autologous bone marrow transplantation therapy for hematopoietic and solid tumors.[174,176–178]

Clinical trials in the treatment of malignancies to date have had only mixed findings of some partial response or transient falls in circulating tumor cells.[179] The populations receiving benefit appear to be the same as those benefiting from radiotherapy targeted with MoAbs (i.e., patients with diffuse leukemia or lymphoma). Toxicities, which have been dose related and similar, include capillary leak syndrome, low serum albumin, and weight gain. Rarely has pulmonary edema been reported. A more serious toxicity of profound sensory motor peripheral neuropathy was noted in three patients treated for breast cancer with a ricin A immunoconjugate.[180] Consequently, MoAbs used in immunotoxin conjugates may have a greater role in tumor therapy; however, research is needed to increase the specificity of the immunotoxin for the tumor in vivo.

Perhaps the most encouraging in vivo use of an immunotoxin is in the treatment of steroid-resistant acute GVHD. Zolimomab aritox (Orthozyme CD5 Plus®) is an immunotoxin with ricin A conjugated to a murine MoAb directed against the CD5 antigen. This antigen is expressed primarily on mature T lymphocytes. In a multicenter trial of 34 steroid-resistant GVHD patients, 16 of 32 evaluable patients had either a complete or a partial response.[181] This study suggests that this immunotoxin may be an effective immunosuppressive agent for treating acute GVHD. Currently, zolimomab aritox has orphan drug approval from the FDA.

The concept of attaching an antineoplastic drug to antibodies for therapeutic use is not new. Chlorambucil had been conjugated to polyclonal goat antibodies for investigational therapeutic use well before MoAbs were developed.[182,183] The combination of antineoplastic agents with MoAbs should direct the drug to the specifically targeted tumor cells, improving the therapeutic-to-toxic ratio compared with the shotgun approach of systemic chemotherapy. As before, the requirements for conjugating drugs to MoAbs are: (1) conjugates should be stable enough to prevent indiscriminate release of drugs and exposure to normal tissue but be able to act once they reach the targeted cell; (2) conjugation should neither interfere with the specificity of the antibody nor reduce the effectiveness of the drug; and (3) conjugates may or may not have the same mechanisms of action, side effects, or pharmacokinetics as their individual components. A number of trials are under way to evaluate these antineoplastic conjugates to MoAbs.[184,185] The most common agents used as conjugates are antimetabolites and antibiotics, such as doxorubicin and daunorubicin.[186–191]

Several studies with various antineoplastic conjugates have demonstrated cytotoxicity in cell cultures and in animal tumors.[190,192,193] From animal studies, it is not clear what doses of conjugates are necessary; however, it appears that more drug per antibody is needed to kill the cell than with immunotoxins. This problem of drug potency may be approached by increasing the amount of active drug per milligram of immunoglobulin or using agents with higher intrinsic potencies on a molar basis, such as the vinca alkaloids. Another approach has been to couple liposomes filled with chemotherapeutic drugs to a MoAb. However, studies thus far have not been able to provide response rates that compare with systemic chemotherapy, although they have decreased toxicity.[184]

A new approach in applying MoAbs to cancer therapy is to use MoAbs to deliver enzymes to tumor cell surfaces. The chosen enzyme conjugate would be able to convert relatively noncytotoxic drug precursors into active drugs. The prodrug is then activated at the tumor site and can penetrate the nearby tumor cells.[194] MoAbs conjugated to the enzyme alkaline phosphatase (AP) have been developed and used to convert the prodrug mitomycin phosphate to mitomycin alcohol in both in vitro and in vivo models.[195] Antitumor responses were observed in animals treated with the MoAb-AP conjugated to carboxypeptidase G2 enzyme, which has been used for the prodrug activation of nitrogen mustard 1 to form active benzoic acid mustard 2.[196] Antibody enzyme conjugates may overcome the limitations of other MoAb conjugates. These limitations include antibody internalization, release of the immunotoxin or drug once in the cell, low potency of many cytotoxins, tumor heterogeneity, and physiological barriers. However, the MoAb-enzyme conjugates may have a new set of limitations: immunogenicity, availability of enzymes and prodrugs, and development of chimeric or recombinant antibodies. Overcoming these limitations will bring these new antibody-enzyme conjugates to clinical trial.

Problems and Possible Solutions for MoAb Therapy in Oncology—The targeted antigen can be secreted or shed into the extracellular fluid by the tumor. Free tumor antigens would be valuable in increasing the sensitivity of assays to detect tumor marker. However, in treatment, these free tumor antigens can bind the MoAb or MoAb conjugates, consuming the antibodies or preventing the desired distribution of the MoAbs to tumor cells. The excess free tumor antigens have been associated with shortened half-life of the infused MoAbs because of an increased clearance of the complex.[196] As with HAMAs, the formation of large amounts of immune complexes of free tumor antigen and MoAb may produce toxicity. Possible solutions to this problem include plasmapheresis before therapy to remove free tumor antigens, scheduling multiple MoAb treatments, and using large doses to overcome free tumor antigen binding.

Antigenic modulation is the disappearance of antigen from the surface of cells targeted with MoAb. The modulated cell lacks the targeted surface antigen, making it resistant to serotherapy by the specific MoAb. This property may not limit the use of immunoconjugates, in which it is desirable to have the conjugate enter the cell. Not all antigens modulate, nor do all antibodies cause modulation.

Administered MoAbs do not always distribute and concentrate in the targeted tissues. The MoAbs can be concentrated by the reticuloendothelial system, exposing these organs to toxicity. Tumors located in tissue distal from the circulatory system may not be accessible to the MoAbs, rendering them less susceptible to the antibody therapy. Approaches for overcoming such problems include selecting and using antibody classes, subclasses, or fragments that will give a more desirable distribution. Moreover, administering cold unlabeled antibodies to saturate nonspecific uptake sites before administering cytotoxic MoAbs may enhance binding of the targeted cells.

Subpopulations of the tumor may lack the surface

antigen targeted by the MoAb because of tumor heterogeneity and may escape therapy. This lack can be overcome with the use of MoAb cocktails[197] for different tumor antigens on the tumor cell or radioisotope conjugates that kill the cells within their radiation fields. Enzyme-linked MoAbs that convert prodrugs to the active form may also overcome this problem. In addition, MoAb localization to the tumor may also be improved by changing administration routes (e.g., subcutaneous administration in melanoma[197] or intraperitoneal administration in ovarian cancer).[198]

Ongoing studies will examine these limitations and methods of managing them in the next several years. New problems with the use of MoAbs will undoubtedly be discovered; however, MoAbs will also be applied more widely as these limitations are overcome and techniques are developed for increasing the efficacy while reducing the toxicities of MoAb therapy.

Autoimmune Diseases

MoAbs have long been recognized as useful research tools in the study of autoimmune diseases.[199,200] MoAbs to human T-cell surface antigens are useful for studying the T cells, their subpopulations, and their functions. There are a number of clinical conditions (e.g., systemic lupus erythematosus, Sjögren's syndrome, juvenile rheumatoid arthritis, and multiple sclerosis) associated with disorders of T lymphocytes. MoAbs are also being used to study the nature of such autoimmune diseases as myasthenia gravis,[201] type I diabetes mellitus,[202] and autoimmune thyroid diseases.[203] Potential exists for applying MoAbs in the therapy of autoimmune diseases, including T-cell disorders.[204–207] As discussed in the transplantation section, immune modulation with antibodies may be able to induce tolerance in autoimmune diseases. In vitro and autoimmune animal model studies show that inhibition of the CD28 pathway can decrease autoantibody production and induce tolerance.[208] The B7:CD28 pathway has also been shown to be important in potentiating T-cell stimulation in the synovial fluid of patients with rheumatoid arthritis.[209] Clinical trials are now being organized to see if antibody can provide improvement in humans.

Toxin Reversal

An area of considerable interest is the use of MoAbs to treat gram-negative bacteremia and septic shock.[210] The sepsis syndrome seems to be the result of the release of endotoxins from the bacterial cell wall. The lipid A component of the lipopolysaccharide molecule appears to be responsible for most endotoxic activities. Animal studies[211,212] and human studies[213,214] have shown the effectiveness of immunoglobulins in providing some protective activity against septic shock and death. However, further trials to evaluate the ability of MoAbs to limit mortality due to sepsis revealed that they were ineffective.[215]

The pathogenesis of septic shock also involves the release of cytokines, including TNF and IL-1, in response to endotoxin and other mediators. MoAbs have been prepared against these cytokines, and several MoAbs directed against TNF have been evaluated in clinical trials. Unfortunately, studies to date have shown anti-TNF MoAbs to be ineffective in preventing mortality due to sepsis.[215,216]

Other approaches, such as an IL-1–receptor antagonist produced by recombinant DNA techniques, are also being studied.[217] A large phase III trial that evaluated 893 patients with sepsis showed no clinical benefit using an anti-IL-1–receptor MoAb.[215] The reason for the failure is unclear at this time.

MoAbs are being prepared for a variety of other infectious organisms, including HSV[218] and group B streptococcus.[219] Trials are under way to evaluate the protective activity of these antibodies.

Vaccines

In addition to providing passive immunity, MoAbs may be a source for the production of vaccines for active immunization.[220,221] An antibody has a specific antigen-binding site. Anti-antibodies may be produced against the idiotype (the binding portion of an antibody) and other parts of the antibody. The antibodies formed against the idiotype are known as anti-idiotype antibodies. Any given anti-idiotype antibody will be structurally similar to the antigen against which the MoAb was originally developed. In other words, the anti-idiotype is an internal image of the original antigen. This anti-idiotype antibody should thus be antigenic (i.e., capable of inducing immunity). For example, an anti-idiotype antibody could be produced against the idiotype of a MoAb specific for a parasite,[222] and this anti-idiotype antibody would then be used as a vaccine to induce immunity (Figure 11-9). This technique may have advantages over the current method of purifying antigens and producing them in large quantities, because the anti-idiotype antibody would serve as a nonpathogenic antigen. This method of vaccine production is now undergoing research.[223]

MoAbs as reagents may replace the current polyclonal antisera used in serology because of their advantages in specificity, reproducibility, and unlimited availability. MoAbs have been produced against a variety of viruses,[224–226] bacteria,[210,223,227] and parasites.[47,228] Applications for these MoAbs are being evaluated for the treatment or prevention of infectious diseases.[224,229] Human MoAbs have been shown to protect mice from 10 times the 50% lethal dose (LD_{50}) of tetanus toxin.[230] This capability may have future applications in the treatment of human tetanus toxin exposures. MoAbs against various stages of malarial parasites can induce protective immunity. Protective MoAbs have been produced against merozoites of *Plasmodium yoelii, P. knowlesi, and P. falciparum.* In studies with mice infected with *P. yoelii*, injections of

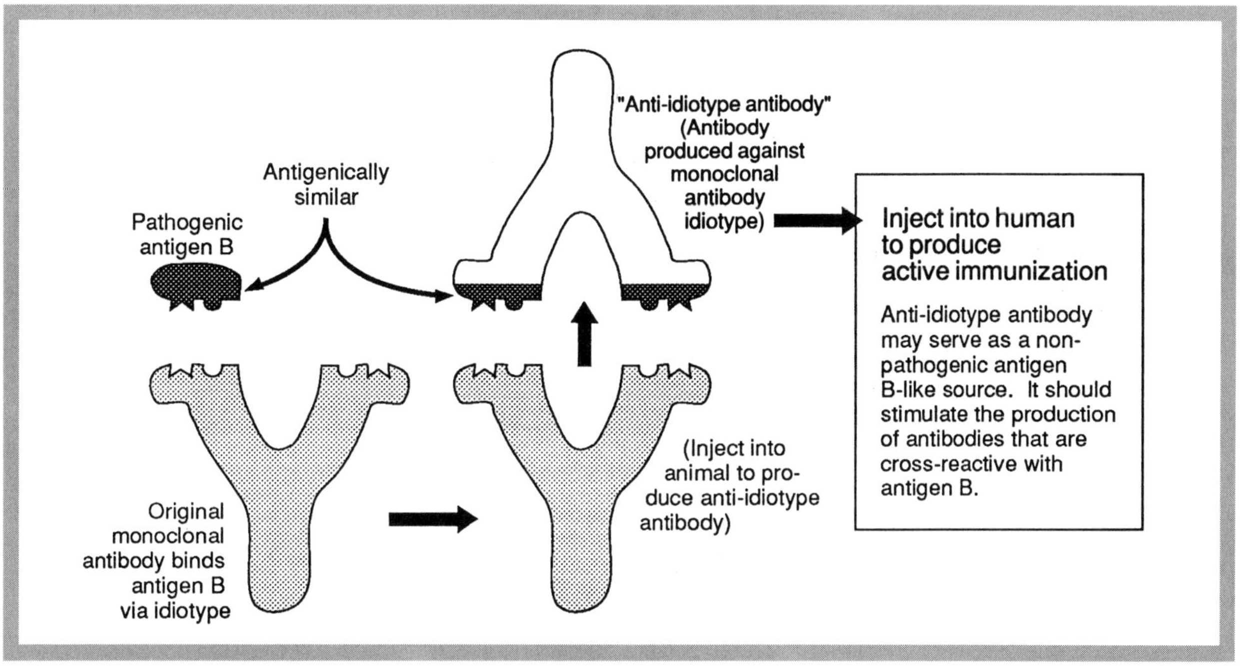

Figure 11-9. Anti-idiotype antibody for active immunization

MoAbs specific for *P. yoelii* reduced the level of infection (although extent of control over the infection was not the same for all mice infected). MoAbs against *P. falciparum* are capable of inhibiting parasite reinvasion and intraerythrocytic development in vitro. Passive protection has been demonstrated with MoAbs to the promastigote stage of *Leishmania mexicana* and to the schistosomula of *Schistosoma mansoni*. Thus, MoAbs against specific antigens on these parasites may be useful as reagents to treat these infections passively.[222]

SUMMARY

Monoclonal antibodies (MoAbs) are created by fusing antibody-secreting B lymphocytes to an immortal myeloma cell. The MoAb can be produced in cell cultures, mouse ascites, and bioreactors. A single MoAb is cloned to produce a colony of identical cells that can be frozen for storage.

Murine MoAbs are predominantly produced and are the mainstay for in vitro assays. However, in vivo human antimurine antibodies have been identified in patient serum, leading researchers to seek ways of producing human or human-like MoAbs. Human MoAbs are difficult to produce, primarily due to the lack of sufficient human myeloma cell lines and desired lymphocytes. Hybrid MoAbs have been created and include interspecies MoAbs, Epstein-Barr virus-transformed MoAbs, lymphoblastoid derivatives, chimeric antibodies, and those produced by recombinant DNA techniques. These hybrid MoAbs are less antigenic than murine MoAbs but are not as easy to produce.

MoAb fragments are created by cleaving the immunoglobulin molecule at the hinge region, resulting in Fab and $F(ab')_2$ fragments. Recombinant DNA fragments are produced by combining genes that encode for the heavy and light chains or the variable regions. MoAb fragments may prove to be more effective and have fewer side effects than whole MoAbs.

Most of the research efforts have originated in the oncology field, but several medical specialties have been able to take advantage of MoAb technology. Currently, MoAbs are approved for in vivo administration in transplantation, cardiology, and oncology. There remains a great amount of interest in applying MoAbs to oncology, autoimmune diseases, and infectious diseases.

Although MoAb technology has advanced in the past decade, limitations associated with their production and effective applications remain. Many of these limitations are being identified in studies.

MoAbs have become an essential tool in laboratories around the world. Hundreds of clinical studies have resulted in disappointing outcomes; however, this data has helped identify obstacles that are being overcome. In the recent past, a few new MoAbs have reached the market, and several are in phase II and III clinical trials, indicating the success researchers have had overcoming problems. Given the current state of MoAb research, it is likely that the role of MoAbs in pharmaceutical care will expand.

REFERENCES

1. Kohler G, Milstein C. Continuous cultures of fused cells

secreting antibody of predefined specificity. *Nature* 1975; 256:495–7.
2. Lewis DE, Rickman WJ. Methodology and quality control for flow cytometry. In: Rose NR, Friedman H, Fahey JL, editors. *Manual of Clinical Laboratory Immunology*. 3rd ed. Washington, DC: American Society for Microbiology; 1992. p. 164–73.
3. Fleeger CA, editor. *USP Dictionary of USAN and International Drug Names 96*. Rockville, MD: United States Pharmacopeial Convention; 1996.
4. Milstein C. Monoclonal antibodies. *Cancer* 1982;49:1953–7.
5. Diamond BA, Yelton DE, Scharff MD. Monoclonal antibodies: a new technology for producing serologic reagents. *N Engl J Med.* 1981;304:1344–9.
6. Chisholm R. On the trail of the magic bullet. *High Technol Bus*. 1983;3:61.
7. Meyer L. Construction of human T-cell hybridomas. In: Schook LB, editor. *Monoclonal Antibody Production Techniques and Applications*. New York: Infotechnology Publishing; 1987. p. 35–48.
8. Birch JR, Bonnerjea J, Flatman S, *et al*. The production of monoclonal antibodies. In: Birch JR, Lennox ES, editors. *Monoclonal Antibodies: Principles and Applications*. New York: Wiley-Liss; 1995. p. 231–65.
9. Kagan JN, Fahey JL. Tumor immunology. *JAMA* 1987; 258:2988–92.
10. Zimmerman U, Vienken J. Electric field-induced cell fusion. *J Membr Biol*. 1982;62:165–85.
11. Posillico EG. Microencapsulation technology for large scale antibody production. *Biotechnology* 1986;4:114–7.
12. Moro AM, Rodrigues MTA, Gouvea MN, *et al*. Multiparametric analyses of hybridoma growth on glass cylinders in a packed-bed bioreactor system with internal aeration. Serum-supplemented and serum-free media comparison for MAb production. *J Immunol Methods* 1994; 176:67–77.
13. Levy JA, Lee HM, Kawahata RT, *et al*. Purification of monoclonal antibodies from mouse ascites eliminates contaminating infectious mouse type C viruses and nucleic acids. *Clin Exp Immunol*. 1984;56:114–20.
14. Schroff RW, Steven HC. Human immune responses to murine monoclonal antibodies. In: Foon KA, Morgan AC, editors. *Monoclonal Antibody Therapy of Human Cancer*. Boston, MA: Martinus Nijhoff; 1985. p. 121–38.
15. De-Jager R, Abdel-Nabi H, Serafini A, *et al*. Current status of cancer immunodetection with radiolabeled human monoclonal antibodies. *Semin Nucl Med*. 1993;23:165–79.
16. Abrams PD, Knost JA, Clark G, *et al*. Determination of the optimal human cell lines for the development of human hybridomas. *J Immunol*. 1983;131:1201–4.
17. Ostberg L, Pursch E. Human x (mouse x human) hybridomas stably producing human antibodies. *Hybridoma* 1983; 2:361–7.
18. Campling BG, Cole SPC, Atlaw T, *et al*. The EBV hybridoma technique and its applications. In: Strelkauskas AJ, editor. *Human Hybridomas: Diagnostic and Therapeutic Applications*. New York: Marcel Dekker; 1987. p. 3–22.
19. Glassy M, Handley H, Hagiwara H, *et al*. UC-729-6: a human lymphoblastic B-cell line useful for generating antibody secreting human/human hybridomas. *Proc Natl Acad Sci USA* 1983;80:6327–31.
20. O'Hare MJ, Edwards PAW. Human monoclonal antibodies and LICR-LONHMy2 system. In: Strelkauskas AJ, editor. *Human Hybridomas: Diagnostic and Therapeutic Applications*. New York: Marcel Dekker; 1987. p. 47–64.
21. Kudo T, Saeki H, Katayose Y, *et al*. Construction of a human B cell line, TKHMY, suitable for production of stable human hybridomas. *J Immunol Methods* 1994;177:17–22.
22. Morrison SL. Transfectomas provide novel chimeric antibodies. *Science* 1985;229:1202–7.
23. Jones P, Dear PH, Foote J, *et al*. Replacing the complementarity determining regions in a human antibody with those from a mouse. *Nature* 1986;321:522–5.
24. Edwards PAW, O'Hare MJ. The production of human monoclonal antibodies. In: Beverley PCL. *Methods in Hematology: Monoclonal Antibodies*. Edinburgh: Churchill Livingstone; 1986. p. 60–96.
25. Morrison SL, Johnson MJ, Herenberg LA, *et al*. Chimeric human antibody molecules: mouse antigen-binding domains with human constant region domains. *Proc Natl Acad Sci USA* 1984;312:643–6.
26. Boulianne GL, Hozumi N, Shulman MJ. Production of functional chimeric mouse/human antibody. *Nature* 1984;312:643–6.
27. Neuberger MS, William GT, Fox RO. Recombinant antibodies possessing novel effector functions. *Nature* 1984; 312:604–8.
28. Hartman N, Gill LL, De Winter RFC, *et al*. Generation of a recombinant mouse-human chimeric monoclonal antibody directed against carcinoembronic antigen. *Int J Cancer* 1989;44:424–33.
29. Sun LK, Curtis P, Rakowicz-Szulczynska E, *et al*. Chimeric antibody with human constant regions and mouse variable regions directed against carcinoma associated antigen 17-1A. *Proc Natl Acad Sci USA* 1987;84:214–8.
30. Riechmann L, Clark M, Waldmann H, *et al*. Reshaping human antibodies for therapy. *Nature* 1988;332:323–7.
31. Junghans RP, Waldmann TA, Landolfi NF, *et al*. Anti-Tac-H, a humanized antibody to the interleukin-2 with new features for immunotherapy in malignant and immune disorders. *Cancer Res*. 1990;50:1495–502.
32. Liu AY, Robinson RR, Hellstrom KE, *et al*. Chimeric mouse-human IgG1 antibody that can mediate lysis of cancer cells. *Proc Natl Acad Sci USA* 1987;84:3439–43.
33. Clark M. General introduction. In: Birch JR, Lennox ES, editors. *Monoclonal Antibodies: Principles and Applications*. New York: Wiley-Liss; 1995. p. 1–43.
34. Staez UD, Bevan MJ. Hybrid hybridoma producing a bispecific monoclonal antibody that can focus effector T-cell activity. *Proc Natl Acad Sci USA* 1986;83:1453–75.
35. Gruber M, Schodin BA, Wilson ER, *et al*. Efficient tumor cell lysis mediated by a bispecific single chain antibody expressed in escherichia coli. *J Immunol*. 1994;152:5368–74.
36. Orland I, Gussow DH, Jones PT, *et al*. Cloning immunoglobulin variable domains for expression by polymerase chain reaction. *Proc Natl Acad Sci USA* 1989;86:3833–7.
37. Huse WD, Sastry L, Iverson SA, *et al*. Generation of a large combinatorial library of the immunoglobulin repertoire in phage lambda. *Science* 1990;246:1275–81.
38. Buchegger F, Haskell CM, Schreyer M, *et al*. Radiolabeled

fragments of monoclonal antibodies against carcinoembryonic antigen for the localization of human colon carcinoma grafted into nude mice. *J Exp Med.* 1983; 158:413–27.
39. Mach JP, Carrel S, Forni M, *et al.* Tumor localization of radiolabeled antibodies against carcinoembryonic antigen in patients with carcinoma: a critical evaluation. *N Engl J Med.* 1980;303:3–10.
40. Delaloye B, Bischof-Delaloye A, Buchegg F, *et al.* Detection of colorectal carcinoma by emission computerized tomography after injection of I-123 labeled Fab or $F(ab')_2$ fragments from monoclonal anti-carcinoembryonic antigen antibodies. *J Clin Invest.* 1986;77:301–11.
41. Ward ES, Gussow D, Griffiths AD, *et al.* Binding activities of a repertoire of a single immunoglobulin variable domains secreted from Escherichia coli. *Nature* 1989;341: 544–6.
42. Chaudhary VK, Batra JK, Gallo MG, *et al.* A rapid method of cloning functional variable region antibody genes in Escherichia coli as single chain immunotoxins. *Proc Natl Acad Sci USA* 1990;82:1066–70.
43. Hiatt A, Cafferkey R, Bowdish K. Production of antibodies in transgenic plants. *Nature* 1989;342:76–8.
44. Denis F, Leonard G, Mounier M, *et al.* Efficacy of five enzyme immunoassays for antibody to HIV in detecting antibody to HTLV-IV. *Lancet* 1987;1:324–5.
45. Batzer FR. Tests kits for ovulation and pregnancy. *Contemp OB/Gyn.* 1986;28:7–16.
46. Nowinski RC, Tam MR, Goldstein LC, *et al.* Monoclonal antibodies for diagnosis of infectious diseases in humans. Science 1983;219:637–44.
47. Lange JV, Walker DH. Production and characterization of monoclonal antibodies to Rickettsia rickettsii. *Infect Immun.* 1984;46:289–94.
48. Tam MR, Stamm WE, Handsfield H, *et al.* Culture-independent diagnosis of chlamydia trachomatis using monoclonal antibodies. *N Engl J Med.* 1984;310:1146–50.
49. DeYoung HG. The greening of biotechnology. *High Technol.* 1984;4:59–67.
50. Bell TA, Kuo C, Stamm WE, *et al.* Direct fluorescent monoclonal antibody stain for rapid detection of infant chlamydia trachomatis infections. *Pediatrics* 1984;74:224–8.
51. Kiviat N, Peterson M, Kinney-Thomas E, *et al.* Cytologic manifestations of cervical and vaginal infections. II. Confirmation of chlamydia trachomatis infection by direct immunofluorescence using monoclonal antibodies. *JAMA* 1985;253:997–1000.
52. Guenthner SH, Linnemann CG Jr. Indirect immunofluorescence assay for rapid diagnosis of influenza virus. *Lab Med.* 1988;19:581–3.
53. Schuster EA, Benke JS, Tegtmeier GE, *et al.* Monoclonal antibody for rapid laboratory detection of cytomegalovirus infections: characterization and diagnostic application. *Mayo Clin Proc.* 1985;60:577–85.
54. Van de Berg AP, von Son WJ, Jiwa NM, *et al.* Recent advances in the diagnosis of active cytomegalovirus infection after organ transplantation. *Transplant Proc.* 1990;22: 226–8.
55. Sarngadharan MG, Popovic M, Bruch L, *et al.* Antibodies reactive with human T-lymphocytropic retroviruses (HTLV-111) in the serum of patients with AIDS. *Science* 1984;224:506–8.
56. Lawrence J. Diagnostic test for HIV infection. *Infect Surg.* 1987;6:339–44, 368.
57. Dopel SH, Porstmann T, Grounow R , *et al.* Application of human monoclonal antibody in a rapid competitive anti-HIV ELISA. *J Immunol Methods* 1989;116:229–33.
58. Davey RD Jr., Vasudevachari MB. Serologic evaluation of patients with human immunodeficiency virus infection. In: Rose NR, De Macario EC, Fahey JL, *et al.*, editors. *Manual of Clinical Laboratory Immunology*. 4th ed. Washington, DC: American Society for Microbiology; 1992. p. 364–70.
59. Dubarry M, Luilier M, Malot N, *et al.* Enzyme immunoassay for detection of malarial antigens in human plasma by Plasmodium falciparum monoclonal antibodies. *Am J Trop Med.* 1990;43:116–23.
60. Stout C, Murphy MD, Lawrence S, *et al.* Evaluation of a monoclonal antibody pool rapid diagnosis of respiratory infections. *J Clin Microbiol.* 1989;27:448–52.
61. Covington TR, Lawson LC, Young LL, editors. *Handbook of Non-prescription Drugs*. 10th ed. Washington, DC: American Pharmaceutical Association; 1993.
62. Smith LH, Teng NN. Clinical applications of monoclonal antibodies in gynecological oncology. *Cancer* 1987;60: 2068–74.
63. Colcher D, Hand H, Wunderlich D, *et al.* Monoclonal antibodies to human mammary carcinoma associated antigens and their potential uses for diagnosis, prognosis, and therapy. *Immunodiagnostics* 1983:215–58.
64. Papsidero LD, Croghan GA, Asirwatham J, *et al.* Immunohistochemical demonstration of prostate-specific antigen in metastases with the use of monoclonal antibody F5. *Am J Pathol.* 1985;121:451–4.
65. Raubitcheck A, Senyk G, Larrick J, *et al.* Human monoclonal antibodies against group A red blood cells. *Vox Sang.* 1985;48:305–8.
66. Whiteside TL. Monoclonal antibodies in tissue section diagnosis. In: Gordon DS, editor. *Monoclonal Antibodies in Clinical Diagnostic Medicine*. Tokyo: Igaku-Shou; 1985. p. 19–43.
67. Kung PC, Goldstein G, Reinherz EL, *et al.* Monoclonal antibodies defining distinctive human T-cell surface antigens. *Science* 1979;206:24–79.
68. [Anonymous]. 1993 revised classification system for HIV infection and expanded surveillance case definition for AIDS among adolescents and adults. *MMWR* 1992;41(RR-17):1–19.
69. McMichael AJ. Monoclonal antibodies to HLA antigens: new approaches to the study of structure, genetics and function. In: McMichael AJ, Fabre JW, editors. *Monoclonal Antibodies in Clinical Medicine*. London: Academic Press; 1982. p. 335–64.
70. Chamberlin J. *The Analysis of Drugs in Biological Fluids*. 2nd ed. Boca Raton, FL: CRC; 1995. p. 163–90.
71. Secher DS, Burke DC. A monoclonal antibody for large scale purification of human leukocyte interferon. *Nature* 1980;285:446–50.
72. Tsung YK, Milkunsky A, Alpert E. Derivation and characterization of a monoclonal hybridoma antibody specific for human alpha-fetoprotein. *J Immunol Methods* 1980;

39:363–8.

73. USAN Council. Monoclonal antibodies: guidelines for nomenclature of monoclonal antibodies. *Clin Pharmacol Ther.* 1993;54:114–6.
74. Mach J, Chatal J, Lumbroso J, *et al.* Tumor localization in patients by radiolabeled monoclonal antibodies. *Cancer Res.* 1983;43:5593–600.
75. Murry J, Rosenblum N, Sobol R, *et al.* Radioimaging in malignant melanoma with ^{131}I-labeled monoclonal antibody. *Cancer Res.* 1985;45:2376–80.
76. Berger HJ. Myocardial imaging new radiotracers aid diagnosis. *Diagn Imaging* 1987;9:78–89.
77. Halpern SE, Dillman RO, Hagen PL. The problems and promise of monoclonal antitumor antibodies in diagnostic imaging. *Diagn Imaging* 1983;5:40–7.
78. Esteban JM, Schlom J, Gansow OA, *et al.* New method for the chelation of indium-111 to monoclonal antibodies: biodistribution and imaging of athymic mice bearing human colon carcinoma xenografts. *J Nucl Med.* 1987;28: 861–70.
79. Mears CF. Chelating agents for the binding of metal ions to macromolecules. *Nucl Med Biol.* 1986;13:311–5.
80. Krejcarek GE, Tucker KL. Covalent attachment of chelating groups to macromolecules. *Biochem Biophys Res Comm.* 1977:581–5.
81. Carrasquillo JA, Mulshine JL, Bunn PA, *et al.* Indium-111 T101 monoclonal antibody is superior to iodine-131 T101 in imaging of cutaneous T-cell lymphoma. *J Nucl Med.* 1987;28:281–7.
82. Eary JF, Schroff RW, Abrams PG, *et al.* Successful imaging of malignant melanoma with technetium-99m-labeled monoclonal antibodies. *J Nucl Med.* 1989;30:25–32.
83. Serafini AN. From monoclonal antibodies to peptides and molecular recognition units: an overview. *J Nucl Med.* 1993:533–6.
84. Goodwin DA. Pharmacokinetics and antibodies. *J Nucl Med.* 1987;28:1358–62.
85. Moldofsky PJ, Powe J, Mulhern CB, *et al.* Metastatic colon carcinoma detected with radiolabeled F(ab′)$_2$ monoclonal antibody fragments. *Radiology* 1983;149:549–55.
86. Wilbanks AB, Peterson LA, Miller S, *et al.* Localization of mammary tumors in vivo with I-131-labeled Fab fragments of antibodies against mouse mammary epithelium (MME) antigens. *Cancer* 1981;48:1768–75.
87. Ford CHJ, Cason AG. Antibody mediated targeting in the treatment and diagnosis of cancer: an overview. *Cancer Chemother Pharmacol.* 1986;17:197–208.
88. Wahl RL, Parker CW, Philpott GW. Improved radioimaging and tumor localization with monoclonal F(ab′)$_2$. *J Nucl Med.* 1983;24:316–25.
89. Olin BR, Hebel SK, Dewein AC, *et al.*, editors. *Drug Facts and Comparisons*. St. Louis, IL: Facts and Comparisons; updated monthly. p. 765–6.
90. Khaw BA, Yasuda T, Gold HK, *et al.* Acute myocardial infarct imaging with indium-111-labeled monoclonal antimyosin Fab. *J Nucl Med.* 1987;28:1671–8.
91. Khaw BA, Strauss HW, Moore R, *et al.* Myocardial damage delineated by indium-111 antimyosin Fab and technetium-99m pyrophosphate. *J Nucl Med.* 1987;28:76–82.
92. Tamaki N, Yamada T, Matsumor IA, *et al.* Indium-111-antimyosin antibody imaging for detecting different stages of myocardial infarction comparison with technetium-99m-pyrophosphate imaging. *J Nucl Med.* 1990;31:136–42.
93. Williamdec G, Palacio I, Yasuda T, *et al.* Antimyosin antibody cardiac imaging: its role in diagnosis of myocarditis. *J Am Coll Cardiol.* 1990;11:97–104.
94. Alavi A, Gupta N, Dalevsky HI, *et al.* Detection of thrombophlebitis with ^{111}In-labeled anti-fibrin antibody: preliminary results. *Cancer Res.* 1990;50(*Suppl*):958S–61S.
95. Rosenbrough SF, Mcalee JG, Grossman ZD, *et al.* Thrombus imaging: a comparison of radiolabeled GC4 and T2G1S fibrin specific monoclonal antibodies. *J Nucl Med.* 1990; 31:1048–54.
96. Oster ZH, Srivastava SC, Som P, *et al.* Thrombus radioimmunoscintigraphy: an approach using monoclonal antiplatelet antibody. *Proc Natl Acad Sci USA* 1985; 82:3465–8.
97. Peter AM, Lavender LD, Needham SG, *et al.* Imaging thrombus with radiolabel monoclonal antibody to platelets. *Br Med J.* 1986;293:1525–7.
98. Jung M, Kletter K, Dudczak R, *et al.* Deep vein thrombosis: scintigraphic diagnosis with In-111 label monoclonal antifibrin antibodies. *Radiology* 1989;173:469–75.
99. Oster ZH, Som P, Zamora PO. Mesenteric vascular occlusion: a diagnostic method using a radiolabeled monoclonal antibody reactive to platelet. *Radiology* 1989;171:653–6.
100. DeLand FH, Goldberg DM. Diagnosis and treatment of neoplasms with radionuclide-labeled antibodies. *Semin Nucl Med.* 1985;25:2–11.
101. Larson SM. Radiolabeled monoclonal anti-tumor antibodies in diagnosis and therapy. *J Nucl Med.* 1985;26:538–45.
102. Moldofsky PJ, Sears HF, Mulhern CB, *et al.* Detection of metastatic tumor in normal sized retroperitoneal lymph nodes by monoclonal antibody imaging. *N Engl J Med.* 1984;311:106–7.
103. Larson SM, Carrasquillo JA, Krohn KA, *et al.* Diagnostic imaging of malignant melanoma with radiolabeled antitumor antibodies. *JAMA* 1983;249:811–2.
104. Foster CS, Neville AM. Monoclonal antibodies to the human mammary gland. *Human Pathol.* 1984;15:502–13.
105. Halpern SE, Dilman RO, Witztum KF, *et al.* Radioimmunodetection of melanoma utilizing ^{111}In-96.5 monoclonal antibody: a preliminary report. *Radiology* 1985; 155:493–9.
106. Larson SM, Carrasquillo JA, McGuffin RW, *et al.* Use of ^{131}I-labeled, murine Fab against a high molecular weight antigen of human melanoma: preliminary experience. *Radiology* 1985;155:487–92.
107. Rainsbury RM. Localization of human breast carcinomas by radiolabeled monoclonal antibodies. *Br J Surg.* 1984;71: 805–12.
108. Neal CE, Meis LC. Correlative imaging with monoclonal antibodies in colorectal, ovarian, and prostate cancer. *Semin Nucl Med.* 1994;24:272–85.
109. Horne T, Granowska M, Dicks-Mireaux C, *et al.* Neuroblastoma imaged with ^{123}I-meta-iodo-benaylguanidine and with ^{123}I-labeled monoclonal antibody, UJ13A, against neural tissue. *Br J Radiol.* 1985;58:476–80.
110. Leyden MJ, Thompson CH, Lichtenstein M, *et al.* Visualization of metastases from colon carcinoma using an iodine 131-radiolabeled monoclonal antibody. *Cancer*

1986;57:1135–9.
111. Allum WH, MacDonald F, Anderson PO, *et al.* Localization of gastrointestinal cancer with a ^{131}I labeled monoclonal antibody to CEA. *Br J Cancer* 1986;57:1135–9.
112. Pateisky N, Phillipp K, Skodler WD, *et al.* Radioimmunodetection in patients with suspected ovarian cancer. *J Nucl Med.* 1985;26:1369–76.
113. Hirayama K, Chung YS, Sawada T, *et al.* Characterization and biodistribution of a mouse/human chimeric antibody directed against pancreatic cancer mucin. *Cancer* 1995;75(*Suppl* 6):1545–53.
114. Kovacs JA, Ng VL, Hasur H, *et al.* Diagnosis of pneumocystis carinii pneumonia improved detection in sputum with use of monoclonal antibodies. *N Engl J Med.* 1988; 318:589–93.
115. Weinstein JN, Eger RR, Covell DG, *et al.* The pharmacology of monoclonal antibodies. *Ann New York Acad Sci.* 1987;507:199–210.
116. Murray J, Rosenblum MG, Lamki L, *et al.* Clinical parameters related to optimal tumor localization of indium-111-labeled mouse antimelanoma ZME-018. *J Nucl Med.* 1987; 28:25–33.
117. Scheinberg DA, Chapman PB. Therapeutic applications of monoclonal antibodies for human disease. In: Birch JR, Lennox ES, editors. *Monoclonal Antibodies: Principles and Applications.* New York: Wiley-Liss; 1995. p. 45–107.
118. Beatty JD, William LE, Yamaguchi D, *et al.* Presurgical imaging with indium-labeled anticarcioembryonic antigen for colon cancer staging. *Cancer Res.* 1990;50:922–6.
119. Ellis G, Ferguson M, Yamanak D, *et al.* Monoclonal antibodies for the detection of occult carcinoma cells in bone marrow of breast cancer patients. *Cancer* 1989;63:2509–14.
120. Hooks MA, Wade C, Millikan WJ. Muromonab CD-3: a review of its pharmacology, pharmacokinetics, and clinical use in transplantation. *Pharmacotherapy* 1991;11:216–37.
121. Scheinberg DA, Chapman PB. Therapeutic applications of monoclonal antibodies for human disease. In: Birch JR, Lennox ES, editors. *Monoclonal Antibodies: Principles and Applications.* New York: Wiley-Liss; 1995. p. 41–105.
122. Guinan EC, Gribben JG, Boussiotis VA, *et al.* Pivotal role of the B7:CD28 pathway in transplantation tolerance and tumor immunity. *Blood* 1994;84:3261–82.
123. Haber E. In vivo diagnostic and therapeutic uses of monoclonal antibodies in cardiology. *Ann Rev Med.* 1986;37:249–61.
124. Faulds D, Sorkin EM. Abciximab (c7E3 Fab): a review of its pharmacology and therapeutic potential in ischemic heart disease. *Drugs* 1994;48:583–98.
125. Coller BS, Scudder LE, Berger HJ, *et al.* Inhibition of human platelet function in vivo with a monoclonal antibody. *Ann Intern Med.* 1988;109:635–8.
126. Bode C, Matsueda GR, Hui KY, *et al.* Antibody-directed urokinase: a specific fibrinolytic agent. *Science* 1985;229: 765–7.
127. Wenger TL, Butler VP, Haber E. Treatment of 63 severely digitalis-toxic patients with digoxin-specific antibody fragments. *J Am Coll Cardiol.* 1985;5(*Suppl* A):118a–23a.
128. Rose DR, Seaton BA, Petsko GA, *et al.* Crystallization of the Fab fragment of a monoclonal anti-digoxin antibody and its complex with digoxin. *J Mol Biol.* 1983; 165:203–6.
129. Koprowski H, Herlyn M, Steplewski Z, *et al.* Specific antigen in serum of patients with colon carcinoma. *Science* 1981;212:53–5.
130. Steplewski Z, Chang TH, Herlyn M, *et al.* Release of monoclonal antibody-defined antigens by human colorectal carcinoma and melanoma cells. *Cancer Res.* 1981;41:2723–7.
131. Herlyn M, Sears HF, Steplewski Z, *et al.* Monoclonal antibody detection of a circulating tumor associated antigen: presence of antigen in sera of patients with colorectal, gastric and pancreatic carcinoma. *J Clin Immunol.* 1982:135–40.
132. Dillman RO. Antibodies as cytotoxic therapy [review]. *J Clin Oncol.* 1994;12:1497–515.
133. Berstein ID, Tam MR, Nowinski RC. Mouse leukemia: therapy with monoclonal antibodies against a thymus differentiation antigen. *Science* 1980;207:68–71.
134. Scheinberg DA, Strand M. Leukemic cell targeting and therapy by monoclonal antibody in a mouse model system. *Cancer Res.* 1982;42:44–9.
135. Masui H, Kawamoto T, Sato JD, *et al.* Growth inhibition of human tumor cells in thymic nude mice by anti-epidermal growth factor receptor monoclonal antibody. *Cancer Res.* 1984;44:1002–7.
136. Brady LW, Woo DV, Karlsson U, *et al.* Radioimmunotherapy of human glioma using I-125-labeled monoclonal antibody to epidermal growth factor receptor. *Proc Am Soc Clin Oncol.* 1988;7:82. Abstract 319.
137. Cuttitta F, Carney DN, Mulshine J, *et al.* Bombesin-like peptides can function as autocrine growth factors in human small cell lung cancer. *Nature* 1985;316:823–6.
138. Harris DT, Mastrangelo MJ. Serotherapy of cancer. *Semin Oncol.* 1989;16:180–98.
139. Shawler DL, Beauregard J, Halpern SE, *et al.* Tissue distribution and serum kinetics of T101 monoclonal antibody during passive anticancer therapy. *Clin Immunol Immunopathol.* 1986;41:43–54.
140. Brown SL, Miller RA, Levy R. Antiidiotype antibody therapy of B-cell lymphoma. *Semin Oncol.* 1989;16:199–210.
141. Brown SL, Miller RA, Horning SJ, *et al.* Treatment of B-cell lymphomas with anti-idiotype antibodies alone and in combination with alpha interferon. *Blood* 1989;73:651–61.
142. Masucci G, Wershall P, Nielsen J, *et al.* Lymphokine activated killer (LAK) cells in antibody-dependent cellular cytotoxicity (ADCC) using Mab 17-1A: a combination of potential usefulness in tumor therapy. *Hybridoma* 1989;8:507–16.
143. Tong AW, Lee JC, Wang RM, *et al.* Augmentation of lymphokine activated killer cell cytotoxicity by monoclonal antibodies against human small cell lung carcinoma. *Cancer Res.* 1989;49:4103–8.
144. Eisenthal JA, Cameron BB, Uppenkamp I, *et al.* Effects of combined therapy of lymphokine-activated killer cells, interleukin-2 and specific monoclonal antibody on established melanoma lung metastases. *Cancer Res.* 1988;48: 7140–5.
145. Masucci G, Wershall P, Raghammer P, *et al.* Granulocyte

monocyte colony-stimulating factors augments the cytotoxic capacity of lymphocytes and monocytes in antibody-dependent cellular cytotoxicity. *Cancer Immunol Immunother.* 1989;29:288–92.

146. Foon KA, Schroff RW, Bunn RA, *et al.* Effects of monoclonal antibody therapy in patients with chronic lymphocytic leukemia. *Blood* 1984;64:1085–93.
147. Dillman RO, Beauregard JC, Cutter M, *et al.* Toxicities and efficacy of 24 hour infusion of T 101 monoclonal antibody in chronic lymphocytic leukemia. *Proc Am Soc Clin Oncol.* 1985;4:230.
148. Dillman RO, Beauregard JC, Halpern SE, *et al.* Toxicities and side effects associated with intravenous infusions of murine monoclonal antibodies. *J Biol Response Modif.* 1986;5:73–84.
149. Dillman RO. Human antimouse and antiglobulin responses to monoclonal antibodies. *Antibody Immunoconj Radiopharmaceut.* 1990;3:1–15.
150. Shawler DL, Miceli MC, Wormslely SB, *et al.* Induction of in vitro and in vivo antigenic modulation by the anti-human T cell monoclonal antibody T101. *Cancer Res.* 1984;44:5921–7.
151. Meeker T, Lowder J, Cleary MI, *et al.* Emergence of idiotype variants during the treatment of B-cell lymphoma with anti-idiotype antibodies. *N Engl J Med.* 1985;312:1658–65.
152. Nadler LM, Staswhenko P, Hardy R, *et al.* Serotherapy of a patient with a monoclonal antibody directed against a human lymphocyte-associated antigen. *Cancer Res.* 1980;40:3147–54.
153. Bloomer WD, Lipsztein R, Dalton JF. Antibody-mediated radiotherapy. *Cancer* 1985;55:2229–33.
154. Pectaside D, Stewart S, Courtenay-Luck N, *et al.* Antibody-guided irradiation of malignant pleural and pericardial effusion. *Br J Cancer* 1986;53:727–32.
155. Keenan AM, Harbert JC, Larson SM. Monoclonal antibodies in nuclear medicine. *J Nucl Med.* 1985;26:531–7.
156. Hantowich DJ, Virzi F, Doherty PW. DTPA-coupled antibodies labeled with yttrium-90. *J Nucl Med.* 1985;26:503–9.
157. Schoff HP, Weiden PL, Appelbaum J, *et al.* Rhenium-186 labeled antibody inpatients with cancer: report of a pilot phase 1 study. *Antibody Immunoconj Radiopharmaceut.* 1990;3:99–111.
158. Strand M, Scheinberg DA, Gansow OA, *et al.* Monoclonal antibody conjugates for diagnostic imaging and therapy. In: Bous BD, Langman R, Trowbridge I, *et al.*, editors. *Monoclonal Antibody and Cancer.* Orlando, FL: Academic; 1983. p. 125–31.
159. Kozak RW, Atcher RW, Gansow OA, *et al.* Bismuth-212-labeled Anti-Tac monoclonal antibody: particle emitting radionuclides as modalities for radioimmunotherapy. *Proc Natl Acad Sci USA* 1986;83:474–8.
160. Humm JL. Dosimetric aspects of radiolabeled antibodies for tumor therapy. *J Nucl Med.* 1986;27:1450-97.
161. Lashford LS, Davies AG, Richardson RB, *et al.* A pilot study of 131-I monoclonal antibodies in the therapy of leptomeningeal tumors. *Cancer* 1988;61:857–68.
162. Kemshead JT, Hopkins K. Uses and limitations of monoclonal antibodies (MoAbs) in the treatment of malignant disease: a review. *J R Soc Med.* 1993;86:219–24.
163. Esteban JM, Colcher D, Sugarbaker P. Quantitative and qualitative aspects of radiolocalization in colon cancer patients of intravenously administered MoAb B72.3. *Int J Cancer* 1987;50–9.
164. Bertram JH, Gill PS, Levin AM, *et al.* Monoclonal antibody T101 in T-cell malignancies: a clinical, pharmacokinetic and immunologic correlation. *Blood* 1986;68:752–61.
165. Frankel AE, Houston LL, Issell BF. Prospectives for immunotoxin therapy in cancer. *Ann Rev Med.* 1986;37:125–42.
166. Vitetta ES, Uhr JW. Immunotoxins. *Ann Rev Immunol.* 1985;3:197–212.
167. Neville DM Jr. Immunotoxins for in vivo therapy: where are we? *Ann NY Acad Sci.* 1987;507:155–64.
168. Marsh JW, Neville DM Jr. Development of an immunotoxin with in vivo efficacy for murine systems. *Ann NY Acad Sci.* 1987;507:165–77.
169. Raso V, Watkins SC, Slayter H, *et al.* Intracellular pathways of ricin A chain cytotoxins. *Ann NY Acad Sci.* 1987;507:172–86.
170. Bregni M, De Fabritiis P, Raso V, *et al.* Elimination of clonogenic tumor cells from human bone marrow using a combination of monoclonal antibody: ricin A chain conjugates. *Cancer Res.* 1986;46:1208–13.
171. Epenetos AA, Hooker G, Krausz T, *et al.* Antibody-guided irradiation of malignant ascites in ovarian cancer: a new therapeutic method possessing specificity against cancer cells. *Obstet Gynecol.* 1986;68(*Suppl*):71–4.
172. Gilliland DG, Steplewski Z, Collier RJ, *et al.* Antibody directed cytotoxic agents: use of monoclonal antibodies to detect the action of toxin A chains to colorectal carcinoma cells. *Proc Natl Acad Sci USA* 1980;77:4539–43.
173. Muirhead M, Martin P, Torok-Storb B, *et al.* Use of antibody-ricin A chain conjugate to deplete neoplastic cells from human bone marrow. *Blood* 1983;62:327–32.
174. Ramsay NK, Kersey JH. Bone marrow purging using monoclonal antibodies. *J Clin Immunol.* 1988;8:81–8.
175. Byers V, Henslee J, Antin J, *et al.* Safety and therapeutic response to a pan-T-lymphocyte monoclonal antibody ricin A chain in graft versus host disease (GVHD) [abstract]. *Proc Am Soc Clin Oncol.* 1988;7:190.
176. Ramsay N, LeBein T, Nesbit M, *et al.* Autologous bone-marrow transplantation for patients with acute lymphoblastic leukemia in second or subsequent remission: results of bone marrow treated with monoclonal antibodies BA-1, BA-2, and BA-3 plus complement. *Blood* 1986;66:508–13.
177. Baumgartner C, Imbach P, Luthy A, *et al.* Autologous bone marrow transplantation for stage IV abdominal non-Hodgkin's lymphoma after in vitro purging with anti-y 29/55 monoclonal antibody and complement. In: Boss BD, Langman RE, Trowbridge IS, *et al.*, editors. *Monoclonal Antibody and Cancer.* Orlando, FL: Academic; 1983. p. 73–9.
178. Gorin NC, Dousay L, Paportye JP, *et al.* Autologous bone marrow transplantation with marrow decontamination by immunotoxin T 101 in the treatment of leukemia and lymphoma: first clinical observation. *Cancer Treat Rep.* 1985;69:953–9.
179. Hertler AA, Frankel AE. Immunotoxins: a clinical review

of their use in the treatment of malignancies. *J Clin Oncol.* 1989;7:1932–42.

180. Gould BJ, Borowitz MJ, Groves ES, *et al.* Phase I study of an anti-breast cancer immunotoxin by continuous infusion: report of a targeted toxic effect not predicted by animal studies. *J Natl Cancer Inst.* 1989;81:775–81.
181. Byers VS, Henslee PJ, Kernan NA, *et al.* Use of anti-pan T-lymphocyte ricin A chain immunotoxin in steroid resistant acute graft-versus-host disease. *Blood* 1990;75:1426–32.
182. Ghose T, Norvell ST, Guclu A, *et al.* Immunochemotherapy of human malignant melanoma with chlorambucil-carrying antibody. *Eur J Cancer* 1975;11:321–6.
183. Ghose T, Norvell ST, Guclu A, *et al.* Immunochemotherapy of cancer with chlorambucil carrying antibody. *Br Med J.* 1972;26:495–9.
184. Ford CHJ, Newman CE, Johnson JR, *et al.* Localization and toxicity study of a vindesine-anti-CEA conjugate in patients with advanced cancer. *Br J Cancer* 1983;47:35–42.
185. Takashi T, Yamaguchi T, Kitamura K, *et al.* Clinical application of monoclonal antibody-drug conjugates for immunotargeting chemotherapy of colorectal carcinoma. *Cancer* 1988;61:881–8.
186. Lagueux J, Page M, Delorme F. Daunorubicin-albumin copolymer targeting to leukemic cells in vitro and in vivo. *Semin Oncol.* 1984;11:59–63.
187. Page M, Delorme F, Lafontaine F, *et al.* Chemotherapy with daunorubicin-anti-CEA conjugates in human colon adenocarcinoma grafted in nude mice. *Semin Oncol.* 1984;11 (*Suppl* 3):56–8.
188. Arnon R, Sela M. In vitro land in vivo efficacy of conjugates of daunomycin with anti-tumor antibodies. *Immunol Rev.* 1982;62:5–27.
189. Primm MV, Jones JA, Price MR, *et al.* Tumor localization of monoclonal antibody against a rat mammary carcinoma and suppression of tumor growth with adriamycin-antibody conjugates. *Cancer Immunol Immunother.* 1982;12: 125–34.
190. Dillman RO, Shawler DL, Johnson DE, *et al.* Preclinical trials with combination and conjugates of T101 monoclonal antibody and doxorubicin. *Cancer Res.* 1986;46: 4886–91.
191. Greenfield RS, Dausesa A, Edson HA, *et al.* Optimization of immunotherapy with adriamycin (hydrazone)-immunoconjugates in human B-lymphoma xenografts. *Antibody Immunoconj Radiopharmaceut.* 1991;4:107–19.
192. Garnett MC, Baldwin RW. An improved synthesis of a methotrexate albumin-T791/36 monoclonal antibody conjugate cytotoxic to human osteogenic sarcoma cell lines. *Cancer Res.* 1986;46:2407–12.
193. Mueller BM, Reisfeld RA, Silveria MH, *et al.* Pre-clinical therapy of human melanoma with morpholino-doxorubicin conjugated to monoclonal antibody directed against an intergrin on melanoma cells. *Antibody Immunoconj Radiopharmaceut.* 1991;4:99–106.
194. Senter PD. Activation of prodrugs by antibody-enzyme conjugates: a new approach to cancer therapy. *FASEB J.* 1990;4:188–93.
195. Senter PD, Schreiber GJ, Hirschberg DL, *et al.* Enhancement of in vitro and in vivo tumor activities of phosphorylated mitomycin-c and etoposide derivatives by monoclonal antibody-alkaline phosphatase conjugates. *Cancer Res.* 1989;49:5789–92.
196. Bagtshawe KD, Springer CJ, Searle F, *et al.* A cytotoxic agent can be generated selectively at cancer sites. *Br J Cancer* 1988;58:700–3.
196. Meeker TC, Lowder JN, Maloney DG, *et al.* A clinical trial of anti-idiotype therapy for B-cell malignancy. *Blood* 1985;65:1349–63.
197. Wahl RL, Lieber TM, Headington J, *et al.* Lymphoscintigraphy in melanoma: initial evaluation of a low protein dose monoclonal antibody cocktail. *Cancer Res.* 1990;50: 941–8.
198. Stewart JS, Hird V, Snook D, *et al.* Intraperitoneal radioimmunotherapy of ovarian cancer, pharmacokinetic, toxicity and efficacy of I-131 labeled monoclonal antibodies. *Int J Radiat Oncol Biol Phys.* 1989;16:405–13.
199. Chiorazzi N. Human monoclonal antibodies as probes to study autoimmune and allergic disorders. *Biotechnology* 1986;4:210–7.
200. Morimoto C, Schlossman SF, Reinherz EL. Use of monoclonal antibodies in the study of autoimmunity and immunodeficiency. In: Hayes BF, Eisenbarth GS, editors. *Monoclonal Antibodies: Probes for the Study of Autoimmunity and Immunodeficiency.* Orlando, FL: Academic; 1983. p. 116.
201. Lindstrom J. Use of monoclonal antibodies in the study of myasthenia gravis. In: Hayes BF, Eisenbarth GS, editors. *Monoclonal Antibodies: Probes for the Study of Autoimmunity and Immunodeficiency.* Orlando, FL: Academic; 1983:259–98.
202. Eisenbarth GS, Jackson R, Srikanta S. Type I diabetes: autoimmunity and immunodeficiency. In: Hayes BF, Eisenbarth GS, editors. *Monoclonal Antibodies: Probes for the Study of Autoimmunity and Immunodeficiency.* Orlando, FL: Academic; 1983. p. 197–219.
203. Kohn LD, Yavin E, Yavin Z. Autoimmune thyroid disease studied with monoclonal antibodies to the thyrotropin receptor. In: Hayes BF, Eisenbarth GS, editors. *Monoclonal Antibodies: Probes for the Study of Autoimmunity and Immunodeficiency.* Orlando, FL: Academic; 1983. p. 221–58.
204. Christadoss P, Dauphinee M. Immunotherapy for myasthenia gravis: a murine model. *J Immunol.* 1986;136:2437–40.
205. Schoenfeld Y, Raugh J, Massicotte H, *et al.* Polyspecificity of monoclonal lupus autoantibodies produced by human/human hybridomas. *N Engl J Med.* 1983;24:414–20.
206. Billingham MEJ, Hicks C, Carney S. Monoclonal antibodies and arthritis. *Agents Action* 1990;29:77–87.
207. Mathieson PW, Cobbold SP, Hale G, *et al.* Monoclonal antibody therapy in systemic vasculitis. *N Engl J Med.* 1990; 323:250–3.
208. Milich DR, Linsley PS, Hughes JL, *et al.* Soluble CTLA-4 can suppress autoantibody production and elicit long term unresponsiveness in a novel transgenic model. *J Immunol.* 1994;153:429–35.
209. Verwilghen J, Lovis R, De Boer M, *et al.* Expression of functional B7 and CTLA4 on rheumatoid synovial T cells. *J Immunol.* 1994;153:1378–85.
210. Teng NNH, Kaplan HS, Herbert JM, *et al.* Protection against gram-negative bacteremia and endotoxemia with

human monoclonal IgM antibodies. *Proc Natl Acad Sci USA* 1985;82:1790–4.

211. Pier GB, Thomas D, Small G, *et al*. In vitro and in vivo activity of polyclonal and monoclonal human immunoglobulins G, M and A against Pseudomonas aeruginosa lipopolysaccharide infections. *Immunology* 1989;57:174–9.
212. Salles MF, Mandine E, Zalisz R, *et al*. Protective effects of murine monoclonal antibodies in experimental septicemia E. coli antibodies protect against different serotypes of E. coli. *J Infect Dis*. 1989;159:641–9.
213. Ziegler EJ, MuCutchan JA, Fierer J, *et al*. Treatment of gram-negative bacteremia and shock with human antiserum to mutant of Escherichia coli. *N Engl J Med*. 1982;307:1225–30.
214. Dunn D, Priest BP, Condie RM. Protective capacity of polyclonal and monoclonal antibodies directed against endotoxin during experimental sepsis. *Arch Surg*. 1988; 123:1389–93.
215. Suffredini AF. Current prospects for the treatment of clinical sepsis. *Crit Care Med*. 1994;22:S12–8.
216. Abraham E, Wunderink R, Silverman H, *et al*. Efficacy and safety of monoclonal antibody to human tumor necrosis factor alpha in patients with sepsis syndrome. A randomized, controlled, double-blind, multicenter clinical trial. TNF-alpha MAb Sepsis Study Group. *JAMA* 1995; 273:934–41.
217. Ohisson K, Bjork P, Bergenfeblt M, *et al*. Interleukin-1 receptor antagonist reduces mortality from endotoxin shock. *Nature* 1990;348:550–2.
218. Mester JC, Glorioso JC, Rouse BT. Protection against zosteriform spread of herpes simplex virus by monoclonal antibodies. *J Infect Dis*. 1991;163:263–9.
219. Hill HR, Gonozales LA, Knappe WA, *et al*. Comparative protective activity of human monoclonal and hyperimmune polyclonal antibody against group B streptococci. *J Infect Dis*. 1991;163:792–8.
220. Steinitz M, Tamir S, Frodin JE, *et al*. Human monoclonal anti-idiotypic antibodies. *J Immunol*. 1988;141:3516–22.
221. Hiernaux JR. Idiotypic vaccines and infectious diseases. *Infect Immun*. 1988;56:1407–13.
222. Daiv JR. The immunology of parasites. In: Braunwald E, Isselbacher KJ, Petersdorf RG, *et al*, editors. *Harrisons's Internal Medicine*. 11th ed. New York: McGraw-Hill; 1987. p. 771–3.
223. Steinitz M, Tamir S, Goldfarb A. Human antipneumococci antibody produced by an Epstein-Barr virus (EBV) immortalized cell line. *J Immunol*. 1984;132:877–82.
224. Emanuel D, Peppard J, Chenimi J, *et al*. The diagnostic, prophylactic, and therapeutic uses of monoclonal antibodies to human cytomegalovirus. *Transplant Proc*. 1987;19(*Suppl* 7):132–7.
225. Emanuel D, Gold J, Colacino, *et al*. A human monoclonal antibody to cytomegalovirus (CMV). *J Immunol*. 1984;133: 2202–5.
226. Foung SK, Perkins S, Koropchak C, *et al*. Human monoclonal antibodies neutralizing varicella zoster virus. *J Infect Dis*. 1985;52:280–5.
227. Hunter K Jr, Fisher G, Hemming V, *et al*. Antibacterial activity of a human monoclonal antibody against Haemophilus influenzae type B capsular polysaccharide. *Lancet* 1982;2:798–9.
228. Udomsangpetch R, Lungren K, Berzins K, *et al*. Human monoclonal antibodies to Pf155: a major antigen of malaria parasite Plasmodium falciparum. *Science* 1986;231: 57–9.
229. Engleberg NC, Eisenstein BI. The impact of new cloning techniques on the diagnosis and treatment of infectious diseases. *N Engl J Med*. 1984;311:892–901.
230. Fremark BD, Ozer H. Construction of a stable protective human monoclonal antibody to the C fragment of tetanus toxin. In: Strelkauskas AJ, editor. *Human Hybridomas: Diagnostic and Therapeutic Applications*. New York: Marcel Dekker; 1987. p. 81–94.

SELF-ASSESSMENT QUESTIONS

1. Monoclonal antibodies are produced by injecting the desired antigen into a mouse, and then isolating and purifying the antibodies from the serum.

   a. true
   b. false

2. What two types of cells are used to create an antibody-secreting hybridoma cell?

   a. B lymphocyte and B lymphocyte
   b. B lymphocyte and myeloma
   c. myeloma and myeloma
   d. virus and myeloma

3. Murine MoAbs are less antigenic and more effective than chimeric antibodies.

   a. true
   b. false

4. Which of the following is an advantage of Fab MoAb fragments?

   a. They are more cytotoxic.
   b. They can bind to two different antigens.
   c. They have better tissue penetration.
   d. They have greater antigen specificity than whole MoAbs.

5. Covalent conjugation of radioisotopes to MoAbs requires binding of fresh isotopes to the antibody before every treatment.

   a. true
   b. false

6. In which of the following diseases is imciromab (Myoscint®) used to help with the diagnosis?

   a. colon cancer
   b. myocardial infarction
   c. ovarian cancer
   d. malignant melanoma

7. OncoScint is approved for imaging for which of the following malignancies?

   a. colorectal cancer
   b. ovarian cancer
   c. prostate cancer
   d. a and b

8. Abciximab is a(n):

   a. immunotoxin to reverse allograft rejection.
   b. ^{111}In-labeled MoAb to alpha-fetoprotein.
   c. MoAb Fab to platelet glycoprotein IIIb/IIa.
   d. chimeric human-murine antibody Fab that binds platelet glycoprotein IIb/IIIa.

9. MoAbs that bind the lipid A component of lipopolysaccharide prevent mortality associated with gram-negative sepsis.

   a. true
   b. false

10. Which of the following is the most cytotoxic when attached to a MoAb?

    a. ^{111}In
    b. ^{99}mTc
    c. doxorubicin
    d. ricin A chain

11. Which of the following is an advantage of MoAb therapy?

    a. Antitumor MoAbs respond only to antigens expressed on the surface of tumor cells.
    b. Murine MoAbs can compensate for antigenic modulation.
    c. Murine MoAbs are inexpensive and easy to produce.
    d. Murine MoAbs have limited toxicities.

12. Chimeric antibodies consist of which of the following combinations?

    a. mouse Fc and human Fab
    b. mouse Fc and mouse Fab
    c. mouse Fab and human Fc
    d. human Fab and human Fc

13. Which of the following techniques provides the greatest yield of monoclonal antibodies in large-scale production? Cell development in:

    a. bioreactors
    b. human ascites
    c. mice ascites
    d. tissue culture

14. Which type of MoAb can have antitumor effects without entering the cell?

    a. radioisotope conjugates
    b. murine MoAbs
    c. immunotoxins
    d. chimeric antibodies

15. Monoclonal antibodies are being developed to diagnose infections with viruses, bacteria, and parasites.

    a. true
    b. false

16. Which of the following forms of MoAbs is the most useful for in vivo imaging?

    a. unconjugated MoAbs
    b. ^{111}In-labeled MoAbs
    c. ^{90}Y-labeled MoAbs
    d. ^{212}B-labeled MoAbs

17. All of the following problems have been encountered with the therapeutic use of MoAbs in cancer *except:*

    a. binding of free tumor antigens (antigens shed from tumor cells).
    b. antibodies taken up by the reticuloendothelial system rather than bind tumor.
    c. patients forming an antibody response to the MoAb (human antimurine antibody response).
    d. cellular internalization of receptor-antibody complex (antigenic modulation) when using an immunotoxin.

Answers to Self-Assessment Questions

Chapter 1

1. a
2. b
3. d
4. d
5. a
6. b
7. a
8. d
9. b
10. a
11. b

Chapter 2

1. c
2. a
3. a
4. b
5. a
6. b
7. b
8. a
9. c
10. a
11. a
12. b
13. a
14. d
15. a
16. a
17. c
18. a
19. d

Chapter 3

1. b
2. a
3. d
4. d
5. c
6. b
7. a
8. a
9. c
10. d
11. a
12. b
13. d
14. c
15. a
16. c
17. a
18. d

Chapter 4

1. d
2. a
3. d
4. c
5. b
6. c
7. a
8. b
9. a
10. b
11. c
12. d
13. d
14. a
15. d
16. b
17. b
18. d
19. c
20. d

Chapter 5

1. b
2. c
3. e
4. d
5. b
6. d
7. molecular mimicry
8. a
9. e
10. c
11. selective IgA deficiency
12. to decrease frequency and severity of infections
13. intravenously
14. 200–500 mg/dl
15. 350–500 mg/dl
16. severe combined immunodeficiency disease with ADA deficiency
17. viral infections, malignancies, malnutrition, advanced age, pharmacologic agents
18. influenza
19. d
20. e

Chapter 6

1. c
2. c
3. c
4. c
5. d
6. b
7. d
8. b
9. c
10. b
11. d
12. d
13. a
14. b
15. d
16. a
17. b
18. b
19. c

Chapter 7

1. d
2. c
3. a
4. b
5. d
6. a
7. b
8. c
9. b
10. b
11. c
12. b

13. c
14. a
15. d
16. c
17. c

Chapter 8
Part I

1. b
2. c
3. b
4. c
5. a
6. b
7. a
8. b
9. c
10. d
11. a
12. b
13. d

Part II

1. c
2. c
3. b
4. b
5. c
6. c
7. c
8. a
9. c
10. b
11. b
12. b
13. 3 months
14. c
15. c
16. b
17. c
18. c
19. a

Chapter 9

1. b
2. a
3. e
4. c
5. d
6. b
7. e
8. a
9. e
10. e

Chapter 10

1. inhibition of RNA, DNA, and protein synthesis
2. f
3. e
4. f
5. acute flu-like syndrome, consisting of fever, chills, headaches, myalgias, nasal congestion, dizziness, and tachycardia.
6. e
7. a
8. renal cell carcinoma and melanoma
9. a
10. aldesleukin (Proleukin) and teceleukin (Tecin)
11. e
12. a
13. b
14. f
15. bone pain, myalgias, and skin rash
16. a
17. GM-CSF and IL-3
18. d
19. f
20. e

Chapter 11

1. b
2. b
3. b
4. c
5. a
6. b
7. d
8. d
9. b
10. d
11. c
12. c
13. a
14. a
15. a
16. b
17. d

Glossary

ABO system—the major blood grouping system in humans.

Active immunization—inducing immunity against harmful agents by exposure to antigens (also known as vaccination).

Adaptive (acquired) immunity—immunity that develops as a result of exposure to an antigen.

Adoptive immunotherapy—the transfer of active immunologic reagents to a tumor-bearing host (such as the transfer of cells with antitumor reactivity to mediate antitumor effects).

Adjuvant—material, usually an aluminum salt, capable of nonspecifically enhancing an immune response.

Affinity—the strength of attraction between one binding site on the antigen or epitope and a single binding site on the antibody; an expression of strength of binding between two entities.

Affinity chromatography—a method used to isolate pure proteins by coupling either antibody or antigen to an inert solid phase, such as dextran beads in a column. A solution containing the antigen or the antibody of interest is run through the column, where the specific antigen or antibody will bind. The specific antigen or antibody can then be eluted from the column in a concentrated pure form.

Agammaglobulinemia—a deficiency of all classes of serum immunoglobulins.

Agglutination—the process by which particles (e.g., red blood cells or bacteria) complex to form clumps; specific immunoglobulins sometimes cause this effect.

AIDS-related complex—a term encompassing a variety of conditions, including unexplained weight loss, oral candidiasis, unexplained fever, extrainguinal lymphadenopathy, oral hairy leukoplakia, unexplained night sweats, herpes zoster, and unexplained diarrhea.

Allele—one of two or more alternate genes present at a given locus on a chromosome.

Allergen—an antigen capable of causing an allergic reaction.

Allergy—an immunologic hypersensitivity.

Alloantigens—allelic forms of antigens present in some, but not all, individuals in a given species.

Allogenic—molecules or cell types within a species that have identical functions but are antigenically distinct.

Allograft—grafted tissue of genetically nonidentical individuals of the same species.

Alpha-fetoprotein—an embryonic globulin, similar to serum albumin, that can be detected in the serum of adults with primary liver cancer tumors.

Anaphylatoxins—complement fragments C4a, C3a, and C5a, which can induce mast cell degranulation, resulting in increased vascular permeability and smooth muscle contraction.

Anaphylaxis—an immediate allergic reaction mediated by IgE-sensitized mast cells.

Anergy—diminished cell-mediated reactivity as shown by the inability to react to a battery of common skin-test antigens.

Antibody—an immunoglobulin produced by mature B cells or plasma cells in response to an antigenic stimulus and capable of binding with a specific antigen.

Antibody affinity—a measure of the strength of the bond between a single antigen-combining site (Fab) and an antigenic determinant.

Antibody avidity—a measure of the antigen-antibody binding strength that is dependent on the affinity to the epitope and the effective number of binding sites on the antibody. Avidity is enhanced by the number of bonds formed and is usually much greater than affinity.

Antibody-dependent cell-mediated cytotoxicity—a means of destroying target cells by coating them with antibody that attracts Fc receptor–bearing immune effector cells (killer cells, natural killer cells, macrophages, and neutrophils).

Antigen—a substance capable of reacting with products

of the immune system (i.e., the target of an immune response).

Antigen-binding sites—locations on the antibody molecule that combine specifically with the corresponding antigenic determinant.

Antigenic modulation—a phenomenon in which cells lose or internalize their surface antigens after interactions with the immune system.

Antigen-presenting cell—a specific type of cell (e.g., macrophage, dendritic cell, or B cell) that stimulates T lymphocytes by displaying processed antigen to them in conjunction with major histocompatibility complex class II molecules.

Anti-idiotypic antibodies or anti-idiotypes—antibodies directed against the surface determinants of the antigen-combining site of other antibodies.

Antilymphocyte globulins—antibodies directed against lymphocytes, usually used as an immunosuppressive agent. Commonly produced by hyperimmunizing animals with human lymphocytes.

Antiserum—serum from any animal that contains antibodies against a specific antigen.

Antithymocyte globulins—polyclonal antibodies directed against human thymus lymphocytes, typically used as an immunosuppressive agent. Commonly produced by hyperimmunizing horses with human thymocytes.

Antitoxin—an antibody or antiserum prepared in response to a toxin or toxoid.

Ascites—serous fluid that collects in the peritoneum of an animal; this fluid may contain antibodies produced by an injected hybridoma.

Atopy—the state of being allergic to normal environmental antigens.

Attenuated—made less virulent.

Attenuated vaccine—a preparation composed of live microbes of low virulence that can induce immunity against highly virulent microbes.

Autoantibody—an antibody to normal self antigens.

Autoantigen—a host's self antigen.

Autoimmunity—an immune response to autoantigens.

Autologous antigen—an antigen that is found in the host and that does not normally elicit an immune response; also called a self antigen.

Avidity—the functional combined strength of all the interactions between an antigen and the entire antibody (multiple Fab sites). *See* **Antibody avidity.**

Azathioprine—a purine analogue converted to 6-mercaptopurine in vivo, useful as an immunosuppressant.

Bacillus Calmette-Guérin—a strain of live, attenuated *Mycobacterium bovis* that may induce resolution of some local tumors, probably through enhanced macrophage- or T cell–mediated activity.

Basophils—a granulocytic cell that releases histamine and other inflammatory mediators when stimulated by an antigen.

β_2-microglobulin—a protein associated with HLA class I antigens.

Biological response modifiers—a heterogeneous group of substances that, in a specific or nonspecific manner, promote immune interactions with malignant cells.

Blotting—a technique of transferring DNA, RNA, or protein separated in gels onto a reactive membrane, such as nitrocellulose.

B lymphocytes—cells derived from the bone marrow in mammals that are the precursors of plasma cells, which respond to antigenic stimulation by producing antibodies.

Bursa of Fabricius—lymphoid tissue found in the hind gut of birds that is responsible for B-lymphocyte maturation.

Cachectin—a monokine, also referred to as tumor necrosis factor, that is an endogenous pyrogen and catabolic substance.

Carcinoembryonic antigen—an antigen normally found in the fetal gut that may be present in the serum of patients with cancer (primarily of the colon or lung) as well as in smokers and patients with inflammatory conditions.

Cell-mediated immunity—specific immunity dependent principally on the presence of T lymphocytes.

Chemotaxis—the chemical attraction of phagocytic cells to the site of inflammation or infection; the attraction of living protoplasm to chemical stimuli.

Chimeric antibody—an antibody made up of fragments from different species (e.g., an antibody with mouse Fab and human Fc segments).

Class I genes—genes of the major histocompatibility complex responsible for compatibility of tissues and organs (also known as histocompatibility or transplantation genes); *HLA-A*, *-B*, and *-C* loci encode for the class I HLA molecules in humans.

Class II genes—genes of the major histocompatibility complex that participate in the immune response (also known as *Ir* genes); *HLA-D* loci encode for the class II HLA molecules in humans.

Class III genes—genes of the major histocompatibility complex that contribute to the complement system and tumor necrosis factor.

Clone—one of a group of genetically identical cells derived from a single original cell.

Clusters of differentiation (CD)—a nomenclature system that categorizes cell surface molecules of human leukocytes; also used to categorize monoclonal antibodies according to the antigens they recognize.

Codominance—equal expression of alleles inherited from each parent.

Colony-forming unit (CFU), granulocyte-monocyte—a term used to describe the in vitro production of a colony of cells of granulocytic and monocytic lineage within a semisolid medium, such as methylcellulose.

Colony-stimulating factors (CSFs)—a group of substances that increase production and activity of various types of hematologic cells. Granulocyte-macrophage CSF stimulates granulocytes and macrophages; granulocyte CSF stimulates primarily granulocytes (neutrophils).

Complement—a group of plasma proteins that may induce cell lysis when a stimulus initiates their sequential activation.

Conjugate—a product obtained by joining two or more dissimilar molecules (e.g., radioisotopes, drugs, or toxins covalently coupled to an antibody).

Cytokines—a generic term for soluble substances produced by cells to communicate with other cells to trigger or suppress cellular activity after interaction with an antigen. *See also* **Soluble mediators** (synonym).

Cytotoxicity—the process of killing cells.

Delayed hypersensitivity reactions—a specific inflammatory immune reaction elicited by an antigen and mediated by primed T cells; does not usually appear until 24 hours after contact with an antigen.

Demargination—the movement of cells from the endothelial walls of blood vessels into circulation.

Determinant—a three-dimensional site on an antigen to which antibody is specifically able to become attached by its antigen-binding site. A single antigen may have several antigenic determinants (epitopes).

Diapedesis—the active amoeba-like movement of blood cells, including phagocytes, through the endothelial cells lining the walls of capillaries into the tissue.

Differentiation—a process during hematopoiesis in which cells take on functions and abilities different from their predecessors.

Effector cells—cells (lymphocytes, phagocytes) that directly function to achieve the end result, as opposed to regulatory cells.

***env* gene**—the gene that encodes for the envelope protein of human immunodeficiency virus.

Enzyme-linked immunosorbent assay (ELISA)—an immunoassay in which antibody or antigen is detected by the binding of an enzyme coupled to either anti-immunoglobulin or antibody specific for the antigen.

Enzyme-multiplied immunoassay technique (EMIT)—a quantitative competitive immunoassay that uses an enzyme detection system. The enzyme-coupled antigen retains its enzymatic activity when unbound but loses its activity when bound to the antibody. The enzyme activity is inversely proportional to the amount of antibody-antigen binding.

Eosinophils—a granulocytic cell capable of phagocytosis. Eosinophils also ingest immune complexes and clear parasitic organisms from the host.

Epitope—a single antigenic determinant; the smallest structural portion of an antigen to which antibody can specifically attach by its antigen-binding site.

Fab—fragment of antigen binding—the single antigen-binding site of an antibody formed by the cleaving of the antibody to fragments with papain.

$F(ab')_2$—a dimeric fragment that contains two antigen-binding sites formed by the cleaving of the antibody to fragments with pepsin.

Fc—crystallizable fragment—the portion of an immunoglobulin that binds to macrophages, lymphocytes, and mast cells via Fc receptors. Also carries sites for fixation of complement.

Fc receptors—receptors located on cell surfaces that bind the Fc portion of an immunoglobulin.

Fluorescence—absorption of light at one wavelength and the emission of light at another wavelength.

Fluorescence immunoassay—an immunoassay technique that uses fluorescent-labeled antibodies or antigens to detect the presence of the antibody-antigen complex.

Fusion—a technique by which the cellular membranes of two or more cells are combined to form one cell; the resulting hybrid cell contains many of the chromosomes of the fusion partners.

***gag* gene**—the gene that encodes for the core protein of human immunodeficiency virus.

Gene—a unit of DNA that encodes for a single polypeptide chain.

Genotype—all alleles detected in a given individual; a genetic "portrait."

Graft-versus-host disease—a pathological reaction caused by the transplantation of competent donor T cells into an incompetent host (that is, one unable to reject them). This reaction occurs when the donor cells attack the host.

Graft-versus-leukemia effect—the decreased incidence of leukemic relapses seen in patients receiving allogenic transplants in comparison with autologous transplants.

Granulocytes—a group of antigen-nonspecific cells capable of phagocytosis. Granulocytes include neutrophils, eosinophils, and basophils.

Granulocytopenia—decreased numbers of granulocytes in the peripheral blood.

Group-specific—common to all the members of a group of viruses.

Haplotype—the set of genes present on any one chromosome; they are inherited as a unit. Each somatic cell will have two haplotypes, one of paternal origin and one of maternal origin.

Haptens—small molecules that are not immunogenic unless conjugated to a larger carrier molecule.

HAT—acronym for a selective cell culture medium containing hypoxanthine, aminopterin, and thymidine; used in monoclonal antibody technology to select for fused myeloma and B-lymphocyte cells (hybridomas).

Helper ($CD4^+$) T cell—a subclass of T cells responsible for stimulating other T cells and B cells; also called helper T lymphocytes.

Hematopoiesis—the formation and development of blood cells.

Hematopoietic growth factor—*see* **Colony-stimulating factor.**

Hemolytic disease of the newborn—a disease of newborns characterized by anemia and jaundice and caused by incompatibilities of the Rh phenotype of mother and fetus (also known as erythroblastosis fetalis).

High endothelial venule—a section of the circulatory system in which the specific structure is designed to allow some lymphocytes to cross from the lymphatic system to the blood.

Histiocyte—a synonym for macrophage.

Histocompatibility—the ability to accept grafts between individuals.

Human antimurine antibody (HAMA) response—antibody response produced in humans against infused immunogenic murine antibodies (usually monoclonal antibodies); also called human antibodies to mouse antibodies, or human antimouse antibodies.

Human immunodeficiency virus (HIV)—believed by most investigators to be the cause of acquired immunodeficiency syndrome.

Human leukocyte antigens (HLA)—the major histocompatibility antigens in humans.

Humoral immunity—specific immunity; immunity mediated principally by immunoglobulins, which are secreted by plasma cells and found in plasma, lymph, and other tissue fluids.

Hybridoma—a cell or cell line obtained by the fusion of two different cells. A hybridoma cell contains chromosomes from each of the fusion partners. A B-cell hybridoma results from the fusion of a B lymphocyte and a tumorous plasma cell. It is capable of prolonged survival and can secrete antibody.

Hyperchimeric antibody—a monoclonal antibody in

which the hypervariable regions come from a non-human source (such as a mouse) and the rest of the antibody structure is derived from human sources. Also known as a humanized antibody.

Hypergammaglobulinemia—an excess of gamma globulin in the blood.

Hypervariable region—a subsection within the variable region of an antibody responsible for the antigen specificity of the antibody. Denoted for the high variance of amino acid sequences between antibodies of different specificity.

Idiotypes—surface determinants in the variable domain of antibodies that are typically the binding sites for the target antigen.

Immune complexes—antigen-antibody complexes.

Immunization—the process of inducing active or passive specific immunity by administering antigenic substances or antigen-specific antibodies.

Immunodeficiency—a partial or total deficiency of cellular immunity, humoral immunity, or both.

Immunogen—any substance able to provoke an immune response.

Immunoglobulin—a glycoprotein consisting of heavy chains and light chains linked together, often synthesized in response to the presence of a foreign substance. *See also* **Antibody.**

Immunomodulator—an agent capable of enhancing, suppressing, or restoring an immune system either directly or indirectly.

Immunotoxin—the conjugate of an antibody and a naturally occurring toxic substance, such as ricin.

Inflammation—a consequence of a nonspecific immune response causing tissue damage, characterized by tissue pain, swelling, and warmth.

Interferon—a glycoprotein that exerts virus-nonspecific but host-specific antiviral activity.

Interleukin—a soluble factor released from leukocytes or other cells with defined biological effects. Protein composition and DNA sequence of encoding gene are defined. (*See* chapter 2 for specific interleukins.)

J chain—joining chain normally found in polymeric immunoglobulins (IgM and IgA).

K cell—killer cell, responsible for antibody-dependent cellular cytotoxicity.

Kupffer cells—mononuclear phagocytes that are fixed within the sinusoids of the liver.

Langerhans cell—a macrophage fixed in the skin responsible for antigen presentation to lymphocytes.

Leukotrienes—lipoxygenase metabolites of arachidonic acid with multiple biological activities.

Levamisole—anthelmintic drug with possible immunostimulating effects.

Linkage-associated antigens—surface antigens, each of which is commonly associated with one or more specific diseases.

Lipopolysaccharide—any compound in which lipid is linked to polysaccharide. Often refers to an endotoxin derived from the cell wall of gram-negative bacteria.

Liposome—a spherical microstructure consisting of concentric phospholipid bilayers. Liposomes are hollow in the center and may be filled with drugs.

Locus—position on the chromosome where a specific gene is found.

Lymphokine-activated killer (LAK) cells—a type of lymphocyte that develops an increased antitumor effect when stimulated by interleukin 2.

Lymphokines—soluble secretory products of lymphocytes that stimulate or suppress the activity of other cells.

Lymphopoiesis—the development of lymphatic tissue.

Lysosomes—intracellular organelles containing digestive enzymes (lysozymes).

Lysozyme—a muramidase capable of hydrolyzing structural bonds in the cell walls of certain bacteria, particularly gram-positive cocci.

Macrophage—a phagocytic cell found in tissue and believed to be derived from blood monocytes; may act as an antigen-presenting cell.

Major histocompatibility complex (MHC)—a collection of genes found in all vertebrate species that encodes for the production of cell surface proteins associated with transplantation, immune response, and the complement system. In humans, the MHC is also known as the human leukocyte antigen complex. *See* **Human leukocyte antigens.**

Mast cells—granulocytic cells that leave the bone marrow more quickly than basophils, mature in connective tissue, and retain the capacity to differentiate. There are two types of mast cells—connective tissue–type mast cells and mucosal-type mast cells.

Mitogen—a substance that induces proliferation of lymphocytes.

Mixed lymphocyte reaction—the in vitro proliferative response of lymphocytes after exposure to lymphocytes of differing haplotypes.

Modulation—the disappearance of cell surface receptors after combining with specific antibodies.

Monoclonal antibodies (MoAbs)—homogeneous antibodies produced by a single clone. MoAbs can be of any class of antibodies; however, most murine MoAbs are of the IgG or IgM class.

Monocytes and macrophages—mononuclear phagocytic cells.

Monokines—biologically active substances secreted by monocytes and macrophages, such as interleukin 1 and tumor necrosis factor.

Mononuclear phagocyte system—mononuclear phagocytic cells found primarily in the reticular connective tissue of immune and other organs. *See also* **Reticuloendothelial system.**

Mucositis—inflammation of the mucosal membrane.

Mucus—a clear, viscid secretion of mucous membranes consisting of mucin, epithelial cells, and leukocytes.

Muramyl dipeptide—a substance derived from mycobacterial cell walls, used as an immunostimulant, similar to Bacillus Calmette-Guérin.

Myeloma cell line—a category of tumorous plasma cells with the sustained ability to grow in culture.

Natural killer cells—lymphocytes that preferentially kill virally infected or malignant cells in the absence of prior immunization.

Neutralization—the process by which antibody, either with or without complement, neutralizes the infectivity of microorganisms such as viruses.

Nude mice—a hairless strain of mice that congenitally lack a thymus and have a marked deficiency in T lymphocytes but do possess natural killer cells.

Oncofetal antigens—cell surface markers normally present on fetal, but not adult, tissue that are also found on malignant cells.

Oncogene—a gene of mammalian or viral origin that is capable of causing neoplastic transformation of cells.

Ontogeny—the development of the individual organism.

Opsonin—a substance that binds to antigens and enhances phagocytosis by macrophages and neutrophils (e.g., complement and antibodies).

Opsonization—the process by which particles, microorganisms, or immune complexes become coated with complement or antibodies that make them more easily phagocytosed.

Paratope—a site on an antibody or a T-cell receptor that binds to the epitope of an antigen.

Passive immunization—inducing immunity by introduction of protective agents (e.g., preformed antibodies or specific cells) derived from extrinsic sources into a nonimmune host.

Perforins—proteins found in the cytoplasmic granules of natural killer cells that promote pore formation in nonself cells, leading to leakage of cell contents and cell death.

Peyer's patches—discrete colonies within gut mucosal-associated lymphoid tissue that contain mature B and T cells.

Phagocytes—cells capable of phagocytosis.

Phagocytosis—the process by which cells ingest and digest solid substances, such as bacteria and foreign particles.

Phagolysosome—a product of the fusion of a phagosome with a lysosome.

Phagosome—a vesicle that forms around a particle engulfed by a phagocyte.

Phenotype—a description of all the alleles detected in a given individual by serologic testing.

Plasma cell—the mature B lymphocyte, which is capable of secreting antibody.

Pluripotent cell—a primitive cell that has the potential to differentiate into any mature, functional cell.

Polyclonal activation (PCR)—activation of many clones of nonspecific lymphocytes.

Polymerase chain reaction—a process that enables the amount of a particular DNA sequence or gene to be greatly amplified.

Prostaglandins—cyclooxygenase metabolites of arachidonic acid with many biological activities.

Proto-oncogene—a normal gene that is usually involved in cellular growth or regulation and that, when altered or mutated, can become an oncogene.

Regulatory cell—a cell that has the primary function of stimulating or suppressing the production or activation of other cells, such as effector cells.

Reticuloendothelial system—a term, perhaps inaccurate, used to describe the mononuclear phagocyte system, a collection of cells that share the common function of phagocytosis and digestion of particulate material.

Retrovirus—a virus capable of transcribing viral RNA to DNA by means of the enzyme reverse transcriptase.

Rheumatoid factor—an antibody directed at human IgG that is present in patients with rheumatoid arthritis and other connective tissue diseases.

Rh system—a blood grouping system based on Rh antigens.

Self-renewal—a process by which some early bone marrow progenitor cells replenish their population rather than allowing all cells to undergo differentiation.

Serologic typing—a method of detecting cell surface antigens by using antisera.

Serotherapy—administration of antisera or specific immunoglobulins that are targeted for a specific antigen. *See also* **Passive immunization**.

Soluble mediators—secreted regulatory proteins, including all proteins or glycoproteins (such as interleukins, interferons, and cytokines) that mediate immune function.

Specificity—selective reactivity; the ability to distinguish among different determinants or sections of antigens.

Stem cell—a cell capable of self-replication and differentiation into various kinds of secondary cells.

Stroma—the supporting cells within the bone marrow, including fibroblasts, endothelial cells, adipocytes, and macrophages. The stromal cells produce many of the growth factors that promote hematopoiesis.

Suppressor T cell ($CD8^+$)—a subclass of T cells responsible for suppressing the immune response to a stimulus; also called suppressor T lymphocytes.

Swine flu—the name given to a type of influenza that broke out in 1976 and stimulated a nationwide vaccination program.

Syngenic—genetically identical (as in identical twins or inbred strains of animals).

T-cell receptor (TCR)—a molecule on the surface of T lymphocytes specifically capable of recognizing antigen in association with major histocompatibility complex molecules. TCRs consist of two polypeptide chains (alpha and beta or gamma and delta) associated with the CD3 complex.

Thymus—the small immunologic organ found in the anterior mediastinal cavity, responsible for T-cell growth and development.

T lymphocytes—cells derived from the bone marrow that differentiate within the thymus; they play a major role in the activity of the cell-mediated immune system. *See also* **Helper T cell** and **Suppressor T cell.**

Tolerance—an immunologic response of nonreactivity to a particular antigen, although responses to other antigens are normal.

Toxoid—a pharmacologically inactive toxin preparation that retains the ability to stimulate production of antitoxin.

Transfection—the process by which a DNA segment may be introduced into another cell, incorporated, and read to produce a protein.

Transfectoma—a continually renewing cell (e.g., a hybridoma or a myeloma cell) that has been transfected with a foreign DNA segment.

Tumor necrosis factor alpha (TNF-α)—a substance produced by host monocytes and macrophages that is capable of killing tumorous cells and eliciting inflammatory responses; also referred to as cachectin.

Type-specific—distinct for each virus within the group.

Vaccination—active immunization with modified attenuated or killed microorganisms to provide resistance and to prevent infectious disease (also known as active immunization).

Vaccine—a product consisting of attenuated or killed microbial agents used as an antigen to provide immunity.

Variolation—injection of live smallpox virus from disease pustules to protect against smallpox.

Virion—formed virus particle.

Virulence—the degree of pathogenicity of various strains of organisms.

Western blot—an immunoblotting method used for identifying specific proteins recognized by antibodies.

Wheal-and-flare—a cutaneous reaction in response to an injected antigen consisting of a raised edematous lesion surrounded by erythema.

Xenogenic—derived from tissues of individuals of different species. *See* **Allogenic**.

Index

A

Abciximab 280
Active immunization 86, 108
Acute rejection 187
Acyclovir 189, 190
ADCC. *See* Antibody-dependent cell-mediated cytotoxicity
Adoptive cellular immunotherapy 256
AIDS, CDC clinical definition of 127
ALG. *See* Antilymphocyte globulin
Allele 36
Allergens 55
Anaphylactic reactions 54
  antiallergy agents 59
  antihistamines 59
  corticosteroids 59
  leukotriene inhibitors and antagonists 59
  pharmacologic therapies 59
  sympathomimetic agents 59
Androgens 73
Anergy 64
Antibody 23
  affinity 24
  anti-idiotype 285, 290
  avidity 25
  bivalent 275
  cross-reactivity 25
  Fab 23
  Fc 23
  heavy chains 23
  IFN-α 25
  IgA 23
  IgD 23
  IgE 23
  IgG 23
  IgM 23
  IL-2 25
  killer (K) and natural killer (NK) cells 25
  light chains 23
  memory cells 25
  non-B and non-T lymphocytes (null cells) 25
  perforins 25
Antibody deficiency diseases 76
  therapy for 78
Antibody-dependent cell-mediated cytotoxicity (ADCC) 232, 233
Antigen-binding site 39
Antigen-presenting cell (APC) 19
  B lymphocytes 19
  dendritic cells 19
  follicular dendritic cells 19
  Langerhans cells 19
  microglial cells 19
Antigen-specific (adaptive) immunity 6
  antigens and antigen presentation 6
Antigenic modulation 273
Antilymphocyte globulin (ALG) 184
Antisera 42
Antithymocyte globulin (ATG) 175, 180, 184
Antiviral therapy 130
  antiretroviral resistance 132
  combination therapy 133
  inhibitors of viral binding 130
  integrase inhibitors 133
  non-nucleoside reverse transcriptase inhibitors 132
  protease (proteinase) inhibitors 133
  reverse transcriptase inhibitors 131
APC. *See* Antigen-presenting cell
ATG. *See* Antithymocyte globulin
Atopy 58
Attenuated live vaccines 91, 99
Autoimmune diseases 72, 290
  autoantigens 72
Autoimmunity 10, 72
  immunopathologic mechanisms 75
  treatment of autoimmune diseases 75
Azathioprine (AZA) 153, 162, 163, 171, 175–7, 179, 183, 184, 190–2, 194, 195

B

Basophils 17, 19, 56
  basophilia 20
  basophilopenia 20
Biological response modifiers 236
  interferons 236
Bioreactor 273
Bivalent antibodies 275
Bone and muscle disorders 193
Bone marrow 16, 27
  stroma 17
Bone marrow transplantation (BMT) 214, 252
  allogenic 214
  autologous 214
  neutropenia 252
  preparative regimens 216
  syngenic 214
Bone marrow transplantation, complications after 217
  acute GVHD 217
  GVL effect 217
Brequinar 161, 165
Bruton's disease 76

C

Cancer antigen 125 (CA125) 231, 232
Cancer immunotherapy 233
  Bacillus Calmette-Guérin (BCG) 234, 235
  immunostimulants 234
  levamisole 235
  tumor vaccines 234
  viral antigens 234
Capromab pendetide 280
CD2 166
CD3 166
CD3⁺ T cells 166, 167
CD4 154, 166
CD4⁺ T cells 156, 157, 168
CD4⁺/CD8⁺ ratio 120, 278
CD8 166
CD8⁺ T cells 157
Cell and tissue typing 278
  anti-Rh factors 278
  blood typing 278
Cell-mediated reactions 63
Cellular immune response 8
Cellular immunodeficiency with immunoglobulins (Nezelof's syndrome) 78
Childhood Immunization Initiative (CII) 91
Chlamydia trachomatis 276
Chronic GVHD. *See* Graft-versus-host disease, chronic
Chronic lymphocytic leukemia (CLL) 285
Chronic rejection. *See* Rejection, chronic
Clusters of differentiation (CD) 278
Colony-stimulating factors (CSFs) 17
  G-CSF 249
  GM-CSF 249
  IL-1 249, 255
  IL-3 (multi-CSF) 249, 255
  IL-4 249
  IL-5 249
  IL-6 249, 255
  IL-11 249, 256
  M-CSF 18, 249, 255
  multipotential CSF (multi-CSF or IL-3) 249
  PIXY-321 255
  tumor necrosis factor (TNF) 256
Complement 5

deficiencies 79
Complications after bone marrow transplantation 217
acute GVHD 217
GVL effect 217
Complications after solid organ transplantation 186
infectious complications 187
Corticosteroids 156, 157, 193, 194
CsA. *See* Cyclosporine
CTL. *See* Cytotoxic T lymphocyte
Cyclophosphamide (CTX) 153, 163, 176, 190, 195
Cyclosporin A. *See* Cyclosporine
Cyclosporin G 159
Cyclosporine (cyclosporin A or CsA) 153, 156–9, 161, 169–71, 175–7, 179, 180, 183, 184, 189–95
Cytokine release 286
Cytomegalovirus (CMV) 188–90, 277
infection 183, 223
pneumonia 185
Cytotoxic reactions 60
Cytotoxic T lymphocyte (CTL) 231, 232
viral TAAs 231

D

Dacliximab (Zenapax) 280
DCH. *See* Hypersensitivity, delayed cutaneous
Deoxyspergualin 161, 162
Diabetes mellitus 193
Diagnostic kits, commercial MoAb immunofluorescence (IF) 276
Digibind, digoxin-immune Fab fragment 284
Dosimetry 287
Drug-induced reactions 61
Drug interactions 168
management of 170
minor interactions 171
moderately serious interactions 171
serious interactions 171

E

Edobacomab 280
Enzyme-linked immunosorbent assay (ELISA) 58, 124, 272
Eosinophil chemotactic factor 57
Eosinophils 19
eosinophilia 19
Epstein-Barr virus 189
Erythroblastosis fetalis (hemolytic disease of the newborn or HDN) 46, 48
Erythropoietin 249
Estrogens 73

F

Fab 275
$F(ab')_2$ 275
FK506. *See* Tacrolimus
Forward grouping 47

G

G-CSF. *See* Granulocyte colony-stimulating factor
Ganciclovir 189, 190
Genotype 37
GM-CSF. *See* Granulocyte-macrophage colony-stimulating factor
Graft-versus-host disease (GVHD) 20, 186
anticytokine antibodies 221
ATG 219
corticosteroids 220
cyclosporine (CsA) 220, 221
GVL effect 218
immunosuppressive agents 219
OKT3 219
pathophysiology of acute GVHD 217
staging and grading 218
tacrolimus 220, 221
Graft-versus-host disease, chronic 221
bacterial infections 222
fungal infections 222
management of infectious complications 221
viral infections 222
Granulocyte colony-stimulating factor (G-CSF) 19, 249–54
Granulocyte colony-stimulating factor, recombinant (rG-CSF) 251–4
bone marrow transplantation 251
Granulocyte-macrophage colony-stimulating factor (GM-CSF) 18, 19, 249–54
bone marrow transplant 250
myelodysplastic syndrome 254
toxicities 254
Granulocyte-macrophage colony-stimulating factor, recombinant (rGM-CSF) 251–4
bone marrow transplantation 251
Gusperimus. *See* Deoxyspergualin
GVHD. *See* Graft-versus-host disease

H

HAMA. *See* Human antimurine antibodies
Haplotype 36
Heart transplantation 181
chronic rejection 183
immunologic complications 183
immunosuppressive treatment 183
indications and candidate selection 181
mechanical bridging 182
postoperative complications 183
transplantation technique 182
Heat shock proteins 74
Hemolytic disease of the newborn (HDN or erthyroblastosis fetalis) 46, 48
Hepatitis C 277
Herpes simplex virus (HSV) 222
herpes simplex viruses 1 and 2 276
High endothelial venule 29
Histamine 57
Histiocyte. *See* Macrophages
HIV. *See* Human immunodeficiency virus
HIV infection 117
acute 126
asymptomatic 127
etiology 117
immunopathogenesis 119
persistent generalized lymphadenopathy 127
prevention 123
HIV testing 124
saliva and urine tests 126
HLA. *See* Human leukocyte antigen
HLA phenotype 37
class I proteins 37
class II genes 38
HLA system
$CD4^+$ (helper) T cells 215
$CD8^+$ T cells 215
MHC 215
HLA typing 42
Home testing kits 126
Human anti-human antibodies (HAHAs) 273
Human antimurine antibodies (HAMAs) 273
formation (xenosensitization) 167
response 286
Human immunodeficiency virus (HIV) 116
culture 125
infection. *See* HIV infection
quantitation of HIV RNA 126
testing 124
transmission 121
type 1 (HIV-1) 277
viral replicative cycle 117
Human leukocyte antigen (HLA) 36, 154, 279
Humoral immune response 7
primary 8
secondary 8
Hybridoma 270
Hyperlipidemia 192
Hypersensitivity 54
delayed cutaneous hypersensitivity (DCH) 63
Hypersensitivity reactions
type I (anaphylactic or immediate) 9, 54
type II (cytotoxic) 54, 60, 61
type III (immune complex–mediated) 54, 62
type IV (delayed) 20, 54, 63

I

Idiopathic thrombocytopenic purpura (ITP), chronic 61
Idiotypes 72
  anti-idiotype antibodies 72
IFN. *See* Interferon
IL. *See* Interleukin
Imaging, with labeled MoAbs 280
  99mTc-labeled MoAbs 281
  cardiac imaging 282
  imaging of infectious diseases 282
  iodine compounds (^{123}I, ^{131}I) 281
  radioisotope conjugate 281
  tumor imaging 282
IMIG. *See* Intramuscular immune globulin
Immune complex–mediated reactions 62
Immune factors 74
  cross-reacting antigens 75
Immunodeficiency 10
  common variable 77
  primary 76
  secondary 79
Immunodeficiency disease, severe combined (SCID) 78
  therapy for cellular deficiencies 79
Immunodeficiency diseases 76
Immunogenicity, approaches to increasing 100
  adjuvants 100
  anti-idiotypes 101
Immunoglobulin A (IgA) deficiency 105
Immunologic therapy 133
  ampligen 136
  autologous CD8⁺ T-cell transfusions 134
  bone marrow transplantation 134
  corticosteroids 137
  cyclosporine 137
  cytokine modulation 137
  cytokines 135
  hydroxyurea 137
  immune enhancement 134
  immune replacement 134
  immune suppression 136
  IVIG and passive immunotherapy 134
  therapeutic immunization 135
Immunosuppression, nonpharmacological means of 172
  apheresis 173
  blood transfusion 173
  irradiation 173
  photopheresis 173
  splenectomy 173
Immunosuppressive agents 219–21
  ATG 219
  anticytokine antibodies 221
  corticosteroids 220
  cyclosporine (CsA) 220
  OKT3 219
  tacrolimus 220
Immunosuppressive treatment, for transplantation
  heart 183
  kidney 175
  liver 175
  lung and heart-lung 184
  small intestine 186
Immunotherapy 60
Indium In 111 altumomab pentetate 280
Indium In 111 imciromab pentetate 280
Indium In 111 satumomab pendetide 280
Infections, opportunistic. *See* Opportunistic infections
Infectious complications 187
  bacterial infections 187
  fungal infections 191
  hepatotrophic viruses 190
  herpes group viruses 188, 190
  opportunistic infections 191
  viral infections 188
Inflammation 8
Inhibitors of cell proliferation
  azathioprine (AZA) 162
  cyclophosphamide (CTX) 163
  methotrexate (MTX) 164
  mycophenolate mofetil 164
Inhibitors of early T-cell activation
  cyclosporine (CsA) 157
  tacrolimus 159
Inhibitors of late T-cell function
  deoxyspergualin (Gusperimus) 162
  leflunomide 162
  sirolimus 161
Interferon (INF)
  alpha 236, 237, 239–42, 248
  beta 236, 242
  gamma 18, 154, 155, 157, 236, 242
Interferon alpha
  chronic myelogenous leukemia (CML) 238, 239
  colorectal cancer 242
  hairy cell leukemia 237
  hepatitis B 239, 240
  hepatitis C 239, 240
  Kaposi's sarcoma 239
  melanoma 240, 241
  multiple myeloma 241, 242
  renal cell carcinoma 240
Interferon beta
  toxicities 242
Interferon gamma
  toxicities 242
Interleukin (IL) 243
  IL-1 19, 154, 179, 243
  IL-2 154, 157, 160, 243, 244
  IL-3 18, 19, 155, 243
  IL-4 56, 155, 243
  IL-5 19, 56, 155
  IL-6 56, 154, 155, 243
  IL-11 243
Interleukin 2
  metastatic renal cell carcinoma 244
Interleukin 2, recombinant 246–9
  biological response modifier combinations 247
  BMT 248
  melanoma 247, 248
  metastatic renal cell carcinoma 246
  toxicities 246
Intramuscular immune globulin (IMIG) 102
  hepatitis B immune globulin 103
  prophylaxis of viral infections 102
  serotherapy 102
  toxin-induced diseases 102
  varicella-zoster immune globulin 103
Intravenous immune globulin (IVIG) 78, 103
  IgG subclasses 104
  selection variables 107
  side effects 105
  subclass deficiency 105
  therapeutic uses 106
Irradiation 173
ITP. *See* Idiopathic thrombocytopenic purpura
IVIG. *See* Intravenous immunoglobulin

K

Kidney transplantation 152, 174
  de novo and recurrent renal disease 176
  immunologic complications 175
  immunosuppressive treatment 175
  indications and candidate selection 174
  postoperative complications 175
  transplantation technique 174
Killer (K) cells 232

L

LAK cells. *See* Lymphokine-activated killer cells
Leflunomide 161, 162
Leukemia, chronic lymphocytic (CLL) 285
Leukotrienes 57
Linkage disequilibrium 38
Liver transplantation 178
  immunology of the transplanted liver 179
  immunosuppressive treatment 179
  indications and candidate selection 178
  organ allocation 179
  postoperative complications 180
Lung and heart-lung transplantation 183
  CMV pneumonia 185
  immunosuppressive treatment 184

indications and candidate selection 184
Pneumocystis carinii pneumonia 185
postoperative complications 184
Luteinizing hormone (LH) 277
Lymph nodes 16, 27
Lymphocytes 20
B lymphocytes (humoral immunity) 22
cytotoxic T lymphocyte (CTL) 21
GM-CSF 21
helper T lymphocytes 20
IFN-γ 20, 21
IL-2 20, 21
memory T lymphocytes 21
plasma cell 22
suppressor T lymphocytes 20
T lymphocytes (cell-mediated immunity) 20
Lymphocytotoxicity assay 42
Lymphoid cells 16
Lymphokine-activated killer (LAK) cells 232, 233

M

Macrophage colony-stimulating factor (M-CSF) 18, 249, 255
Macrophages 17, 232
fixed 17
Kupffer cells 17
Langerhans cells 17
mesangial cells 17
microglial cells 17
osteoclasts 17
reticular cells 17
wandering 17
Major histocompatibility complex (MHC) 36, 154, 279
Malignancy 79, 194
Malnutrition 79
MALT. *See* Mucosal-associated lymphoid tissue
Mast cells 17, 20, 56
Megakaryocytes 20
Memory, immunologic 29
Methotrexate (MTX) 164
Methylprednisolone 183
MHC. *See* Major histocompatibility complex
Minor histocompatibility genes 38
Mixed lymphocyte culture (MLC) 43
Mixed lymphocyte reaction (MLR) 43
Mizoribine 161, 165
MoAb fragments
Fab and $F(ab')_2$ fragments 275
pharmacology and pharmacokinetics 275
Monoclonal antibodies (MoAbs) 21, 166–9
abciximab 270
affinity column 279
anti-CD4 278
anti-CD8 278
anti-IL-1–receptor 290
anti-TNF 290
cardiac disease 283
clusters of differentiation (CD) 22
diagnostic kit, immunofluorescence 276
drug assays 279
flow cytometry techniques 270
guidelines for nonproprietary naming 279
HAMA formation (xenosensitization) 167
home testing kits 277
imaging with 280–2
in vitro diagnostic reagents 276
in vivo applications 279
infectious disease diagnosis 276
medium containing HAT 272
names adopted by the USAN Council 279, 280
OKT (Ortho) series 278
OKT3 166
Oncoscint CR/OV 270
protein purification 279
therapeutic uses 283
to CD28
to treat cancer 284
to treat gram-negative bacteremia 290
transplantation 283
xenosensitization (HAMA formation) 167
Monoclonal antibodies, chimeric
gene transfection 274
human-murine Fab 283
recombinant DNA techniques 274
Monoclonal antibody fragments
Fab and $F(ab')_2$ fragments 275
pharmacology and pharmacokinetics 275
Monocytes 17
Mononuclear cells 17
macrophages 17
Mononuclear phagocytes 17
MTX. *See* Methotrexate
Mucosal-associated lymphoid tissue (MALT) 28
Muromonab-CD3 280
Mycophenolate mofetil 161, 164, 165, 183
Myeloid cells 16

N

Natural killer (NK) cells 232
Nebacumab 280
Neisseria gonorrhea 276
Neoplasms 130
Kaposi's sarcoma 130
non-Hodgkin's lymphoma 130
Neutrophil chemotactic factor 57
Neutrophils 19
demargination 19
neutropenia 19
neutrophilia 19
Nezelof's syndrome (cellular immunodeficiency with immunoglobulins) 78
Nonspecific (innate) immunity 4
physical and chemical barriers 4

O

OKT3 166–8, 175, 177, 180, 184, 190, 195, 278
ATG 189
lymphocyte subsets 167
Oncofetal antigens 231
alpha-fetoprotein (AFP) 231
carcinoembryonic antigen (CEA) 231
Oncologic diagnosis 278
Oncology 284
antigenic modulation 286
B-cell lymphoma 285
enzyme conjugate 289
immunoconjugates 287–9
immunotoxins 287
MoAbs to treat cancer 284
radioisotope conjugates 287
Opportunistic infections 128
candidiasis 129
CMV 129
cryptococcal meningitis 129
herpesvirus 129
Mycobacterium avium complex 129
Mycobacterium tuberculosis 129
Pneumocystis carinii pneumonia 128
toxoplasmosis 129
Opsonization 61
Organ transplants 153
Ovulation tests 277

P

p24 antigen assay 125
p24 core antigen 277
Pancreas transplantation 176
immunologic complications 177
immunosuppressive treatment 177
indications and candidate selection 176
islet cell transplantation 177
postoperative complications 177
transplantation technique 177
Passive immunization 101, 108
PCP. *See Pneumocystis carinii* pneumonia
PCR. *See* Polymerase chain reaction
Peripheral stem cell transplantation 214
Phagocytosis 5
Pharmacodynamic interactions 170
Pharmacokinetic interactions 169
Plasmodium falciparum 277
Platelet-activating factor (PAF) 57

Platelets 17, 20
Pluripotent stem cell 16
Pneumocystis carinii 277
  Pneumocystis carinii pneumonia (PCP) 185
Polymerase chain reaction (PCR) 45, 125
Polymorphonuclear leukocyte (PMN) 17, 19
Prednisone 175, 177, 184
Pregnancy tests 277
  Human chorionic gonadotrophin (HCG) 277
Preparative regimens 216
  donor lymphocyte depletion 217
  immunosuppressive agents 217
Prostaglandins 57
Prostate-specific antigen (PSA) 231, 232

R

Radioallergosorbent test (RAST) 58
Radioimmunoassay (RIA) 272
Rapamycin. *See* Sirolimus
Rejection
  acute 187
  chronic 187
  of solid organ or bone marrow graft 20
Restriction fragment length polymorphism (RFLP) 45
Reticuloendothelial system 17
Reverse grouping 47
  rG-CSF. *See* Granulocyte colony-stimulating factor, recombinant
  rGM-CSF. *See* Granulocyte-macrophage colony-stimulating factor, recombinant
  Ricin A immunoconjugate 288
  Rickettsia rickettsii 277
  rIL-2. *See* Interleukin 2, recombinant

S

Saliva and urine tests 126
Selective IgA deficiency 77
Sequence-specific oligonucleotide (SSO) 45
Serologic crossmatch 42, 43
  complement-dependent cytotoxicity assay 43
  flow cytometry crossmatch 43
Serum sickness reactions 62
Severe combined immunodeficiency disease (SCID) 78
Sevirumab 280
Sirolimus 161, 189
Skin testing 58
Small intestine transplantation 186
  immunosuppressive treatment 186
  indications and candidate selection 186
  postoperative complications 186
Spectrum of disease 126
Spleen 16, 28
Steroids 191
Superantigens 74

T

Tacrolimus 156, 159–61, 170, 171, 186, 189, 191–4
Technetium Tc 99m biciromab 280
Thymus 16, 27
TNF. *See* Tumor necrosis factor
Tolerance 21, 30, 74
Toxin reversal 290
Transplant complications
  hypertension 191
Transplant immunology 154–5
  acute cellular rejection 155
  adhesion molecules 155
  CD4 receptors 154
  CD8 receptors 154
  cytokine mediators 154
  major histocompatibility complex 154
  T-cell receptor (TCR) 154
Transplant immunotherapy 155–72
  antilymphocyte globulin (ALG) 165
  antithymocyte globulin (ATG) 165
  azathioprine (AZA) 155, 162, 163
  corticosteroids 155, 156
  cyclophosphamide (CTX) 163
  cyclosporine (CsA) 155, 157
  cyclosporine analogues 159
  deoxyspergualin (Gusperimus) 162
  drug interactions 168
  inhibitors of cell proliferation 162
  inhibitors of early T-cell activation 157
  inhibitors of late T-cell function 161
  leflunomide 162
  management of drug interactions 170
  methotrexate (MTX) 164
  minor interactions 171
  miscellaneous antiproliferatives 165
  MoAbs 166–8
  moderately serious interactions 171
  mycophenolate mofetil 164
  OKT3 155, 166–8
  pharmacodynamic interactions 170
  pharmacokinetic interactions 169
  polyclonal antilymphocyte antibodies 155, 165
  serious interactions 171
  sirolimus 161
  tacrolimus 159–61
Tumor immunology 230
Tumor lysis 286
Tumor-associated antigen (TAA) 231, 278
Tumor necrosis factor (TNF) 179
Tumor necrosis factor alpha 154
Tuvirumab 280
Type and cross 47
Type and screen 47

U

United Network for Organ Sharing (UNOS) 153, 154
University of Wisconsin solution 180

V

Vaccines 87, 290
  adjuvants 100
  allergenicity 87
  anti-idiotypes 101
  attenuated live microorganisms 91, 99, 100
  biotechnological approaches to vaccine development 96
  carrier organisms: the vaccinia model 99
  cloned proteins 96
  development 138
  inactivated (killed) vaccines 91, 94, 95
  influence of socioeconomic benefits 87
  innactived microbial products 91
  legislation and initiatives 89
  National Childhood Vaccine Injury Act (NCVIA) 89
  resurgence of disease without vaccination 87
  subunit vaccines 96
  synthetic peptides 96, 98
  traditional approaches to vaccine development 91
  Vaccine Adverse Event Reporting System (VAERS) 89
Vaccines, attenuated live 91, 99
  carrier organisms (the vaccinia model) 99
Vaccine development
  biotechnological approaches 96
  cloned proteins 96–8
  subunit vaccines 96
  synthetic peptides 96, 98, 99
Vaccines, inactivated (killed) 94, 95
  H. influenzae 95
  HAV vaccine 95
Votumumab 280

W

Western blot 125

X

X-linked agammaglobulinemia 76

Z

Zenapax. *See* Dacliximab
Zolimomab aritox 280